OCCUPATIONAL THERAPY

Performance, Participation, and Well-Being

Senior Editors

Charles H. Christiansen, EdD, OTR, OT(C), FAOTA

Chief Academic Officer
Dean of the School of Allied Health Sciences
Professor, Department of Occupational Therapy
University of Texas Medical Branch
Galveston, Texas

Carolyn M. Baum, PhD, OTR/L, FAOTA

Professor, Occupational Therapy and Neurology and
Elias Michael Director, Program in Occupational Therapy
Washington University School of Medicine
St. Louis, Missouri

Contributing Editor

Julie Bass-Haugen, PhD, OTR/L, FAOTA

Professor and Chair
Department of Occupational Science and Occupational Therapy
The College of St. Catherine
St. Paul, Minnesota

An innovative information, education, and management company
6900 Grove Road • Thorofare, NJ 08086

MT

Don't miss the important companion Web site to *Occupational Therapy: Performance, Participation, and Well-Being, Third Edition.*
Please visit us at http://www.cb3e.slackbooks.com

ISBN-10: 1-55642-530-9
ISBN-13: 9781556425301

The work SLACK Incorporated publishes is peer reviewed. Prior to publication, recognized leaders in the field, educators, and clinicians provide important feedback on the concept and content that we publish. We welcome feedback on this work.

Printed in the United States of America.

Library of Congress Cataloging-in-Publication Data

Occupational therapy : performance, participation, and well-being
/ senior editors, Charles H. Christiansen, Carolyn M. Baum ;
contributing editor, Julie Bass-Haugen. -- 3rd ed.
p. ; cm.
Includes bibliographical references and index.
ISBN 1-55642-530-9 (alk. paper)
1. Occupational therapy. I. Christiansen, Charles. II. Baum, Carolyn Manville. III. Bass-Haugen, Julie.
[DNLM: 1. Occupational Therapy. 2. Employment--psychology.
WB 555 O1489 2004]
RM735.O366 2004
615.8'515--dc22

2004012306

Published by: SLACK Incorporated
6900 Grove Road
Thorofare, NJ 08086 USA
Telephone: 856-848-1000
Fax: 856-853-5991
www.slackbooks.com

Contact SLACK Incorporated for more information about other books in this field or about the availability of our books from distributors outside the United States.

Last digit is print number: 10 9 8 7 6 5 4 3 2 1

3/1/06

Dedication

We take pride in dedicating this third edition to Gail S. Fidler, OTR, FAOTA,
Pompano Beach, Florida
with thanks for her inspiration, intellect, and support for us and for the profession of occupational therapy.

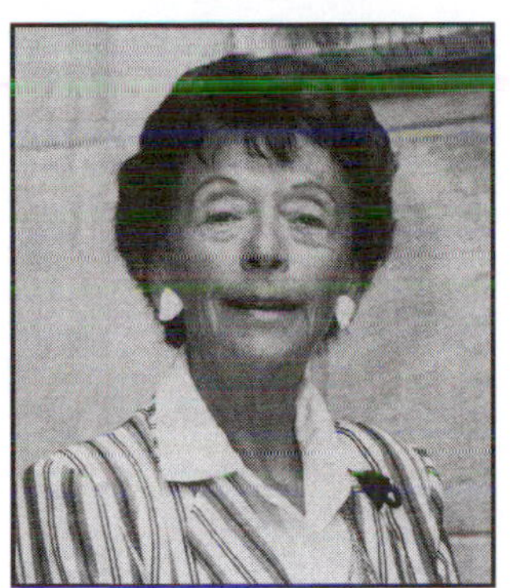

Contents

ACKNOWLEDGMENTS

We would like to acknowledge the efforts of the following contributing authors to the first and second editions of *Occupational Therapy*, without whose efforts this volume would not have been possible:

Karin J. Barnes
James Berger
Paula Bohr
Betty Bonder
Barbara Borg
Carolyn Brayley
Catherine E. Bridge
Mary Ann Bruce
Barbara Acheson Cooper
Mary Corcoran
Harriet Davidson
Janet Duchek
Winnie Dunn
Elizabeth DePoy
Elizabeth Devereaux
Janet Duchek
Winnie Dunn
Shereen D. Farber
Patrick Fougeyrolas
Nancy Gerein
Laura Gitlin
Davod Grau
Harlan Hahn
Betty Hasselkus
Douglas Hobson
Margo Holm
Kathy Kniepmann
Ellen Kolodner
Douglas V. Krefting
Laura H. Krefting
Lori Letts
Ruth E. Levine
Lela Llorens
Leonard Matheson
Marian Minor
Karin Opacich
Kenneth J. Ottenbacher
Janet L. Poole
Patricia Rigby
Joan C. Rogers
Susan Ayres Rosa
Barbara Boyt Schell
Janette K. Schkade
Sally Schultz
Richard K. Schwartz
Roger O Smith
Jean Cole Spencer
Debra Stewart
Susan Strong
Mary Sladky Struthers
Elaine Trefler
Robyn L. Twible
Fraser Valentine
Mary Warren

About the Authors

Charles H. Christiansen, EdD, OTR, OT(C), FAOTA is the George T. Bryan Distinguished Professor and Dean of the School of Allied Health Sciences at the University of Texas Medical Branch at Galveston. He earned his Occupational Therapy degree from the University of North Dakota in 1970 and later received an MA in Counseling Psychology from Ball State University. He received his Doctor of Education degree from the University of Houston in 1979. He became a Fellow of the American Occupational Therapy Association (AOTA) in 1983 and served as treasurer from 1986 to 1989. He was elected Vice-President in 2003. He was awarded the Eleanor Clarke Slagle Lectureship in 1999. He is the founding editor of *OTJR: Occupation, Participation and Health*. Dr. Christiansen is interested in health promotion and the contribution of occupations to health, well-being, and quality of life. He is an active member of the Society for the Study of Occupation: USA and other international occupational science societies.

Carolyn M. Baum, PhD, OTR/L, FAOTA is the Elias Michael Director and Professor of Occupational Therapy and Neurology at Washington University School of Medicine in St. Louis, Missouri. Dr. Baum has served as President of the AOTA and is the current president, and President of the American Occupational Therapy Certification Board (now NBCOT). She served on the National Center for Medical Rehabilitation Research at the National Institute of Health and the Institute of Medicine's Committee to Assess Rehabilitation Science and Engineering Needs. In those capacities, she contributed to reports to Congress. Dr. Baum's research is on the relationship of occupation and participation in older persons with chronic neurological diseases. She is editor of *OTJR: Occupation, Participation and Health* and consistently contributes to scholarly journals and text books.

Julie Bass-Haugen, PhD, OTR/L, FAOTA is a professor and chair of the Department of Occupational Science and Occupational Therapy at the College of St. Catherine. She received her BS in Occupational Therapy from the University of Minnesota and her MA and PhD in Educational Psychology—Statistics and Research Methods from the University of Minnesota. Dr. Bass-Haugen's expertise and interests include motor behavior, occupation and health, and research methods in occupational therapy. She has authored chapters on the occupational therapy task-oriented approach in Trombly's *Occupational Therapy for Physical Dysfunction* and has made numerous presentations to national and international audiences. Dr. Bass-Haugen has also served on the editorial board of the *American Journal of Occupational Therapy*.

CONTRIBUTING AUTHORS

Rondell Berkeland, EdD, OTR/L is chair of the Department of Occupational Therapy at The College of St. Scholastica in Duluth, Minnesota. He received a BS in Occupational Therapy from the University of Minnesota, a MPH in Public Health from the University of Minnesota, and a EdD in Educational Leadership from St. Thomas University. Dr. Berkeland's expertise and interests include community mental health, homeless populations, and the integration of service learning and applied research in professional education. He is also an active member of the professional community, having served on the Committee of State Association Presidents, the Representative Assembly, National Conference Committee, the State Association Board, and numerous other committees and task forces.

Robert K. Bing, EdD, OTR, FAOTA was Founding Dean Emeritus and Professor Emeritus of Occupational Therapy at the University of Texas Medical Branch at Galveston at the time of his death in 2003. He earned his occupational therapy degree at the University of Illinois College of Medicine and later received Master's and Doctoral degrees in Human Development from the University of Maryland at College Park. During his distinguished career, Dr. Bing served as President of the AOTA from 1984 to 1986. He became a Fellow of AOTA in 1975 and received the Award of Merit in 1987. As a noted expert in the history of occupational therapy and medicine, Dr. Bing was invited to deliver the Eleanor Clark Slagle Lecture in 1983. He continued to volunteer, lecture, and write until his death following a long illness. A scholars program and professorship have been named in his honor at UTMB.

Catana Brown, PhD, MA, OTR, FAOTA is an associate professor at the University of Kansas Medical Center. She received her BS in Occupational Therapy from Colorado State University, her MA in Occupational Therapy from New York University, and her PhD in Psychology and Research in Education from the University of Kansas. Dr. Brown's expertise and interests are in promoting satisfying and successful community living for people with psychiatric disabilities. She is part of an interdisciplinary team, the Psychiatric Disabilities Research Program, that has federal funding to examine the efficacy of a skills training program and train allied health professionals to provide health promotion services to people with psychiatric disabilities.

Carol Brownson, MSPH, PHLC serves as Deputy Director of the Robert Wood Johnson Foundation Diabetes Initiative National Program Office at Washington University in St. Louis. She received her Masters in Public Health degree from the University of Missouri—Columbia. Ms. Brownson has experience in community health, health education theory and practice, needs assessment methods, program development, and coalition building. Her background includes 16 years of chronic disease prevention and control program development and management in the Missouri Department of Health, and five years experience developing the community practice program for the Program in Occupational Therapy at Washington University School of Medicine in St. Louis. She is a contributing author to *Occupational Therapy in Community-Based Practice Settings* and a co-author of the AOTA Commission on Practice's position paper, *Occupational Therapy in the Promotion of Health and the Prevention of Disease and Disability Statement.*

Jane A. Davis, PhD (Candidate), MSc, OTReg(Ont), OT(C), OTR is a doctoral student in the Department of Public Health Sciences, in collaboration with the Institute of Human Development, Life Course and Aging at the University of Toronto. Her research interest is in occupational development across the life course, and she has coauthored a book chapter on the subject, which was published in *Introduction to Occupation* in 2003. For her PhD dissertation, Jane is examining how the work-life balance discourse, as presented by media, is taken up or resisted by executives throughout their careers. Jane is a co-editor of the *Sense of Doing* column in *OT Now* published by the Canadian Association of Occupational Therapists.

Winnie Dunn, PhD, OTR, FAOTA is professor and chairperson of the Occupational Therapy Program at Kansas University Medical Center in Kansas City, Kansas. Dr. Dunn is known for her research that seeks to understand how people process sensory information. She is widely published, including texts on pediatric occupational therapy practice. She has done hundreds of workshops to establish best practices in pediatrics. She has received many honors, including the Eleanor Clarke Slagle Lectureship, the highest academic honor of the AOTA. Dr. Dunn and her colleagues at the University of Kansas are the authors of the occupational therapy model, The Ecology of Human Performance.

Dorothy Edwards, PhD is associate professor of occupational therapy and neurology at the School of Medicine at Washington University in St Louis. She earned her BS in Psychology at Loyola University, New Orleans, Louisiana and her Doctor of Philosophy degree in Aging and Development at Washington University in St. Louis in 1980. In addition to her faculty roles, Dr. Edwards is currently a senior investigator in Washington University's Alzheimer's Disease Research Center. Her research is focused on the impact of cognitive impairment on community participation and quality of life in healthy older adults and persons with Alzheimer's disease and stroke. Her research has been supported by several funding agencies, including the James S. McDonnell Foundation, the American Heart Association, and the National Institutes of Health. Dr. Edwards is a member of the editorial board of *OTJR: Occupation, Participation and Health.*

Nancy Flinn, PhD, OTR/L is an an associate professor in the Department of Occupational Science and Occupational Therapy at The College of St. Catherine in St. Paul, Minnesota. She received her BS in Occupational Therapy from the University of Minnesota and her MA and PhD in Educational Psychology from the University of Minnesota. Dr. Flinn's expertise and interests include stroke rehabilitation and application of motor control to clinical practice. Her current work is in the area of constraint-induced movement therapy. Dr. Flinn has also been active in the Minnesota Occupational Therapy Association.

Mary Lou Henderson, MS, OTR/L is associate professor and occupational science program director in the Department of Occupational Science and Occupational Therapy at the College of St. Catherine. She received her BS in Occupational Therapy from the University of Kansas and her MS in Education from the University of Kansas. Ms. Henderson's expertise and interests are in pediatrics and school-based therapy and curriculum in occupational science and occupational therapy education. She has served on many organizations and boards, including secretary of the Society for the Study of Occupation and the roster of accreditation evaluators for the Accreditation Council of Occupational Therapy Education (ACOTE) of the AOTA.

Staffan Josephsson, PhD, OT(Reg) is associate professor in the Department of Occupational Therapy at Karolinska Institutet, Stockholm, Sweden. He earned his occupational therapy degree at the University College of Health Science in Stockholm, Sweden in 1985 and is licensed as a registered occupational therapist in Sweden. He received his doctoral degree in medical sciences in the area of geriatrics from the Karolinska Institutet in Stockholm, Sweden in 1994 . He is interested in narrative reasoning in occupational therapy and chronic disease. Dr. Josephsson is a member of the editorial board of the *American Journal of Occupational Therapy*.

Hans Jonsson, PhD, OT(Reg) is associate professor and head of the masters program in occupational therapy in the Department of Occupational Therapy, Karolinska Institutet, Stockholm, Sweden. He earned his occupational therapy degree at the University College of Health Science in Stockholm, Sweden in 1977 and is licensed as a registered occupational therapist in Sweden. He received his doctoral degree in medical sciences in the area of occupational therapy from Karolinska Institutet in Stockholm, Sweden in 2000. He is interested in occupational transitions, especially retirement and narrative methodology in research. Dr. Jonsson is a member of the editorial board of *OTJR: Occupation, Participation and Health*.

Shelly J. Lane, PhD, OTR/L, FAOTA holds a BS in Allied Health, Occupational Therapy from The State University and a PhD in Anatomy/Neuroscience from the University of Texas Health Sciences Center, San Antonio. She is currently Professor and Chair of Occupational Therapy at VCU Health Systems in VA. She has focused her clinical, teaching, and research interests in two areas: infants at risk for developmental delay and learning disabilities and neuroscience applications to occupational therapy. Dr. Lane's current research focuses on examining the effectiveness and feasibility of the "Let's Play!" model, a family-centered, play-focused, and assistive technology supported early intervention service model. Dr. Lane has published and lectured locally, nationally, and internationally on topics related to those above. Recent publications include those from her research related to assistive technology, play, and infants, and the second edition of *Sensory Integration: Theory and Practice*, a book on which she is both chapter author and secondary editor.

Jennifer Landry, PhD (Candidate), MSc, OTReg(Ont), OT(C) is a doctoral student in Public Health Sciences and Aging at the University of Toronto, and works part-time doing community-based occupational therapy. She is interested in enabling principles and processes for working with communities and consumer groups as well as with individuals. Publications from her master's thesis focused on qualitative methodology and a social perspective on disability and women.

Barbara A. Larson, MS, OTR/L, FAOTA is the director of Internet Clinical Applications for Isernhagen Work Systems, a division of WorkWell Systems, Inc. She received her BS in Occupational Therapy from the University of Minnesota and her MA in Health and Human Services Administration and Management from St. Mary's University. Her interests and expertise include work programs and ergonomics. She has been active in local, regional, and national organizations and has served as a consultant and instructor.

Mary Law, PhD, OT(C) is professor and associate dean of Rehabilitation Science and Codirector of CanChild Centre for Childhood Disability Research at McMaster University, Hamilton, Canada. Dr. Law's research centers on the environmental factors that support daily life and participation of children with disabilities. She is part of a team that developed the Canadian Occupational Performance Measure and in addition to the Person, Environment, Occupation Model, is an author of the Canadian Occupational Therapy Guidelines, *Enabling Occupation*. Dr. Law is the editor of *PT and OT in Pediatrics*. She is widely published, including major texts on client-centered practice, evidence-based practice, and occupation-based practice. She also serves a review function with many funding agencies, including the National Institutes of Health. She holds many national awards, including the Muriel Driver Lectureship, the highest academic honor of the Canadian Occupational Therapy Association.

Jennie Q. Lou, MD, MSc, OTR is an associate professor in Public Health Program and Department of Occupational Therapy at Nova Southeastern University in Ft. Lauderdale, Florida. Dr. Lou has been working in the fields of medicine, neuroscience, and occupational therapy, and her recent scholarly work includes randomized clinical trials and other outcome studies in the fields of neurorehabilitation and wellness. Dr. Lou has served as principal investigator and research consultant on many research projects, and she has been the author and editor for many scientific publications. In 2000, Dr. Lou, along with nine other occupational therapists, represented the AOTA at the Human Genome Educational Model Project (HuGEM II) where they received training on the Human Genome Project and genetics. In 2001-2002, Dr. Lou was the AOTA's representative to the Human Genetic Model Curricula Project. During her service, Dr. Lou worked with experts from other health care disciplines on developing model curricula to integrate genetic education into the curriculum.

Kathleen Matuska, MPH, OTR/L is associate professor in the Department of Occupational Therapy at the College of St. Catherine. She received her BS in Occupational Therapy from the University of Minnesota and her MPH in Public Health Administration from the University of Minnesota. Her expertise and interests include health promotion and community-based wellness programs for the elderly and individuals with multiple sclerosis. Other interests include lifestyle balance and its influence on quality of life. She has served on many organizations and boards and is currently treasurer of the Society for the Study of Occupation.

Mary Ann McColl, PhD, BSc is the associate director of research at the Centre for Health Services and Policy Research at Queen's University. She received her BSc in Occupational Therapy from Queen's University and her PhD in Epidemiology and Biostatistics from the University of Toronto. Dr. McColl has expertise and interests in health service utilization among people with disabilities, aging and disability, spirituality and occupational therapy, community integration and social support, and acquired brain injury and spinal cord injury. She has authored numerous publications in occupational therapy and disability studies. Dr. McColl is the recipient of many awards and distinctions, including the Outstanding Scholar Award of the National Honour Society of Occupational Therapy by AOTF, the Lifetime Fellowship Award, and the Muriel Driver Memorial Lectureship by the CAOT.

Penelope Moyers, EdD, OTR, FAOTA is professor and dean of the School of Occupational Therapy at the University of Indianapolis, Indianapolis, Indiana. Dr. Moyers is a Fellow of the AOTA and currently serves as Chair of AOTA's Commission on Continuing Competence. She is recognized for her expertise in substance abuse disorders, evidence-based practice, and continuing competence. Dr Moyers is the author of the AOTA's *Guide to Occupational Therapy Practice* and numerous publications that guide occupational therapy practice in ethical and effective practice.

Helene J. Polatajko, PhD, OTReg(Ont), OT(C), FCAOT is professor and chair in the Department of Occupational Therapy at the University of Toronto. She was the 1992 recipient of the Muriel Driver Memorial Lectureship awarded by the CAOT and is a member of the American Occupational Therapy Foundation Academy of Research. She is a consistent contributor to the literature. Her work centers on human occupation and the enablement of occupational performance and occupational competence. She has a particular interest in the use of cognitive approaches to enable occupational performance in children with development coordination disorder. She is an author of both the Canadian Occupation Performance Measure and the Canadian Model of Occupational Performance, and is the editor of *OTJR: Occupation, Participation, and Health.*

Kathlyn L. Reed, PhD, OTR, MLIS, AHIP is Visiting Professor at the School of Occupational Therapy, Texas Woman's University-Houston Center, Houston, Texas. She received her BS in Occupational Therapy at the University of Kansas and MA in Organization and Administration of Occupational Therapy at Western Michigan University. Her PhD was earned in Special Education at the University of Washington in Seattle. Additionally she has her MLIS in Library and Information Studies from the University of Oklahoma. Dr. Reed became a fellow of the American Occupational Therapy Association in 1975. She holds the Association's two highest awards, the Award of Merit in 1983 and the Eleanor Clarke Slagle Lectureship in 1986. She has consistently presented at national and international conferences since the early 1970s, has coauthored six textbooks, and been published in both occupational therapy and library science journals. Dr. Reed's interests are in the terms and concepts of the profession, models of practice developed in the profession, and the history of the profession. She is truly the profession's keeper of terms and concepts—a task that she enjoys and one that is a true gift to the profession.

Jon A. Sanford, MArch is a Research Architect at the Rehab R&D Center at the Atlanta VAMC and Co-Director of the NIDRR-funded Rehabilitation Engineering Research Center on Workplace Accommodations within the Center for Assistive Technology and Environmental Access at Georgia Tech. He is also the Director of Research for Extended Home Living Services, Wheeling, IL, the nation's largest provider of home modifications for older adults with disabilities. Mr. Sanford is one of the few architecturally-trained researchers engaged in accessibility and design for aging. He serves as Principal Investigator on numerous projects related to home modification interventions, including best practices in assisted toileting and bathing. In addition, he has developed two assessment protocols for home modifications to provide home assessments through telerehabilitation technology for rehab inpatients prior to discharge.

Marjorie E. Scaffa, PhD, OTR, FAOTA is an Associate Professor and Chairperson of the Department of Occupational Therapy at the University of South Alabama in Mobile, an occupational therapy program she founded in 1993. She received her MS in Occupational Therapy from Virginia Commonwealth University and a PhD in Health Education from the University of Maryland. Dr. Scaffa has worked in a number of clinical and community settings and is the editor of *Occupational Therapy in Community-Based Practice Settings*, which was published in 2001. She has served as a member of the editorial board for the *American Journal of Occupational Therapy* and has been a member of the American Occupational Therapy Foundation's Task Force on Occupation in Societal Crises since its inception in October 2001.

Susan L. Stark, PhD, OTR/L is a faculty member at Washington University School of Medicine, Program in Occupational Therapy. Dr. Stark has served as the representative from the AOTA to the World Health Organization for the International Classification of Impairment Disability and Handicap and is currently contributing to the development of the clinical manual for the International Classification of Functioning, Disability and Health. Dr. Stark is the principal investigator in the Environment and Occupational Performance Laboratory at Washington University School of Medicine, where she conducts studies of the outcome of environmental modification interventions on the lives of older adults and persons with disabilities and the influence of contextual factors on the participation of individuals with disabilities. Currently, she is a coinvestigator on a study of community accessibility, funded by the Centers for Disease Control and Prevention.

Gretchen Van Mater Stone, PhD, OTR/L, FAOTA holds a BS in Occupational Therapy from Indiana University, a Master's in Special Education as well as a doctoral degree in Educational Psychology from the University of Texas at Austin. She currently holds a dual appointment as Professor in the Occupational Therapy Program and the Department of Psychology at Shenandoah University. She serves as an ongoing consultant to an occupational therapy program at Kocaeli Medical University in Izmit, Turkey. Dr. Stone maintains a strong interest in cross-cultural clinical education, with an emphasis on developing curricula that increases awareness of the impact of the physical environment as well as the cultural environment on the choices people have available to them in daily life. Through sponsorship of Project HOPE, she works in communities at the international level to develop programs that enable people with limited resources to accomplish their goals.

Elizabeth Townsend, PhD, MAdEd, OTReg(NS), OT(C), FCAOT is a Professor and the Director of Dalhousie University's School of Occupational Therapy. She was Canada's Muriel Driver Lecturer in 1993, and is particularly known for her leadership in writing Canadian guidelines for client-centered occupational therapy, now known as *Guidelines for Enabling Occupation*. With a focus on critical analysis of systems and society, she has also published on institutional ethnography, notable in her book on *Good Intentions Overruled*, a critical analysis of enabling client empowerment in mental health services. With Dr. Charles H. Christiansen, she was coeditor of the book, *Introduction to Occupation: The Art and Science of Living*.

Ann A. Wilcock, PhD, RegOT(SA) is the Professor of Occupational Science and Therapy in the School of Health and Community Development at Deakin University, Geelong, Victoria, Australia. She completed undergraduate studies in occupational therapy in the United Kingdom and at the University of South Australia. Her graduate diploma and PhD in Public Health were earned at the University of Adelaide. She has delivered invited keynotes for the WFOT World Congress in Montreal and the Sylvia Docker Lecture for OT:Australia. She is founding president of the International Society of Occupational Scientists and the recipient of an honorary doctorate from the University of Derby. She is founding editor of the *Journal of Occupational Science*, and author of several books and numerous scholarly articles on occupational therapy and occupational science. Dr. Wilcock is internationally recognized as an expert in the role of human occupation as a determinant of health, and has interests in the history of occupational therapy, neuroscience, and population health.

Mary Jane Youngstrom, MS, OTR/L, FAOTA is a clinical instructor at the University of Kansas Medical Center. She received her BS in Occupational Therapy from the University of Kansas and her MS in Business Management—Focus Health Care, School of Business Administration, from the University of South Florida. Ms. Youngstrom's expertise and interests are in management and development of occupational therapy services with a focus on provision of services for older adults and defining occupational therapy's contribution to the health and health care needs of our communities. She has served on the AOTA's Executive Board and recently completed a 4-year term as chair of AOTA's Commission on Practice. Ms. Youngstrom has also held state leadership positions and served on numerous committees and task forces for AOTA and the National Board for Certification in Occupational Therapy (NBCOT).

PREFACE

Of all the professions dedicated to the health of people, none perhaps can lay as much claim to being oriented toward quality of life than occupational therapy. Occupations are the very essence of life, and being enabled to participate in them is, ultimately, the aspect of functioning that most contributes to life's quality. The founders of the field, influenced by consumers in the beginning, understood the power of occupation. They recognized the magic of participation in life and how this was necessary for well-being.

Sometimes it is not clear that the health care system fully appreciates quality of life as an indicator of health. Movement, strength, and endurance do not constitute adequate proxies for the richness of engaging in a task that has personal and symbolic meaning. Occupational therapists have tools to record the impact of engagement in meaningful occupations and the relationship that engagement has on perceived well-being and quality of life. As we become more visible in the use of occupation in therapy, we become more visible in a health care system that is asking people to take more responsibility to manage their health conditions. The focus of the health care system on function and participation matches with *Occupational Therapy's* knowledge, skill, and values.

For years, some occupational therapy educators and practitioners have been lobbying for a practice orientation that truly incorporates the idea of occupation into the therapy that is delivered on a daily basis. This has been more consistently possible, perhaps in pediatrics than in other specialty areas of practice, owing largely to reimbursement policies. We have taken the challenge in this text to provide useful guidance regarding how those in practice can think "occupationally" as they attend to the functional problems of their patients and clients. Occupation must be the focus of treatment in children, adults, and older adults.

The world has changed greatly in the nearly 15 years since the first edition of this textbook was published. Occupational therapy has changed greatly also. The pace and demands of practice are daunting. The present needs clear, relevant guidance (and evidence) for thinking through intervention choices. The future will need more attention to how occupational therapy can be delivered to organizations and, indeed, populations.

With these thoughts in mind, this third edition was organized around a template for decision making that helps the practitioner deliver services with an improved understanding of what occupation is and can be, and how its many dimensions can be used to inform intervention decisions. It is our hope that it provides both the framework and the tools that will support occupational therapy practitioners as they use occupation as both a means and an end to addressing the real issues facing people with functional deficits and disabilities.

We welcome Julie Bass-Haugen to our editorial team. She has added her genius for taking difficult concepts and translating them into learning exercises that clarify concepts and engage readers in the material. Her participation has enriched the occupation of preparing this edition, and we are grateful that she was willing to share her weekends with us.

We thank the many contributors to this volume, who each in her or his own way, brought a unique gift of intellect and experience to help us explain the PEOP model. The volume is designed to move the reader through a basic understanding of humans as occupational beings. This is followed by a section that explains the Person-Environment-Occupation-Performance model and provides templates for planning intervention. The third and final section addresses intervention and the outcomes that should reasonably be expected through application of the model. New to this edition of the book is an important companion Web site that has the learning exercises found in this book. To view this Web site, please visit http://www.cb3e.slackbooks.com.

Once again we have added a page that lists contributors to earlier editions who are not authors for this current volume. We appreciate the many students, consumers, and colleagues whose ideas have helped us in the formulation of this book. We also thank our family members and friends whose support was essential to the completion of this revision.

Most importantly, we would like to acknowledge and dedicate this third edition to our dear friend and colleague, Gail Fidler. Gail has been a force in the profession for many years; she has been a constant crusader for higher standards of practice, for adhering to the founding principles of our profession, and for recognizing the unique and important role occupational therapy has in promoting lifestyles that engender high level wellness. We take pride in this dedication, recognizing that it is a small tribute to a woman who has had such a great influence on our work and in promoting and developing the profession of occupational therapy.

CC/CB/JBH
Galveston, Texas
St. Louis, Missouri
St. Paul, Minnesota

Humans as Occupational Beings (Understanding Human Occupation)

Section I

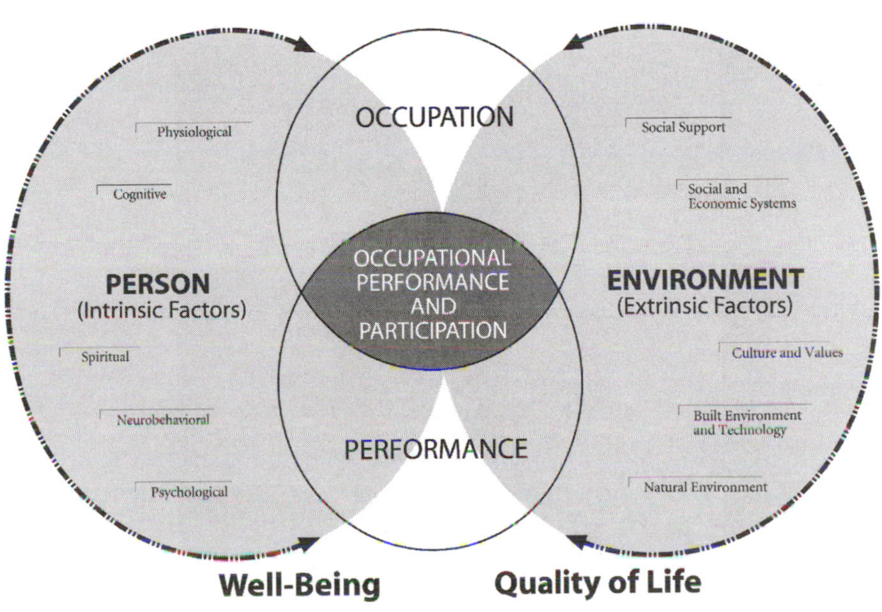

Chapter One Objectives

The information in this chapter is intended to help the reader:

1. Define occupation and identify its many dimensions.
2. Appreciate that occupations are complex phenomena.
3. Understand the distinction between obligatory and discretionary occupations.
4. Appreciate the importance of taxonomies for understanding phenomena.
5. Identify approaches for classifying occupations.
6. Define work, play, leisure, self-care, and sleep.
7. Describe habits, routines, and lifestyles.
8. Describe how most working people generally allocate time.
9. Understand the types and meanings of occupational patterns.
10. Appreciate how life stories contribute to coherence and meaning.

Key Words

archetypal places: Propose the idea that space and furnishings should be designed to support the fundamental types of activities that people do in various built environments (Spivak, 1973).

basic self-care: Personal activities such as eating, grooming, hygiene, and mobility that are necessary for maintenance of the self within the environment.

function: Reflects an individual's performance of activities, tasks, and roles during daily occupations (Baum & Edwards, 1995).

habits: Influence behavior in a semiautomatic way without need for conscious, deliberate action.

instrumental activities of daily living (IADL): Include telephone, food preparation, housekeeping, laundry, shopping, money management, use of transportation, and medication management as important occupations necessary for living independently in the community (Lawton, 1971).

leisure: A particular class of activity involving discretionary time and a state of mind (Gunter & Stanley, 1985; Witt & Goodale, 1982).

lifestyles: Defined by habits, routines, and occupational preferences to address personal needs and the demands of the environment (Elliott, 1993).

narrative: Refers to the autobiographical stories that provide a sense of unity and purpose through which lives are described and interpreted to the self and others (Mancuso & Sarbin, 1985; McAdams, 1992).

obligatory activities: Refer to required activities, including self-care, employment, and sleep (Csikszentmihalyi & Larson, 1984).

occupational perseverance: Perceived progress toward meeting an important or valued goal (Carlson, 1995, p. 145).

occupations: Human pursuits that are goal-directed or purposeful, are performed in situations or contexts that influence them, can be identified by the doer and others, and are meaningful to the individual.

play: The primary occupation of childhood; also a term often used interchangeably with leisure to describe the nonwork activities of adults.

productivity: "Activities and tasks which are done to enable the person to provide support to the self, family and society through the production of goods and services" (Canadian Association of Occupational Therapy [CAOT], 1995, p. 141).

routines: Provide an orderly structure for daily living that extends over time and pertains to a particular set of activities within a defined situation (Bond & Feathers, 1988).

sleep: Obligatory and necessary for self-maintenance. Current theories suggest that sleep provides important restorative functions by repairing tissue, allowing for the consolidation of memory traces and information, and conserving energy (Horne, 1988; Meddis, 1983; Webb, 1983).

taxonomy: A method for organizing objects or events in nature.

work: An activity required for subsistence.

A human being must have occupation if he or she is not to become a nuisance to the world.
Dorothy I. Sayers

Chapter One

THE COMPLEXITY OF HUMAN OCCUPATION

Charles H. Christiansen, EdD, OTR, OT(C), FAOTA and Carolyn M. Baum, PhD, OTR/L, FAOTA

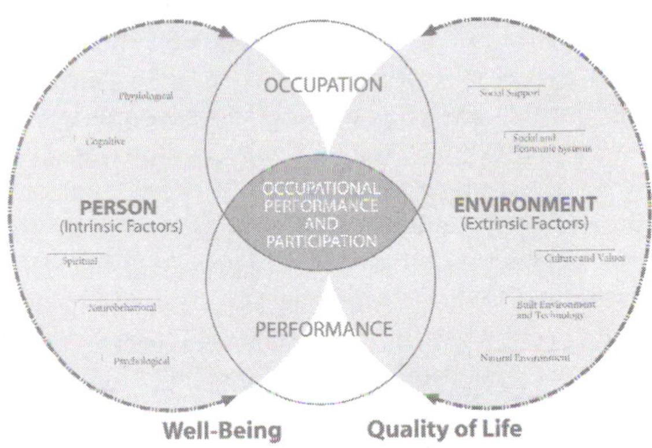

Setting the Stage

In this chapter, the task of understanding people as occupational beings begins with an exploration of the many dimensions of daily human activities. First, the complexity of the nature and meaning of what people do is illustrated. A description of the characteristics of human occupation is provided, along with a discussion of how those characteristics enable us to name and categorize different activities using taxonomies, including the *International Classification of Functioning, Disability and Health*. The chapter then proceeds with an analysis of activities from the standpoint of the factors influencing what people do, how they do it, why they pursue one activity over another, where people undertake activities, and the times during which some activities are customarily undertaken. Descriptions of some major categories of daily activity, such as work, play, personal care, and sleep, are provided. The chapter concludes with a brief discussion of the meanings people attach to activities and events; that is, how daily occupations are understood within the context of the lives (and life stories) of the people participating in them.

Don't miss the companion Web site to *Occupational Therapy: Performance, Participation, and Well-Being, Third Edition.*
Please visit us at http://www.cb3e.slackbooks.com.

Christiansen, C. H., & Baum, C. M. (2005). The complexity of human occupation. In C. H. Christiansen, C. M. Baum, and J. Bass-Haugen (Eds.), Occupational therapy: Performance, participation, and well-being (3rd ed.). Thorofare, NJ: SLACK Incorporated.

Occupations are what we do. They provide the basis for feelings about ourselves. They engage us in the world around us and, in so doing, enable us to survive and maintain ourselves. They develop our abilities and skills, allow us to pursue our interests, allow us to relate with other people, and allow us to express our values.

Mary Catherine Bateson, a well-known anthropologist and author, wrote:

> The capacity to do something useful for yourself or others is key to personhood, whether it involves the ability to earn a living, cook a meal, put on shoes in the morning, or whatever other skill needs to be mastered at the moment. (Bateson, 1996)

The routines of daily living mentioned by Bateson may often seem simple and mundane, but what seems simple is often complex. This is because daily occupations are often not just about doing, but about doing for a particular reason that is usually part of a larger picture. Occupations are done for ourselves and for others, and their connection with the social world imbues them with personal meaning. For this reason, putting on shoes is sometimes not just an act of dressing. On a particular morning, it may be part of an act of preparing for a job interview that represents the first opportunity to realize the advantages of the graduate degree that took nearly 20 years of formal education to attain. On such a morning, getting dressed is an important part of a day full of promise, of longstanding dreams, of future opportunity, and of the potential for pride in accomplishment. In fact, every occupation performed on that day may have an added importance beyond just being able to fulfill the task at hand. Other mornings may entail routines that may be equally important for other reasons. On the morning of the interview, the important goal is to succeed in making a good impression and to be hired for that position.

Because occupations encompass the many facets of life itself, they are by nature elaborate and difficult to understand. Much like a puzzle, their various pieces must be identified and arranged before a recognizable picture is apparent. But while the many dimensions of occupations contribute to their complexity, they also explain their rich, important role as the means through which we express our uniqueness. Each action and interaction with the world around us provides an opportunity to define ourselves. Much like a sculptor shaping clay, occupations are the means through which, over time, we shape our identities.

What Are Occupations?

John Dewey described occupations as continuous activities having a purpose (Dewey, 1916). Occupations have also been defined as the ordinary and familiar things that people do every day (Christiansen, Clark, Kielhofner, & Rogers, 1995). It follows, then, that if an activity is an occupation, it must be recognizable (or it would not be familiar). When phenomena are recognizable, they quickly become part of the working language of the culture. This enables people to describe and communicate about them.

With this thought in mind, Clark and colleagues (Clark et al., 1991) define occupations as "chunks of daily activity that can be named in the lexicon of [the] culture" (Christiansen, Backman, Little, & Nguyen, 1999). Kielhofner (1995) describes human occupation as "doing culturally meaningful work, play, or daily living tasks in the stream of time and in the contexts of one's physical and social world."

Each of these definitions contains elements, ranging from the goal directedness and the use of time to the influence of culture and the environment. Collectively, these multiple dimensions serve to underscore the complexity of occupation as a human concern.

Appreciating the Complexity of Occupations

To fully understand the complexity of occupation, we begin with a passage from *A River Runs Through It* by Norman Maclean. This beautiful story is one man's memory of growing up in Montana as the son of a Presbyterian minister who had a passion for fly-fishing. In this family, fly-fishing became a teaching metaphor for teaching the lessons of life and was a central leisure activity in family outings.

To many people, fly-fishing is one of life's most pleasant and challenging leisure pursuits. The passage below, from Maclean's beautiful story, serves as a particularly good example for beginning this section (Figure 1-1):

> ...in a typical week of our childhood Paul and I probably received as many hours of instruction in fly fishing as we did in all other spiritual matters. After my brother and I became good fishermen, we realized that our father was not a great fly caster, but he was accurate and stylish and wore a glove on his casting hand. As he buttoned his glove in preparation to giving us a lesson, he would say 'It is an art that is performed on a four-count rhythm between ten and two o'clock.' (Maclean, 1976)

As the passage by Maclean suggests, to truly understand fly-fishing, one must appreciate that it has many dimensions. First, it requires a capacity to plan, to organize, to sequence, and to move, according to a particular technique that requires much practice. But it also has subtle creative and expressive qualities, so that casting a rod properly can be viewed as an art form as well as a skill.

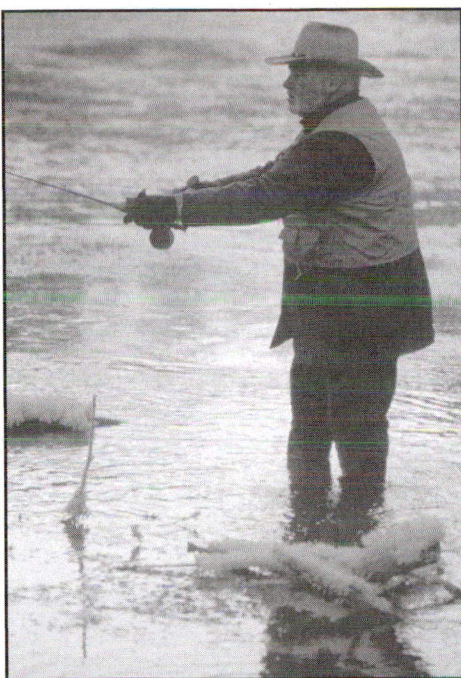

Figure 1-1. Fly-fishing—an occupation with many dimensions. (Reproduced with permission of Photos.com.)

The purpose of fly-fishing is to provide enjoyment through doing it and doing it well, rather than simply "catching a fish." In fact, when fly-fishing, people "get hooked" in the sense that what they do, how they do it, and where they do it seem to come together to create a special experience, described by Maclean as almost spiritual in nature. Finally, in Maclean's passage, fly-fishing is remembered as a boyhood activity that calls forth memories with special meaning. In *A River Runs Through It*, fly-fishing symbolizes special relationships, growing up, and meeting and mastering challenge.

The many facets of fly-fishing illustrate the complexity of occupations. Occupations have dimensions related to performing them, involving abilities, skills, and tools. Occupations have dimensions related to where they are done and under what circumstances, thus forming an important part of our experiences and life stories. In this sense, occupations also have dimensions related to their personal importance and meaning. They shape our identity and contribute to our sense of self. Finally, occupations have a social dimension in that how we describe them, how we value them, and how they provide us with meaning can often depend on our relationships and experiences with other people.

Occupations as Doing, Occupations as Meaning

Many descriptions of human occupation focus on what is done, or the performance of tasks. From a biological perspective, the term *function* is often used to describe an individual's performance of activities, tasks, and roles during daily occupations (Baum & Edwards, 1995). Still others have suggested that the important characteristic that distinguishes occupations from other human activities is the social and symbolic context that gives them meaning.

Nelson (1988, 1996) has recognized that people use the term *occupation* to refer to the process of doing as well as the situations in which occupations are done. In so doing, he provides a view that brings doing and meaning together. In Nelson's view, occupational performance describes the "doing" of occupation, whereas occupational form concerns the context of the doing or the background elements of a "doing situation" that provide it with purpose and meaning.

Consider, for example, the occupation of baking an apple pie for a special occasion using your grandmother's recipe. Using Nelson's concept, occupational performance would describe the steps and actions involved in following the recipe as the pie is prepared. The "occupational form" in this instance consists of the circumstances that give the act special meaning. The pie baking could call forth special memories of previous occasions, recollections of family traditions and relationships, and anticipations of good experiences to come (Figure 1-2).

In the illustration used above, it is easy to imagine that baking a pie for a friend's homecoming could bring about a different quality of action and attention than what might be found if the same person was baking a pie to contribute to a charity fundraiser. This is because it is likely that there would be different meaning associated with the two situations, even though the recipes and acts required for completing the task would be exactly the same.

Occupations have purposes, they have task-related or doing characteristics, and they have situations in which they are done. Most importantly of all, they have meaning for the person engaged in them. Occupations are given form by doing something in a particular place and at a particular time that imbues them with meaning.

While there are many definitions of occupation, some consistent characteristics can be found in them. Occupations are human pursuits that (a) are goal-directed or purposeful, (b) are performed in situations or contexts that influence how and with whom they are done, (c) can be identified by the doer and others, and (d) have individual meaning for the doer as well as shared meaning with others.

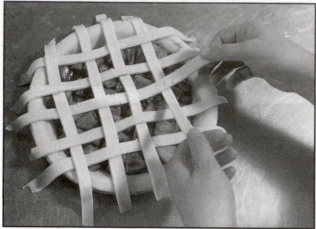

Figure 1-2. Form and performance. Baking an apple pie involves objects, processes, and contexts. (Reproduced with permission of Photos.com.)

In the following section, various approaches to describing the nature of occupation are presented. When we describe or classify a phenomenon, we are really speaking of how that phenomenon can be understood in terms of its similarities and differences with related phenomena. Through comparison, we relate the unknown to the known, thus increasing our understanding.

TAXONOMIES

Taxonomy is a method for organizing objects or events in nature. In their everyday use of language, people describe and classify based on the differences they observe. These primitive classification systems have been called *folk taxonomies*, and their purpose is to facilitate communication (Cormack, 1971).

One example of a folk taxonomy is the common classification for produce at a farmers' market. People classify produce as either fruits or vegetables, mostly unaware of the logic that creates this classification. Scientists, however, recognize a much broader array of edible plants, with various precise distinctions less important to the market shopper, but very important to science.

Folk taxonomies also exist for describing occupations. The most elementary folk taxonomy divides daily occupations into work and leisure, often viewed as work or nonwork. Other approaches have described occupations based on the degree of skill or practice required to engage in them (amateur versus professional), whether they are typically done alone or with others (individual versus group), and whether they are chosen or necessary.

The 18th century biologist Carl Linneaus (1735) created one of the best known taxonomies for classifying plants and animals (Figure 1-3). In this hierarchical system, each descending level becomes more precise as the plants or animals grouped and named share more characteristics in common. In a similar way, the classification of everyday occupations requires that they be identified and grouped according to their properties or characteristics. If researchers hope to study, compare, and understand daily occupations in a logical manner, then useful methods for classifying them will need to be developed.

Kingdom	Animal
Phylum	Chordate
Subphylum	Vertebrate
Class	Mammals
Order	Primates
Family	Hominids
Genus	Homo
Species	Sapiens

Figure 1-3. Example of classification of humans by Carl Linneaus.

Folk classifications used in everyday language are often not useful for science because they lack the precision and logic necessary in scientific classification. Just as folk taxonomies facilitate communication in everyday language, scientific taxonomies assist scientists and scholars in their communication by providing a means for identifying, labeling, grouping, and comparing the characteristics of phenomena under study. Science is often concerned with understanding and explaining differences, and taxonomies permit such differences to be described and categorized according to rules and the application of logic.

CLASSIFYING OCCUPATIONS

Approaches to classifying occupations have evolved from anthropology, sociology, psychology, human factors engineering, and medicine, particularly rehabilitation. These approaches have considered daily occupation from the standpoint of five questions:

1. What is done?
2. How is it done?
3. Why is it done?
4. Where is it done?
5. When is it done?

Each of these questions has implications for describing and comparing human occupations in a way that leads to greater understanding of occupational phenomena. In the following sections, we consider each of these questions as a convenient way of describing some of the characteristics that can be used to differentiate one category of occupations from another.

What Is Done?

A common approach to the classification of occupations involves describing what is done. This method groups occupations based on the nature of the tasks involved and is a frequent approach used to classify work-related occupations. These types of classification systems are used to facilitate efforts by government agencies concerned with workforce issues and the labor market. Because work has important implications for the productivity and economic status of nations and groups, far more attention has been devoted to the classification of work-related occupations than any other aspect of daily activity.

For example, in the United States, the development of the *Dictionary of Occupational Titles* (United States Department of Labor, 1991) was based on a task description approach that considered the extent to which a particular job required the use of objects, information, or interaction with people. Its successor, O*NET, or the Occupational Information Network, is a comprehensive database organized around the key attributes and characteristics of workers and occupations. The content model has six major domains, including worker experience, characteristics, and requirements; occupation requirements; occupational characteristics; and occupation-specific information (Peterson et al., 1997). The structure of the database enables the user to focus on areas of information that specify the key attributes and characteristics of workers and occupations. Each of the 1,122 work-related occupations in the database has requirements that include a combination of 52 abilities and skills (Fleishman & Reilly, 1992). This approach is similar to the *International Standard Classification of Occupations* (International Labor Organization, 1991), adopted in 1988 by the International Labour Organization, a specialized agency of the United Nations, and used in many countries. ISCO-88 classifies work and workers based on the nature, range, and complexity of the tasks performed (International Labor Organization, 1991).

The How of Occupations: Abilities and Skills

All occupations require specific abilities and skills if they are to be performed competently. For example, driving requires that the performer also have an acceptable level of attention, good visual acuity and reaction time, satisfactory knowledge of traffic laws and signage, and sufficient dexterity or coordination necessary to operate a vehicle.

Although these abilities and skills are necessary, they are not sufficient to ensure that a person can drive from home to work. Driving is also subject to environmental conditions. The roads must be passable, the car must be operational, and the directions to work must be known or shown on a map.

Fleishman, a human factors engineer, and Fisher, an occupational therapist, have done research aimed at understanding the ability and skill requirements for tasks and occupations (Fisher, 1997; Fleishman, 1972, 1975; Fleishman & Quaintance, 1984; Fleishman & Reilly, 1992; Fleishman et al., 1996). Fleishman and his colleagues have identified 52 abilities that can be used to classify the requirements of thousands of tasks. In theory, every purposeful occupation can be classified according to the abilities and skills required in its performance. Fisher has identified the skilled movement and cognitive characteristics of common household tasks as a way of measuring functional independence following medical rehabilitation.

Occupational taxonomies developed in biology and medicine tend to focus on abilities and skills required to perform tasks because this permits the targeting of rehabilitation efforts necessary to resume daily occupations despite physical or cognitive limitations. In biology and medicine, abilities and skills are often referred to as *functions*.

Because occupations involve more than just doing, a complete taxonomy of occupational performance should include not only human factors, such as abilities and skills, but task requirements and environmental factors as well. A new classification system developed by the World Health Organization (2001), called the *International Classification of Functioning, Disability, and Health*, recognizes the importance of factors other than abilities and skills (or their absence) and identifies environmental and social dimensions as important ways to categorize what people do (Figure 1-4). Activities describe performance of a task or action by an individual. Participation classifies an individual's involvement in life situations that occur in society. Each of these dimensions provides a greater understanding of occupations as transactions between people and environments. The body function/structure dimension helps us understand the factors that must be

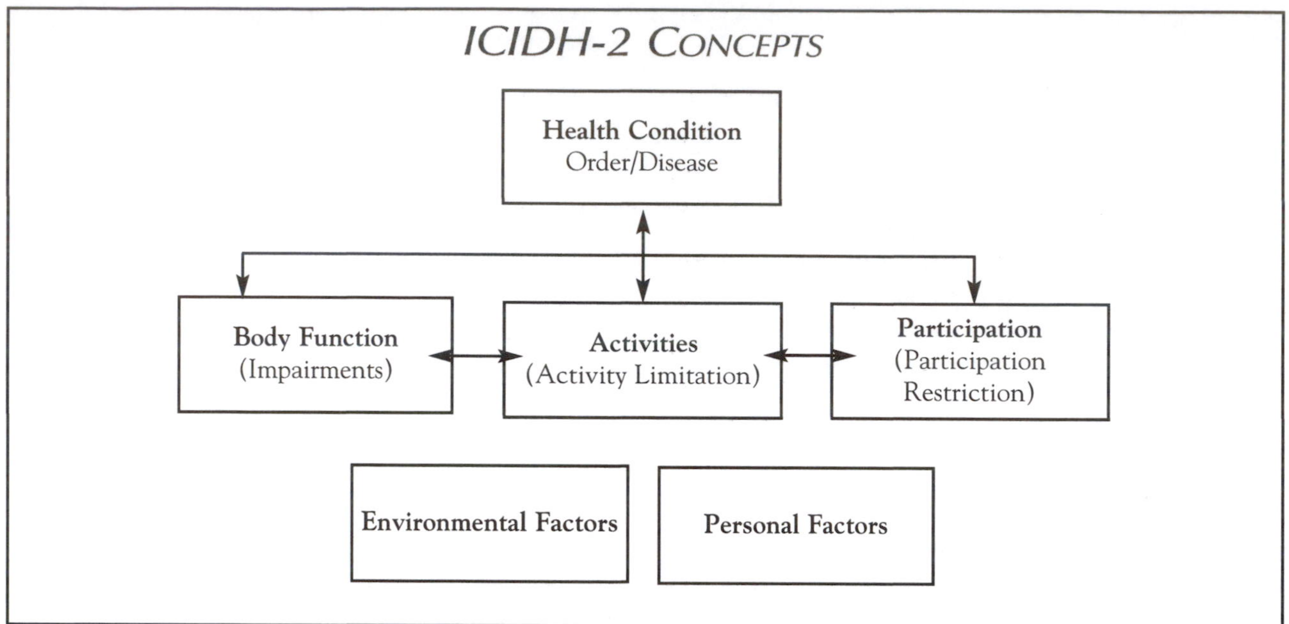

Figure 1-4. ICIDH-2 concepts.

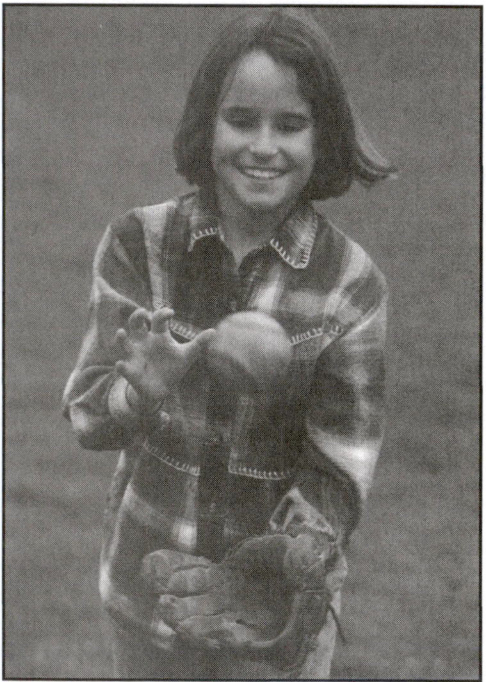

Figure 1-5. Playing catch is a leisure activity that represents more than mere movement. (Reproduced with permission of Photos.com.)

present to support the occupations of individuals. For example, to engage in throwing a ball, the individual must be able to initiate the action, attend to the target, and have the ability to grip and throw the ball—all while maintaining an upright position. These are body functions. The throwing of the ball is the activity. The participation is involvement of the child on a little league team or the adult playing catch with his or her child. Each of these involves meaningful engagement in occupation (Figure 1-5). Impairments can limit activities and thus limit participation in occupations.

The Why of Occupations: Grouping Occupations by Purpose

Although what people do during a typical day defines their "round" of daily occupations, the purposes of these activities constitute another approach to their classification. Studies of time use have used various taxonomies to categorize daily activities and have allowed researchers to describe how a typical day is spent when grouped according to the purpose of a given activity. These have varied according to the purposes for studying time use, which can range from economic purposes (as in measuring the value of goods and services) to lifestyle trends and public health. In recent years, efforts have been made to address the complexities of time use measurement through the formulation of more detailed time use surveys. These typically have as many as 12 major groups or categories and many subgroupings. For example, recent national time use surveys in Australia and Canada use major categories that include employed work, work at home, caring for household members, shopping, personal care, school and education, community participation, active leisure, entertainment, and passive leisure (Pentland, Harvey, Lawton, & McColl, 1999; Robinson, 1999).

Each major category may have several subcategories. For example, showering, eating, and getting dressed pertain to personal care; windsurfing, soccer, and running are types of active leisure; and stamp collecting, reading, and watching television are types of passive leisure.

In distinguishing among general categories of occupation, the most common classification used in everyday discourse identifies the domains of paid work, household work, leisure, personal care, and sleep. These categories have been convenient as general labels for communicating about and studying human occupation, largely because they account for the cycle of activities that constitutes the typical day, regardless of the culture being studied (Moore, 1995). Each of these general classifications will be briefly discussed in the following sections.

Work

Work has been defined traditionally as activity required for subsistence. Primeau (1995) provided a useful review of the domain of work, noting that definitions of this category of occupation vary from that of paid employment to that which is the opposite of rest or nonwork. She illustrates one of the difficulties in classifying occupation by noting that household work that is unpaid has discretionary characteristics. That is, the worker typically has great choice in determining what is done, and such discretionary choice is usually typical of play, rest, or leisure activities. Moreover, she points out that some people may derive relaxation and enjoyment from performing household chores, thus exhibiting another characteristic typical of nonwork activities. Another example is the sports "played" by professional athletes. These individuals often are paid generous salaries to exhibit their skills in tennis, baseball, soccer, hockey, and other sports for admiring audiences. Amateurs pursue these same occupations as freely chosen pastimes for recreation and leisure.

The term *productivity* has been proposed as a more useful alternative to the term *work*, recognizing that much productive activity is done outside of paid employment (Canadian Association of Occupational Therapists, 1995). The definition proposed for this category is, "Those activities and tasks that are done to enable the person to provide support to the self, family and society through the production of goods and services" (p. 141).

Leisure and Play

The characteristics of choice, expression, and development are often attributed to activities described as leisure. As a primary occupation of children, play is also a leisure category; however, the term is also used interchangeably with leisure to describe the nonwork activities of adults.

There is no agreement on whether or not play constitutes a classification similar to or different from leisure. Some activities pursued as leisure activities, such as reading or gardening, are not considered play or playful in nature according to some definitions. Given these and other similar examples, it may be appropriate to classify play as a special category of leisure activity.

Leisure has been defined as a particular class of activity, as discretionary time, and as a state of mind (Gunter & Stanley, 1985). Freedom of choice in participation without a particular goal other than enjoyment seems to be the defining characteristic of leisure activity. This "state of mind" philosophy dates back to the Greek philosophers Aristotle and Plato, who viewed leisure in terms of its opportunity for expression and self-development.

According to theorists, leisure participation fulfills important psychological needs. Attempts to classify specific leisure occupations have been reported (Holmberg, Rosen, & Holland, 1990; Overs & Taylor, 1977), but the validity of these classification systems has not been studied. Taxonomy of leisure based on need gratification (Tinsley & Eldredge, 1995) has been proposed that identifies 11 clusters of leisure pursuits that fulfill identified needs.

A more recent taxonomy (Stebbins, 1997) describes two types of leisure, serious and casual, each of which provides individuals with a distinct type of experience resulting in different states of mind. Serious leisure is described as the systematic pursuit of an amateur, hobbyist, or volunteer activity that becomes so engaging that the participant devotes considerable time and energy toward acquiring the skills, knowledge, and experience associated with it (Stebbins, 1997). In contrast, casual leisure is aimed at more immediate, short-term, and pleasure-inducing experiences that require little or no special training to enjoy them (Figure 1-6). Examples of casual leisure would include a walk in the park, window shopping, or going on a picnic.

Personal Care

Those activities that are necessary for maintenance of the self within the environment constitute the category of personal care. Often included in this category are activities related to basic self-care, such as eating, grooming, and hygiene. Other terms found in the literature for this broad category include *self-maintenance* (Reed, 1984) and *activities of daily living* (American Occupational Therapy Association [AOTA], 1994).

Personal tasks are viewed as necessary from a societal point of view (Christiansen, 2000). While eating and hygiene tasks are essential for survival and health, dressing and grooming are important to social interaction. This is because societies and cultures have many expectations for how people will present themselves. These role expectations influence an individual's acceptance and standing in the social community. If expectations are not met, people are at risk of losing their social standing. This

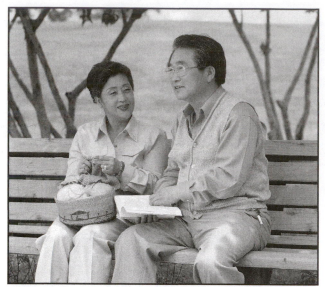

Figure 1-6. Knitting and other needlecrafts are popular leisure activities for both young and old alike. (Reproduced with permission of Photos.com.)

influences the degree of support and cooperation they receive from others. Social acceptance is essential to a healthy self-concept and success in many aspects of daily life, ranging from mate selection to career advancement (Hogan & Sloan, 1991) (Figure 1-7).

Sleep

Sleep is a specific personal-care occupation that is necessary for health (Kryger et al., 1995). Because humans spend approximately one-third of their lives in sleep, it is an important time use category. Despite decades of study, little is known with certainty about the function of sleep. Sleep is defined by behavioral and electrophysiological conditions. When asleep, organisms are quiet and devoid of movement. Brain waves indicate five distinct stages as evidenced by electroencephalographic (EEG) monitoring. The final stage is characterized by the presence of rapid eye movement (REM). In this stage, the EEG pattern is similar to wakefulness, yet the body has low muscle tone and is unresponsive to stimuli (Siegel, 1994).

From an evolutionary perspective, scientists are puzzled at how sleep has survived as a behavior. During sleep, animals cannot do any of the adaptive behaviors necessary for survival of the species, such as procreation, self-protection, or getting nourishment. Current theories suggest that sleep provides important restorative functions by repairing tissue, allowing for the consolidation of memory traces and information, and conserving energy (Aronoff, 1991; Hobson, 1995) (Figure 1-8).

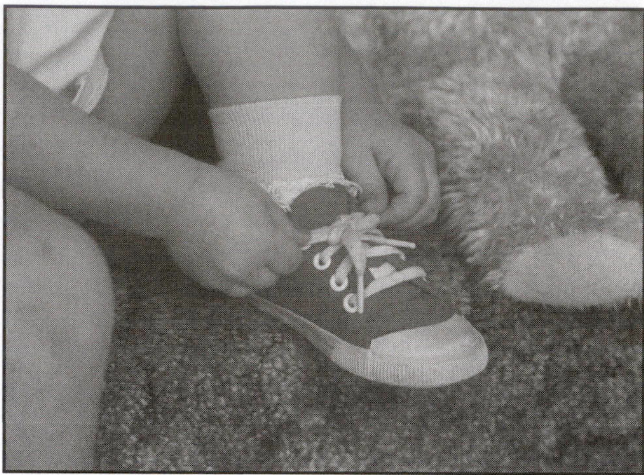

Figure 1-7. The mastery of self-care tasks by children has special meaning. (Reproduced with permission of Photos.com.)

The Where of Occupations

Occupations happen in places, and these places are often specific to the activity being pursued. In the built environment, rooms are designed around activities. Thus, self-care and sleep take place in bathrooms and bedrooms, cooking takes place in kitchens, and recreation takes place in gymnasiums and parks. The geographic location of activities has significant implications for individual mobility, public transportation, opportunities for participation and experience, and the development of social relationships.

Spivak (1973) used the term *archetypal places* to propose the idea that space and furnishings should be designed to support the fundamental types of activities that people do in various built environments. These concepts have been extended in ecological models of architecture, which propose that design of the built environment should be influenced significantly by concepts in psychology. Of particular interest is the symbolic communication that occurs through signs, symbols, and artifacts in environmental design. For example, it has been claimed that architectural designs can be improved to support human activity through improved understanding of transactions involving people and objects in homes, workplaces, and other environments (Altman & Werner, 1985; Lang, 1992a, 1992b).

Both built and natural environments have characteristics that influence behavior through the ways that they are perceived or experienced (Gibson, 1979; Murray, 1938). These characteristics of environments influence levels of arousal and motivation (Berlyne, 1960; Eysenck, 1982).

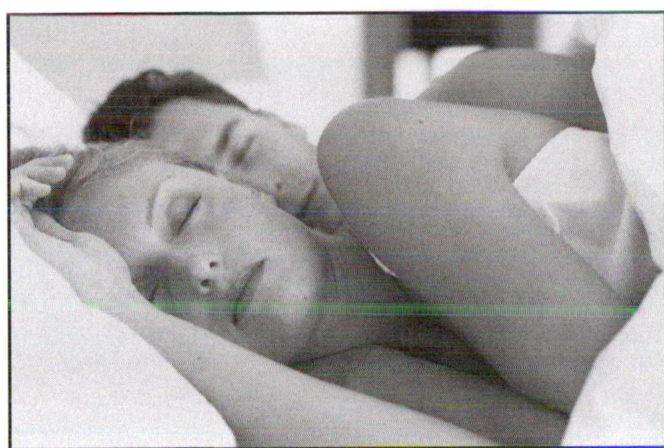

Figure 1-8. Despite the large amount of time devoted to this occupation, sleep is still poorly understood. (Reproduced with permission of Photos.com.)

The When of Occupation: Time Use and the Hierarchy of Acts

Occupation and time use are two sides of the same coin. Occupations have a temporal (time-related) dimension that is experienced over the lifetime as a continuous stream of time, interrupted by the requirement of sleep, and marked by the experience of significant events. As lives are lived over time, they are experienced as stories with a definite sequence because they have beginnings, middles, and ends.

Occupations are sometimes described as nested or embedded within each other as segments strung together over time (Bateson, 1996; Christiansen, 1991; Christiansen et al., 1995; Harre, Clark, & DeCarlo, 1985; Little, 1989; Trombly, 1995). For example, a picnic outing can be viewed as a whole event, but this event can be explained or identified by the many occupations comprising the excursion. These can range from preparing the food, to driving to the location, to eating hamburgers and potato salad, and so on. In turn, each of these occupations can be further subdivided into necessary tasks, such as collecting the items in preparation for packing. Each task has several steps or actions that can be further analyzed and described as acts. A fishing outing can be viewed as part of a summer vacation, as part of an eventful year with a loved one, or as part of a lifetime of such outings. As we move up the hierarchy, the behavior described is more complex, accounts for greater periods of time, and—it can be argued—is potentially more meaningful to the individual. Unfortunately, there are as yet no conventions for precisely naming or defining the levels of this unfolding hierarchy of time use.

Occupations may also be done concurrently. It is widely recognized that childcare often involves the performance of simultaneous activities. Studies of time use account for this enfolded nature of occupations by describing them as primary or secondary. For example, one may be driving to work, listening to the radio, and drinking coffee. Driving to work would be the primary activity, while drinking coffee and listening to the radio would be considered secondary activities.

Time Use

In this section, we begin with a review of literature that describes how time is used when activities are grouped into some of the main categories we have previously defined. This will lead logically to a discussion of other patterns of time use, including patterns of occupation over time, which are called *lifestyles*.

Much of the current information on time use comes from consumer research, although governmental agencies and scientists studying gerontology and leisure have also made useful contributions to our general understanding of how people "spend" their time.

General Patterns of Time Use

Time use studies indicate that for adults in the United States, on average, approximately 30% of a typical 24-hour day is spent sleeping; 10% is allocated to personal care activities (including eating); and another 10% is allocated to household work, such as cooking, laundry, and cleaning.

For those who are employed, approximately 25% of one's daily time is spent on actual paid work (excluding breaks). Thus, nearly 60% of the waking day is devoted to obligatory or required activities, including employment, for a typically employed adult. This proportion of obligatory activity has also been found for adolescents (Csikszentmihalyi, 1990).

There is international consistency in time allocation. Percentages reported for the United States are similar to data collected in other countries, showing remarkably consistent patterns, both for obligatory and discretionary categories of occupation, as well as in more specific areas of occupation, such as self-care and household maintenance (Baltes, Wahl, & Schmid-Furstoss, 1990; Castles, 1994; Mercer, 1985; Sjoberg, 1990).

Patterns of Occupation

Part of the predictability of living from day to day reflects the consistency of occupations. Obligatory occupations, such as self-care and sleep, are typically repeated as part of daily routines. Yet, some occupations, such as watching television or playing computer games, become so engaging they are pursued obsessively, sometimes with negative health consequences. Other occupations seem to have a self-perpetuating quality, which encourages the individual to continue pursuing them. A preliminary study involving university students suggested that one important element of this phenomenon, which Carlson (1995) terms *occupational perseverance*, was the individual's perceived progress toward meeting an important or valued goal. This tendency to continue pursuing an activity seems to be distinct from habits.

Habits

Some behaviors are repeated so often that they become habitual, performed on an automatic, preconscious level. In the extreme, recurring behavior may meet a strong physiological and psychological need, which is described as an addiction.

Habits influence behavior in a semiautomatic way without need for conscious, deliberate action. They are established through prior repetition of a series of acts and thus serve to enable higher occupations. Habits are more likely to occur in familiar environments and serve the purposes of conserving energy needed for attention and decision making while enabling us to do things we must do regularly without requiring high levels of motivation or energy.

Routines

Routines are occupations with established sequences, such as the morning ritual surrounding showering and dressing for the day. Routines provide an orderly structure for daily living as suggested in this description by Bond and Feathers (1988), who write that "a routine has a stability about it that extends over time and pertains to a particular set of activities within a defined situation" (p. 328).

Studies have supported the idea that certain activities naturally take place at certain times of the day. For example, a study of the daily lives of older adults in Germany (Baltes et al., 1990) observed that work and self-maintenance activities tended to predominate in the morning and early afternoon, whereas leisure and restful activities were associated with late afternoon and evening periods. Similar activity rhythms have been found in studies of higher-order group living animals, such as mountain gorillas (Harcourt, 1977).

Studies of biological rhythms tend to support the idea that routines are highly influenced by internal clocks. Routines are also provided structure by social and environmental factors that provide behavioral expectations. For example, working for an employer imposes the routine of a workday, while business hours at a favorite store may dictate shopping routines, just as religious services influence the times when spiritual occupations occur on days of worship.

Viewed over extended periods, habits and routines comprise important dimensions of lifestyles, components of which have been shown to influence health and well-being. For example, regular exercise, rest, and appropriate dietary habits are known as lifestyle behaviors that can be influenced by daily routines. Additionally, adherence to therapeutic regimens, such as eating or taking medications at prescribed times, can also be influenced by habits and routines. Unfortunately, the extent to which habits and regular routines contribute to healthful consequences (independent of specific practices) is not yet well understood.

Lifestyles

Habits, routines, and occupational preferences help define lifestyles. Lifestyles can be defined as a distinctive modes of living that are both observable and recognizable, and over which the individual has choice. Elliott (1993) notes that a routine or established way of dealing with personal needs and the demands of the environment, as well as an established and consistent pattern of involvement in a particular type of behavior, are also important characteristics of lifestyles (Figure 1-9).

Most studies of lifestyle have concentrated on behaviors related to maintaining health or well-being or preventing disease or injury. Behaviors in both areas often occur in clusters. That is, people who wear seat belts also tend to get adequate amounts of sleep, eat regular meals, exercise, and get regular medical and dental check-ups (Kulbock, Earls, & Montgomery, 1988). Conversely, people who abuse substances are often involved in delinquent behavior (Osgood, 1991).

Current theories of lifestyle intervention emphasize the importance of environments, including communities, social networks, values, norms, social sanctions, and opportunities for alternate behaviors, as factors important to influencing lifestyles. Work in anthropology and psychology shows that people understand their lives best as part of an unfolding story (Klinger, 1977). The importance of stories in creating life meaning constitutes an important concluding section in our survey of the complexities of occupation (Figure 1-10).

Life Stories

Viewing the past, present, and future as part of an unfolding story is an important mechanism in the meaning of everyday occupation and is known as narrative. Narrative refers to the autobiographical stories through which lives are described and interpreted to the self and others. These stories provide a sense of unity and purpose (Mancuso & Sarbin, 1985; McAdams, 1992). Jerome

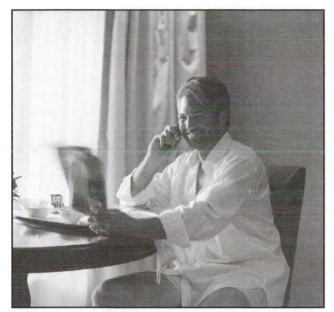

Figure 1-9. Lifestyles are partially explained by regular routines. Here, the morning routine illustrates embedded or nested activities. (Reproduced with permission of Photos.com.)

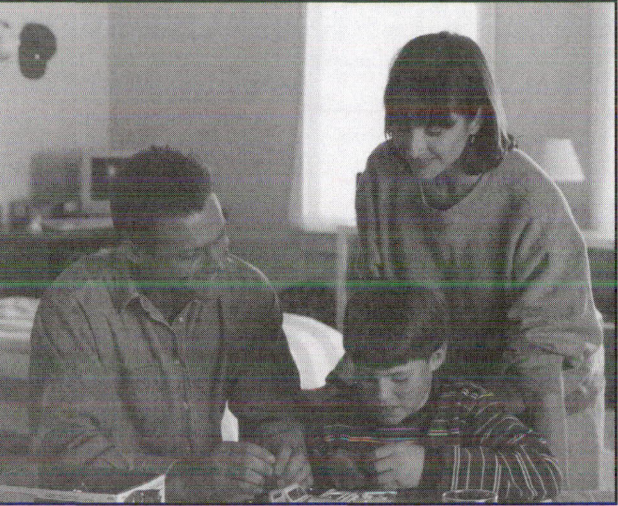

Figure 1-10. Parenting is a role that embodies many important dimensions of life meaning. Doing homework is an occupation filled with opportunities for symbolic meaning. What are some possible meanings that could be derived from this interaction? (Reproduced with permission of Photos.com.)

Bruner (1990) is convinced that the ability to make meaning of life events is so dependent on stories that he theorizes an innate or biological disposition to interpret events in the world through language.

It is believed that our sense of self, or social identity, is very much influenced by our ongoing interpretation of events through our life stories (Christiansen, 1999; Gergen & Gergen, 1988). Because our life stories are constantly being written and revised to incorporate new experiences, narrative can also serve as a motivational influence. That is, as we develop our life stories, we are guided by many possible scripts depending on the opportunities and options available to us (Markus, 1986).

Summary

This chapter began with a review of definitions and a description of the complexity of human occupation. Our examination of occupation proceeded with a description of its many dimensions. We observed that occupations can be classified as variations in the use of time. Traditional approaches to describing and classifying occupations were reviewed. In the traditional grouping by type and purpose, the categories of work, play, self-maintenance, leisure, and sleep were defined. Other approaches to classification include those based on the questions related to what, how, why, where, and when occupations are performed.

The information in this chapter provides an important backdrop for viewing occupation and appreciating its immense complexity. People in environments undertake occupations. These three elements—people, occupations, and environments—and the dynamic relationships among them helps to explain why understanding the nature of occupations can become so complex.

Occupations are also key to creating identities and establishing meaning in lives, and this adds to the complexity. As a result, information in this chapter can illustrate key concepts surrounding occupation for people in general, but it cannot explain the importance and meaning of occupations in a particular life. To begin to do this would require a familiarity with the concepts in the first section of this book and an in-depth interview and case study.

In the years ahead, more sophisticated information technologies will enable the collection and analysis of much additional data that will add to the body of knowledge in occupational science and permit the identification of options for enabling each person to pursue a lifestyle that brings well-being and life satisfaction.

Evidence Worksheet

Author(s)	*Year*	*Topic*	*Method*	*Conclusion*
Baum & Edwards	1995	Occupational engagement in persons with Alzheimer's disease	Descriptive	People with dementia of the Alzheimer type who remain actively engaged in meaningful occupations require less help with their daily self-care and show less disturbing behaviors thus reducing stress on their caregivers
Christiansen	1999, 2000	Occupations and life satisfaction in healthy community dwelling adults	Descriptive	Engagement in occupations perceived as more self-fulfilling and identity-related resulted in greater life satisfaction and happiness
Jonsson et al.	2000	Adaptation to retirement through occupational engagement	Descriptive	Retirement requires new temporal structures and must provide satisfactory meaning and rhythm for optimal transition from working roles
McGregor & Little	1998	Meaning through valued occupations	Descriptive	Goal achievement and efficacy are related to happiness, while identity dimensions of occupations are associated with measures of meaning
Primeau	2000	Household work routines and child care	Case study	Shared routines resulted in synchronized child care. Traditional routines resulted in maternal responsibility and paternal assistance with child care
Wood et al.	2000	Environment, time use, and adaptation in primates	Case study	Environmental opportunities and time interacted to produce press and channeling that limited behavioral expression

References

Altman, I., & Werner, C. (1985). *Home environments. Human behavior and environment: Advances in theory and research.* New York: Plenum.

American Occupational Therapy Association. (1994). Uniform terminology for occupational therapy—third edition. *American Journal of Occupational Therapy,* 48(11), 1047-1054.

Aronoff, M. S. (1991). *Sleep and its secrets: The river of crystal light.* Los Angeles: Insight Books.

Baltes, M. M., Wahl, H. W., & Schmid-Furstoss, U. (1990). The daily life of elderly Germans: Activity patterns, personal control, and functional health. *The Journals of Gerontology,* 45(4), 173-179.

Bateson, M. C. (1996). Enfolded activity and the concept of occupation. In R. Z. F. Clark (Ed.), *Occupational science: The evolving discipline.* Philadelphia: F. A. Davis.

Baum, C. M., & Edwards, D. (1995). Position paper: Occupational performance: Occupational therapy's definition of function. *American Journal of Occupational Therapy,* 49(10), 1019-1020.

Berlyne, D. E. (1960). *Conflict, arousal and curiosity.* New York: McGraw-Hill.

Bond, M. J., & Feathers, M. T. (1988). Some correlates of structure and purpose in the use of time. *Journal of Personality and Social Psychology, 55*(2), 321-329.

Bruner, J. (1990). *Acts of meaning.* Cambridge, MA: Harvard University Press.

Canadian Association of Occupational Therapists. (1995). *Guidelines for client-centred practice of occupational therapy.* Toronto: Author.

Carlson, M. (1995). The self perpetuation of occupations. In R. Z. F. Clark (Ed.), *Occupational science: The emerging discipline* (pp. 143-158). Philadelphia: F. A. Davis.

Castles, I. (1994). *How Australians use their time.* Canberra: Australia Bureau of Statistics.

Christiansen, C. H. (1991). The perils of plurality. *Occupational Therapy Journal of Research, 10*, 259-265.

Christiansen, C. (1999). Occupation as identity. Competence, coherence and the creation of meaning. *American Journal of Occupational Therapy, 53*(6), 547-558.

Christiansen, C. H. (2000). The social importance of self-care intervention. In C. H. Christiansen (Ed.), *Ways of living: Self-care strategies for special needs* (pp. 1-12). Bethesda: American Occupational Therapy Association.

Christiansen, C. H., Backman, C., Little, B. R., & Nguyen, A. (1999). Occupations and well-being: A study of personal projects. *American Journal of Occupational Therapy, 53*(1), 91-100.

Christiansen, C. H., Clark, F. A., Kielhofner, G., & Rogers, J. (1995). Position paper: Occupation. *American Journal of Occupational Therapy, 49*(10), 1015-1018.

Clark, F. A., Zemke, R., Frank, G., Jackson, J., Pierce, D., Wolf, R., et al. (1991). Occupational science: Academic innovation in the service of occupational therapy's future. *American Journal of Occupational Therapy, 45*, 300-310.

Cormack, R. M. (1971). A review of classification. *Journal of the Royal Statistical, 34*(3), 321-367.

Csikszentmihalyi , M. (1990). *Flow—The psychology of optimal experience.* New York: Harper and Row.

Csikszentmihalyi, M., & Larson, R. (1984). *Being adolescent: Conflict and growth in the teenage years.* New York: Basic Books.

Dewey, J. (1916). *Democracy and education.* New York: MacMillan.

Elliott, D. S. (1993). *Health enhancing and health compromising lifestyles.* New York: Oxford University Press.

Eysenck, M. N. (1982). *Attention and arousal.* New York: Springer-Verlag.

Fisher, A. (1997). Multifaceted measurement of daily life task performance: Conceptualizing a test of instrumental ADL and validating the addition of personal ADL tasks. *Physical medicine and rehabilitation: State of the art reviews, 11*, 289-303.

Fleishman, E. A. (1972). On the relation between abilities, learning and human performance. *Journal of the American Psychologist, 27*, 1017-1032.

Fleishman, E. A. (1975). Toward a taxonomy of human performance. *Journal of the American Psychologist, 30*(12), 1127-1149.

Fleishman, E. A., et al. (1996). Abilities: Evidence for the reliability and validity of the measures. In N. G. Peterson, M. D. Mumford, & W. C. Borman (Eds.), *O*Net Final Technical Report.* Salt Lake City, Utah: Department of Employment Security.

Fleishman, E. A., & Quaintance, M. K. (1984). *Taxonomies of human performance: The description of human tasks.* Orlando: Academic Press.

Fleishman, E., & Reilly, M. (1992). *Handbook of human abilities: Definitions, measurements, and job task requirements.* Bethesda: Management Research Institute.

Gergen, K. J., & Gergen, M. M. (1988). *Narrative and the self as relationship. Advances in experimental and social psychology* (pp. 17-55). New York: Academic Press.

Gibson, J. J. (1979). *The ecological approach to vision perception.* Boston: Houghton-Mifflin.

Gunter, B. G., & Stanley, J. (1985). Theoretical issues in leisure study. In B. G. Gunter & R. St. Clair (Eds.), *Transitions to leisure: Conceptual and human issues* (pp. 35-51). Lanham, MD: University Press of America.

Harcourt, A. H. (1977). Activity periods and patterns of social interaction: A neglected problem. *Behavior, LXVI*, 1-2:121-134.

Harre, R., Clarke, D., & DeCarlo, N. (1985). *Motives and mechanisms: An introduction to the psychology of action.* London: Methuen.

Hobson, J. (1995). *Sleep.* New York: Scientific American Library.

Hogan, R., & Sloan, T. (1991). Socioanalytic foundations for personality psychology. *Perspectives in Personality, 3*(Part B), 1-15.

Holmberg, K., Rosen, D., & Holland, J. L. (1990). *The leisure activities finder.* Odessa, FL: Psychological Assessment Resources.

Horne, J. A. (1988). *Why we sleep. The functions of sleep in humans and other mammals.* Oxford: Oxford University Press.

International Labor Organization. (1991). *International standard classification of occupations.* Geneva: International Labour Organization (United Nations).

Jonsson, H., Borell, L., & Sadlo, G. (2000). Retirement: An occupational transition with consequences for temporality, balance and meaning of occupations. *Journal of Occupational Science, 7*(1), 29-37.

Kielhofner, G. W. (1995). *A model of human occupation: Theory and application.* Baltimore: Williams & Wilkins.

Klinger, E. (1977). *Meaning and void: Inner experience and the incentives in people's lives.* Minneapolis: University of Minnesota Press.

Kryger, M., Roth, T., et al. (Eds.). (1995). *Principles and practice of sleep medicine*. Philadelphia: W. B. Saunders.

Kulbock, P., Earls, F., & Montgomery, A. (1988). Lifestyle and patterns of health and social behavior in high risk adolescents. *Advances in Nursing Science, 11*, 22-35.

Lang, A. (1992a). Toward a mutual interplay between psychology and semiotics. *Journal of the Society for Accelerated Learning and Teaching, 18*(3), 45-66.

Lang, A. (1992b). On the knowledge in things and places. In M. Cranach, W. Doise, & G. Mugny (Eds.), *Social representations and the social basis of knowledge* (pp. 76-83). Bern: Huber.

Lawton, M. P. (1971). The functional assessment of elderly people. *Journal of the American Geriatric Society, 19*(6), 465-481.

Linneaus, C. (1735). *Systema naturae*. Stockholm: Laurentis Salvii Holmiae.

Little, B. R. (1989). Personal projects analysis: Trivial pursuits, magnificent obsessions and the search for coherence. In D. B. N. Cantor (Ed.), *Personality psychology: Recent trends and emerging directions* (pp. 15-31). New York: Springer-Verlag.

Maclean, N. (1976). *A river runs through it*. Chicago: University of Chicago Press.

Mancuso, J. C., & Sarbin, T. R. (1985). The self-narrative in the enactment of roles. In T. R. Sarbin & K. E. Scheibe (Eds.), *Studies in social identity* (pp. 233-253). New York: Praeger Publishers.

Markus, H. (1986). Possible selves. *American Psychologist, 41*, 954-969.

McAdams, D. (1992). *Unity and purpose in human lives: The emergence of identity as a life story. Personality Structure in the Life Course* (pp. 323-376). New York: Springer.

McGregor, I., & Little, B. R. (1998). Personal projects, happiness and meaning: On doing well and being yourself. *Journal of Personality and Social Psychology, 74*(2)m 494-512.

Meddis, R. (1983). *The evolution of sleep. Theories in modern sleep research. Sleep mechanisms and functions in humans and animals-an evolutionary perspective* (pp. 57-106). Wokingham, England: Van Nostrand-Reinhold.

Mercer, D. (1985). Australians' time use in work, housework and leisure: Changing profiles. *Australian and New Zealand Journal of Sociology, 21*(3), 371-394.

Moore, A. (1995). The band community: Synchronizing human activity cycles for group cooperation. In R. Z. F. Clark (Ed.), *Occupational science: The emerging discipline* (pp. 95-106). Philadelphia: F. A. Davis.

Murray, H. A. (1938). *Explorations in personality*. New York: Oxford University Press.

Nelson, D. L. (1988). Occupation: Form and performance. *American Journal of Occupational Therapy, 42*(10), 633-641.

Nelson, D. L. (1996). Therapeutic occupation: A definition. *American Journal of Occupational Therapy, 50*(10), 775-782.

Osgood, D. W. (1991). *Covariation among adolescent health problems*. Background paper for U.S. Congress Office of Technology Assessment. Washington, D.C.: U.S. Government Printing Office.

Overs, R. P., & Taylor, S. (1977). Avocational counseling instrumentation. In D. M. Compton & J. E. Goldstein (Eds.), *Perspectives of leisure counseling* (pp. 89-105). Alexandria, VA: National Recreation and Park Association.

Pentland, W. E., Harvey, A. S., Lawton, M. P., & McColl, M. A. (Eds.). (1999). *Time use research in the social sciences*. New York: Kluwer Academic/Plenum Publishers.

Peterson, N., Mumford, M., Borman, W., Jeanneret, P., Fleishman, E., & Levin, K. (1997). *O*NET final technical report* (Vols. 1-3). Salt Lake City, UT: Department of Workforce Services.

Primeau, L. A. (1995). Work versus non-work: The case of household work. In R. Z. F. Clark (Ed.), *Occupational science: The evolving discipline* (pp. 57-70). Philadelphia, F. A. Davis.

Primeau, L.A. (2000). Household work: When gender ideologies and practices interact. *Journal of Occupational Science, 7*(3), 118-127.

Reed, K. L. (1984). *Models of practice in occupational therapy*. Baltimore: Williams & Wilkins.

Robinson, J. P. (1999). The time-diary method. In W. E. Pentland, A. S. Harvey, M. P. Lawton, & M. A. McColl (Eds.), *Time use research in the social sciences* (pp. 47-89). New York: Kluwer Academic Plenum Publishers: .

Siegel, J. M. (1994). *Brainstem mechanisms generating REM sleep. Principals and practice of sleep medicine* (pp. 125-144). New York: W. B. Saunders.

Sjoberg, L. M. R. (1990). Action and emotion in everyday life. *Scandinavian Journal of Psychology, 31*, 9-27.

Spivak, M. (1973). Archetypal place. *The Architectural Forum, 140*, 44-49.

Stebbins, R. A. (1997). Casual leisure: A conceptual statement. *Leisure Studies, 16*, 17-25.

Tinsley, H. E., & Eldredge., B. D. (1995). Psychological benefits of leisure participation: A taxonomy of leisure activities based on their need gratifying properties. *Journal of Counseling Psychology, 42*(2), 123-132.

Trombly, C. A. (1995). Purposefulness and meaningfulness as therapeutic mechanisms. *American Journal of Occupational Therapy, 49*, 960-972.

United States Department of Labor. (1991). *Dictionary of Occupational Titles (Revised)*. Washington, D.C.: United States Employment Service.

Webb, W. B. (1983). *Theories in modern sleep research. Sleep mechanisms and functions in humans and animals-an evolutionary perspective* (p. 1-17). Wokingham, England: Van Nostrand-Reinhold.

Witt, P. A., & Goodale, T. (1982). Stress, leisure and the family. *Recreation Research Review, 9*(3), 28-32.

Wood, W., Towers, L., & Malchow, J. (2000). Environment, time-use and adaptedness in prosimians: Implications for discerning behavior that is occupational in nature. *Journal of Occupational Science*, *7*(1), 5-18.

World Health Organization. (2001). *International classification of functioning, disability and health*. Geneva, Switzerland: Author.

Chapter One: The Complexity of Human Occupation Reflections and Learning Activities

Julie Bass-Haugen, PhD, OTR/L, FAOTA

REFLECTIONS

When we think about occupation after reading this chapter, we realize that the idea of occupation is both beautiful in its simplicity and amazing in its complexity. Let's think about some of our occupations from childhood (e.g., coloring, swinging upside down on a bar, building sandcastles, riding a bike). Remember how totally lost or absorbed we could be in them. Life (and occupations) seemed so simple then. If we allow ourselves to re-experience these occupations in our minds, it hardly seems like there is any more to them than just the "doing." Now, when we look at those same occupations again after reading this chapter, we begin to appreciate the complexity of occupations and their effect on all aspects of life.

I remember coloring a lot as a child. Let's think about different ideas introduced in the chapter and see how they relate to my childhood occupation of coloring. This chapter introduced different classification systems and the meaning of occupations. How would I classify my coloring? In some ways, it must have been part of the work of childhood. After all, it couldn't have been all fun to master holding the crayon and learn to stay within the lines. On the other hand, I remember how coloring allowed me to express myself through different colors and develop my artistic interests. Isn't this play? Here, we can begin to appreciate why it has been so difficult to develop a classification system for the things we call occupations. The meaning of this occupation is also difficult to describe. Furthermore, the meanings I attribute to coloring are unique to me. Some words I associate with coloring are success, creativity, peacefulness, and comfortable. How might my meanings be different than another person with different experiences?

In this chapter, we also had a beginning discussion on the personal abilities and skills that are needed for successful occupational performance. Different occupations require different abilities and skills. The abilities and skills that I need for inline skating are obviously quite different than those I need for coloring. An analysis of an occupation can help us understand the underlying structures and functions that support a given occupation. For my coloring (at its best), I was able to sit erect, hold a pencil, see the page, conceptualize a plan, initiate smooth and continuous movements, and evaluate my final product. The list I generated only contains a few of the many skills and abilities I used in coloring!

This chapter also discussed the influence of environment on occupations. In my example of coloring, did having "my own little corner" in the house (the natural/built environment) influence my experience? Did the periodic interjections from my mom ("that is your most beautiful picture yet") or the sharing of a page with my sister who was my best buddy (social environment) shape my occupation? Did the values regarding artistic accomplishments held by my extended family (cultural environment) influence my passion for coloring?

Temporal or time-related dimensions of occupations were also identified as important to consider. Sometimes, my coloring was the only occupation I was doing at a given time. But, if I think about it, my coloring was often being done at the same time (concurrently) as another occupation, say watching TV. Sometimes, coloring was the main occupation (primary), and sometimes coloring became secondary as I began to watch my favorite TV show. The necessity of my coloring also varied. At school, I am sure that coloring was obligatory if I was going to get a passing grade in kindergarten. At home, however, coloring was discretionary in that I could choose to do it or not do it at a given point in time.

The nature of my coloring had certain characteristics at a certain point in time and has been evolving ever since. There was the period of time when coloring with crayons in a coloring book was a predominant occupation in my life and one of which I was particularly proud. I then have vague recollection of a time when I realized it wasn't cool anymore to be coloring unless I used an easel, colored pencils, or the front of my 5th grade math notebook. This coloring of mine has evolved further yet into doodling during meetings and a mother-daughter activity. How will the passage of time continue to influence my coloring?

The temporal dimension of coloring likely influenced my coloring in other ways as well. Is my coloring as a child in some small way connected to (or embedded in) who I am as an adult? Did coloring connect to my printing and cursive writing in elementary school? Did coloring then connect to an interest in expressing myself through written and artistic forms? When we reflect on some of these possible temporal connections in our lives, how can we not be amazed at the power of occupation?

The last topic area in this chapter addressed the relationships between occupations and habits, routines, and lifestyles. This topic was used to examine and characterize the patterns of occupations we have in our lives. After all, we are not very interesting or complete if all we have is a single occupation. It is the constellation of occupations that make me, me and you, you. For example, you know very little about me if all I tell you is that I colored as a child. However, you would begin to get a clearer picture if I told you coloring was one of many similar occupations that included magnetic sketch pads and art projects. You would know even more about my patterns if I told you I had quite a variety of occupations as part of my daily routine. My day also consisted of outdoor occupations including wading in the creek, biking around the neighborhood, playing basketball in the driveway, and playing hide and seek on the big hill near our house. And this is only a small sample of my childhood occupations and the patterns they formed!

In summary, this chapter provided a foundation for understanding the simplicity and complexity of our occupations. The meanings we attach to our occupations were introduced in the many dimensions of occupation and the influence of personal and environmental characteristics on our performance.

Journal Activities

1. Look up and write down two dictionary definitions of occupation. Highlight the components of the definition that are most related to the descriptions of occupation in Chapter One.
2. Identify the most important new learning for you in this chapter.
3. Identify one question you have about Chapter One.
4. Generate possible synonyms or related words for the following key terms introduced in Chapter One. Use information in the chapter and your own ideas.
   - Occupation
   - Work
   - Leisure or play
   - Personal care

Technology/Internet Learning Activities

1. Use a discussion database to share assigned journal entries.
2. Use an Internet search engine (e.g., google, dogpile, mamma, yahoo, excite) to conduct a general and specific search related to topics in this chapter.

- General Search
  - ✧ Enter each key word from Journal Activity #4 (occupation, work, leisure or play, personal care). You may want to add other words to your search line as well (e.g., definition, theory, classification, taxonomy, research).

    What types of sites did your search engine find for each word?

    Evaluate the quality of the Internet sites.

    Give an example of a site that has useful information for each term.

    What surprises did you encounter in these searches?

    Try a different search engine. Do you get different results?
  - ✧ Enter some of your synonyms or related words from journal activity #4. You may want to add other words to your search line as well (e.g., definition, theory, classification, taxonomy, research).

    What types of sites did your search engine find for each word?

    Evaluate the quality of the Internet sites.

    Give an example of a site that has useful information for each term.

    What surprises did you encounter in these searches?

    Try different search engines and add other keywords. What are your results?
- Specific Search
  - ✧ Conduct a search on the following phrases:

    Dictionary of Occupational Titles or Occupational Information Network (or O*Net)

    International Standard Classification of Occupations

    World Health Organization International Classification of Function

    Time use surveys

Human performance taxonomy
Leisure Tinsley or Leisure Stebbins
Archetypal places

- ✧ Try different search engines and add other keywords. What are your results?
  What information on these topics is available on the Internet?
  What topics interest you?
  Document these interest areas and Internet sites for future interest.
- ✧ What other technology-based searches might be helpful in the general and specific searches?

Individual Learning Activities

Individual Learning Activity #1: Reflection on an Occupation

- Reflect on an occupation in your life using a process similar to the one discussed in the reflection. This occupation may be from your childhood or a current occupation. Follow the instructions below.
  1. Describe one of your occupations.
  2. How would you classify this occupation?
  3. Describe the meanings of this occupation to you.
  4. What skills and abilities do you have that support performance of this occupation?
  5. What are some of the environmental factors that support performance of this occupation?
  6. How has this occupation changed over time?
  7. What other occupations are done concurrently with this occupation?
  8. How is this occupation embedded in other aspects of your life?
  9. How does this occupation relate to your habits, routines, or lifestyles?

Individual Learning Activity #2: An Occupational Profile of 2 Days

- Develop an occupational profile of 2 days in your life. If possible, try to pick days that are typical rather than extraordinary. Follow the instructions to complete the grid on p. 21.
  1. Pick one weekday and one weekend day to record your use of time in terms of occupations.
  2. Identify the time from the beginning to the end of each change in occupation.
  3. Identify the primary occupation you are doing at that time.
  4. Indicate whether the primary occupation is obligatory or discretionary.
  5. Categorize your primary occupations as work, play, self-care, or rest and write the total time spent on that occupation in the category (e.g., 15 minutes = 0.25, 6½ hours = 6.5).
  6. Identify any secondary occupations you are doing at that time (e.g., your primary occupation is studying, your secondary occupation is listening to music).
  7. Describe each day in terms of hours of time for each of the four categories of your primary occupations.

Sample

Time	*Primary Occupation*	*Obligatory or Discretionary*	*Work*	*Play*	*Personal Care*	*Rest/ Sleep*	*Secondary Occupation*
12:00 am to 6:30 am	Sleep	Obligatory				6.5	None

Time Use Survey

Time	*Primary Occupation*	*Obligatory or Discretionary*	*Work*	*Play*	*Personal Care*	*Rest/ Sleep*	*Secondary Occupation*
From To							
From To							
From To							
From To							
From To							
From To							
From To							
From To							
From To							
From To							
From To							
From To							
From To							
From To							
From To							
From To							
From To							
From To							
From To							

Group Learning Activities

Group Activity #1: Representing Occupations in a Collage

Preparation: Read Chapter One
Time: 45 minutes to 1 hour
Materials:

- Poster board (at least 18 X 24)
- Magazines
- Craft supplies
- Tape, glue, scissors

Instructions:

- Individually:
  - ✧ Use the materials above to create a collage that represents the array of occupations in your life. In addition to depicting actual occupations, try to communicate meaning and patterns of occupation.
- In small groups:
  - ✧ Present your collage to a small group of peers. Listen to the presentations of collages by your peers.

Discussion:

- Summarize how you would describe the occupations and patterns of occupations of each group member.
- Discuss the similarities and the differences in your occupational lives.

Group Activity #2: Sharing Descriptions of One Occupation

Preparation:

- Read Chapter One.
- Complete Individual Activity #1.

Time: 30 to 45 minutes
Materials: Journal entries
Instructions:

- Individually:
  - ✧ Bring Individual Activity #1
- In small groups:
  - ✧ Use the table below to identify the different occupations for your group members and to answer the following questions. After you have filled in the table, complete the discussion below.

    Identify one of your occupations.
    What is (are) the classification(s) of this occupation in your life?
    What are the meanings of this occupation to you?
    What skills and abilities do you have that support performance of this occupation?
    What are some of the environmental factors that support performance of this occupation?

Person	*Occupation*	*Classification(s)*	*Meanings*	*Skills/Abilities*	*Environment Influences*
1.					
2.					
3.					
4.					

Discussion:

- Summarize the occupations for each group member.
- Tell one story regarding your occupation to the rest of the group.
- Discuss how the classification(s), meanings, and stories of one occupation might be different for different group members.
- Discuss the similarities and the differences in your responses.
- Discuss some hypothetical skills and abilities (or limitations) that could make performance of the occupation easier? more difficult?
- Discuss some hypothetical environmental factors that could make performance of the occupation easier? more difficult?
- How might the variation in and complexity of your responses to each of the questions make it challenging to do research studies on human occupation?

Group Activity #3: Sharing Results of Internet Searches

Preparation:

- Read Chapter One.
- Complete Technology/Internet Activity #2.

Time: 30 to 45 minutes

Materials:

- Notes from Technology/Internet Activity #2
- Internet access (optional)

Instructions:

- Discuss strategies used for Internet search.
- Discuss findings from Internet search.
- Discuss questions from Technology/Internet Activity #2.

Chapter Two Objectives

The information in this chapter is intended to help the reader:

1. Understand the changes in human occupation in Western civilization during the span of recorded history.
2. Appreciate how the relationship between work and leisure changed through history as the result of technological developments.
3. Explain how religion influenced work and leisure.
4. Understand how patterns of work and leisure influenced cultural attitudes and behaviors.
5. Describe how beliefs about work changed over time.
6. Appreciate how attitudes toward leisure changed through history.

Key Words

agricultural age: The period of history when farming or crop production was the primary form of human work.

capitalism: An economic system based on a belief in private ownership of the means of production and distribution of goods and characterized by a free competitive market and profit as an incentive.

Civilian Conservation Corps: An agency created by the government during the Depression to create employment opportunities in the service of conservation projects to enhance and preserve the natural environment.

conspicuous consumption: Spending lavishly to impress others.

Industrial Revolution: The social and economic changes in Great Britain, Europe, and the United States that began in the second half of the 18th century and involved widespread adoption of industrial methods of production.

Medieval Period: The period in European history between antiquity and the Italian Renaissance, often considered to be between the end of the Roman Empire in the 5th century and the early 15th century.

postindustrial age: The period following industrialism where service-oriented work rather than production of goods created most employment opportunity.

Puritan ethic: A belief in strict moral or religious principles with emphasis on the value of work and diminished respect for pleasurable activity.

work ethic: A belief in the moral value of hard work.

Work Progress Administration: An agency created during the Depression to provide work through commissioned projects in the arts and humanities.

Man's activity is either a making or a doing.
Both of these aspects of the active life depend... on the contemplative life.
Coomaraswamy

Chapter Two

THE EVOLUTION OF OCCUPATION

Robert K. Bing, EdD, OTR, FAOTA

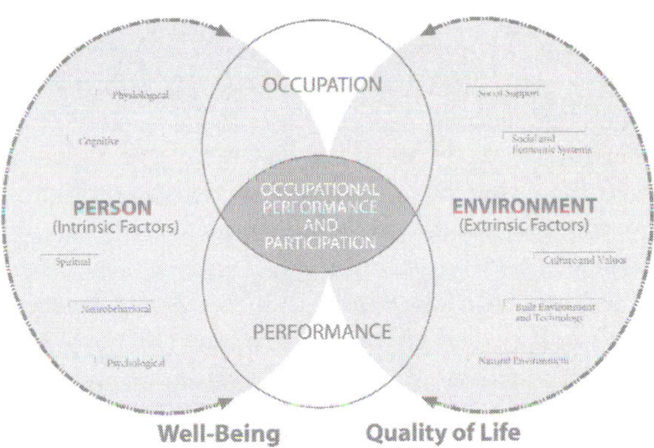

Setting the Stage

In this chapter, the historical evolution of goal-directed human time use is described. Recorded accounts and archaeological findings have provided a glimpse of the daily round of occupations from early times through the present, stretching from agrarian and preindustrial ages through postindustrial and modern (information age) eras. This chapter illustrates how technological advances accounted for changes in the types of occupations undertaken and the time devoted to them.

One consequence of technological development was the relative amount of time devoted to work and leisure (or play). Despite differences in the types of occupations pursued, characteristics of each age support the underlying theme that humans undertake occupations to meet basic needs for security, safety, emotional satisfaction, and novelty.

Bing, R. K. (2005). The evolution of occupation. In C. H. Christiansen, C. M. Baum, and J. Bass-Haugen (Eds.), Occupational therapy: Performance, participation, and well-being *(3rd ed.). Thorofare, NJ: SLACK Incorporated.*

THE BEGINNINGS

The earliest humans occupied their time with the need to survive. Work was divided: men were hunters and gatherers and women, because of their child-bearing responsibilities, were the preservers and fashioners of materials for consumption. With the perfection of these tasks, the greatest of man's transformations of the environment began. Hunting and planting cultures became dominant. Animal husbandry was added, along with fashioning various artifacts, such as tools, pottery, textiles, and basketry, useful in accomplishing more complex tasks. As humans collected themselves into settlements, more specific divisions of labor occurred, and valued specialists emerged as artisans. Surpluses in the production of food and artifacts allowed humans to engage in trade between nearby settlements. The Agricultural Age had arrived and would last for several thousands of years (Roberts, 1993).

THE CLASSICAL PERIOD

Traditional Judeo-Christian beliefs provide an explanation of how labor was to become an all-absorbing element of human life. Adam and Eve were created to cultivate and guard the Garden of Eden, but they were admonished by God not to taste the fruit of the tree that gives knowledge of what is good and evil (Genesis 2:15). The disobedience of this commandment, known as original sin, caused the couple to be banished, with the declaration: "Because of what you have done, the ground will be under a curse. You will have to work hard all your life to make it produce enough for you" (Genesis 3:17-18).

The Hebrews recognized the burden of original sin, yet they held a reverence for work and the contemplative life. Several scriptures in the Old Testament attest to the belief that labor is necessary to prevent poverty and destitution (Proverbs 10:15-16; Proverbs 13:3; Proverbs 14:20; Proverbs 20:13). The Talmud states that labor is a holy occupation, and even if one does not need to work to survive, one must nevertheless labor, for idleness causes an early death. Further, those who truly revere heaven must eat from the labor of their hands. These individuals are far above those who devote their entire time to studying God's work and depend upon others for sustenance (Rapaport, 1910). Labor was the way of expiating original sin and regaining spiritual dignity.

Some centuries later, the Greeks made clear distinctions between work and leisure. Like the Hebrews, they regarded work as God's curse, and it was performed by slaves (Maywood, 1982). Mental labor, thought to be a part of work, was condemned, along with the mechanical arts, such as pottery or weaving. The philosophers Plato and Aristotle declared that the reason the majority of men labored was "in order that the minority, the elite, might engage in pure exercises of the mind—art, philosophy, and politics" (in other words, leisure) (Tilgher, 1930). Plato asks, "What is the right way of living? Life must be lived as play, playing certain games... singing and dancing, and then a man will be able to propitiate the gods..." (Huizinga, 1950). Aristotle's concept has been summarized as "freedom from the necessity of being occupied" (deGrazia, 1962).

Class stratification developed, with slaves, peasants, and craftsmen; a middle class of merchants who concentrated on bartering and exchanging goods; and a wealthy upper class indulged in the luxuries of living, such as teaching, discovering, thinking, and composing music. Braude (1975) states that if one worked when it was *not necessary*, there was a risk of compromising the distinctions between slave and master. Leadership was based on the work a person *did not have to do*. From these roots, leisure became a foundation stone of Western culture. Leisure in Greek is *skole*, and in Latin, *scola*, the English, *school*. The term used to designate the place for learning is derived from the word that originally meant *leisure*.

The Romans adopted the Greek work ethic. Along with nearly unlimited manpower, the Romans held their empire together through technology, particularly in constructing edifices and organizing useful activities for the benefit of the populace (Lipset, 1990). For instance, baths were elaborately designed to include cool, warm, and hot rooms, using both water and fire. These baths were places of leisure for the wealthy and nobility. A wide variety of afternoon pleasures were available: including exercise, massage, and hair plucking (because body hair was thought to be in poor taste). Evening meals were artful events for pleasure seekers. The Romans thought there were only two occupations suitable for the free man—agriculture and business, particularly if these led to an honorable retirement as a country gentleman (Tilgher, 1930).

EARLY CHRISTIANITY AND ISLAMIC BELIEFS

The early Christians followed the Hebrew thinking of work as God's curse. Work did take on some positive values. Bodily and spiritual health was maintained through labor, particularly when it crowded out idleness and sloth, both considered forms of evil. The Apostle Paul, in his letters to the Ephesians and Thessalonians, mentioned the value of work. It gains self-respect, respect from others; keeps one from being dependent upon others; and provides one with something to share with others in need (Good News Bible, 1971).

Islam, meaning submission or surrender in Arabic, first appeared in the latter years of the first century, common era, and was the latest of the three great monotheistic religions (the others being Judaism and Christianity). The Qur'ran (Koran) is considered the last revelations from God and provides a complete view of all life, including activity for man.

Muslims' work ethic is exemplified by a door sign found in Senegal: *Work as if you will never die; pray as if you will die tomorrow.* A fundamental belief is that the earth was created for the benefit of man, and God has given him control over it. Man's duty is to profit from this gift and to be generous in helping those who are less fortunate. Yet:

> It is not permitted... to avoid working for a living on the pretext of devoting his life to worship or trust in Allah... The Prophet taught his companions that the whole of a human being's dignity is tied up with his work—any sort of work ... [however] always take the middle path (balance between work and leisure, a balanced lifestyle). (Al-Qaradawi, 1960)

Qur'anic verses mention that man acts according to his own will and desires, including the pursuit of happiness and pleasure, but within the context of specific laws, customs, and behavior.

THE MEDIEVAL PERIOD

With the collapse of the Roman Empire, the western world descended into what came to be known as the Dark or Middle Ages. The all encompassing mood was one of pessimism and gloom. "Life, to borrow Hobbe's phrase, was 'solitary, poor, nasty, brutish, and short';... mankind was being punished for its sins and sinners, and everyone had better repent because the end was near" (Goodale & Godbey, 1988). The prevailing survival tasks returned, and a two-tier civilization became evident: peasants and the nobility, made up of wealthy merchants and royalty.

There were long breaks from the day's drudgery, particularly during the nongrowing season. Popular leisure in medieval rural areas borrowed a Roman principle, *saturnalia*, and converted it into a "binge," an unrestrained indulgence in food and drink. It served well as an emotional release for those who knew scarcity all too well (Cross, 1990).

A movement, founded by St. Augustine, created communal monastic living, wherein adherents dissociated themselves from worldly affairs to concentrate on a spiritual life. St. Benedict added labor to the traditional vows of poverty, chastity, humility, obedience, and silence. Monks were never inactive because idleness was considered an enemy of the soul; 7 hours were given to occupations and 2 hours to reading (Bennett, 1926). This movement grew throughout Europe, until there were at least 40,000 monasteries under Benedictine rule.

A remarkable machine had been invented within the monasteries—the clock. Goodale and Godbey (1988) state, "Days and lives became divided into increasingly precise units, and human activity became synchronized not by song but by an endless stream of tics and tocks." Work and leisure were never again to be quite the same. Alfred The Great, King of Wessex (849-899 AD) was given one of the contraptions by the local abbot. He was so impressed by its significance that he offered the right of the freeborn to a three-twentyfourths division of the day into work, leisure, and rest.

During the medieval period, leisure primarily centered on seasonal, pagan, and church-related celebrations or feast days. Fairs were popular as opportunities for nearby communities to display and exchange the results of their labors. One secular holiday was the *Feast of Fools*, usually celebrated about January 1. Cox (1969) describes the festival:

> Even ordinarily pious and serious townsfolk donned bawdy masks, sang outrageous ditties, and generally kept the whole world awake with revelry and satire. Minor clerics painted their faces, strutted about in the robes of their superiors, and mocked the stately rituals of the church and court.

Remnants can be seen in today's Halloween and New Year's Eve celebrations.

The work ethic had evolved so that labor was seen as a way of delaying or avoiding despair. It was a preferred method for the expiation of sin. Hard labor in the fields was considered the antidote for pride and the wantonness of the flesh. In the 13th century, Thomas Aquinas, Italian philosopher and Doctor of the Church, using Aristotelian logic, categorized work as it was to be valued. Farming was first; then handcrafts; and, last, commerce. Financial enterprises were not included because Aquinas felt that interest earned was not work. Profit was earned only through work or inheritance. Work was a necessity, and it should be organized through various guilds—all part of a providential plan (Roberts, 1993).

During this era, families tended to include several children. The size of the family was influenced by the kinds of work to be performed within the family. In order for farms to be successful, children were introduced to a variety of agricultural tasks at the earliest age possible, when their coordination and strength could be put to use. In the "cottage industries," where handcrafts were a primary source of income, young children, particularly girls, were put to work learning the required skills. Play time was incidental, seasonal, and allowed only when there was no significant work to be performed.

Among middle-class youth, apprenticeships became the chief source of education and were the best means of rising to a position of respectability and influence in the community. It was not uncommon for a father to apprentice his own son and another man's son, whom he treated as his own. This apprenticeship generally lasted 7 years and included moral, religious, and civic instruction. He taught "all the mysteries of his craft, including recipes, rules, and applications of science, mathematics, and art as might be involved in the craft" (Bennett, 1926).

Slavery became a serious issue in accomplishing needed, but undesirable, work. During the first millennium, Arabs transported eastern European Slavs (who gave their name to this kind of forced labor) to northern Africa. Italian merchants sold slaves from Germany and central Europe to the Arabs. Black African slaves were first brought to Europe in the mid-15th century and within 100 years, merchants from several nations were shipping Black Africans across the Atlantic to Brazil, the Caribbean islands, and North America. Roberts (1993) concludes, "The trade thus entered upon a long period of dramatic growth whose demographic, economic, and political consequences are still with us."

The Protestant (Work) Ethic

The Reformation arrived in the early years of the 16th century in western Europe. This upheaval created significant changes in the ethics of occupations. Martin Luther, an Augustinian friar, became discontent with Roman Catholic practices. Within 3 years, he was excommunicated, and the Protestant Reformation was underway.

Luther felt work was natural, a way out of the curse of original sin. It was the universal base of society; all those who can work must work; working and serving God were synonymous. He fostered the idea of the "calling," wherein one dutifully performs the work God has called him or her to do. Luther believed that all occupations had equal spiritual dignity; thus, manual labor was acceptable. He did not approve commerce as an occupation because it did not involve real labor. This put him at odds with Aquinas' value hierarchy. Further, Luther believed that everyone should work enough to meet basic living needs; to acquire wealth was sinful.

Within the next century, the Protestant Work Ethic was materially altered by John Calvin, a Frenchman. He brought to fruition capitalism, which had been introduced just prior to the Reformation. Everyone must work, that was the will of God. A fair price for one's efforts and a reasonable profit were acceptable. Calvin believed in predestination, a revolutionary idea that said that the Elect were chosen by God to inherit eternal life. All others were damned. The "chosen" were not to lust after the fruits of their labor; rather, to apply their sweat and toil toward profit, which was to be used in helping establish the Kingdom of God on earth. Miserly hoarding, usury, idleness, and anything that softens the soul were signs of damnation.

Modern capitalism came into being with labor not being casual, but "methodical, disciplined, rational, uniform, and hence specialized work" (Tilgher, 1962). These were essential characteristics if one were to please God. Calvin broke with Luther over the issue of "the calling." Everyone has a duty to seek a station in life that will bring greatest satisfaction and profit. Success is the certain indication that one has been chosen. Profit was to be invested in even greater works.

During this same period, work-free days were ever-increasing in numbers, and most were tied to the religious calendar. At one time, Paris had 103 holidays, while the rural areas celebrated 84 days, not including those days off because of inclement weather. In the mid-16th century, the English Parliament attempted to restrict holidays to 27 per year, but met with considerable resistance from rural areas. During days following a religious holiday, there would be several kinds of secular fun: horse parades; processions of various trade guilds; circuses and traveling shows; and various sports, such as running, wrestling, boxing, cricket, and even trying to climb a greased pole with some kind of trophy on top (Cross, 1990).

A tradition among urban craft people (i.e., tailors, mechanics) was "St. Monday," usually a whole day off. Women's trades, such as lace and laundry, did not fare as well, because they did not earn sufficient wages and were not as well organized as the men's guilds.

The Puritan Ethic

One of the more significant movements of the 16th and 17th centuries in England was the Puritans. They appeared during the Elizabethan Age and strongly objected to the Anglican church's hierarchy and propensity for ceremonial lavishness. They were Calvinist in their learnings and wanted to purify the church along lines suggested by Luther and Calvin. They objected to the prevailing customs and morals, which they believed to be vain, wanton, and wasteful in ostentatious display.

By the time the Puritans had immigrated to North America, they had developed a strict code that covered their views of occupation. Work was essential to survival of the community. One was to save and to use the profits for the benefit of themselves and others. Borrowing from Calvin, prosperity was evidence of God's grace, not only in the here and now, but would lead toward eventual salvation. Ostentatious dress, gluttony, idleness, and lust were immoderate pleasures and, thus, sinful. Thus arose the God-fearing middle-class businessperson.

On the other hand, they were not joyless fanatics. "Eating, relaxing pastimes, and sexual gratification, the Puritan ministers argued, all gave refreshing pleasures that when practiced in moderation benefited the individual and hence the community" (Daniels, 1995). Nearly every community had a tavern where alcohol was served, but inebriation was abhorred. Moderate amounts of alcoholic libations were provided at town expense to attract unpaid workers to house-raisings and to provide the necessary courage to walk out on a stringer or ridgepole (Morison, 1930).

Drama and art were thought to be sensuous display. Instrumental music, even in church, was denied for the same reason. "Simple, functional beauty and art they produced and appreciated as being closest to God's design" (Goodale & Godbey, 1988).

Puritans had a somber view of childhood. Laws were passed enjoining parents and masters to teach children to read (Hall, 1982). The seeking of knowledge by reading was an important activity. Children were not to be humored or encouraged in family play because that would eventually lead to perverseness and aberrant behavior in their later years. No toys were manufactured in 17th century New England. Children often attempted to make toys out of their surroundings, but parents discouraged their use in play (Mergen, 1980).

Puritans did enjoy themselves, despite the external trappings of asceticism. "H. L. Mencken quipped that Puritanism was 'the haunting fear that someone, somewhere, may be happy'; that view seems destined to live forever" (Daniels, 1995). They went about their fun both boisterously and spiritually, within the family and in the community. Much of today's sense of human and personal responsibility is inherited from the Puritans. They believed that their material and spiritual welfare was dependent upon their own efforts. Worldly wealth and personal pleasures were far less important than intellectual and spiritual pleasures (Goodale & Godbey, 1988).

The Industrial Revolution

The Agricultural Age gave way, slowly, to what came to be known misleadingly as the *Industrial Revolution*. It lasted at least two centuries, first in Europe, then in North America. The historian Charles A. Beard (1901) defines it as "that great transformation which has been brought about... by discoveries and inventions which have altered fundamentally all methods of production and distribution by means of life, and consequently revolutionized all economic functions of the society." The initial phase consisted of producing articles through the use of simple, hand-operated machines, progressing to later phases using sophisticated and complex power-driven machinery (Tierney, 1968).

What was revolutionary was the impact the new technology had upon people's lives. The idea that work came from a *calling* fell away, and Calvin's notions about capitalism took on a new meaning. The modified Protestant Work Ethic now included the "moral sanction to profit making through hard work, organization and rational calculation" (Yankelovitch, 1981a). People were warned to work hard; otherwise, poverty was in their future, and moralists stressed the social duty of everyone to be productive. Nelson (1981) states that "man became a producer of things and his social well-being became secondary to the production of marketable goods."

By the mid-19th century, the apprentice system was considered inadequate for preparing workers for the new labor, so trade and training schools emerged, first in Europe and later in America. A pioneer proponent was the Swiss educator and social reformer Johann Pestalozzi. He saw special skill training as a way for young people to avoid poverty and to gain self-sustaining employment. He contended that preparation for a vocation must include a broad range of human education (Nelson, 1982).

Pestalozzi's views resulted in the establishment of technical institutes and "manual training schools," generally in large cities. The first institution in America devoted to manual training was established at Washington University, St. Louis, in 1879. It was a 3-year program, admitting boys at least 14 years old. The curriculum included a wide variety of hand and machine tool instruction, as well as mathematics, drawing, and English. Other similar schools were created for girls, with emphases upon textiles, commerce (typewriting, shorthand), and domestic sciences (Bennett, 1937). All of these institutes and schools had to continuously update the courses of study to keep current with the expanding technology.

Industrial capitalism brought about a familiar class stratification. Those living in rural areas and former slaves did not adapt well to the industrial setting. A large working class, primarily of immigrants, increasingly became available. Jewish communities established special training programs to "Americanize" immigrants' skills. A small leisure class emerged, known as captains of industry. Thorstein Veblen in 1899 published his *Theory of the Leisure Class* in which he describes their tendency toward conspicuous consumption, vicarious consumption, conspicuous leisure, and conspicuous waste (Veblen, 1994). Cross (1990) states:

> What drove these men was the hope of winning status through the possession of wealth and the display of freedom from work. Leisure was not valued as an opportunity for self-expression or growth so much as a means of demonstrating social status.

Goodale and Godbey (1988) describe this generation as being at opposite ends of the scale: "one with plenty of money and plenty of free time but little experience in how to use either; the other with long hours of enforced, standardized, unfulfilling work, but with little of the communal leisure they had previously experienced." In time, the working class sorted out most of its problems and came to desire and consume the goods it was producing. A middle class emerged, made up of managers, supervisors, owners of small- and medium-sized businesses, and they adopted many of the habits of the leisure class.

Although work dominated everyday life, free time was available and consisted of a variety of leisure pursuits. Many middle-class Americans, living by the Puritan ethic, felt they could not play unless they were improving themselves or preparing for more work. For many, the annual vacation was a stay at a Chautauqua resort or health spa. The length of a vacation was debated. "President Howard Taft recommended two to three months, New York Supreme Court Judge Henry Bischoff suggested two months for professional men, one month for businessmen, and two weeks for clerks" (Schlereth, 1991).

Railroads realized that vacationers were a lucrative business. They created tours and built elaborate resorts on their rail lines, for even those of moderate means. With the coming of the automobile and a highway system, middle-class Americans, at long last, had found a way to meet their wanderlust needs.

Closer to home, family fun was varied with girls spending time with their mothers doing needlecrafts while boys were building tree houses or indulging in a variety of sports. Lawn games, such as croquet, archery, and lawn tennis, were played by both sexes. Most parlors had a "Victrola," a piano, or an organ. Solitary and family reading of novels and adventure stories were popular. Holidays included elaborate meals and picnics.

Physical fitness became a craze, ranging from calisthenics and tumbling to intense gymnastics. Bicycles were popularized, with cycle clubs having their distinct uniforms and colors. Spectator sports became a trend, with track, field, and ball games. Baseball, football, and boxing became professionalized, which "put skilled players on the field and unpracticed spectators in the stands" (Schlereth, 1991).

Times of Crises

The Industrial Revolution received a severe jolt a decade following World War I. Complex, interrelated, and unresolved issues, such as reparations and protective tariffs, contributed to world economic collapse. By the early 1930s, half of German men between 16 and 30 were out of work. The unemployment rate in Australia went from less than 10% in 1929 to more than 30% in 1932 (Reader's Digest, 1977). In the United States, unemployment was 19% by 1938. Despair was everywhere. One jobless father lamented, "During the Depression, I lost something. Maybe you call it self-respect, but in losing it, I also lost the respect of my children, and I'm afraid I am losing my wife" (Kennedy, 1999).

Two U.S. notable government programs were the Works Progress Administration (WPA) and the Civilian Conservation Corps (CCC). In its 8 years, WPA employed more than 8.5 million people at a total cost of $11 billion. Highways, bridges, public buildings, and parks were constructed. Thousands of artists, musicians, actors, and writers were put to work in their crafts (Kennedy, 1999). During its decade of life, the CCC put to work more than 3 million idle young men in reforestation, flood control, river and shoreline projects, and disaster relief. The men earned $30 a month and were required to send $25 home for their families (McElvaine, 1993).

Free time was limited and generally revolved around the family and the community. For most, monies were not available for new toys. Children and youth accepted hand-me-down objects or constructed their own out of scrap materials and played games, often making up the rules as they went. Cereal box tops and a dime (earned from chores) brought, through the mail, many simple, but cherished, treasures. Radios, table and lawn games, activities in parks, and the movies were staples. Brief Sunday afternoon auto rides were popular diversions. The traditional Puritan ethic held fast and proved a lifesaver to those savaged by the Great Depression.

World at War and Peace

The world depression came to an end with the advent of World War II. America quickly became the *arsenal for democracy*: "an abundantly endowed and uniquely privileged sanctuary where economic mobilization could proceed free from most supply problems, safe from enemy harassment, and therefore with maximum efficiency" (Kennedy, 1999). Unprecedented numbers of women in the Allied nations left their homes to work in war industries or to perform support services. The Puritan work ethic, coupled with the resolve to win the war, brought unprecedented success.

While many material shortages prevailed, leisure was considered essential to the war effort. The family and community found plenty with which to be amused: the radio, dances, sports, the movies, teen canteens, choral and band groups. Family events at home and in parks provided respite from work. Chatty V-mail letters to those in service was a favorite pastime.

With World War II ending in 1945, a peace time economy emerged, with certain immediate goals: reclamation of Europe and the Far East and reconstruction of the world's industries, to meet the pent-up needs for goods. In 1948, the United Nations adopted the "Universal Declaration of Human Rights." Among these was "the right to work, to free choice of employment, to just and favorable conditions of work... the right to equal pay for equal work." In another article, "everyone has the right to rest and leisure, including reasonable limitation of working hours and periodic holidays with pay" (General Assembly of the United Nations, 1948a, 1948b).

The commercialization of leisure became a dominant feature of the postwar lifestyle: professional sports, television, movies, the local pub, or cocktail lounge. Hobbies and pastimes took on great importance and were hugely financed. The joke that the only difference between boy's and men's toys is the price became quite true. Colleges and universities realized that to recruit students they would have to be able to adequately answer an important question: "Other than attending class and studying, what are the students doing on campus?" Intramural sports, pep rallies, intercollegiate games, fraternity/sorority dances, and visits to the local hangouts were essentials. The young adult culture centered on leisure through socialization.

On October 4, 1957, the world was stunned by the news that the Soviet Union had successfully placed in orbit an object that came to be known as "sputnik." This event set off a gigantic race for technological superiority, with the goal of leapfrogging over the Soviet Union to place a man on the moon and return him safely to earth, within a decade. With the Puritan Work Ethic firmly tucked under their arms, North American scientists, industrialists, and entrepreneurs went to work.

The Postindustrial Age

Suddenly, everything was in flux. The advancements, many of them having to do with communications technology, were accompanied by a shift in ways of thinking and feeling. Ferguson (1980) describes the social ferment of the 1970s and the consciousness-raising of the 1980s as:

> ...a social transformation resulting from personal transformation change from the inside out... Change can only be facilitated, not decreed. It seems to speak to something very old. And perhaps by integrating magic and science, art and technology, it will succeed...

Naisbitt and Aburdene (1982) popularized the transformation by declaring that Western society was reluctantly leaving behind the Industrial Age and entering the "Information Age," in which the new wealth was know-how: "The occupational history of the United States tells a lot about us. For example, in 1979, the number-one occupation became clerk, succeeding laborer, succeeding farmer. Farmer, laborer, clerk—that is a brief history of the United States." Louv (1983) prefers "Postindustrial Age" to describe the new era, in which he sees two conflicting cultures. Traditionalists are caught in the present and are highly distrustful of the new technologies. Others exuberantly see a transformation "into something new and fresh: [they] perceive the future as a new technological frontier to be conquered and won."

A revised Puritan Work Ethic evolved. In Yankelovitch's study of basic American values (1981b), there are four themes: (1) *the good provider*: the family's breadwinner is the real man or woman; (2) *independence*: by standing on one's own two feet, one avoids dependence upon others; work is equated with autonomy; (3) *success*: "hard-work always pays off"; it comes in the form of home ownership in a select neighborhood, a rising standard of living, conspicuous consumption of leisure, a secure retirement; and (4) *self-respect*: one can feel good about one's self by keeping faith with the precept, "work hard at something and do it well"; hard work, menial or exalted, has dignity.

The most portentous change was the rapid increase of women in the work setting outside the home. Putnam (2000) indicates, "The fraction of women who work outside the home doubled from fewer than one in three in the 1950s to nearly two out of three in the 1990s." This has resulted in significant shifts in shared responsibilities for housework, child care, and community volunteer work. There has been no general decline in free time; however, changes have occurred. Robinson and colleagues (1999) note that less educated people gained free time, whereas their college-educated counterparts, for the most part, have lost it. Dual-career families are spending more time at work than they used to, averaging 14 more hours at work each week in 1998 than in 1969. Time diary studies "show that, unsurprisingly, people who spend more time at work do feel more rushed, and these harried souls do spend less time eating, sleeping, reading books, engaging in hobbies, and just doing nothing" (Putnam, 2000).

Electronic and communication devices, derived from the space race, altered not only the workplace, but how free time is spent. The computer has become a focal point in both locales. News and entertainment have become individualized. Putnam (2000) declares:

> In 2000, with my hi-fi Walkman CD, wherever I live I can listen to precisely what I want when I want and where I want. As late as 1975, Americans nationwide chose among a handful of television programs. Barely a quarter century later, cable, satellite, video, and the Internet provide an exploding array of individual choice.

At an accelerating pace, the electronic transmission of information, news, and entertainment have virtually changed all features of living.

Conclusion

Throughout history, humans have been true to their nature to grow and develop, which is an ability to increase in capacity and complexity, in order to not merely survive, but to thrive in an ever-changing, unpredictable life. Critical to these processes is the drive toward work and its balancer, leisure or play. When judiciously blended, they continuously help meet the universal needs of emotional response from others; security of a long-term sort; and novelty of experience (Linton, 1945).

Some of the most deep-seated values one holds collect around work and leisure or play. Gibran (1951) says it well when he wrote:

> When you work, you fulfill a part of earth's furthest dream, assigned to you when that dream was born, and in keeping yourself with labor you are in truth loving life, and to love life through labor is to be intimate with life's inmost secret... It is to charge all things you fashion with a breath of your own spirit.

Of equal significance are the values expressed by Godbey (1985): "Leisure is living in relative freedom... so as to be able to act from internally compelling love in ways that are personally pleasing, intuitively worthwhile, and provide a basis for faith."

Acknowledgments

The author wishes to express his profound appreciation to Ilham Kahlil, OTS, for her invaluable assistance in gathering information about Islam.

References

Al-Qaradawi, Y. (1960). *The lawful and prohibited in Islam.* Indianapolis, IN: American Trust Publications.

Beard, C. A. (1901). *The industrial revolution.* London: George Allen & Unwin, Ltd.

Bennett, C. A. (1926). *History of manual and industrial education up to 1870.* Peoria, IL: The Manual Arts Press.

Bennett, C. A. (1937). *History of manual and industrial education: 1870-1917.* Peoria, IL: The Manual Arts Press.

Braude, L. (1975). *Work and workers.* New York: Praeger.

Cox, H. (1969). *The feast of fools: A theological essay on festivity and fantasy.* New York, NY: Harper & Row.

Cross, G. (1990). *A social history of leisure since 1600.* State College, PA: Venture Publishing, Inc.

Daniels, B. C. (1995). *Puritans at play: Leisure and recreation in colonial New England.* New York, NY: St. Martin's Griffin.

deGrazia, S. (1962). *Of time, work and leisure.* New York, NY: Twentieth Century Fund.

Ferguson, M. (1980). *The Aquarian conspiracy: Personal and social transformation in the 80s.* Los Angeles, CA: JP Tarcher.

General Assembly of the United Nations. (1948a). Universal Declaration of Human Rights, Resolution 217 A (III), Article 23(1).

General Assembly of the United Nations. (1948b). Universal Declaration of Human Rights, 1948, Resolution 217 A (III), Article 24.

Gibran, K. (1951). *The prophet.* New York, NY: Alfred A. Knopf.

Godbey, G. (1985). *Leisure in your life* (2nd ed.). State College, PA: Venture Publishing.

Goodale, T. L., & Godbey, G. C. (1988). *The evolution of leisure: Historical and philosophical perspectives.* State College, PA: Venture Publishing, Inc.

Good News Bible. (1971). New York: American Bible Society, Ephesians 4:28; I Thessalonians 4:11-12; 2 Thessalonians 3:6-13; Genesis 2:15; Genesis 3:17-18; Proverbs 10:15-16; Proverbs 13:3; Proverbs 14:20; Proverbs 20:13.

Hall, D. D. (1982). Literacy, religion and the plain style. In J. Fairbanks (Ed.), *New England begins the seventeenth century* (p. 102). Boston, MA: Museum of Fine Arts.

Huizinga, J. (1950). *Homo ludens: A study of the play-element in culture.* Boston, MA: Beacon Press.

Kennedy, D. M. (1999). *Freedom from fear: The American people in depression and war, 1929-1945.* New York, NY: Oxford University Press.

Linton, R. (1945). *The cultural background of personality.* New York, NY: Appleton-Century-Crofts, Inc.

Lipset, S. M. (1990). The work ethic—Then and now. *Public Interest, winter,* 61-69.

Louv, R. (1983). *America II.* Los Angeles, CA: J. P. Tarcher.

Maywood, A. G. (1982). Vocational education and the work ethic. *Canadian Vocational Journal, 18,* 7-12.

McElvaine, R. S. (1993). *The great depression: America, 1929-1941.* New York, NY: Times Books.

Mergen, B. (1980). Toys and American culture: Objectives as hypotheses. *Journal of American Culture, 3,* 746-750.

Morison, S. E. (1930). *Builders of the Bay Colony.* Boston, MA: Houghton Mifflin.

Naisbitt, J., & Aburdene, P. (1982). *Megatrends.* New York, NY: Avon Books.

Nelson, L. P. (1981). Background: The European influence. In R. Barella & T. Wright (Eds.), *An interpretive history of industrial arts. 30th Yearbook, American Council on Industrial Arts Teacher Education* (p. 25). Bloomington, IL: McKnight & McKnight.

Putnam, R. D. (2000). *Bowling alone: The collapse and revival of American community.* New York, NY: Touchstone.

Rapaport, S. (1910). *Tales and maxims from the Talmud.* London: George Routhledge Sons.

Reader's Digest. (1977). *Great events of the 20th century: How they changed our lives.* Pleasantville, NY: Reader's Digest Association, Inc.

Robinson, J. P., Godbey, G., & Jacobson, A. J. (1999). *Time for life: The surprising ways Americans use their time.* State College, PA: Pennsylvania State University Press.

Roberts, J. M. (1993). *History of the world.* New York, NY: Oxford University Press.

Schlereth, T. J. (1991). *Victorian America: Transformations in everyday life, 1876-1915*. New York, NY: HarperPerennial.

Tierney, W. F. (1968). The industrial revolution. In J. F. Luetkemeyer (Ed.), *A historical perspective of industry. 17th Yearbook, American Council on Industrial Arts Teacher Education* (p. 91). Bloomington, IL: McKnight & McKnight.

Tilgher, A. (1930). *Homo faber: Work through the ages*. New York, NY: Harcourt Brace.

Tilgher, S. (1962). Work through the ages. In S. Nosow & W. H. Form (Eds.), *Man, work, and society: A reader in the sociology of occupations* (pp. 10, 19, 20). New York, NY: Basic Books.

Veblen, T. (1994). *The theory of the leisure class*. New York, NY: Penguin Books.

Yankelovitch, D. C. (1981a). *New roles: Searching for self-fulfill-ments in a world turned upside down*. New York, NY: Random House.

Yankelovitch, D. C. (1981b). The meaning of work. In J. O'Toole, J. L. Scheiber, & L. C. Wood (Eds.), *Working: Changes and choices* (pp. 34-35). New York, NY: Human Science Press.

Chapter Two: The Evolution of Occupation
Reflections and Learning Activities
Julie Bass-Haugen, PhD, OTR/L, FAOTA

REFLECTIONS

This chapter introduced the highlights of occupational evolution, especially as it relates to Western civilization. In a sense, it is about the history of occupational engagement over the centuries. Some readers might wonder, can't we just skip the history stuff? One of the things I have learned over the years is that the best way to understand who we are and where we are going is to look at where we have been. This also holds true for understanding who we are as occupational beings. A detailed examination of the evolution of occupations in one culture is also a good way to begin to explore the occupational evolution of another culture.

There were two themes in this chapter that are important to note. These themes are evident in every period of history that was examined in the chapter. Both of these themes related to the delicate interplay between our patterns of work and our patterns of leisure.

The first theme was that patterns of work and leisure have the characteristic of both changing and recurring over the ages. The expression "what goes around, comes around" is often used to describe things like fashion, that appear, disappear, and re-appear over time. You only have to look at several decades of photographs to see that the jeans we call flares in this decade once had a life as bell-bottoms in the 1960s and 1970s. This is also true of occupations. Some creative arts, like needlework, were almost disappearing in the latter half of the 20th century. In recent years, these and other occupations have made a huge comeback in many areas of the country. This is evident in the large number of craft stores that are appearing on the scene. The case was made in this chapter that patterns of work and leisure occupations (habits, routines, lifestyle) also "go around, come around." Each period of history makes some changes from the previous period and reclaims some characteristic of a bygone era.

The second theme was that religion and patterns of work and leisure have played a large role in shaping a society's values and behaviors. Let's think about each of these ideas separately. Religion has always had a major influence in defining a culture. In the last couple of decades, any discussion of Northern Ireland, Afghanistan, or the Middle East has included a commentary on the religions of the area. While these examples might seem a little too obvious, if we look carefully, we can see religious influences on the celebrations of a small town in Brazil and the exercise practices in an urban area of China.

Patterns of work and leisure also shape a society. Even if we don't live in an agricultural area, we have heard that the work life of a farmer is from "sun up to sun down" and 7 days a week. We might also guess that leisure on a farm is woven into the fabric of each day in small ways. In urban areas, we may find that most work life is based on the 40+ hours per week, Monday through Friday schedule. Leisure is done around this schedule and is generally assigned specific blocks of time. Tuesday and Thursday evenings may be scheduled for going to the athletic club. Saturday evenings may be reserved as a time for a movie or dinner with friends. This chapter helped us understand how occupations have evolved from these two influences, religion and work/leisure patterns.

From the description of each time period, we saw people had beliefs about work. Some of these beliefs changed, and some recurred at various intervals. These beliefs considered the nature of work, the purpose of work, the benefits of work, and who should do certain kinds of work. We learned that the role of work has been tied to specific religious beliefs about a person's relationship with God. We also saw that certain aspects of work were viewed as important for the health and welfare of people. Finally, each period consisted of certain types of work, and sometimes these types of work were classified as part of a hierarchy.

Leisure was also valued from the beginning of Western civilization. However, we learned that the characteristics and uses of leisure time have changed over time. In fact, we might conclude that the leisure of one era became the work of another era, and the work of one era became the leisure of another era. Plato and Aristotle characterized exercise of the mind as leisure. Today, some workers look to gardening or baking as a means of leisure and being free from exercises of the mind. One common thread of leisure through the ages is that it often includes the occupations that are considered discretionary, not obligatory.

As I read this chapter, I reflected on the evolution of occupations in my own family. I have fairly reliable information on some aspects of work and leisure for each generation back to my great-grandparents. It is clear the values, beliefs, and practices that my family and I have regarding work and leisure have roots from several time periods discussed in this chapter. I expect many readers will have similar insights.

Journal Activities

1. Look up and write down two dictionary definitions of evolution. Highlight the component of the definition that is most related to the descriptions of these terms in Chapter Two.
2. Identify the most important new learning for you in this chapter.
3. Identify one question you have about Chapter Two.
4. Reflect on one subgroup of Western culture today. Describe one current work and leisure pattern of this culture and identify possible evolutionary influences on this pattern from the periods discussed in this chapter.
   - Identify the culture.
   - Describe the work and leisure pattern of the culture.
   - Identify the values and beliefs associated with work and leisure for the culture.
   - What characteristics of this pattern have changed from previous periods of time?
   - What characteristics have recurred or reappeared from previous periods of time?
   - What are some possible religious influences on this pattern?
   - How has this pattern influenced the values and behaviors of this culture?

   (Possible cultures: sandwich generation (mid-life) women, two-worker families, over-scheduled children, aging workers with delayed retirement, people working in professional sports or entertainment industry, workers with disabilities, etc.)
5. Imagine you are going to conduct an investigation of the evolution of occupations over time in a culture or the patterns of occupations at one point in history. What strategies would you use to find information? Where would you begin? What disciplines might you include? What key words might lead you to the relevant literature?

Technology/Internet Learning Activities

1. Use a discussion database to share assigned journal entries.
2. Examine the work and leisure patterns and values/beliefs of a culture not discussed in Chapter Two.
3. Select a non-Western culture or a Western culture not discussed in Chapter Two that is of interest.
4. Discuss possible technology-based strategies for finding information with your peers.
5. Use at least two technology-based strategies to obtain basic information on this culture as it relates to work and leisure patterns and values/beliefs (e.g., Internet searches, online encyclopedias, online full text journals).
6. Summarize your findings on a discussion database. Include the culture, the era, the primary religious influences, work occupations and patterns, leisure occupations and patterns, values/beliefs, and technology-based resources used.
7. Review the findings posted by your peers. Discuss those search strategies that worked and those that didn't.

Applied Learning

Individual Learning Activity #1: Patterns of Work and Leisure in One Family

Document the patterns of work and leisure in a specific family.

Instructions:

- Select a family to study that would have general information on several generations of family members. (This may be your own family or any other family).
- Document the characteristics of and occupational evolution for several generations of this family. (Use the format on the next page to summarize information).

	Youngest Generation	*Parent of Youngest Generation*	*Grandparent of Youngest Generation*	*Great-Grandparent of Youngest Generation*
Approximate Dates of Birth and Death				
Geographic Information (country, region, urban/rural, etc.)				
Personal Information (socioeconomic class, ethnic or cultural group, education, religion)				
Work (occupations and patterns)				
Leisure (occupations and patterns)				
Values and Beliefs				

For example, I might document a grandmother who lived from about the 1880s to 1970s. She lived in the United States' Midwest region, in a medium-size town. She grew up in a middle-class, German Protestant household; graduated from high school; and had some postsecondary education. Her parents had emigrated from Germany to the United States. She had several work occupations as an adult, but the primary one was a small business owner of a flower shop/greenhouse. Because she and her husband were the only employees, this work required multiple general and specific skills, long hours, sacrifice, self-sufficiency, and long-term commitment. Leisure occupations included those that could be done when physically tired, were short in duration, could be integrated during the day, and could be scheduled during times when the business was closed. Her most frequent occupations were crossword puzzles, jigsaw puzzles, television, and holiday dinners for extended family. Some of the values and beliefs transmitted included dedication, thriftiness, humor, perseverance, pride in work, and family commitment.

Individual Learning Activity #2: Patterns of Work and Leisure for a Character in a Biography/Novel

Read a biography or novel (or reflect on one you've read previously) that represents a period of time discussed in this chapter. Document the characteristics of one or more people, work and leisure patterns, and values/beliefs using the grid below.

	Person One	*Person Two*	*Person Three*
Approximate Dates of Birth and Death			
Geographic Information (country, region, urban/rural, etc.)			
Personal Information (socioeconomic class, ethnic or cultural group, education, religion)			
Work (occupations and patterns)			
Leisure (occupations and patterns)			
Values and Beliefs			

Active Learning

Group Learning Activity #1: Exploring the Occupational Evolution of Different Families and Their Values and Beliefs

Preparation:
- Read Chapter Two.
- Complete Individual Learning Activity #1.

Time: 45 minutes to 1 hour

Materials:
- Completed grid from Individual Learning Activity #1
- Flip chart, chalk board, white board, or virtual discussion space

Instructions:
- Individually:
  - ✧ Grid from Individual Learning Activity #1.
- In small groups:
  - ✧ Share the information on one or two members of the family you studied. Summarize the information on the grid below. Whenever possible, try to summarize the information for an individual's primary working years as 1900 to 1960 or 1960 to present.
  - ✧ Analyze the grid for themes related to work, leisure, and beliefs/values for each era.

	Working Adult Years 1900 (or before) to 1960	*Working Adult Years 1960 to present*
Geographic Areas		
Personal Characteristics		
Work (occupations and patterns)		
Leisure (occupations and patterns)		
Values and Beliefs		

Discussion:

- What trends do you see for work occupations and patterns for the two time periods?
- What trends do you see for leisure occupations and patterns for the two time periods?
- What trends do you see in values/beliefs about work and leisure for the two time periods?
- What questions do you have after this activity? What did you learn?

Group Learning Activity #2: Exploring Values and Beliefs About Work and Leisure as Discussed in Chapter Two

Preparation:

- Read Chapter Two.
- Select Individual Learning Activity #1 or Individual Learning Activity #2 as the basis for this activity.
- Complete Individual Learning Activity #1 or Individual Learning Activity #2.

Time: 45 minutes to 1 hour

Materials:

- Completed grid from Individual Learning Activity #1 or #2
- Flip chart, chalk board, white board, or virtual discussion space

Instructions:

- Individually:
  - ✧ Grid from Individual Learning Activity #1 or #2.
- In small groups:
  - ✧ Share the information on values/beliefs from the grids for Individual Learning Activity #1 or #2.
  - ✧ Review the list of values/beliefs below about work and leisure (from Chapter Two).
  - ✧ For each value/belief on your Individual Activity grids, identify a corresponding value/belief from the list below. Keep a running tally of the values/beliefs below that are reflected in Individual Activity grids.

Discussion:

- What are some of the values/beliefs from the list below that were evident in your grids? Were there any surprises? Why do you think these values/beliefs are held?
- What are some of the values/beliefs from the list below that were not evident in your grids? Were there any surprises? Why do you think these values/beliefs are not held?
- Pick several values/beliefs from the list below that were evident in your grids. Use Chapter Two to determine the era these values/beliefs were held.

A Summary of Values/Beliefs Discussed in Chapter Two

- Work should be divided.
- Work should be perfected.
- Work is a means to prevent poverty or destitution.
- Work is a means to prevent early death.
- Work is a means of expiating sin.
- Work is a means of regaining/maintaining dignity.
- Work is a curse.
- Leisure is all the things you don't have to do.
- Work is good for the health of the body and spirit.
- Work helps avoid evil, idleness, or sloth.
- Work limits dependency on others.
- Work helps one gain self-respect.
- Work allows one to share with others.

- There should be a balance between work and leisure.
- Leisure is important for periodic emotional release.
- Work is a way to avoid despair.
- Work is a way to expiate sin.
- Some types of work are best for some types of people.
- Some work has more importance than others.
- Some types of work should have influences on size of family.
- Work is natural.
- Work is the universal base of society.
- Work is a way to serve God.
- All types of work have dignity.
- Everyone should work enough to meet basic needs.
- Acquiring wealth is sinful.
- The type of work chosen represents a calling.
- One should expect to make a reasonable profit by work.
- Some people are chosen or predestined for certain types of work.
- Work should be methodical, disciplined, rational, uniform, and specialized.
- It is important to have sufficient work-free days.
- Religious holidays should be followed by secular fun.
- Work is essential to survival.
- One should save and use profits from work.
- Prosperity is evidence of God's grace.
- Leisure that is ostentatious, idle, gluttonous, or sensuous is sinful.
- Leisure that brings refreshment when done in moderation is encouraged.
- One's material and spiritual welfare is dependent on one's own efforts.
- Intellectual and spiritual pleasures are more important than wealth and personal pleasures.
- It is one's social duty to be productive and make a profit.
- Leisure is a means to demonstrate social status.
- Leisure is a way to improve self and prepare for more work.
- Some people need/deserve more leisure time than others.
- Leisure should revolve around family and community.
- All people have a right to work.
- One has a right to rest, leisure, and control of work hours.
- Work allows one to be a good provider, independent, successful, and self-respecting.
- Work at home should shared.

Chapter Three Objectives

The information in this chapter is intended to help the reader:

1. Understand occupation as both a product and process of development.
2. Review historical and philosophical views of the developmental process.
3. Review developmental stages or phases of life.
4. Appreciate the biological, social, and psychological links between development and occupational engagement.
5. Review the arguments underlying classic controversies surrounding human development, including nature versus nurture and linear versus pyramidal theories.
6. Review concepts related to stage views of development.
7. Review developmental concepts from psychological, psychoanalytic, and cognitive theories of development.
8. Understand the basic propositions of selection, optimization, and compensation underlying the theory of development proposed by Baltes.
9. Understand the basic concepts underlying the self-determination theory by Deci and Ryan.
10. Understand the role of plasticity in development across the lifespan.

Key Words

competence: Having the ability and skill to do a required task or occupation according to expectations set by the self and others.

development: The process of growth and maturation occurring across the lifespan.

linear theories of development: View the developmental process as comprised of sequential stages, such as connecting the links in a chain.

nature versus nurture: An age old controversy about human development that questions the relative influences of genetics and environment in determining what people are like.

plasticity: Capable of being molded or shaped.

pyramidal theories of development: View the developmental process as the formation of levels of function and capacity that support the later development of more sophisticated and elaborate behaviors and capacities.

self-determination theory: Theory of motivation by Edward Deci and Richard Ryan in which drives for competence, autonomy, and relatedness influence development and well-being.

SOC theory: Theory by Baltes that views development as a process of responding to environmental demands in a way that optimizes gains and minimizes losses.

stages of life: The idea that chronological development from birth to death is marked by distinct age periods with common developmental life tasks and concerns associated with the stage.

All growth depends upon activity.
There is no development physically or intellectually without effort, and effort means work.
Calvin Coolidge

Chapter Three

Occupational Development

Dorothy Edwards, PhD and Charles H. Christiansen, EdD, OTR, OT(C), FAOTA

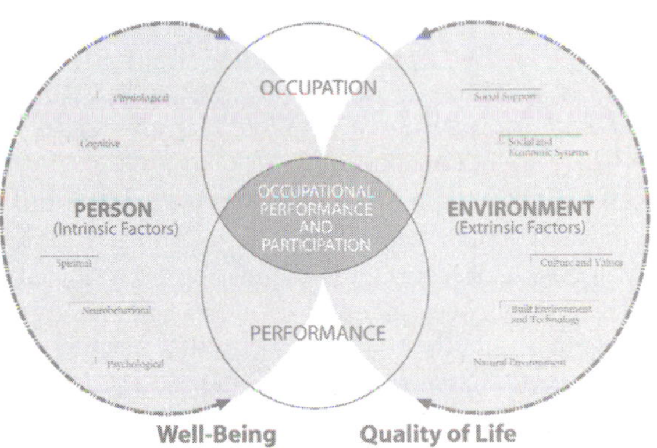

Setting the Stage

This chapter will discuss the central function of occupation in human development. Occupations serve as both the product and process for development. By guiding a person's performance of significant roles and responsibilities, occupational engagement enables the person to grow physically, intellectually, emotionally, and socially. New theories, such as those proposed by Baltes (emphasizing selection, optimization, and compensation) or Deci (emphasizing self-determination and competence), support this view of development and its application within an occupational performance framework for practice.

Edwards, D., & Christiansen, C. H. (2005). Occupational development. In C. H. Christiansen, C. M. Baum, and J. Bass-Haugen (Eds.), Occupational therapy: Performance, participation, and well-being *(3rd ed.). Thorofare, NJ: SLACK Incorporated.*

Introduction

How do people develop and become unique individuals similar to their siblings and friends, but different from anyone else in history? The answer to this question can be found in our everyday experiences, yet it remains difficult to describe and explain. The evidence of a person's progression from infant to elder is clearly visible in physical and social changes, but the underlying process of development remains less obvious. Over the centuries, scholars, poets, philosophers, and scientists have all addressed the process, trying to fathom its deep mysteries. However, much remains to be learned.

The Bible addresses child-rearing practices and the roles of parents in the moral lives of children. The Greek and Roman philosophers were very curious about the nature of learning and growth of individual awareness and social responsibility. The first scientific findings related to differences in strength, auditory perception, and reaction time (Gillham, 2001). Formal descriptions of child development appeared in the 17th century as children began to be seen as qualitatively different from adults (Aries, 1962a, 1962b; Papalia, 2001).

The first psychological studies of adolescence were published in the early 1900s by G. Stanley Hall (Hall, 1904). Research on adult life and aging followed in the 1930s. Most developmental scientists agree that there is a fundamental order in the human life course. Research conducted by many different disciplines ranging from the biological sciences such as genetics and physiology to the social sciences including psychology, sociology, and anthropology support this point of view.

We know more about development today than at any other time in history. Studies of the brain and the human genome are expanding our knowledge of the biological forces that shape human experience across the lifespan. However, biology alone cannot explain how and why humans change over the course of their lives. The development of the human as a social being requires the nurturing of parents and communities. Through experiences with the world around them, children mature into adults. Similarly, the experiences throughout life lead to the wisdom of older age. These experiences most often come in the context of daily human occupations, those activities, tasks, or roles related to self-care, play or leisure, work, and other productive pursuits (such as education) that comprise the routines of everyday life. Because occupations constitute the experiences through which learning occurs, either directly or indirectly, the study of occupation helps us understand the factors that influence development over time.

Thus, everyday doing provides the means through which development occurs. Evidence for the relationship between occupation and human development can be drawn from the work of scientists in the social and behavioral sciences, such as psychology, sociology, and anthropology, as well as from the emerging discipline known as occupation science. The purpose of this chapter is to draw selectively from this work to examine the dynamic and reciprocal relationship between development and human occupation across the lifespan. The term *reciprocal* is used because humans are open systems whose experiences change them. At the same time, age and other factors related to development influence the choice and nature of experiences (Figure 3-1).

Development Defined

Developmental psychologists refer to the behaviors that are associated with life experiences as roles, tasks, and activities. Development can be defined as the changes in these behaviors over time. The goal of the scientific study of development is to describe, explain, and ultimately predict behaviors that occur at different stages of life (Papalia & Olds, 1998). These observable behaviors reflect the underlying physical, cognitive, and emotional states of the individual. Studies of human development have shown that these changes over time generally occur in a systematic and orderly manner (Green, 2002).

Growth, Maturation, and Learning

Three basic mechanisms are associated with behavioral changes over time. These are growth, maturation, and learning. While these terms are often used interchangeably, each actually represents a separate and distinct process (Short-Degraff, 1988). Growth is defined as the biological proliferation of cells, leading to an additive increase in the size or number of cells (Malina & Bouchard, 1991). Maturation is the emergence or unfolding of the individual's unique genetic potential (Rice, 2001). Genetic and biological factors, including hormones, propel growth, while maturation occurs on a more individualistic and variable schedule. Learning theorists believe that new skills and behaviors are acquired through modeling, shaping, and social reinforcement. These three processes (growth, maturation, and learning) interact to influence human biological, cognitive, emotional, and social development (Table 3-1).

Occupations and Development

The study of development provides a foundation for understanding occupation. Although most developmental theories do not specifically address occupational perform-

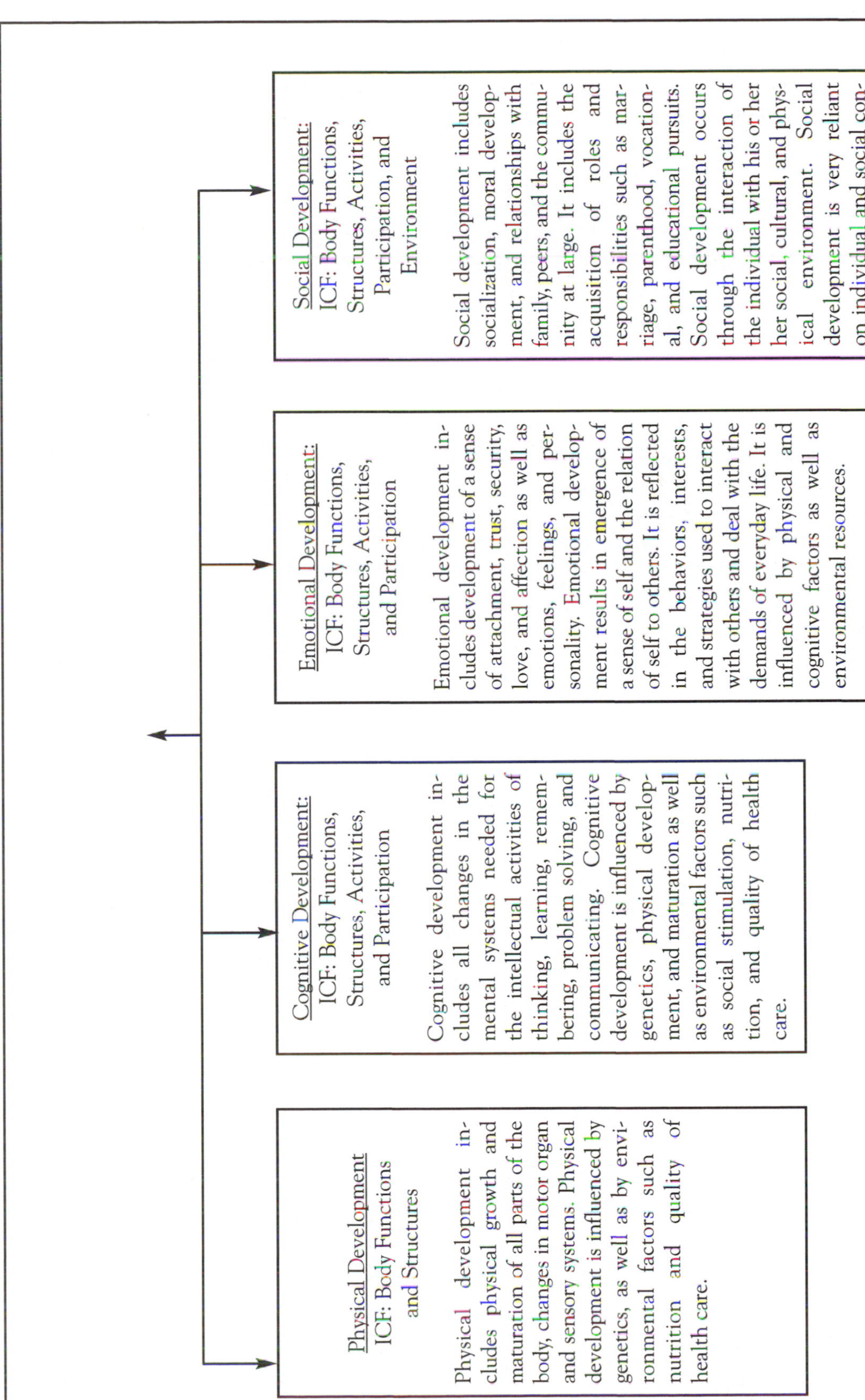

Physical Development
ICF: Body Functions and Structures
Physical development includes physical growth and maturation of all parts of the body, changes in motor organ and sensory systems. Physical development is influenced by genetics, as well as by environmental factors such as nutrition and quality of health care.
Cognitive Development:
ICF: Body Functions, Structures, Activities, and Participation
Cognitive development includes all changes in the mental systems needed for the intellectual activities of thinking, learning, remembering, problem solving, and communicating. Cognitive development is influenced by genetics, physical development, and maturation as well as environmental factors such as social stimulation, nutrition, and quality of health care.
Emotional Development:
ICF: Body Functions, Structures, Activities, and Participation
Emotional development includes development of a sense of attachment, trust, security, love, and affection as well as emotions, feelings, and personality. Emotional development results in emergence of a sense of self and the relation of self to others. It is reflected in the behaviors, interests, and strategies used to interact with others and deal with the demands of everyday life. It is influenced by physical and cognitive factors as well as environmental resources.
Social Development:
ICF: Body Functions, Structures, Activities, Participation, and Environment
Social development includes socialization, moral development, and relationships with family, peers, and the community at large. It includes the acquisition of roles and responsibilities such as marriage, parenthood, vocational, and educational pursuits. Social development occurs through the interaction of the individual with his or her social, cultural, and physical environment. Social development is very reliant on individual and social context.

Figure 3-1. Domains of human development.

Table 3-1

Changing Behavior Through Learning: Key Terms

- **Conditioning:** Changes in behavior that occur after responses to specific stimuli are rewarded. Learning theories based on conditioning hypothesize that new learning occurs as a result of positive reinforcement or rewards, and old patterns are abandoned as a result of negative punishment reinforcement.
- **Shaping:** Changes in behavior associated with feedback. Feedback involves providing learners with information about their responses. Feedback can be positive (increases the response) or negative (decreases the response). Shaping procedures are based on principals of operant conditioning.
- **Modeling:** Changes in behavior that occur through observing and imitating the behaviors of others. Social learning theory emphasizes the role of learning through observation and interaction with others.
- **Social reinforcement:** Changes in behavior associated with the positive or negative consequences of others.

ance, the concepts presented by developmental researchers and scholars are very relevant for students of occupational therapy. Occupational scientists are contributing important knowledge for the understanding of development at all stages and periods of life (Hershberger, Plomin, & Pedersen, 1995; Turkheimer & Waldron, 2000).

In addition, many notable occupational therapy scholars have studied development. Historically, they have been particularly interested in the issues associated with infant and child development, but there are also some investigators studying occupational performance in adults and the elderly. In 1970, Llorens proposed a developmental theory of occupational therapy that described many of the same factors addressed in the 1980s and 1990s by life-span developmental psychologists. Her theory is grounded in the work of developmental psychologists such as Gessell, Erikson, and Havinghurst and occupational therapy investigators such as Ayres and Mosey. She constructed a schema that incorporated the work of many theorists to provide a context for viewing development. This theory suggests that development occurs horizontally through the growth of physical, cognitive, linguistic, and psychosocial skills and longitudinally through the maturation and extension of these skills, abilities, and behaviors. Mastery of these skills, abilities, and relationships are necessary for achievement of successful coping behaviors and adaptive relationships.

In her Eleanor Clarke Slagle Lecture, Llorens (1970) defined nine postulates describing development and the role of occupational therapy in facilitating normal development and restoring mastery when disease, injury, or environmental insufficiencies disrupt development at any stage of life (Table 3-2).

Her theory also addresses environmental influences on mastery and the role of the environment in mediating the growth of skills and abilities. Interaction with social, civic, and community groups supplement the contributions of the family as the individual matures. Work, leisure, and self-care activities all promote growth and adaptation regardless of chronological age, maturational level, or stage of life. Llorens also applied these principles to occupational therapy practice. Interventions need to be geared to the developmental level of the client to be successful. Therapies that require skills and abilities beyond the capacity of the client increase stress and decrease the benefits of treatment.

Differing Approaches to Understanding Development: Questions and Controversies

Philosophers and scientists have been puzzling over the forces that influence development since the beginning of time. Given the complexity of the topic, it is not surprising that these questions are still debated today. Are the basic characteristics of an individual influenced more by genes or by that person's experiences? This controversy is fundamental to the formulation of developmental theories. It is useful to review some of the unresolved but important questions underlying the study of development.

Nature Versus Nurture

The oldest debate has focused on the contributions of heredity (nature) and the environment (nurture) on behavior. Supporters of the nature perspective attribute behavioral characteristics and age-related change primarily to internal forces such as genetics, biological processes, and physical maturation. The proponents of the nurture perspective suggest that the most powerful determinants of development are external to the individual (i.e., development is the result of learning through interaction with the external environment).

Table 3-2

A Developmental Theory of Occupational Therapy

Basic Assumptions of Lloren's Theory of Development

- Humans develop horizontally in areas of neurophysiological, physical, and psychosocial growth, acquiring skills at specific periods of time.
- Humans develop longitudinally in a continuous process in each of these areas as they age.
- Mastery of particular skills both horizontally and longitudinally is necessary for achievement of satisfactory coping behaviors and adaptive relationships.
- Mastery is achieved naturally in the course of development.
- The fundamental capacity of the individual is stimulated within the supportive environment of the family, community, and social groups to promote development and the acquisition of skills.
- Physical or psychological trauma related to disease, injury, or environmental insufficiency can interrupt the growth and development process.
- Growth interruption causes gaps in the developmental cycle, resulting in a disparity between expected coping behaviors, adaptive capacities, and skills and abilities.
- Occupational therapy through the skilled application of activities and relationships can promote growth and development by increasing skills, abilities, and relationships both horizontally and longitudinally.
- Occupational therapy through the skilled application of activities and relationships can provide opportunities to prevent the development of maladaptive neurophysiological, physical, and psychosocial patterns of behavior in the presence of trauma, injury due to disease, or environmental insufficiency.

Adapted from Llorens, L. A. (1970). Facilitating growth and development: The promise of occupational therapy. *American Journal of Occupational Therapy, 24*, 93-101.

This dichotomy between nature and nurture has been described in many ways: maturation versus learning, nativism versus empiricism, and biology versus experience. The Greek philosopher Plato wrote in the *Republic* about the importance of early experience (nurture) on the development of children (Watson, 1963). He taught that knowledge was acquired through hard work, although he did suggest that knowledge was present in the soul at birth (nature). Descartes believed in the existence of innate ideas (nature) (Descartes, 1901). The belief that humans are born with innate ideas is called *nativism*. Nativist philosophers such as Rousseau believed that knowledge unfolded through life, and the goal of education was to provide opportunities for this intrinsic knowledge to appear (Rosseau, 1911). John Locke, on the other hand, was an empiricist. He wrote that a child at birth was a "tabula rasa" or blank slate. Learning occurred only through repeated practice (Lobo, 1998; Locke, 1994). Each of these perspectives recognizes the vital contribution of engagement in activity to the formation of the developing self. The sequencing of the human genome and our rapidly expanding knowledge of behavioral genetics may make these arguments seem old-fashioned today. This new research has changed the question from which factor is most important to how these factors interact to influence behavior. Although research is progressing, it is not known to what extent one's overall health can be attributed to genetics rather than environmental issues. Scientists remain convinced that environment plays a major role as a determinant in health outcomes (Bateson et al., 2004; Lichtenstein et al., 2000). The ultimate goal of developmental research is to facilitate the optimum development of an individual. Only interactionist, holistic, or ecological approaches that recognize the complementary contributions of genetics and environmental factors will be successful. This view is consistent with the Person-Environment-Occupation-Performance (PEOP) model presented in this text.

Linear Versus Pyramidal Theories

Currently, many different theories purport to explain human development. Theories are used to organize data, ideas, and hypotheses and to state them in coherent general propositions, principles, or laws (Rice, 2001). Developmental theories can be categorized by the underlying domain studied (i.e., cognitive theories), the process thought to influence development (i.e., psychoanalytic theories), or the way the theory views development. Linear theories examine the sequential components of development. Hinojosa and Kramer (1999) compare this approach to adding links to a chain. Each link provides an important piece for the completion of the chain. Examples of linear theories include Freud's psychoanalytic theory and Kohlberg's theory of moral development.

Pyramidal theories describe the developmental process as the formation of levels of function and capacity that support the emergence of more sophisticated and elaborate behaviors and capacity in the future. Events early in life provide the foundation or the components for skills needed for roles and responsibilities later in life. This approach suggests that the essential elements of early stages must be present for the next stage to occur. Examples of pyramidal theories include Piaget's theory of cognitive development (Piaget, 1969) and Erikson's psychosocial theory (Erickson, 1994). Both sequential and pyramidal theories recognize that as individuals mature, they encounter certain predictable changes and challenges that are common to their age or stage of life.

Developmental Stages or Phases of Life

The changes that occur because of increasing chronological age or the experience of the individual can also be described in many ways. Historically, developmental researchers have focused on discrete phases or periods of life. Developmental theorists and researchers typically divided the human lifespan into three major periods: childhood, adolescence, and adulthood. Each of these major periods is then subdivided into more discrete stages.

Childhood

Childhood includes the prenatal period, infancy, early childhood, and middle childhood. Infancy extends from birth to toddlerhood, although some researchers have started to examine prenatal behavior in utero before the baby is born (Short-Degraff, 1988). Infancy is a time of rapid change associated with major growth of the cognitive, sensory, and musculoskeletal systems. Considerable social and emotional development is occurring at the same time. Differences in personality and temperament are apparent even in early infancy. Studies in behavioral genetics have sought to determine why children in the same families are so different, and these studies underscore the interplay of both environment and genetics in the early social development of humans (Plomin, DeFries, McClearn, & Rutter, 1994).

Early and middle childhood are associated with the development of the sense of self-identity, reflected in gender roles, play activities, and relationships within the family. Physical growth continues, but changes in cognitive, linguistic, and social skills are even more compelling. The occupations of childhood include physical and imaginary play, self-care activities, school, and family chores and responsibilities.

Adolescence

Adolescence includes early (preteens) and late adolescence. Adolescence marks the transition from child to adult. This transition is filled with challenges related to major changes in all aspects of physical, cognitive, social, and emotional abilities. Many of these changes are associated with sexual maturation and the hormonal changes that influence both physical and emotional status. The formation of a unique sense of self is a major thrust of this stage. Adolescents seek emotional independence from their families, begin to develop intimate relationships, and start the process of career development. Adolescent occupations reflect the transitional nature of this stage. School activities often form the center of adolescent life. Play becomes more structured and formalized through competitive sports, music, dances, and other group experiences. Social relationships are very important. Work and volunteer activities help define productive pursuits that will last for a lifetime (Feldman & Elliot, 1990).

Adulthood

Stages of adulthood are often defined by the developmental tasks and characteristic roles and activities rather than by specific ages. Young adults are often involved in education and career training, decisions about life roles, and establishing social and intimate relationships. In the United States and Canada, there is some blurring of the transition from late adolescence and young adulthood. Thus, blurring occurs for that segment of the population undertaking professional or graduate education, as extended years of education and training delay entry into the workforce. Major shifts in the economy and dramatic changes in the roles of women have had a significant impact on the norms and expectations for young adults in Western industrialized nations. For example, even in the recent past, women were expected to forego careers and assume homemaking and child rearing responsibilities. Today, the shift toward dual-career families, the growing acceptance of same-sex unions, and the loosening of gender-based roles represent some of the significant social and cultural changes influencing young adults. These changes will influence the characteristic occupations of middle age and later life for young adults born during the last three decades of the 20th century. Recent census data in the United States and other developing nations suggests that decisions about marriage and life partners, child bearing, and work are being deferred until later in the

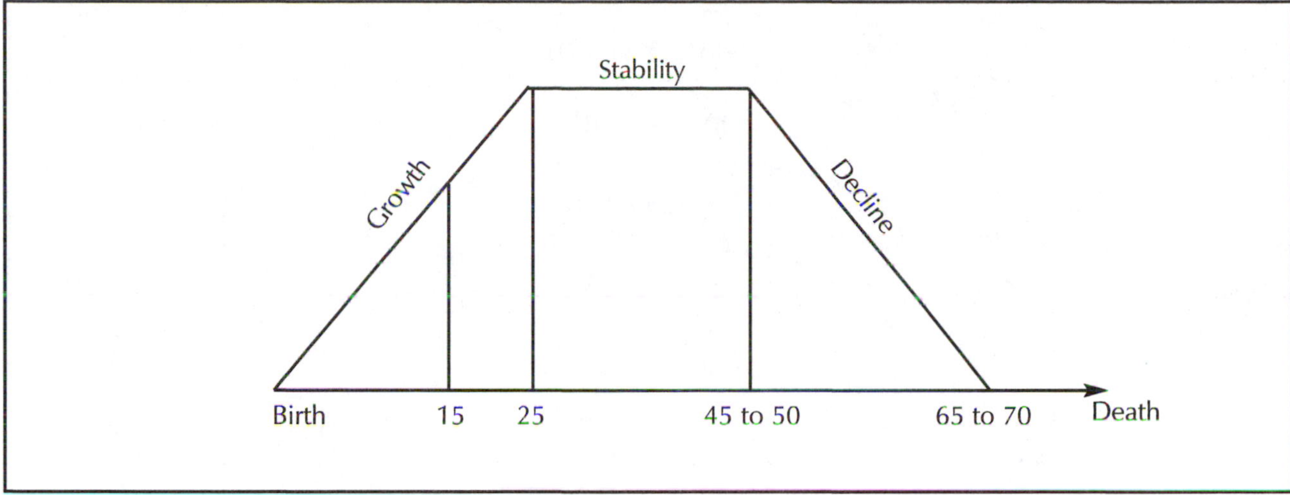

Figure 3-2. Markers of development across the lifespan.

stage of young adulthood than was typical even a few decades ago.

Often, middle age is a time during which adjustment and efforts to "reappraise previous life structures with an eye to making revisions 'while there is still time'" tend to occur (Huyck, 1993). This redefinition of values and lifestyles that sometimes occur often associates middle adulthood with the term *midlife crisis*, but, in fact, some research suggests that few people experience stress at a level that warrants the term *crisis* and such redefinition may not be a universal "marker" event of this stage after all (Kruger, 1994). During middle adulthood, parental responsibilities for children may be decreasing, while responsibilities for one's adult parents may be increasing. Career responsibilities may change, and achievement of significant life goals may become realized. There may be more time and recognition for contributions to community and social activities. Middle adulthood is also marked by a growing awareness of the physical and emotional changes experienced in later life.

Late adulthood is often a time of accommodation of changing physical, emotional, and social status. Physical changes and health issues are very common experiences at this stage. The presence of health and physical problems complicate the lives of older adults. Loss of friends and partners is also a challenge at this time of life. While there are many changes associated with loss of physical capacity, later life may also represent a time of great social and spiritual growth and development. Interpersonal relationships with friends and family may grow richer and more fulfilling, and opportunities to develop and pursue interests and activities that were not available or convenient at earlier stages of life may become possible. Well-being at this stage is often associated with engagement in productive activities and meaningful relationships (Keyes & Ryff, 1998).

How Stages Influence Our Understanding of Development

The "stage of life" view is very dependent on biological processes that focus on the growth, stability, and decline of organisms. Even social scientists used these concepts in their theories and research. Each discrete stage is tied to the underlying biological or physical process. From this perspective, infancy, childhood, and adolescence are periods of significant somatic growth. Young adulthood and the period of reproductive ability were associated with stability. The loss of reproductive ability in middle age marked the onset of decline and regressive ability that ultimately ends in death (Rosow, 1976). Thus, old age from a biological perspective is a time of loss and dysfunction (Figure 3-2).

According to stage theorists, each stage has its own characteristic challenges, adjustments, and achievements. These activities are influenced by stage-related norms, expectations, tasks, and responsibilities that vary according to the social, cultural, economic, and physical environment. For example, the average life expectancy at birth has changed dramatically during the past 200 years (Anderson, 2002). In 1999, the life expectancy at birth was 76.7 years, almost 30 years longer than a baby born in 1900. The opportunities and experiences of a child born in 1800 were very different from those available to a child born in 2000. These differences will be visible across all life stages and all aspects of development. *Longevity* is the term used to describe the expected duration of the lifespan. *Prolongevity*

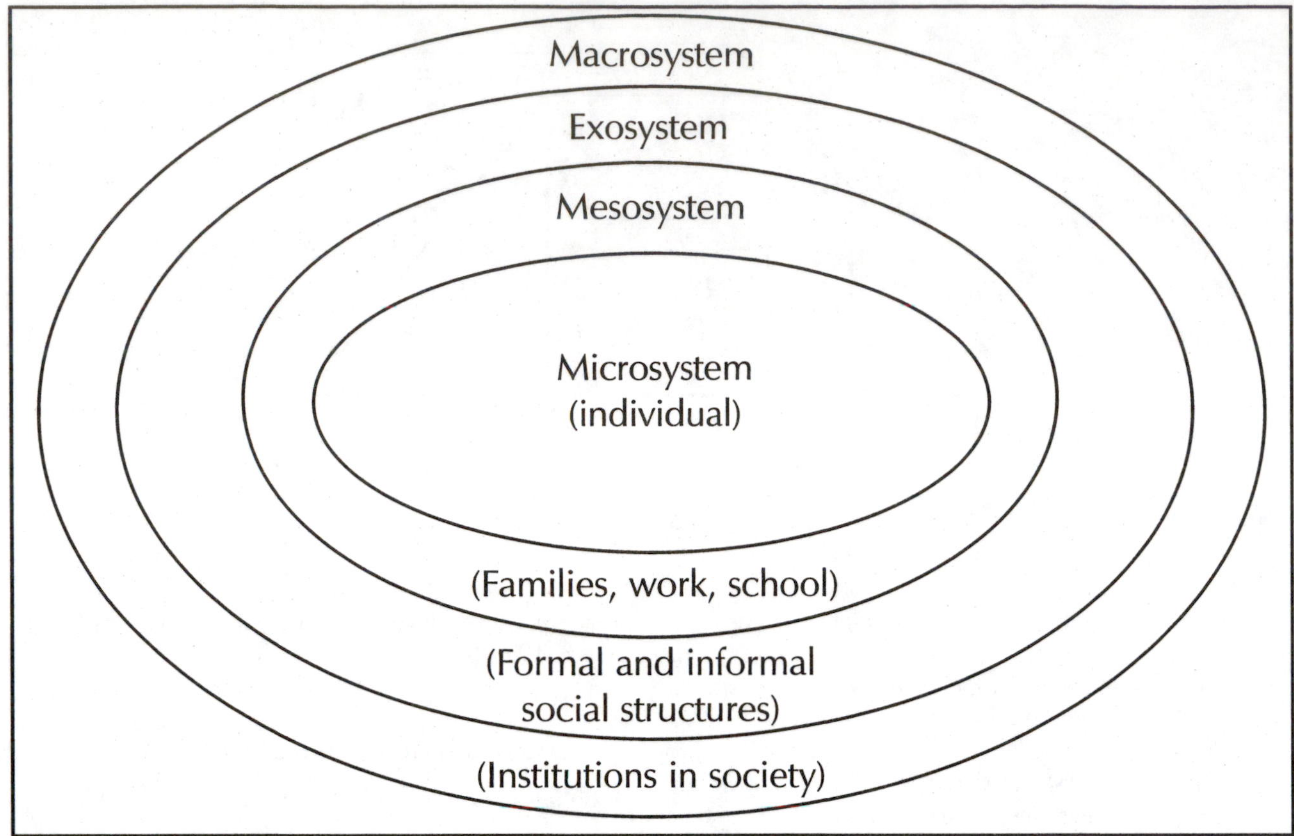

Figure 3-3. Bronfenbrenner's ecological systems model (1977).

is the term proposed by Gruman (1966) to describe the active process of extending the lifespan by eliminating the sources of age-related decline. There is more to prolongevity than the extension of the absolute lifespan. The goal of prolongevity is to improve the overall health and physical capacity of older people to ensure vitality and productive activity in these "extra" years (Rothenberg, Lentzner, & Parker, 1991) (Figure 3-3).

Dimensions or Domains of Occupational Development

Another common strategy for studying development is to examine the dimensions or domains of function important to everyday life. Humans move, think, feel, and learn through interaction with the environment and others. Thus, the four basic dimensions of interest are physical development, cognitive development, emotional development, and social development. Each of these dimensions can be studied separately within discrete stages of life, longitudinally across sequential stages, or interactively within and across these periods. Each of these domains is needed to fully understand occupational development.

While many investigators devote their entire careers to the study of a particular domain, it is important to realize that occupational performance requires the integration of all domains, regardless of the age of the person or the stage of life. All occupational tasks and activities depend on the person's physical state (motor, sensory, and bodily systems), cognitive capacity (awareness, thinking, and communication abilities), emotional responses (feelings, temperaments, and motivations), and social state (roles, relationships, and moral awareness).

Current Models of Occupation-Based Development

Although many models of occupational performance address developmental issues, none of these models specifically present a unified explanation of the role of occupation across the lifespan (Matheson & Bohr, 1997). Despite the absence of a commonly accepted "unifying theory," the literature on occupational performance implicitly acknowledges the developmental consequences of active doing as well as the therapeutic benefits of engagement in occupation. The concepts proposed by Llorens are amplified in these studies.

Law and colleagues (1997) defined occupational performance as the "ability to choose, organize, and satisfactorily perform meaningful occupations that are culturally defined and age appropriate for looking after oneself, enjoying life, and contributing to the emotional social and economic fabric of the community." Studies across a variety of age groups have demonstrated the contributions of engagement in meaningful occupations to health, life satisfaction, and emotional well-being (Law, Steinwender, & Leclair, 1998). The association between occupational performance and development is clear when studies of adults are combined with the findings in the pediatric literature. Primeau and Ferguson (1999) reviewed the literature supporting the occupational performance frame of reference for children. They present assumptions that support the use of this approach in occupational therapy practice. These assumptions also support the value of occupation to people of all ages. These principals are as follows:

- Humans have a drive to engage in occupation.
- Occupation is complex and multidimensional.
- Occupation must be considered within an environmental context.
- Occupation is experienced within the context of time.
- Occupation holds meaning for the person engaged in it.
- Occupation influences health and well-being.
- Occupation is both the product and process of development.

These propositions are similar to the basic principles of lifespan development theory proposed by Baltes and his coinvestigators. The developmental psychologists have devoted their attention to specification of the processes that account for continuity of emotional and intellectual growth across the lifespan. Occupational theorists have used the concept of occupation as the vehicle for achieving these same phenomena. The selection, optimization, and compensation theoretically defined by Baltes and others are supported by the research of occupational scientists who have demonstrated the consequences of engagement in individually determined occupations from infancy to later life.

How can occupation be both the product and process of development? This reciprocal relationship can be observed in the drive to engage in activities that provide opportunities for efficacy, mastery, and meaningful relationships with others (Llorens, 1970; Matheson & Bohr, 1997; Reilly, 1962; Wilcock, 1993). The choice of activities depends on the demands experienced by the individual and the resources available to meet the demands. Activities are highly specific to the individual, although age and the physical and social environment also influence these choices.

The relative allocation of resources available for specific occupations varies across the lifespan. Because occupations are the organized and meaningful tasks and activities of everyday life (Law et al., 1997), the developmental status (i.e., the physical, social, cognitive, and emotional state) of the individual determines the capacity and motivation of the individual to engage in these activities. Although growth and loss occur at every age, traditional developmental theory suggests that, in general, resources are focused on growth in early life, maintenance in midlife, and management of loss or compensation in later life. The balance between the characteristics of the individual, environmental characteristics, and occupational performance shifts over time. Studies of human development have shown that this dynamic interaction is systematic and predictable over specific phases of the lifespan.

Recently, developmental psychologists have been moving toward a synthesis of these two perspectives. Baltes and colleagues (1999) described two approaches to the study of development: person centered (holistic) and functions centered. The holistic approach considers the person a system and attempts to understand development by describing and connecting age periods or states of behavior into an overall pattern of lifetime individual development. The function-centered approach focuses on selecting a particular category of behavior and then describing the mechanisms that change over time in the category selected. They concluded that both perspectives are needed to fully understand age-related changes in behavior.

Developmental Theories Useful to Occupational Therapists

In the following sections, brief overviews of developmental theories most useful to occupational therapists are presented. These include those that are function-centered (i.e., focus on the domains such as thinking, feeling, and interacting), as well as those whose emphasis is on the person contending with contextual factors associated with meeting the everyday challenges of living as individuals move through life (i.e., so-called holistic theories). The following sections present various psychological development theories long with a description of the emerging holistic approach known as lifespan developmental theory (Tables 3-3 and 3-4).

Psychological Development Theories

There are many theories of psychological development. Theorists whose work is relevant to an occupational performance perspective are presented here. As stated previously, occupational engagement provides the experi-

Table 3-3 Developmental Theories of Childhood and Adolescence

Age	Jean Piaget **Cognitive Development Periods**	Sigmund Freud **Psychosexual Development Stages**	Lawrence Kohlberg **Moral Development Levels**
Birth	**Sensorimotor Period** Development focuses on the experience of the self and self in the environment. The child senses and reacts. The first learned social behaviors, crying to communicate needs, is noted at 8 to 12 months.	**Oral Stage** Mouth is the primary area of gratification of impulses. Id is dominant.	
6 mos			
12 mos		**Anal Stage** Gratification results from elimination. Conflict between the id and reality, in the form of parents' demands for control of behavior, begins the development of the ego.	
18 mos			
24 mos	**Preoperational Thinking Period** The use of symbols and formal language begins to appear. Logic is not yet present.		
3 yrs			
4 yrs		**Phallic Stage** Genitals are the primary area of gratification. Superego develops, signaling a conscience.	**Preconventional Morality** The child relies on external controls and the standards of others. Avoiding punishment and receiving reward is characteristic of hedonistic behavior.
5 yrs			
6 yrs			
7 yrs	**Concrete Operations Period** Children begin to develop concepts and to apply logic to problem solving.	**Latency Stage** Calm before the storm of puberty. Diminution of interest in sexual gratification. Identification with parent of the same gender occurs.	
8 yrs			
9 yrs			
10 yrs			**Conventional Morality** Sociocultural awareness and desire to be accepted in the community directs behavior. Concern for law and order is demonstrated.
11 yrs	**Formal Operations Period** The ability to perform abstract thinking and to apply logic to novel experiences develops.	**Genital Stage** Hormonal changes signal the onset of sexual maturity. Focus is on adult modes of sexual expression. Satisfying intimate relationships outside of the family of origin are developed.	
12 yrs			
13 yrs			**Postconventional** Morality is based on the prevailing "social contract." Standards of the community are internalized and judgment to compare one's self to these standards is demonstrated.
14 yrs			
15 yrs			
18 yrs			
21 yrs +			

Table 3-4

Lifespan Developmental Theories

Age	Havighurst **Developmental Tasks**	Erik Erikson **Psychosocial Development Crises**	Daniel J. Levinson **Biopsychosocial Eras**
Birth 2 yrs 4 yrs	**Infancy and Early Childhood** Individual learns to walk, talk, eat, and control elimination. Sex differences are learned. The individual is involved cognitively with language, physical reality and forming concepts, and begins to develop a conscience.	**Basic Trust vs. Mistrust** Learns to trust caretakers. **Autonomy vs. Shame and Doubt** Discovery of sense of autonomy.	**Childhood** Rapid growth and development occur. Individuation of the child begins with gradually increasing biological and psychological separation from the mother.
6 yrs 8 yrs 10 yrs	**Middle Childhood** The individual learns physical skills to achieve competence in play, and is learning to get along with peers in appropriate social and sexual roles. Personal independence begins to be achieved.	**Initiative vs. Guilt** Conscious control of environment. **Industry vs. Inferiority** Determination to achieve mastery develops.	
12 yrs 14 yrs 16 yrs	**Adolescence** The individual begins to have mature relationships with peers of both sexes and learns social and gender roles. Emotional independence from parents begins to be achieved.	**Identity vs. Role Confusion** Childhood crises are mastered. Identity is linked to mastery.	
18 yrs 20 yrs 25 yrs	**Early Adulthood** The individual is selecting and learning to live with a mate and deciding to begin or not begin a family. The individual establishes a home and begins employment.	**Intimacy vs. Isolation** Differentiation in role development. Development of intimate relationships.	**Early Adult Transition** Relationships with family of origin are modified as childhood dependence is replaced with independence and adult identity. **Entering the Adult World**
30 yrs 40 yrs 50 yrs	**Middle Age** The individual achieves social responsibility and satisfactory career performance. Commitment to an intimate relationship occurs. The individual begins to adjust to gradual physiologic changes.	**Generativity vs. Stagnation** Contributions to society overcome self-absorption.	**Age 30 Transition** **Settling Down** **Mid-Life Transition** **Middle Adulthood**
60 yrs 70 yrs 80 yrs	**Later Maturity** Adjusting to deteriorating health, reduced income, and death of spouse. Focus is on establishing satisfactory living arrangements.	**Ego Integrity vs. Despair** Acceptance and integration of one's self and inevitable death.	**Late Adult Transition** **Late Adulthood**

ences needed to foster cognitive and intellectual growth or the opportunity to create a sense of competence and self-esteem. Some theories only address childhood and adolescence, while others take a more comprehensive view and examine development from birth to death. Each of the theories presented provides support for therapeutic intervention. Therapists who use developmental theory as a foundation for treatment are more effective because their interventions support the occupational competence of the individual and help to enhance or preserve the person's sense of self as an active agent with the capacity to master environmental demands or achieve social roles.

Psychoanalytic Theory and Development

Psychoanalytic theory seeks to explain the unconscious forces that shape human experience. Sigmund Freud, a Viennese physician and neuroscientist, described the struggle or conflict that occurs when an individual's natural instincts conflict with the rules and requirements of society. The individual's early experiences of basic psychosexual needs are the basis of personality and behavior in adulthood. Freud proposed five psychosexual stages, and the resolution of each stage advances the child toward a more mature and balanced personality. Healthy personality development is the result of receiving an optimal level of gratification at each stage, enabling the individual to move on to the next stage without fixation. Matheson and Bohr (1997) reviewed psychoanalytic theory from an occupational competence perspective. They concluded, "Freud's notion of the unconscious is a significant contribution to the occupational competence model in that it is the repository of the individual's values which influence role selection."

Cognitive Theory and Development

Piaget introduced the concepts of cognitive development to developmental psychology. Jean Piaget was a Swiss psychologist who wanted to understand how children acquire and use information. This perspective focuses on the contribution of changing and expanding thought processes to the behavior of the child. Piagetian theorists view people as growing and changing beings who actively construct themselves through interactions with the external world (Papalia & Olds, 1998). Although there have been some applications of Piaget's theory to adulthood and later life, the primary emphasis of this work has been on infancy and childhood. Piaget also defined stages of development. At each stage, a child forms a new way of thinking about and understanding the world. Piaget proposed two processes, assimilation and accommodation, as the primary mechanisms of intellectual development (Piaget, 1969). Assimilation is the processing of information in a manner consistent with the individual's perception of reality. Accommodation is defined as changes in the cognitive structures needed to integrate experiences that cannot be assimilated (Matheson & Bohr, 1997). These two primary processes are based on three principles: organization, adaptation, and equilibration. These principles are actively guiding development at all stages and affect all interactions of the person within his or her environment. Development is the result of successfully managing and assimilating environmental challenges.

Learning Theories and Development

Most developmental theories are stage oriented; the general exception to this approach is presented by the learning theorists. Learning theorists propose a different approach. They suggest that development is a continuous process based on quantitative, rather than qualitative, changes. Learning is defined as a "long-lasting change in behavior based on experience or adaptation to the environment" (Papalia & Olds, 1998, p. 26).

Two different approaches to development have been presented: behaviorism proposed by John B. Watson and social learning theory proposed by Albert Bandura. Watson (1930) applied classical stimulus response theories to behavior in children. Watson believed that development, defined as observable consistent changes in behaviors, occurred in response to environmental events. From this mechanistic perspective, the person is only a responder; the control of the behavior exists through the positive and negative stimuli presented by the environment.

The social learning theorists apply principles of learning theory to social behaviors. Albert Bandura (1977, 1982, 2000) is the most prominent proponent of this approach. He claims that children learn in a social context by observing and imitating (modeling) the behavior of others. The social learning theorists reject the mechanistic belief that external stimuli control all behaviors; the person is an active participant in the process. Bandura (1989) has addressed the contributions of cognition to the social learning process. He suggests that individuals influence their own development by choosing future environments as well as the goals they wish to pursue. Self-efficacy, or personal agency, results from the experience of successful mastery of challenging and meaningful tasks.

Psychosocial/Biopsychosocial Theories and Development

These stage theories of personality emphasize the influence of societal norms and expectations on personality.

Erik Erikson was a student of Freud who expanded parts of psychoanalytic theory to the entire lifespan. Unlike Freud, who believed that childhood biological drives determine adult personality, Erikson stressed the role of society in shaping the individual over time. Erikson proposed eight stages of development across the lifespan (1968, 1994). These stages represent "crises" that must be resolved for the person to continue to grow emotionally. The successful resolution of each stage requires the resolution of a positive and opposing negative trait; this resolution leads to the development of a particular virtue or strength. These crises occur according to a predictable maturational timetable, determined in part by the physical maturation of the person interacting with societal norms and expectations. The concept of "identity" is a theme of this theory. Mastery occurs as the individual is able to meet personal and societal demands without losing his or her sense of self at each of the eight stages.

Daniel Levinson (Levinson, 1996; Levinson et al., 1978) is a contemporary developmental theorist who used biographical interviews of men and women to support his biopsychosocial theory of adult development. A person's values, dreams, and experiences interact with biological maturation and societal expectations to influence personality development. Levinson proposed a "life structure" that evolves over time. This structure is based on the roles and relationships that are most important: family, friends, work, and community. Life structures occur during overlapping eras, each lasting about 20 years. These eras have beginning and ending phases. Each phase has its own tasks, goals, and challenges. The eras and phases are linked by transitional periods defined by reappraisal and restructuring, a process that forms the foundation of the next phase. Levinson also uses the term *crises* to describe the tension that moves the person forward toward the next phase. Levinson's original theory was based on in-depth studies of men. He completed a similar study of women in 1996 shortly before his death. He concluded that men and women go through similar eras, phases, and transitions, but that their life structures differ.

Lifespan Developmental Theory

The lifespan approach to the study of human development draws upon the knowledge of many disciplines. One frequently voiced complaint about the early theoretical efforts in this area is that each discipline claimed the primacy of its own domain or area of study, leading to a very fragmented view of the process. The life course is split into unconnected segments (childhood or old age) or isolated domains (personality, intelligence, or muscle strength). This fragmented view leads to underestimating the complexity of the developmental process and the incredible capacity of humans to adapt to change and accommodate obstacles to growth at all points along the continuum from birth to death.

Ontogeny is a scientific term often used to describe human development, or the study of development. Ontogeny, or ontogenesis, is defined as "the origin and development of the individual" (*Oxford English Dictionary*, 1987). Baltes et al. (1999) proposed the following general principals of lifespan human development:

- Growth, stability, and change in behavior occur throughout life.
- There is a continuous interplay between growth (gains) and decline (losses) in ontogeny.
- Selection, optimization, and compensation constitute fundamental elements of development.
- There is age-associated change in adaptive potential (plasticity).

These principals can be translated into an occupational development framework. The study of development helps us to design treatments that reflect the following:

- What an individual needs or wants to do
- The selection of tasks and experiences that support the process of optimization and compensation

According to Baltes (1997), development is embedded in biological, historical, and cultural contexts. Their theory stresses the interplay among these components over time. The influence of different components depends on the particular developmental stage of the individual and the demands of the environment. Development is a lifelong process that is both multidirectional and multidimensional (Baltes et al., 1999). In early life, the gains outnumber the losses, but the balance shifts as the individual grows older. Multidirectionality creates a balance between growth and decline. As some behaviors and capacities are lost, new skills, abilities, and attitudes emerge (Datan, Rodeheaver, & Hughes, 1987). In later life, physical capacities often decline, but wisdom and emotional and creative energy are believed to increase. It is possible to achieve the same goal by the use of different mechanisms. Older adults may maintain important roles by guiding the actions of others rather than by physically performing the specific tasks. For example, a grandmother may share her recipes for holiday foods with her granddaughter rather than prepare the meal herself. Her contribution to the family is not diminished because she doesn't cook the food herself.

Multidimensionality also ensures that the individual has a variety of resources available to support engagement in roles and responsibilities at each stage of life. The relative allocation of physical, cognitive, and emotional resources shifts across the lifespan. In early life, growth functions are prominent, maintenance functions characterize mid-life, and regulation and accommodation of loss occur when maintenance and recovery are no longer possible.

Contextual Factors in Development

According to Baltes and many other lifespan developmental theorists (Lewis, 1999), context is an important determinant of the developmental process. The contextual theorists challenge us to look beyond the individual to the larger systems that influence human experience. The human experience occurs within a specific series of physical, historical, and social environments. Individuals change as they interact with their environments; they also influence their environment and thus play a role in shaping the historical and social context. Urie Bronfenbrenner's ecological approach to development (Bronfenbrenner, 1977, 1994) examines development within different levels of environmental systems. These systems extend from the person and his or her family out to the cultural, political, economic, and religious systems that shape the norms, attitudes, beliefs, and resources that shape society at large. The contextual theorists suggest that individual and group responses to environmental events and demands are highly variable. Personality traits, physical status, and genetics influence response of a given individual to environmental demands. Similarly, cultural, political, and social factors influence societal expectations and the resources available for support of individual needs. Studies of intellectual development and cognitive performance in infancy and later life demonstrate the role of the environment in supporting the capacity of the individual to engage in meaningful activities at later points in time. In childhood, engagement in play and social and physical activities promotes the development of cognitive skills needed for success in later life.

Children reared in situations that are not conducive to health and well-being are at risk for lifelong cognitive, social, and emotional problems (Lerner & DeStefanis, 2000). On a more positive note, toddlers exposed in utero to perinatal stress who were reared in stable families showed fewer developmental delays (Werner, 1989). These findings provide the basis for early intervention programs. We know that normal development cannot occur if the environment does not provide the physical and emotional foundation for growth. Similarly, as older adults lose physical and cognitive ability, environmental support can compensate for loss and allow the individual to maintain a sense of autonomy and mastery.

In addition to facilitating the physical and psychological aspects of development, the environment also provides the framework for evaluating developmental status. For example, Vygotsky (1978) studied the impact of sociocultural characteristics on the development of intellectual abilities (particularly language) in children. To him, language and thought are influenced by everyday experiences. Vygotsky felt that cognitive development was directly related to, and based on, social development (Gage & Berliner, 1988; Ormrod, 1998). What children learn and how they think are derived directly from the culture around them. Vygotsky believed that children begin learning from the world around them, their social world, which is the source of all their concepts, ideas, facts, skills, and attitudes. Our personal psychological processes all begin as social processes, patterned by our culture (Gage & Berliner, 1988). Children are particularly susceptible to culture. As they move into adulthood, they begin to perceive things much differently, and social views are transformed into personal, psychological ones. He cautioned against the imposition of norms and expectations drawn from one culture on children reared in another culture. Cross-cultural studies support the importance of contextual factors on all stages of development.

The Role of Plasticity in Development Across the Lifespan

Perhaps the most significant contribution of the lifespan developmental psychologists to our understanding of occupational performance is the concept of plasticity. *Plasticity* is the term used to describe the ability of an organism to modify or acquire new skills through learning and practice. The high level of human cognitive and behavior capacity requires a very prolonged period of development (Lerner & DeStefanis, 2000). Occupational scientists contribute their unique understanding of the impact of "doing" on the underlying cognitive, physical, and emotional states of the person. Occupation-based treatments of people with physical and cognitive impairments provide important evidence for the role of plasticity in normal development. Newcombe and Learmonth's (1999) studies of infant and child development suggest that plasticity, or the ability to adapt to experiences gained through interaction with the physical and social environment, allow an existing set of strategies to be tuned to greater efficiency and accuracy. Research on plasticity has also shown that, because so many aspects of development are activity dependent, we should not be surprised to observe a broad range of individual differences in response to the same developmental challenges (Abbott & Nelson, 2000). From an evolutionary perspective, the greater plasticity observed in humans when com-

Antecedent Conditions	*Orchestrating Processes*	*Outcomes*
Lifelong development involves a process of selective adaptation and change Demands on the individual change over time, successful development occurs as internal and external resources interact in the context of demands on the individual Selection pressures on development occur with age-related changes in plasticity and associated losses in internal and external resources	**Selection: Goals/Outcomes** Identification of goal domains and directionality of developmental processes **Optimization: Means/Resources** Acquisition/orchestration and enhancement of existing goal-directed means **Compensation: Response to Loss of Means** Acquisition of new goal-directed internal and external means due to loss of available means and resources, changes in adaptive contexts, and readjustment of goal structures	Maximizes gains and minimizes losses Successful growth is based on attainment of salient goals or states of functioning Maintenance of function including resilience/recovery Regulation of loss

Figure 3-4. The lifespan model of selective optimization with compensation. (Adapted from Baltes, P. B. (1997). On the incomplete architecture of human ontogeny: Selection, optimization, and compensation as foundation of developmental theory. *American Psychologist, 52*, 366-380.)

pared to other organisms allows greater flexibility and a wider range of adaptive options available to meet individual and environmental challenges (Lerner & DeStefanis, 2000). This is a real advantage for humans. Evolutionary forces have increased the complexity of our nervous system and our capacity to interact in multidimensional environments. This means that we have a variety of behavioral options at any single point in time; there is no single adaptive reaction or response for any given situation. Each of us is able to influence the course of our own lives. We do this every day through the roles, tasks, and activities that support our occupational choices and interests.

Lifespan theories based on longitudinal studies of large groups of people over time rather than cross-sectional comparisons of different age groups at a single point in time have shown that there is almost as much variability in intra-individual plasticity as there is in stage-related capacity to change. At each stage of life, there is considerable potential for modifying function and developing new strategies. While there is a finite capacity for change, we now know that even the very old can acquire new skills and adapt to physical and emotional losses. The literature suggests that the processes that support skill acquisition in childhood and adolescence are very similar to those used to adapt to change in later life. This process is called selection, optimization, and compensation (Lerner, Freund, DeStefanis, & Habermas, 2001). Thus, the goals of an individual's behavior change across the lifespan, but the process supporting goal achievement is consistent regardless of age.

The Theory of Selective Optimization and Compensation

Selective optimization with compensation (SOC) is a process that unifies the study of development (Baltes & Carstensen, 1996; Baltes & Lindenberger, 1997; Heckhausen, 1998; Schulz & Heckhausen, 1996) (Figure 3-4).

This theory integrates the work of child-adolescent researchers (Hetherington & Parke, 1988; Rutter & Rutter, 1993) with the work of scientists studying aging and midlife development (Schroots, 1996). This theory proposes that successful development results from the simultaneous maximization of gains (desirable goals or outcomes) and the minimization of losses (undesirable goals or outcomes). The choices of goals, the strategies used to achieve these goals, and the behavioral context changes over time. However, longitudinal studies have documented measurable intra-individual stability (conti-

Table 3-5

Principles of Self-Determination Theory

Basic Constructs of Self-Determination Theory

- Human beings are active (rather than passive).
- Humans are naturally inclined toward growth and development rather than being programmed by the social environment.
- Humans have a set of basic psychological needs that are universal rather than being determined by culture.

Motivational Determinants of Behavior

- Desired behaviors occur when individuals feel competent.
- Desired behaviors are more likely to occur when individuals choose to initiate the behavior.
- Desired behaviors are more likely to occur when individuals have satisfying relationships with significant others.

Dimensions of the Social Environment That Influence Motivation

- Structure is the degree to which the relationships between the behavior and important outcomes are understandable, expectations are clear, and positive feedback is provided.
- Autonomy-supporting contexts provide choice, minimize pressure, and encourage individuals to initiate actions themselves.
- Involvement is the extent to which individuals perceive that significant others relevant to the behavior are genuinely interested in them and their well-being.

nuity) despite stage-related physical, social, and emotional changes (discontinuity). Regardless of age, the individual is consciously or unconsciously regulating his or her behavior in response to internal and external stimuli and events. This individual response to developmental demands is called *agency*. Cultural and personal factors, as well as the age of the individual, influence the definition of gains and losses as well as the dynamic interaction between these gains and losses (Lewis, 1999).

The theory of selection, optimization, and compensation is consistent with current views of occupational performance. Baltes and his colleagues (1999) use examples of everyday behaviors, or occupations, to illustrate the meaning of SOC. They describe an interview with Arthur Rubenstein, a famous concert pianist. When Mr. Rubenstein was 80 years old, he was asked how he managed to continue playing the piano so well. He answered that he played fewer pieces (selection); he practiced these pieces more often (optimization); and, to counteract his loss of mechanical speed, he now deliberately plays more slowly before a fast section, to make the latter appear faster (compensation). Even in early infancy, babies produce social behaviors such as smiling or cooing (selection). These behaviors create feelings of attachment in their parents and caregivers (optimization), thus increasing the likelihood that their needs will be met (compensation). Parents, in turn, call upon the resources of society to optimize their child's development and well-being.

Self-Determination and Competence Across the Lifespan

Regardless of age or stage of development, all humans are thought to possess a strong drive to achieve a sense of competence and self-determination (Deci & Ryan, 2000). Self-determination theory (SDT) is a theory of motivation that addresses personality development and function within social contexts. This theory suggests that growth, integrity, and well-being occur through interactions that support three innate psychological needs (competence, autonomy, and relatedness), which, when satisfied, result in health and well-being (Ryan & Deci, 2000). The link between occupational performance, health, and well-being is well established. It is not difficult to extend this research to understanding the contributions of occupation to the development of competence and autonomy (Table 3-5).

At each stage of development, the person, environment, and occupation interactions shape feelings of competence and self-determination. There is a strong relationship between the types of tasks and activities and age-related abilities and interests. Research in this area shows that feelings of competence and well-being vary across the lifespan but that there is no natural decline with age (Ryff, 1989) (Figure 3-5).

According to SDT, age-related social contexts such as school, work, and family life help define the life tasks and challenges that lead first to changes in capacity and then to perceptions of self-efficacy and competence (Deci & Ryan, 2000; Ryff, 1989). These authors also explore the effects of culture on development as well as maintenance of a sense of well-being. Cultural norms and expectations vary greatly across the world and influence the timing and availability of critical roles and responsibilities. Llorens (1970) touched on the same themes in her Slagle lecture: the contributions of self-determination, competence, and culture to development proposed by Deci and Ryan (2000). Deci and Ryan have applied their theory to educational interventions. To date, their work has not been linked to other applications. It is easy to see the relevance of this work to occupational science. Occupational scientists can use this same theoretical perspective to support occupation-based interventions for people with developmental or acquired disabilities. Through task analysis and grading and the use of technology or environmental adaptation, the occupational needs of an individual can be met. Interventions grounded in the life of the individual are more likely to be successful and will lead to enhanced health and well-being.

Summary

This chapter began with the premise that occupation is both the product and process of development. Occupations influence and guide development through the active engagement of the individual in his or her significant roles and responsibilities. Through this active process of engagement, the person grows physically, intellectually, emotionally, and socially. Occupations are also the product of development through the growth, maturation, and modification of the biological, psychological, and social systems that support human activity. Historically, philosophers and biological and social scientists have systematically examined this process. We are the fortunate recipients of this work that began centuries ago. The themes noted in the Bible, debated by Plato and Aristotle, and addressed by contemporary investigators are remarkably consistent. New theories such as those proposed by Baltes (selection, optimization, and compensation) or Deci (self-determination and competence) support the application of the PEOP model to practice and substantiate the perspectives of occupational scientists. The focus on occupation will help all students of human development gain a better understanding of the relationship between occupation, the ever-evolving sense of self, and health and well-being. Occupational scientists have much to contribute to this effort through research and practice.

References

Abbott, L. F., & Nelson, S. B. (2000). Synaptic plasticity: Taming the beast. *Nature Neuroscience*, Nov 3 Suppl, 1178-1183.

Anderson, R. N. D. (2002). *United States Life Tables, 1999*. Hyattsville, MD: National Center for Health Statistics.

Aries, P. (1962a). *Centuries of childhood*. London: Jonathan Cape.

Aries, P. (1962b). *Centuries of childhood: A social history of family life* (R. Baldick, Trans.). New York, NY: Alfred Knopf.

Baltes, M., & Carstensen, L. (1996). The process of successful ageing. *Ageing and Society, 16*, 397-422.

Baltes, P. B. (1997). On the incomplete architecture of human ontogeny: Selection, optimization, and compensation as foundation of developmental theory. *American Psychologist, 52*, 366-380.

Baltes, P. B., & Lindenberger, U. (1997). Emergence of a powerful connection between sensory and cognitive functions across the adult life span: A new window to the study of cognitive aging? *Psychology and Aging, 12*, 12-21.

Baltes, P. B., Staudinger, U. M., & Lindenberger, U. (1999). Lifespan psychology: Theory and application to intellectual functioning. *Annual Review of Psychology, 50*, 191-215.

Bandura, A. (1977). Self-efficacy: Toward a unifying theory of behavioral change. *Psychology Review, 84*, 191-215.

Bandura, A. (1982). Self-efficacy mechanisms in human agency. *Journal of Behavior Therapy and Experimental Psychiatry, 37*, 122-147.

Bandura, A. (1989). Social cognition theory. In R. Vasta (Ed.), *Annals of Child Development. Volume 6: Six Theories of Child Development*. Greenwich, CT: JAL Press.

Bandura, A. (2000). Exercise of human agency through collective efficacy. *Current Directions in Psychological Science, 9*, 75-78.

Bateson, P., Barker, D., Clutton-Brock, T., Deb, D., D'Udine, B., Foley, R. A., et al. (2004). Developmental plasticity and human health. *Nature, 430*, 419-421.

Bronfenbrenner, U. (1977). Toward an experimental ecology of human development. *American Psychologist, 32*, 513-531.

Bronfenbrenner, U. (1994). Ecological models of human development. In T. Husen & T. N. Postlethwaite (Ed.), *The international encyclopedia of education* (pp. 1643-1647). New York, NY: Elsevier Science.

Datan, N., Rodeheaver, D., & Hughes, F. (1987). Adult development and aging. *Annual Review of Psychology, 38*, 153-180.

SOCIETY PHASE	PERSON, ROLE, ENVIRONMENT INTERACTION	CONTRIBUTIONS TO COMPETENCE
Pre-school	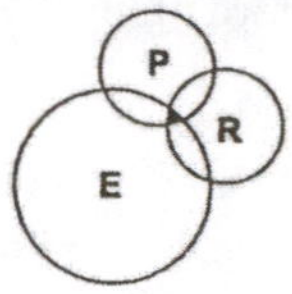 P R E	**Person** - Physical capacities, especially gross motor skills, evolve. Self begins to be expressed as individuality. Assertiveness and communication style are reflected in personality. **Role** - Behaviors emerge to meet parents rule-based demands for self-care & communication. **Environment** - Threats are minimized as the individual learns to manipulate the environment to maximize affordances.
Primary student	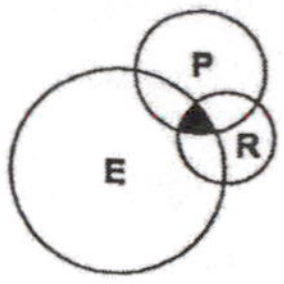 P E R	**Person** - Physical, psychological and sociocultural capacities expand. Competence develops in response to environmental and role challenges. **Role** - Role demands, rules and rewards are prescribed by other individuals and society. **Environment** - Impact of threats are minimized by the individual. Individual integrates the ability to control & use environmental affordances.
Secondary student	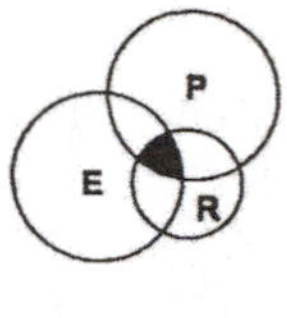 P E R	**Person** - Physical capacities evolve as a result of biological & physical maturation. Individuality & self-efficacy result from self-evaluation of role demands & use of environmental affordances. **Role** - Individual rejects roles prescribed by adults and society & begins to experiment with role behaviors. **Environment** - Individual minimizes environmental affordances to exert "self".
Young careerist	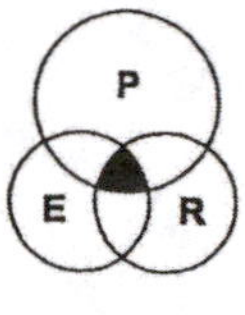 P E R	**Person** - Physical capacities reach their maximum. Individual conforms to cultural and social demands while maintaining a sense of identity and individuality. Individual structures time and environment to maximize competence. **Role** - Individual selects roles consistent with their perception of their abilities & cultural values. Vocational role begins to be established. **Environment** - Individual becomes more adept in utilizing environmental affordances & recognizing or minimizing threats before they impact competence.
Mature careerist	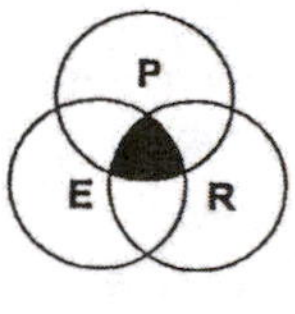 P E R	**Person** - Abilities, diminished as a result of maturation, are optimized through structuring of the environment. Personhood is established within the context of current society and culture. **Role** - Firmly established roles allow individual to gain control over financial, physical and personal environments. **Environment** - Individual minimizes environmental treats to abilities by restructuring or adapting the environment. Individual efficiently and effectively uses environmental affordances to meet role demands.
Active retired	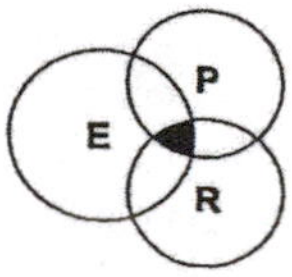 P E R	**Person** - Abilities continue to diminish as a result of maturation. Personhood established within a culture of retirement. **Role** - Primary work role is abandoned. Leisure and other life roles fill time once dominated by work. Individual may continue in a modified work role. **Environment** - Major environmental treats to abilities are handled by restructuring or adapting the environment. Individual becomes less efficient and effective use of environmental affordances to meet role demands.
Frail retired	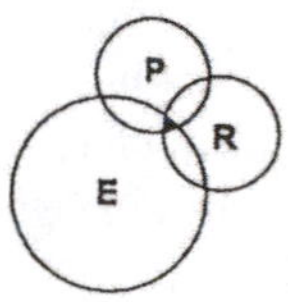 P R E	**Person** - Physical capacities are diminishing with biological and physiological maturation. Personal identify is diminished as the roles which defined the individual are removed. **Role** - Primary life roles are abandoned or are being minimized by society. Individual becomes dependent on others as capacities limit the individuals ability to utilize environmental affordances. **Environment** - Diminished capacities impact the individual's ability to respond to the environment.

Figure 3-5. Occupational competence is role-organized, based on the person's values within the contexts of the environment. As roles change, personal and environmental resources change.

EVIDENCE WORKSHEET

Author(s)	*Year*	*Topic*	*Method*	*Conclusion*
Baltes et al.	1999	Contribution of the process of selective optimization and compensation (SOC) to lifespan development	Theory	Successful development results from the use of SOC to maintain competence by choosing activities (selection) and modifying the task-related demands (compensation) that increase or sustain feelings of well-being and preserve skills (optimization)
Deci & Ryan	2002	Personality development and optimal function occur through engagement in specific types of activities that enhance feelings of competence and self-determination	Theory	Growth, integrity, and well-being occur through engagement in activities that support competence and autonomy. Occupational performance can affect social and emotional development across the lifespan
Keyes & Ryff	1998	Study of factors associated to age-related changes in physical, social, and emotional status	Descriptive	Engagement in productive activities and meaningful relationships is associated with well-being and increased life satisfaction in older adults
Llorens	1970	Role of occupational therapy in facilitating growth and development	Theory	Application of development theory to growth of physical, cognitive, linguistic, and psychosocial skills across the lifespan for persons with a disabling condition
Plomin et al.	1994	Interaction of genetics and social and physical environment on the development of physical characteristics and abilities, personality/temperament, and behaviors on children and adolescents	Theory	The interaction of nature and nurture is reflected in individual differences in children raised in the same family
Primeau & Ferguson	1999	Reciprocal relationship between occupational performance and development	Theory	Occupation is both the product and process of development

Deci, E. L., & Ryan, R. M. (2000). The "what" and "why" of goal pursuits: Human needs and the self-determination of behavior. *Psychological Inquiry*, 11, 227-268.

Descartes, R. (1901). *Meditations on first philosophy* (J. Veitch, Trans.). Amherst, MA: Prometheus Books.

Erikson, E. (1968). *Identity, youth and crisis*. New York, NY: Norton.

Erickson, E. H. (1994). *Identity and the life cycle*. New York, NY: W. W. Norton.

Feldman, S. S., & Elliot, G. (1990). *At the threshold: The developing adolescent*. Cambridge, MA: Harvard University Press.

Gage, N., & Berliner, D. (1988). *Educational psychology* (4th ed.). Boston, MA: Houghton-Mifflin.

Gillham, N. W. (2001). *A life of Sir Francis Galton*. New York, NY: Oxford University Press.

Green, M. P. (2002). *Theories of human development: A comparative approach*. Boston, MA: Allyn & Bacon.

Gruman, G. J. (1966). A history of ideas about the prolongation of life, the evolution of the prolongevity hypothesis to 1800. *Transactions of the American Philosophical Society, 56*, Pt. 9.

Hall, G. S. (1904). *Adolescence, its psychology, and its relation to physiology, anthropology, sociology, sex, crime, religion and education*. New York, NY: Appleton.

Heckhausen, J. S. (1998). Developmental regulation in adulthood: Selection and compensation via primary and secondary control. In J. H. C. S. Dweck (Ed.), *Motivation and self-regulation across the life span*. New York, NY: Cambridge University Press.

Hershberger, S., Plomin, R., & Pedersen, N. L. (1995). Traits and metatraits: Their reliability, stability, and shared genetic influence. *Journal of Personality and Social Psychology, 69*, 673-685.

Hetherington, E., & Parke, R. D. (Eds.). (1988). *Contemporary readings in child psychology* (3rd ed.). New York, NY: McGraw-Hill.

Hinojosa, J., & Kramer, P. (1999). *Theoretical foundations of pediatric occupational therapy* (2nd ed.). Philadelphia, PA: Lippincott Williams & Wilkins.

Huyck, M. H. (1993). *Middle Age. Academic American Encyclopedia* (pp. 390-391). Danbury, CT: Grolier Publishers.

Keyes, C. L. M., & Ryff, C. D. (1998). Generativity in adults' lives: Social structural contours and quality of life consequences. In D. S. A. McAdams (Ed.), *Generativity and adult development*. Washington, DC: American Psychological Association Press.

Kruger, A. (1994). The mid-life transition: Crisis or chimera? *Psychological Reports, 75*, 1299-1305.

Law, M., Cooper, B. A., Strong, S., Stewart, D., Rigby, P., & Letts, L. (1997). Theoretical contexts for the practice of occupational therapy. In C. H. Christiansen & C. M. Baum (Eds.), *Occupational therapy: Enabling function and well-being*. Thorofare, NJ: SLACK Incorporated.

Law, M., Steinwender, S., & Leclair, L. (1998). Occupation, health and well-being. *Canadian Journal of Occupational Therapy, 65*, 81-91.

Lerner, R., & DeStefanis, I. (2000). The import of infancy for individual, family and societal development: Commentary on special section: Does infancy matter? *Infant Behavior and Development, 22*, 475-482.

Lerner, R. M., Freund, A. M., De Stefanis, I., & Habermas, T. (2001). Understanding developmental regulation in adolescence: The use of the selection, optimization, and compensation model. *Human Development, 44*, 29-50.

Lewis, M. (1999). Contextualism and the issue of continuity. *Infant Behavior and Development, 22*, 431-444.

Levinson, D., Darrow, C. N., Klein, E. G., et al. (1978). *The seasons of a man's life*. New York, NY: Alfred A. Knopf.

Levinson, D. J. (1996). *The seasons of a woman's life*. Toronto: Random House of Canada.

Lichtenstein, P., Holm, N. V., Verkasalo, P. K., Iliadou, A., Kapri, J., et al. (2000). Environmental and heritable factors in the causation of cancer. *New England Journal of Medicine, 343*(2), 78-85.

Llorens, L. A. (1970). Facilitating growth and development: The promise of occupational therapy. *American Journal of Occupational Therapy, 24*, 93-101.

Lobo, F. (1998). Social transformation and the changing work-leisure relationship in the late 1990s. *Journal of Occupational Science, 5*, 147-154.

Locke, J. (1994). *An essay concerning human understanding*. Amherst, NY: Prometheus Books.

Malina, R. M., & Bouchard, C. C. (1991). *Somatic growth*. Champaign, IL: Human Kinetic Books.

Matheson, L. N., & Bohr, P. C. (1997). Occupational competence across the life span. In C. H. Christiansen & C. M. Baum (Eds.), *Occupational therapy: Enabling function and well-being* (pp. 429-457). Thorofare, NJ: SLACK Incorporated.

Newcombe, N. S., & Learmonth, A. (1999). Change and continuity in spatial development: Claiming the radical middle. *Infant Behavior and Development, 22*, 457-474.

Ormrod, J. E. (1998). *Human learning*. Upper Saddle River, NJ: Prentice-Hall.

Oxford English Dictionary (Concise Edition). (1987). Oxford, England: Oxford University Press

Papalia, D. (2001). *Human development* (8th ed.). New York, NY: McGraw Hill.

Papalia, D. E., & Olds, S. W. (1998). *Human development* (7th ed.). New York, NY: McGraw-Hill.

Piaget, J. (1969). *The psychology of the child* (H. Weaver, Trans.). New York, NY: Basic Books.

Plomin, R., DeFries, J. C., McClearn, G. E., & Rutter, M. (1994). *Genetics and experience: The interplay between nature and nurture*. Thousand Oaks, CA: Sage Publications.

Primeau, L., & Ferguson, J. M. (1999). Occupational frame of reference. In J. H. P. Kramer (Ed.), *Frames of reference for pediatric occupational therapy* (pp. 469-516). Philadelphia, PA: Lippincott Williams & Wilkins.

Reilly, M. (1962). Occupational therapy can be one of the great ideas of 20th century medicine. *American Journal of Occupational Therapy, 16*, 300-308.

Rice, F. P. (2001). *Human development: A lifespan approach*. Upper Saddle River, NJ: Prentice-Hall.

Rosow, I. (1976). Status and role change through the life span. In R. H. S. Binstock (Ed.), *Handbook of aging and the social sciences*. New York, NY: Van Nostrand Reinhold.

Rosseau, J. J. (1911). *Emile*. London: Dent.

Rothenberg, R., Lentzner, H. R., & Parker, R. A. (1991). Population aging patterns: The expansion of mortality. *Journal of Gerontology, 46*, A66-A70.

Rutter, M., & Rutter, M. (1993). *Developing minds: Challenge and continuity across the life span*. New York, NY: Harper Collins.

Ryan, R. M., & Deci, E. L. (2000). Self-determination theory and the facilitation of intrinsic motivation, social development, and well-being. *American Psychologist, 55*, 68-78.

Ryff, C. D. (1989). Happiness is everything, or is it? Explorations on the meaning of psychological well-being. *Journal of Personality and Social Psychology, 57*, 1069-1081.

Schroots, J. J. (1996). Theoretical developments in the psychology of aging. *Gerontologist, 36*, 742-748.

Schulz, R., & Heckhausen, J. (1996). A life-span model of successful aging. *American Psychologist, 51*, 702-714.

Short-Degraff, M. A. (1988). *Human development for occupational and physical therapists*. Baltimore, MD: Williams & Wilkins.

Turkheimer, E., & Waldron, M. (2000). Nonshared environment: A theoretical, methodological, and quantitative review. *Psychological Bulletin, 126*, 78-108.

Vygotsky, L. S. (Ed.). (1978). *Mind in society: The development of higher psychological process*. Cambridge, MA: Harvard University Press.

Watson, J. B. (1930). *Behaviorism*. New York, NY: Norton.

Watson, R. I. (1963). *The great psychologists from Aristotle to Freud*. Philadelphia, PA: J. B. Lippincott.

Werner, E. (1989). Children of the garden island. *Scientific American, 260*, 102-111.

Wilcock, A. A. (1993). A theory of the human need for occupation. *Journal of Occupational Science, 1*, 17-24.

Chapter Three: Occupational Development Reflections and Learning Activities

Julie Bass-Haugen, PhD, OTR/L, FAOTA

Reflections

It is hard to believe that at one point in time people believed that a human is a human is a human. Children were viewed as adults that were just little in stature. Serious study of the entire lifespan has really only taken place in the past couple of centuries. This chapter discussed the reciprocal influences of development on occupations and occupations on development.

As you read the chapter, there probably seemed to be an overwhelming number of perspectives on development. You might wonder, does it have to be so complex? If you could pretend, however, that there had never been any previous studies of development, where and how would you begin? Think for a moment of a specific person you have known for a number of years. Perhaps it is a child in your family who has moved from infancy to school age. Perhaps it is an adolescent who has gone from puberty to young adulthood. Perhaps it is a grandparent who has gone from middle adulthood to older adulthood. How would you characterize the changes in this person over time? Would you only describe the changes in this person from a biological or physical perspective? How would you account for changes in language, self-concept, or social or cognitive skills? How would you measure development? How would you explain the reasons for change? Would you only look at what was happening within the individual or would you feel a need to look at family, the home, and the community? What terminology would you use to explain your ideas to others? Would you try to explore one specific aspect of development in detail or would you try to propose an overarching explanation of development? Developmental theorists must have wrestled with many of these questions. Because people have different viewpoints and backgrounds, they answered questions like these in different ways. Each viewpoint adds a little more to our understanding of development and the ways in which we study it. In this chapter, we tried to get a handle on the different contributions to the study of development.

One way to describe development is to look at behavioral changes in a person. What do we mean by behavior and how do we study it? Behaviors are linked to our roles, tasks, and activities, and we can study them by looking at growth, maturation, and learning. The definition of growth here focused on genetic and biological factors that occur on a somewhat predictable and uniform schedule. Maturation, on the other hand, is the unique unfolding of a single person. Another way to explain these two terms might be to say that growth is what makes us similar as humans. Maturation is what makes me, me and you, you.

Changes in behavior are evidence of learning specific skills and behaviors. Learning is influenced by a number of mechanisms, including shaping, modeling, and social reinforcement. Say I am trying to learn to play a particular piece of music on the piano. I work with my piano teacher as I practice. After I play it, she gives me specific feedback on the things I did particularly well (e.g., tempo) and things I need to improve (e.g., phrasing). This feedback is shaping my future performance. During the lesson, she also plays the piece for me. I observe her technique and try to imitate her in future efforts. She is modeling the performance she wants me to learn. My warm friendship with my teacher and the enjoyment my family gets when I play provide me with the social reinforcement I need to keep learning.

Developmental theories provide an important foundation for our understanding of human occupation across the lifespan. Although you won't find many developmental theories that explicitly address occupation, it is clear that developmental theories influence our thinking about human occupation and human occupation in turn influences our ideas about development. In the *Developmental Theory of Occupational Therapy*, development is believed to occur horizontally (across different physical, cognitive, linguistic, and psychosocial skills) and longitudinally (toward mastery of skills, abilities, and relationships). Environmental influences and occupational engagement are proposed as important factors in longitudinal development.

Development has been studied using a variety of approaches and in a number of disciplines. It seems from the beginning of time there has been discussion of the nature versus nurture contributions to development. The same question has also been posed using different terms. Do you remember what they were from the chapter? Although we now believe the nature versus nurture argument is too simplistic regardless of its name, there is still interest in the relative contributions of each to human development. For example, explanations of criminal behavior have examined explanations that are genetic in nature and those that are due to environmental influences. Think of the many other characteristics that have been studied in these two ways.

Other common approaches for developmental theories are based on the domain of interest (i.e., the "what"—physical, cognitive, emotional, social), the process influencing development (i.e., the "why"), and the viewpoint on how development occurs (i.e., the "how"). The last approach has resulted in two primary theories that explain how development occurs: linear theories and pyramidal theories. Linear theories propose a definite sequence to development—first this, then that. Pyramidal theories propose that development evolves from a foundation with the highest level depending on the existence of the lowest level—like the Great Pyramids. Do you remember the theories that were provided as examples for linear and pyramidal approaches?

Development can also be described in terms of specific life stages. Childhood, adolescence, and adulthood were introduced as three major stages of development. In turn, each major stage may be broken into substages that have their own characteristics. The characteristics of each stage are most often explained in terms of biological or physical processes. If you look carefully at the description of a stage, you will see specific themes related to growth, stability, or decline. Sometimes, you will see these themes depicted as norms for a certain age.

We also find that some researchers are integrating stage theories and domain theories. The person-centered approach tries to characterize individual development across the lifespan for all dimensions or domains. The functions-centered approach explores particular functions across all stages of life.

Five specific psychological developmental theories were examined in this chapter: psychoanalytic, cognitive, learning, psychosocial, and biopsychosocial. Freud proposed in psychoanalytic theory that early experiences related to psychosexual needs shape later behavior. In cognitive theory, Piaget claimed that development occurs through active engagement with the external world. Intellectual development required ongoing use of the processes of assimilation and accommodation. Learning theories (e.g., behaviorism, social learning theory) introduced development as continuous rather than built on stages. Psychosocial theory, as proposed by Erikson, emphasized societal influences on an individual and introduced eight stages of development with resolution required at each stage before an individual could move on to the next stage. Biopsychosocial theory, as described by Levinson, suggested that life structures evolve over several eras from the interaction of values, dreams, and experiences with biological maturation and societal influences.

A lifespan developmental theory integrates knowledge from many different disciplines and theories in an attempt to integrate the fragments from the many different approaches to development. The key ideas of this approach help us to understand the big picture of development and include the following:

- Growth, stability, and change occur in development.
- Development involves an interplay between growth (gains) and decline (losses).
- Selection, optimization, and compensation occur in development.
- Adaptive potential (plasticity) changes with age.

This theory is an important one as it relates to human occupation, so we will examine it in a little more detail. It claims that development is not just a step-like orderly progression from infancy to old age; it involves periods of growth, stability, and change. This makes perfect sense to me as I look back at the decades of my life so far. There are periods of time that are a blur for me in that there hardly seemed to be anything that stands out in my mind—a period of stability. For example, the period of time from about 2nd to 4th grade all runs together for me. I remember my different teachers and a few other things, but for the most part the other changes in my life during that time seem very gradual. Seventh grade, on the other hand, had enormous ups and downs for me—a period of growth and change. I experienced a significant change in schools and friends, the turmoil of puberty, and a major growth spurt.

Development during periods of growth, stability, and change is best understood by looking at the contexts through the lens of occupations. This idea suggests that my periods of stability and turmoil in childhood can be understood by looking at what was happening to me in the realms of biology, interpersonal relationships, culture, and history. My stable period of time was stable in almost all respects. Changes in my biological make-up were gradual, and my interactions with family and friends were a constant. I don't recall hardly any transitions in my neighbors or classmates during those years. There were no significant losses in my family either. My culture also provided a routine that was predictable and reassuring. On Sunday, we went to church and then had dinner with my grandparents. I had a bath on Saturday. I prepared for a spelling test every week. On the other hand, the contexts during 7th grade provide a backdrop for some of the changes in my development. In addition to the changes discussed above, I had more freedoms, a larger human circle of influence, two brothers who left home and married, and then the addition of my first nephew.

Another idea presented in lifespan developmental theory is that of an interplay between gains and losses as we move through different periods of time. What is meant by this? Let's go back to my memory of 7th grade. What things did I gain during that year? A sense of myself as a woman rather than a girl? A larger view of the world with my new freedoms? Challenges to my intellectual capabilities with new teachers and new classes? What things did I lose during that year? A childhood view of friendships? A comfort with my gross motor movements because of my physical growth? How did these gains and losses interplay? I guess I was the typical teenager in many ways—poised and confident in some situations and hopelessly awkward and uncomfortable in others.

The third idea discussed was selection, optimization, and compensation (SOC). The words may seem foreboding, but the concepts are quite simple. Let's continue with my 7th grade example. As I entered this stage of development, I started formulating goals for myself. I liked learning in school, and I wanted to be a good student even in this big setting. I wanted to make new friends, but I didn't feel it was going to happen easily. I wanted to be active and athletic, but didn't know how to make it happen in this new school with my changing body. Let's take the last goal I had "selected" during this time. I remember doing a lot of activities just for the sake of feeling muscle development, testing my flexibility, and coordinating my movements. Some of these activities were very new to me (e.g., dance), and I remember observing my poses in front of a mirror to "optimize" my performance before the next gym class. I also learned during that year that I was better at athletic activities that had repetitive, endurance requirements (e.g., biking) than I was at activities that required coordination and flexibility (e.g., gymnastics). So over time, I chose to "compensate" for these varied athletic skills by focusing on activities that capitalized on my strengths.

The last idea that Baltes discussed is age-associated change in potential and plasticity. I have learned this concept, too, through my own experience with biking. Over the decades, I have seen significant changes in my potential for biking. In some ways, I have gained potential. I am much more in tune with my body's capabilities and am not nearly so reckless in how I pursue biking. Thus, I have fewer injuries and strains. In other ways, I recognize my areas of declining potential. I am no longer comfortable on a racing bike (especially its seat!) in the typical hunched position. I no longer have good endurance when there is high humidity or heat. If I am not careful, I know I could easily pull a muscle or get tendonitis. So I have adapted my occupation of biking to include pre-biking stretches, regular water intake, a different bike, and stationary bikes in a climate-controlled gym when the outdoor conditions are not optimal. This entire process is an example of my individual response to developmental demands.

It is clear from my biking example that development is hard to discuss without consideration of the influences of context or environment. A number of developmental theories have focused on the contributions of context or environment to our understanding of development. Theories like the ecological approach and Vygotsky's theory of language and cognitive development have studied the interaction between the person and the environment/experience.

Self-determination, a motivation theory, also fits nicely with developmental approaches that support occupational performance across the lifespan. It proposes all people have basic needs related to competence, autonomy, and relatedness. These needs and the degree to which they are supported by the environment influence behaviors or the things people do. And, of course, many of the things that people do are occupations.

One of the key ideas to remember from this chapter is that occupations are a way to measure the outcome of development, and they facilitate the process of development. So take my old, worn out example of biking. As my gross motor movements and eye-hand coordination reached a certain level of skill, ta-da, I could bike (i.e., the occupational product of development). As I biked and biked and biked (i.e., the occupational process of development), my strength, endurance, concentration, and perception improved. It is clear from the complexity of this chapter that development is not quite so simple—even though we wish it was! We have learned much about human development but a lot of questions remain. Who knows—maybe you will answer one of these questions!

Journal Activities

1. Look up and write down a dictionary definition of development and ontogenesis. Highlight the component of the definition that is most related to the definitions in Chapter Three.
2. Identify the most important new learning for you in this chapter.
3. Identify one question you have about Chapter Three.
4. Review the chapter and note other words that were used to represent the nature versus nurture question. Look up dictionary definitions for any words of interest.

Technology/Internet Learning Activities

1. Use a discussion database to share specific journal entries.
2. Use a good Internet search engine to find information on a specific developmental theorist: Freud, Piaget, Watson, Bandura, Erikson, Levinson, Bronfenbrenner, Vygotsky, Baltes. (Note: If you are doing Group Learning Activity #1, please begin this Internet search activity after a theorist has been assigned.)

- Enter the name of the theorist (e.g., "Freud") and "development" in the search line.
- Select several Web sites to review.
- Record the Web sites and evaluate the quality of the Internet sites.
- Obtain the following information:
  - ✧ Personal information about the theorist
  - ✧ Key ideas of theory
  - ✧ Developmental approach (e.g., domain)
  - ✧ Presumed beliefs about occupation

3. Use a good Internet search engine to find information on developmental tests and screening tools.
   - Enter the phrase "developmental screening" in the search line.
   - Select several Web sites to review.
   - Record and evaluate the quality of the Web sites.
   - Record the names and general characteristics of three to five developmental tests.
     - ✧ Name of test
     - ✧ General purpose of test
     - ✧ Target population (i.e., age, demographic characteristics)
     - ✧ Test characteristics (i.e., format, length, cost)
     - ✧ Test reliability and validity (if available)
     - ✧ Examples of test items that relate to occupations

Applied Learning

Individual Learning Activity #1: Narrating Your Story About Occupations and Development

Instructions:

- Select one period of development in your life.
- Describe the characteristics of growth, stability, and change during this period.
- Describe the interplay between gains and losses during this period.
- Describe how selection, optimization, and compensation were evident during this period.
- Describe any changes in your potential during this period.

Individual Learning Activity #2: Interviewing an Older Adult About Occupations Across the Lifespan

Instructions:

- Identify an older adult who is willing to be interviewed about his or her life.
- Practice your interview questions with another person. Use words that the average person would understand.
- Ask the older person to reflect on the major periods of time in life: childhood, adolescence, young adulthood, middle adulthood, older adulthood.
- Ask the following questions for each time period:
  - ✧ Describe a meaningful occupation (or activity) that you did during this stage of life.
  - ✧ Tell a story about a time when you did this occupation.
  - ✧ Describe the place(s) where you typically did this occupation.
  - ✧ Describe other people who did this occupation with you (if applicable).
  - ✧ Describe why this occupation was meaningful to you.

  - ✧ Describe how this occupation was important for this stage of life or your overall development.
  - ✧ Did this occupation influence your development in any special way?
- Summarize your findings from the interview. What was the relationship between occupations and development for this person?

ACTIVE LEARNING

Group Learning Activity #1: Jigsaw Learning of Major Developmental Theories

Preparation:
- Read Chapter Three.
- Complete Technology/Internet Learning Activity #2.

Time: 1 to 1.5 hours

Materials:
- Poster board or PowerPoint display
- Props and costumes

Instructions:
- Individually:
  - ✧ Select a theorist and theory to study: Freud, Piaget, Watson, Bandura, Erikson, Levinson, Bronfenbrenner, Vygotsky, Baltes (every person should select a different theorist).
  - ✧ Research personal information, key ideas, developmental approach, and presumed beliefs about occupation.
  - ✧ Develop a display and obtain props that would be useful in teaching others about your theorist/theory.
  - ✧ Practice portraying yourself as the theorist.
  - ✧ Prepare a 2 to 3 minute "speech" that summarizes your key ideas and presumed beliefs about occupation.
- In the classroom:
  - ✧ Schedule "A Day with Developmental Theorists."
  - ✧ Provide each theorist with 5 minutes to share their display, give speech, and answer questions.

Discussion:
- Discuss new insights that you have regarding specific developmental theories.
- Discuss the contributions of each theory to your understanding of occupations across the lifespan.

Group Learning Activity #2: Collecting Examples of Developmental Screening Tools

Preparation:
- Read Chapter 3.
- Complete Technology/Internet Learning Activity #3.

Time: 30 to 45 minutes

Materials: Internet summaries of Developmental Screening Tools

Instructions:
- Individually
  - ✧ Bring results of Technology/Internet Learning Activity #3.
- In small groups:
  - ✧ Use the table below to summarize developmental screening tools found through Technology/Internet Learning Activity #3.
  - ✧ Record the names and general characteristics of 8 to 10 developmental tests:

    Name of test

    General purpose of test

    Target population—age, demographic characteristics

Test characteristics—format, length, cost
Test reliability and validity (if available)
Examples of test items that relate to occupations

Name of Screening Tool and Internet Site	*General Purpose*	*Target Population*	*Test Characteristics*	*Reliability and Validity*	*Examples of Items on Occupations*

Discussion:

- Discuss the ages of the lifespan that are targeted by most developmental screening tools.
- Discuss how developmental screening tools do/don't address occupation.
- Discuss the items you would include in an ideal occupation-based developmental screening tool for a specific age group.

Chapter Four Objectives

The information in this chapter is intended to help the reader:

1. Understand the relationship between time use and occupation.
2. Appreciate that time is largely a subjective dimension invented by humans as a way of understanding and ordering their environment.
3. Identify influences on time use.
4. Define the term *chronobiology*.
5. List reasons for studying human time use.
6. Identify common approaches to studying and classifying how humans use time.
7. Using major categories of time use, describe how adults typically use time.
8. Identify types of recurring patterns of time use.
9. Distinguish between habits, routines, and rituals.
10. List consequences of disruptions in occupational patterns.

Key Words

chronobiology: The study of the body's physiological clocks.
habit: A recurring, largely automatic pattern of time use within the context of daily occupations.
lifestyle: A distinctive pattern of living that is both observable and recognizable, and over which an individual has choice.
occupational deprivation: A state of prolonged preclusion from engagement in occupations of necessity or meaning due to factors outside the control of the individual.
occupational disruption: A temporary condition of being restricted from participation in necessary or meaningful occupations.
ritual: A prescribed occupation that is intentional in nature and that typically holds special significance and meaning for those performing them.
routine: Habitual, repeatable, and predictable ways of acting.
routinization: A psychological disposition to rely on routines for everyday function.
system of national accounts: An approach used to identify and account for the activities that contribute to the economy of a country.
time use diary: A structured approach for gathering information on how people use time.

The ultimate of being successful
is the luxury of giving yourself the time to do what you want to do.
Leontyne Price

Chapter Four

Time Use and Patterns of Occupations

Charles H. Christiansen, EdD, OTR, OT(C), FAOTA

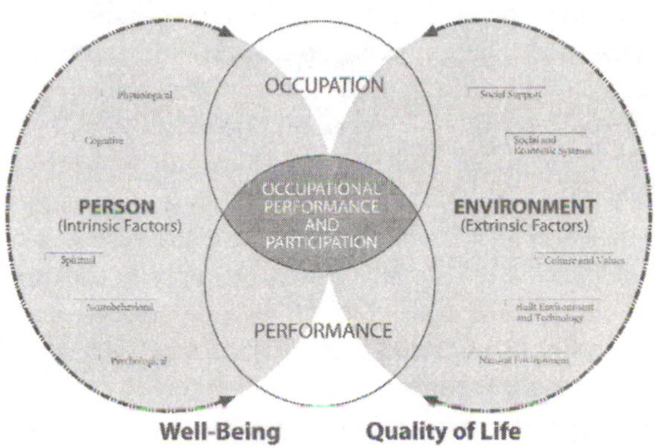

Setting the Stage

This chapter considers the relationship between time and human occupation, presenting time use as another approach for understanding people as occupational beings. The chapter begins with the observation that perceived time is subjective and may be influenced by various environmental and person-related factors that influence attention and action. The body's internal clocks, studied within the field of chronobiology, are identified as an important person-related influence on time use patterns. The chapter proceeds with a discussion of the nature and purpose of habits, routines, rituals, and lifestyles, and the consequences of their disruption.

Don't miss the companion Web site to *Occupational Therapy: Performance, Participation, and Well-Being, Third Edition.* Please visit us at http://www.cb3e.slackbooks.com.

Christiansen, C. H. (2005). Time use and patterns of occupation. In C. H. Christiansen, C. M. Baum, and J. Bass-Haugen (Eds.), Occupational therapy: Performance, participation, and well-being *(3rd ed.). Thorofare, NJ: SLACK Incorporated.*

Introduction

The word *occupation* is derived from the Latin *occupare*, meaning to seize or occupy. The admonition *carpe diem*, meaning "seize the day," refers to the use of time and place to leave a mark on the world. This "leaving a mark" occurs through agency or the active doing through daily human occupations (Emirbayer & Mische, 1998).

From the moment people become aware of their places in the world, they most often experience their lives as an uninterrupted stream of events. Memories of past experiences lead to present activities that encourage anticipations for the future. Events, which consist of recognizable activity experiences, mark the passage of time. The round of daily activities, typically beginning with a morning routine invited by the new light of the day and ending with an extended period of sleep prodded by darkness and fatigue, cycles continuously through lifetimes.[1]

In some parts of the world, the cycles of the seasons are marked by different occupations, providing another indication that time has elapsed. Traditions, celebrations, and rituals may also serve as reminders of time's passage. Examples include birthdays, regular religious services, or New Year celebrations. Clearly, one very important dimension of human occupation is its temporal nature.

Considered together, time and daily occupations are two sides of the same coin. How occupations occupy time determines the patterns and routines of daily life. These are the central concepts of this chapter.

In the following sections, various concepts related to time and human occupation will be reviewed, including how time is customarily perceived and measured, patterns of time use, influences on time use, and recurring habits, routines, and rituals, and their characteristics and purposes (Figure 4-1).

The Relationship Between Time and Occupations

It is possible that we are more precisely aware of the passage of time today than our ancestors were because analog and digital clocks, watches, and timekeepers are widespread in the modern world. Of all inventions used by modern cultures today, the clock may be the most universal and significant. Regardless of when or where they occur, the moment and duration of events can now be described consistently and precisely. This has practical importance for navigation and scheduling. Yet even before technology created these needs, humans were interested in keeping track of time (Whitrow, 1989). Early humans recognized the relationship between time and activities—that time elapsed as activities were undertaken and that occupations needed to occur or recur at particular times. For example, sailors and fishermen found it convenient to know when the tides would be changing. It was also useful to know when the sun would be setting because, before electricity, most outdoor activity could not be undertaken once the darkness of night arrived.

Even today, our dependence on sunlight for everyday activity is made evident in the use of daylight savings time (known in some parts of the world as summer time). This was an idea first conceived by Benjamin Franklin in 1784 in a humorous essay he wrote while living in Paris (Smyth, 1905). Now, with the exception of countries in the tropical regions (where it has no practical benefit), the practice of adjusting clocks (and lifestyles) during the summer months has been adopted around the world. That groups of people would agree to adjust clocks (and their lives) to preserve activity time (and energy) provides an excellent example of the inextricable relationship between time and everyday occupations.

The Experience of Time

How people experience the passage of time has been a topic of interest to both philosophers and scientists for centuries. Despite the standardization of time-keeping, people differ in the manner in which time is perceived. Individual differences appear to be based on age, personality, cultural experiences, and attitudes. Psychophysical and physiological variables, such as the temperature of the body, the state of arousal, and the effect of drugs (Eisler & Eisler, 1994) can also affect time perception. The extent to which accurate perception of the passage of time influences the performance of everyday occupations can be shown among musicians, dancers, and skilled athletes. The skilled performance of music, dance, and sport depends on the precise timing of human movements.

Scientists believe they have now identified areas in the brain that are responsible for time perception. The basal ganglia located deep within the base of the brain and the parietal lobe located on the surface of the right side of the brain are critical areas for this time-keeping system (Rao, Mayer, & Harrington, 2001).

---

[1]The idea that a person moves through time seamlessly as in a stream of consciousness portrays a decidedly Western view of philosophy. The author is aware of Eastern philosophies and religions (Taoism, Confucianism, Buddhism, Hinduism, and others) that interpret time as a number of sequential moments, each distinct in the characteristics and circumstances of what is experienced as the here and now. In this chapter, the experience of time is described in the manner that will be familiar to most readers. This should not be taken to represent a devaluing of the divergent views of time represented in other important philosophies.

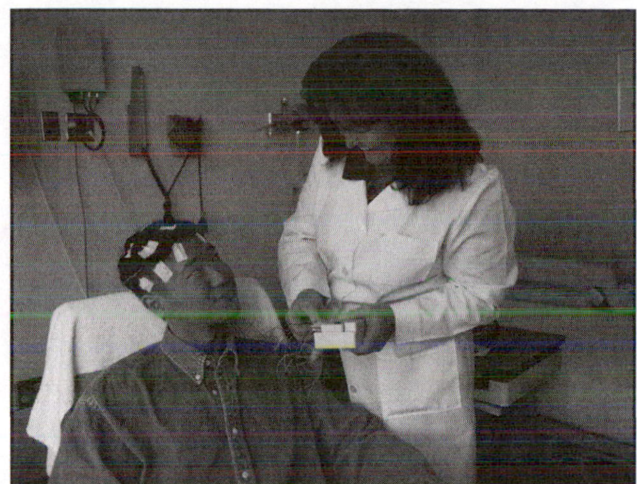

Figure 4-1. Chronobiology is the study of the body's internal clocks. One approach for studying these temporal patterns orchestrated within the brain is through measuring the electrical signals of brain waves. (Reproduced with permission of Getty Images.)

Physiological factors such as lower body temperatures, high levels of arousal, and concentrations of dopamine are thought to influence the perception of time through the body's internal biological clocks (Schleidt & Kien, 1997). Experiments have shown that, as people age, their estimates of the amount of time that has passed, particularly while doing an activity, are higher than people at younger ages. This suggests that as people mature, they perceive that time is moving faster than it actually is, which may explain why there is the nearly universal perception that years get shorter as we get older.

The noted psychologist William James was one of the first people to write about the perception of time in his classic work, *Principles of Psychology*, published in 1890 (James, 1890a). In a chapter on time perception, James discussed a concept widely known as the "specious present," during which he acknowledged that the present is really an interval of time kept in short-term memory because as soon as an event happens and is perceived, it becomes part of the immediate past. Scientists continue to debate the metaphysics of perceived time. Differing points of view include those who argue that there is objective time that exists independently of individual perception (even though the measurement of time is a human invention and units of time are relatively arbitrary and have evolved through consensus) and those who believe that perceived time is a result of how people interpret events in their mind as having an order (Mellor, 1998).

Influences on Time Use

The use of time is influenced by a number of factors. A person's selection of activities may be influenced by habits, social and cultural factors, age, physical status, and role expectations. One obvious influence on time use is available energy. Energy levels in the morning may encourage activities requiring more exertion, such as housecleaning or heavy chores. Societal expectations and worker status also influence time use. For example, retired people may have more time available for discretionary or freely chosen occupations than those employed outside the home or paid through a fixed hour per week schedule.

Activities may also be influenced by environmental factors. For example, in agricultural areas, the different seasons influence the time of year when planting and harvesting take place, so that different kinds of activities may occur at specific times of the year. The recurring pattern of these seasonal variations influences a lifestyle that is highly dependent on nature.

Physiological factors, including hormones, may change levels of arousal, also influencing activity levels and choices. Human activity typically shows recurring patterns, producing a certain daily rhythm. This natural cycle is influenced by internal biological clocks, which are thought to be influenced by hormonal changes and environmental factors. The study of internal clocks is done within a specialized field known as *chronobiology*.

Chronobiology

The term *chronobiology* is derived from the Greek words *chronos* (time), *bios* (life), and *logos* (reason). Although the first known experiment on biological rhythms was done on the heliotrope plant by a French astronomer in the 18th century, serious advances in understanding biological rhythms in humans did not begin until the late 1950s (Pittendrigh, 1960). By then, it was well known that the human body was influenced by many rhythms and that daily patterns of activity were influenced by a rest activity-rhythm that was circadian in nature (i.e., having a 24-hour cycle). The term *circadian* is from the Latin words *circa* (meaning around) and *dia* (meaning day).

During any one day, a person goes through periods of higher and lower arousal or activity. This is known as the rest/activity cycle and has a profound impact on occupational engagement. Environmental changes can disrupt that cycle and can cause physiological disturbances. Scientists are now aware that biological rhythms provide optimal times for human function and can significantly influence the value of medical or therapeutic interventions. This knowledge is the basis for an emerging focus in medicine called *chronotherapeutics* (Decousus, 1994).

Most people know about jet lag, which occurs when travelers cross many time zones. The disruption that sometimes occurs following such travel is called *circadian desynchronization*. This disruption of internal biological clocks can also occur as a result of shift work and can be of limited duration or longer term. Common symptoms of desynchronization include sleep loss, fatigue, diminished performance, loss of appetite, nervous tension, and a feeling of malaise or ill health.

Scientists have now discovered that the biological clocks inside humans depend upon everyday events to "set themselves." Exposure to light, eating meals, and other routines or patterns of social activity are now known to be important to daily rhythms of activity because they serve as time-setters or zeitgebers for internal clocks (Aschoff, 1960; Halberg, 1960). The study of human occupation often shows the connection between internal and external influences (such as social factors) on activity selection and time use (Christiansen, 1993; Halberg, 1994).

The When, What, and Where of Human Occupations

People seldom stop to think about how they actually spend their time. Most people can tell you what they did during the day, and they may recall some of their specific activities during the past week. If they are goal-oriented and structure their time use through careful planning, they will be better informed, but a typical person may develop a routine that varies little unless he or she experiences a significant life change, such as a relocation, new job, marriage or divorce, significant illness or injury, or death of someone close to them. Thus, unless an activity is notable for some reason or changes from the usual routine, it will fade from memory rather quickly. As a result, most people have only a vague idea about how they allocate their time.

Yet, there are practical benefits to understanding time use. Because time allocations for different occupations influence the consumption of goods and services, people who manufacture and sell products are interested in time use data to determine the potential for marketing their products, and people who provide services are interested in tailoring their businesses to the lifestyles of their customers. Because there is often a close association between how time is used and a person's location, city planners and architects may have an interest in this information. Economists are interested in the production of goods and services to measure the wealth of regions and nations and to understand trends in economic development. Public health officials are also interested in time use statistics to determine potential exposure to hazardous substances or pathogens. Psychologists, anthropologists, sociologists, and occupational scientists are interested in time use data as everyday measures of typical behavior, cultural patterns and trends, and lifestyles. How people use time also indicates their underlying beliefs, values, interests, needs, and personality dispositions (Little, Lecci, & Watkinson, 1992).

Purposes for Studying Time Use

Much of the current information on time use comes from studies by governments, often gathered for the purposes of understanding productivity and economic trends. Some consumer research and studies by social scientists have also made useful contributions to the general understanding of how people spend their time. The expression "spending time" is interesting because it conveys a view of time that equates it with other commodities or resources that are consumed. The emphasis on consuming goods and services in many modern societies has influenced time use to the point that individuals may neglect to realize the extent to which they fail to pursue daily endeavors that promote health and/or are meaningful to them (Peloquin, 1990).

Historically, the lack of consistent approaches to classifying or describing everyday time use has made detailed comparisons among these various studies difficult (Harvey, 1990). However, cooperative efforts have been started under the auspices of the United Nations Statistics Division to develop standardized nomenclature and approaches for time use surveys (Bediako & Vanek, 1999). The Trial International Classification of Activities for Time Use Statistics provides a recommended strategy for collecting time use data from large populations (Bediako & Vanek, 1999) and represents an important first step in this global effort (Figure 4-2).

The United Nations uses a conceptual approach known as the System of National Accounts (SNA) to identify and account for the activities that contribute to the economy of a country. Typically, activities that contribute to wealth include both market- and nonmarket-related activities. Therefore, measures other than traditional economic statistics are required to gain a full understanding of the human productivity in a population. Time use studies can help contribute to a more complete overall picture of a nation's economic standing (Ironmonger, 1999).

Of the 10 major groups of the Trial International Classification for Time Use Research Survey, three relate to production and income-producing activities.

Data from time use studies collected for economic purposes are often useful for discerning cultural changes and patterns of work and leisure. Each major group contains subcategories that represent clusters of everyday occupations with related purposes. For example, the major group labeled "personal care and self-maintenance" comprises activities required to meet a person's biological needs, which include sleep, rest periods and naps, personal hygiene, bathing and dressing, meals and self-administered health-related care, and relaxing.

Trial International Classification of Activities for Time Use Statistics (ICATUS)		
01	Work for Organizations	Paid work for corporations, government, non-profits
02-05	Household work	Primary production Non-primary production Construction Services for income
06	Unpaid domestic services	Preparing and serving food Cleaning house and surroundings Clothes care Household management Shopping Travel in relation to these activities
07	Unpaid care giving services	Care of children and adults and travel related to these activities
08	Community services	Voluntary and obligatory services for members of the community and travel related to these activities
09	Learning	Attendance of classes at all levels of instruction including pre-primary, primary, vocational. Higher education and literacy classes, travel related to learning activities
10	Socializing and community participation	Socializing and communicating and participating in community events and related travel
11	Attending/visiting cultural, entertainment and sports evens/venues	Visiting cultural events or venues, exhibitions Watching shows, movie Visiting parks, gardens, zoos Visiting amusement centers, fairs, festivals, circus Watching sports events Travel to and from these places
12	Hobbies, game and other pastime activities	Active participation in arts, music, theatre, dance; engaging in technical hobbies such as collecting stamps, coins, trading cards, Computing, crafts Playing games Taking courses in relation to hobbies Related travel
13	Indoor and outdoor sports participation	Active participation in indoor and outdoors sports Coaching, training Looking for gym, exercise program, trainer Assembling and readying sports equipment Taking courses in relation to sports
14	Mass Media	Includes reading (not related to work, learning); listening to radio or other audio devices; use of computer technology not strictly for work, learning, household management or shopping; going to the library for leisure; Travel to and from places for these purposes
15	Personal care and maintenance	Activities required by the individual in relation to meeting biological needs Performing own personal and health care and maintenance or receiving this type of care Activities in relation to spiritual/religious care Doing nothing, resting relaxing Meditating, thinking, planning

Figure 4-2. Major categories identified within a United Nations sanctioned approach to standardize studies of time use across nations. (Adapted from Statistics Division, Department of Economic and Social Affairs, United Nations.)

Gathering Time Use Data

There are a number of approaches to studying how people spend their time, including observation, structured questions, activity logs, and time diaries. According to information provided by the International Association of Time Use Research (IATUR), nearly 100 countries have sponsored studies of time use during the past 30 years. These government-sponsored studies are done for purposes of understanding economic and social trends and for informing public policy. Other studies, done by social scientists or businesses, seek to understand the time use of individuals for behavioral analysis or marketing purposes (Robinson, 1999; Robinson & Nicosia, 1991). Occasionally, when time logs or diaries are used, the accuracy of these logs or diaries is then checked by random observations or interviews of family members (i.e., proxy reporting) to establish their validity.

However, there is general agreement that time diaries, capturing the flow of daily activity, are the best approach for capturing data to support understanding and theory development in human occupations. This is because time diaries allow the collection of multiple dimensions of human occupation (Robinson, 1999). A limitation of diaries, of course, is that they often fail to capture the context in which a particular daily occupation is being performed.

Szalai (1972) provides an early account of multinational time use studies. More recently, to derive a more complete understanding of how time is used, researchers have asked subjects to report additional data that would provide contextual information about their activities (Harvey, 2000). Thus, subjects may be asked to report where, when, for whom, and with whom a reported activity was being done. In some cases, researchers also collect information on features of time use that would provide distinguishing information, such as whether or not the nature of an occupation was work- or leisure-related. As an example, if a person recorded that he or she was reading a book, the researchers might try, through requesting information on the title of the book, to determine if it was being read for enjoyment or work-related purposes.

Because individuals often are doing more than one activity at a time, scientists are interested in distinguishing between primary and secondary activities. In time use research, primary activities represent those endeavors that constitute the principal pursuit of the moment. Secondary activities are defined as other activities done concurrently with the main or primary activity being reported for a particular interval of activity. For example, a person may be listening to music and talking on a cellular phone while driving to work. In this example, driving to work would be the primary activity, while listening to music and talking on the phone would be secondary because they are nested or enfolded within the primary act of driving to work. Concurrent activities add complexity to the study of time use and increase the importance of discerning the context within which a particular occupation is being performed.

Others studies of time use have collected subjective information, such as the level of perceived tension associated with each daily activity (Michelson, 1985). Although time diaries and structured interviews are the most frequently used approaches to studying the patterns of time use among the general population, other approaches have been used by social scientists interested in the occupations of special populations, such as, for example, those with physical or mental disabilities or retirees. Cynkin (1979) and Neville (1980) each proposed the use of a segmented circle (viewed as a clock or a pie graph) to record a day's activities. Baum and Edwards (1993) developed a card sort to understand time use based on the percent of activities retained as a measure of time use among people with senile dementia.

It is apparent that in cultures where time is viewed in a less structured manner, such as with American Indians, Australian aborigines, and some cultures in the Pacific Islands (to cite a few), the determination of time use may be more difficult, not only for conceptual reasons, but because such cultures may not have access to or use clocks, radios, or other devices that would enable the recollection of exactly when certain activities occurred.

How People Use Time

Just as occupations are influenced by the contextual features of the situations in which they are performed, time use is also subject to the same contexts (Harvey, 2000). Time use statistics are therefore influenced by the social and economic conditions within the countries and regions in which they are conducted. Surveys indicate that, on average, within developed countries, approximately 30% of a typical 24-hour day is spent sleeping; 10% is allocated to self-maintenance and self-care activities (which includes eating); and another 10% is allocated to household maintenance, such as cooking, laundry, housecleaning, and shopping. Approximately 25% of a person's daily time is spent on work or work-related travel. Thus, 60% of the waking day is devoted to what can be termed obligatory or required activities, including productive employment or work, self-care, and household maintenance. Of course, such statistics provide summary descriptions of time use that are typical of the average person. In truth, few individuals will spend their time in a manner exactly as described by this average profile. Examination of individual time use diaries makes it clear that there is infinite variety and scope to the pattern and duration of individual lives.

With this qualification in mind, time use averages seem to demonstrate some international consistency across developed or industrialized nations. An analysis of percentages of time reported in certain activities for adults in Canada and the United States closely resembles data collected in other countries, including Sweden (Sjoberg, 1990), Germany (Baltes, Wahl, & Schmid-Furstoss, 1990), and Australia (Castles, 1994; McLennan, 1997). These data show remarkably consistent patterns, both for required and discretionary categories of daily occupation. Analysis of time use by population subgroups

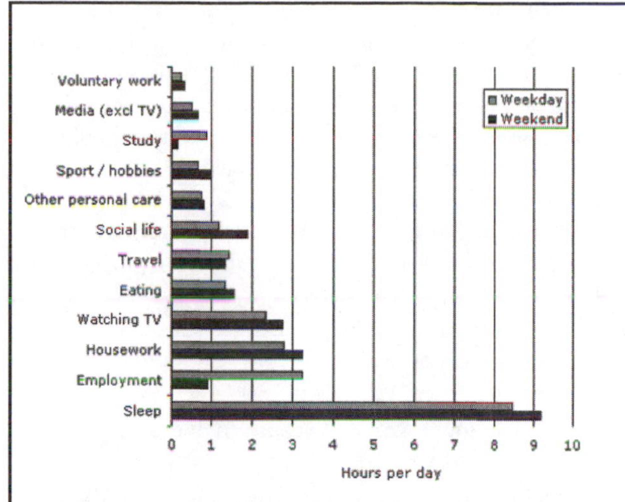

Table 4-1. Time Use Data from the UK Time Use Survey, Year 2000. This graph compiled from a recent time use survey in the United Kingdom shows how people change their time use on weekdays and weekends. The graph depicts time use by persons 8 years old and above. The graph reveals that, on average, people sleep an extra 43 minutes on a weekend day compared to a week day. Employment makes up less than an hour on a weekend day compared to an average of 3 hour and 15 minutes on a weekday. Weekends typically involve more housework, TV watching, social life and sport. (Reprinted with permission of Her Majesty's Stationery Office.)

by age, gender, and educational level may show variations in the amount of time devoted to various activities. Table 4-1 summarizes the average time reported in selected activities for a population sample in the United States (Tsang & Klepeis, 1995).

Studies have shown that the number of activities people perform during any given time segment may differ significantly. Also, the duration of time spent in occupations seems to vary by category and can reveal significant age, gender, cultural, and role differences.

For example, a study of adults in Germany (Baltes et al., 1990) found that, on average, people who reported engaging in more obligatory activities also engaged in a greater number of discretionary activities. Thus, active people tended to be busier than less active people in all aspects of their lives, not just in one area or another. Researchers have theorized that some people have natural tendencies to be active, and this theory seems to be supported by studies of activity frequency (Stones & Kozma, 1989).

Temporal Dimensions of Occupational Behavior

The order and duration of daily occupations often has a familiar pattern, influenced by environmental changes and biological clocks. Thus, the predictability of lives from day to day is derived from the consistency of occupational patterns. Necessary occupations, such as self-care, eating, and sleeping, are typically repeated as part of daily life. Paid employment outside the home also provides a temporal structure that encourages a regular round of occupations. The patterns of daily life, constructed from the order and duration of occupations, can be either healthful or harmful. Included in the various patterns are those whose duration is influenced by attention (resulting in either too much or too little engagement) and those whose order is repeated to a person's benefit or potential harm.

People differ in the frequency with which they engage in certain activities, the length of time they typically spend doing them, and the order in which occupations are pursued. Collectively, these temporal characteristics or dimensions can be described as patterns of occupational behavior. In everyday language, we describe such patterns with words like *habit*, *custom*, *routine*, *ritual*, *ceremony*, *regimen*, *lifestyle*, and *way of life*. These terms specify characteristics relating to duration, frequency, order, and repetition. Scientists have not yet agreed on definitions for these patterns and whether or not some terms currently in use describe distinct characteristics.

Patterns of Duration and Frequency

What compels a person to engage in an occupation with great frequency or for extended periods? Some occupations become so engaging they are pursued continuously to the exclusion of eating, sleeping, or self-care, occasionally leading to negative health consequences. People who become compulsive gamblers exhibit this type of behavior, but there are also people who watch television compulsively, play computer games, or surf the Internet for long durations. The obsessive nature of these patterns may indicate the presence of mental illness.

While there may be biological causes of obsessive behavior, there also seem to be characteristics of activities themselves that impel prolonged engagement. A study involving university students suggested that one important element of this phenomenon, which Carlson (1995) terms *occupational perseverance* (p. 145), was the individual's perceived progress toward meeting an important or valued goal. This tendency to continue pursuing the activity seems to be distinct from habits and is a byproduct of the interests of the individual and the nature of the activity. Some occupations encourage engagement because of the pleasure they bring in balancing challenges and skills. Chess masters of similar levels of skill would probably lose track of time were it not necessary for them to execute their moves within designated intervals. Many hobbyists find a similar escape to interests in their leisure pursuits.

Csikszentimihalyi, a psychologist at the University of Chicago, has studied the characteristics of activities that engage people by providing a level of challenge that encourages the development of higher levels of mastery (Csikszentimihalyi, 1978). His name for this level of attention and the perception of timelessness it engenders is flow. While engaged in flow activities, people frequently lose track of time (Csikszentimihalyi, 1990). Yet, flow as defined by Csikszentimihalyi does not represent a pattern of occupational engagement but rather a property or characteristic of such engagement as experienced by the doer or participant.

At the other end of the continuum are people who spend so little time engaged in what they do that they move seemingly randomly from one activity to the next, doing many things but unable to attend for long to any one activity. This type of behavior suggests the presence of distractibility, either due to anxiety or the presence of a short-term memory disorder that causes people to forget what they were doing in the moments immediately preceding the present.

Patterns of Order and Repetition

It is not uncommon in everyday language to hear people discuss patterns of behavior pertaining to order and repetition. The words *habit*, *routine*, *ritual*, and *lifestyle* are used variously (and sometimes interchangeably) to refer to different instances of these patterns. At this point, however, there is insufficient research and agreement among scientists to provide conclusive definitions for these terms or authoritative descriptions of similarities and differences among them. With this caution in mind, the following sections summarize preliminary thinking about these concepts and their associated phenomena.

Habits

Habit is a concept that embraces notions of both order and repetition in human behavior that has been discussed and studied for a century. Despite this, little consensus has been achieved on the definition of habit. Although habits are typically connected with observed behaviors, it is important to acknowledge that there are habits of thought as well as action. Dewey (1922) defined habits as patterned predispositions that enable individuals to respond to their situations with economy of thought and action: they can act while focusing attention elsewhere. His thoughtful analysis, influenced greatly by the work of William James (James, 1890b), recognized that habits can serve important supportive purposes as humans respond to environmental demands.

The supportive nature of habit has been further discussed by Michael Young (Young, 1988). He proposed the following:

- Habits increase skill in action by enabling a person to focus less on a given action and more on its elaboration.
- Habits reduce fatigue because they require an economy of effort.
- Habits free attention for the unpredictable, enabling a person quickly to detect novel or threatening stimuli.
- Habits enable a person to exercise functions without having to recall and attend to specific elements of a given practice.

These perceived benefits of habit have been extended by Clark, who observes that habits enable attention and energy to be devoted to individual creativity, thereby enriching opportunity for self-expression and creation of identity (Clark, 2000).

Seeking to provide a neurological basis for explaining the performance supporting nature of habit, Dunn (2000) proposed that a continuum exists governed by a person's sensitivity to stimuli and the stability of his or her behavioral responsiveness to such thresholds. According to her formulation, under normal (or habit utility) conditions, repetitive patterns of occupational engagement are balanced to be supportive of human performance as required by varying situations. Her continuum is anchored at one end by habit impoverishment, characterized by over- and under-responsiveness to stimuli, as found in depression and disorders of attention. At the other extreme, habit domination results from over-responsiveness to stimuli as characterized by addictive behaviors (Dunn, 2000). Although the word *habit* has been used to describe behaviors of very short duration (such as biting a fingernail), the term has also been used to describe longer sequences of actions or practices that typify character and personality, such as repeatedly demonstrating initiative or being polite and respectful of others. While such traits are repeated in different situations and may involve similar sequences of specific acts, it is unclear how they would qualify for inclusion in Dunn's continuum. Therefore, the suitability of using the term in this sense is uncertain even if habit is defined in the very general manner proposed by Dewey. The ambiguity surrounding precise definitions may explain why the terms *habit* and *routine* are sometimes used interchangeably. In the next section, we address this apparent confusion.

Routines

Routines have been defined as "habitual, repeatable, and predictable ways of acting" (Corbin, 1999). According to Clark (2000), not all habits are routines and not all routines are habits. Yet, she asserts, all routines consist of actions or occupations:

> Habits are the relatively automatic things a person thinks or does repeatedly. Routines, in contrast, are a type of higher order habit that involves sequencing and combining processes, procedures, steps, or occupations. Routines specify what a person will do and in what order and therefore constitute a mechanism for achieving given outcomes and an orderly life. (Clark, 2000, p. 128S)

Clark offers that routines provide a structure that serves to organize and maintain individual lives and that occupations can be thought of as the building blocks of daily routines (Clark, 2000). This structural, supportive view of the function of routines in daily life is shared by other scientists, including Bond and Feather (Bond, 1988) and Ludwig (1997, 1998) based on qualitative and quantitative studies of individuals in their natural environments.

It is clear that routines are supported by, and perhaps even dependent on, the presence of environmental conditions or situational stimuli. For example, mealtime customs are clearly evident in cultures and influence these behaviors independently of hunger or physiological needs. Businesses and other employers may prescribe working hours that impose a temporal structure that creates necessary routines. This is noted later in the section on occupational deprivation.

Place and Routine

Another aspect of environment that influences routine is the place in which a person lives. Social geographers have studied the impact of place on human behavior and have found that it serves to interconnect the routines of individuals within a location so that a routine of one person may be an important environmental feature that supports the routine of another. For example, Rowles (2000), a social geographer, has extensively studied the routine patterns of behavior of seniors in a small rural town. On a typical day, a resident of the community may make his or her way to a given community destination, such as the store or coffee shop, to be predictably followed by a journey to the community senior center, to converse with friends for a set period, then to return home using a familiar path at the same time each day.

Rowles observed that the elderly participants involved in his study were part of a larger community pattern of events and that a disruption to any one life would become disruptive to the overall patterns of daily life for many of the residents, whose lives had become highly routinized in this place. This "place-related" environmental influence on time use is geographical in the sense that it locates people in proximity, who then adopt routines of occupation that have collective influences on others in the community. Other studies have reported findings similar to those described by Rowles (Cutchin, 2000; Rubenstein, 1986).

Routinization

The term *routinization* is used in the psychological literature to refer to a trait or disposition to depend on routine for everyday function. Reich and Zautra have studied the trait of routinization, which they hypothesize is a characteristic representing the extent to which people (particularly at later stages of life) become so attached to their regular routines that they react aversively to changes in that routine (Reich & Zautra, 1991). They define routinization as the extent to which people are "motivated to maintain the daily events of their lives in relatively unchanging and orderly patterns of regularity" (Reich & Zautra, 1991, p. 161).

There appears to be two factors involved in this disposition sameness, including the need for order and routine in daily life and an aversion or dislike of disruption of such routine. Studies of routinization suggest that they are related to coping styles and the effectiveness of dealing with stressful life events and may have implications for mental health and well-being, particularly for people with chronic illness, disability, or functional declines due to aging (Reich, 2000).

Ritual

A ritual is a type of occupational behavior that shares characteristics with habits and routines but seems clearly distinct. Of the patterned occupations described in the literature, there is most agreement surrounding the concept of ritual. Rituals are prescribed occupations that are intentional in nature and that typically hold special significance and meaning for those performing them. Rituals exist for many purposes and trace their origins to a point before recorded history (Chase & Dibble, 1987). While many rituals are cultural and therefore easily recognizable to others within the culture, others are more personal and may be undertaken privately within specific families or by individuals to commemorate special occasions or events or to accomplish other purposes.

It is not unusual for rituals to mark significant beginnings, such as the commissioning of a ship, the birth or baptism of a newborn, the union of two people who agree to share a life together, or the beginning of a new job. Rituals are also undertaken to mark the end of a period or way of life (such as bachelor parties, divorce parties, funerals, cremations, retirements), the completion of important tasks and the attainment of goals (including graduation ceremonies, negotiated contracts, or extensive projects), and the transition from one state or time period to another (including birthdays, anniversary celebrations, centennials, and days commemorating the birth of certain heroes and celebrities of state). Some rituals, particularly those marking transitions (such as graduations and retirements) may be celebrated for a combination of purposes, such that they simultaneously may mark the completion of one period of life and the beginning of another.

Widely practiced cultural rituals are typically marked by performances that may include prescribed language, symbolic objects and places, ceremonial dress (such as formalwear or uniforms), and attendance by people occupying specific societal positions (such as spiritual leaders, educational officials, particular family members, special friends, or officials sanctioned by the state).

Personal rituals may include language, symbolic objects and place, and certain dress, and may be practiced to celebrate any number of significant events in a person's life, such as a successful surgery, the beginning of a friendship, or the attainment of a personal goal. Whether cultural or personal in nature, the celebration of rituals is often viewed as important to the experience of time and is a characteristic of daily life that can be used to describe lifestyles (Figure 4-3).

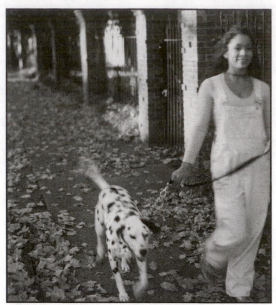

Figure 4-3. One common habit is often part of a daily routine in the morning and afternoon. Walking pets, when done at a consistent time, can also serve as a zeitgeber, or timekeeper, to help entrain biological clocks. (Reproduced with permission of Getty Images.)

Lifestyles

Habits, routines, and rituals help define lifestyles. A lifestyle can be defined as a distinctive mode of living that is both observable and recognizable and over which the individual has choice (Sobel, 1981). Elliott (1993) notes that a routine or established way of dealing with personal needs and the demands of the environment, as well as an established and consistent pattern of involvement in a particular type of behavior, are also important characteristics of lifestyles.

Fidler (1996) suggests that each individual has a unique lifestyle profile that should be understood in terms of the extent to which it permits attention to four essential domains of living, which she identifies as self-maintenance, intrinsic gratification, social contribution, and interpersonal relatedness.

Clearly, lifestyles are associated with cultures, places, histories (and thus age groups), genders, personalities, and other personal characteristics. Attempts to generalize specific patterns are probably optimally done within specific cultural groups or subcultures. Thus, lifestyle research has tended to focus on specific behaviors of interest to urban planners, economists, marketing analysts, and those interested in human development. There has been considerable interest in lifestyles as these pertain to understanding health promotion and disease prevention because links between lifestyle characteristics (such as activity engagement, nutritional habits, and coping behaviors) have been shown to be related to life expectancy, well-being, and health (Amundson, Hart, & Holmes, 1981; Baltes et al., 1990; Bartley, 1994; Dean, Colomer, & Perez-Hoyos, 1995).

Targeted groups for lifestyle studies include segments of the population selected for characteristics such as age, geographic location, gender, ethnicity, economic status, employment, and leisure participation and interests. Time use studies constitute one particular form of lifestyle research.

Disrupted Patterns of Time Use

What happens when established patterns of time use are disrupted? This question is of interest to social scientists and health professionals because of the known relationships between lifestyle, health, and happiness. Disruptions in lifestyle routines can be commonplace and temporary, such as that experienced during travel to different environments, changes in close relationships, experiencing minor illness or injury, disruptions caused by severe weather, construction, or renovation projects, or even the need for car repairs (Whiteford, 2004). More significant disruptions in occupational pattern or lifestyle can be caused by permanent changes of location, through isolated living circumstances, unemployment, retirement, imprisonment, refugeeism, cultural restrictions on participation, or severe illness or injury leading to disability. These more serious restrictions to a person's use of time can have significant consequences and have been described in the literature as forms of occupational deprivation (Whiteford, 2000).

Holmes and Rahe studied the relationship between life events and health in a classical study published in 1967 (Holmes, 1967; Holmes & Rahe, 1967). In their *Social Readjustment Rating Scale* (also known as the schedule or recent events), they identified events that require a change in daily life patterns and viewed these changes as potentially stressful because of their disruption of typical patterns of time use. They found that people who experienced more disruptions in their typical lifestyle during the previous year tended to experience greater numbers of adverse health episodes in the ensuing months, which they attributed to reduced resistance to illness. Their research led to further development of theories viewing life stress as resulting from disruption of ordinary routines and the manner in which individual characteristics permit effective coping and adaptation to such events (Amundson et al., 1981; Antonovsky, 1979).

Some extended changes in environment, such as institutionalization, incarceration, or homelessness, can result in deprived or impoverished conditions for time use. Such occupational deprivation can result in significant physical and psychological consequences (Whiteford, 1995, 1997, 2000). It is possible that sleep difficulties can be viewed as a special category of occupational deprivation because sleep occupies a significant portion of each day and is known as a necessary routine for self-maintenance and survival (Aronoff, 1991; Babkoff, Caspy, Mikulincer, & Sing, 1991). There is also some indication that activity patterns during alert states influence the nature and quality of sleep (Horne, 1985).

Summary

In this chapter, the important relationship between occupations and time use has been examined. It was noted that the experience or perception of time is different from measured or clock time and has an influence on individual behavior. Other influences on time use were described, including cultural, biological, and social factors. Prominent among these are internal clocks or physiological mechanisms that are studied in the field of chronobiology.

Studies of how people use time were described and summarized. It was noted that the purposes of such studies have traditionally ranged from understanding national economic conditions to marketing and public health. Typically, time use studies have not been concerned with specific contexts or qualities of experience during occupational engagement.

Patterns of time use were also described based on characteristics of frequency, duration, sequence, and repetition. Using these characteristics, the concepts of habit, routine, routinization, ritual, and lifestyle were defined and discussed as special approaches to discussing patterns of occupation. It was noted that the relative dearth of research in this area and the variety of disciplines with interest in human time use has precluded the development of consensus surrounding concepts and definitions. The chapter concluded with a brief discussion of disruptions to occupational engagement, including life changes and environments that are occupationally deprived.

References

Amundson, M. E., Hart, C. A., & Holmes, T. H. (1981). About the schedule of recent experience. *Psychiatric Annals*, *11*, 210.

Antonovsky, A. (1979). *Health, stress, and coping: New perspectives on mental and physical well-being.* San Francisco, CA: Jossey-Bass.

Aronoff, M. S. (1991). *Sleep and its secrets: The river of crystal light.* Los Angeles, CA: Insight Books.

Aschoff, J. (1960). Exogenous and endogenous components in circadian rhythms. *Cold Spring Harbor Symposia*, *25*, 11-28.

Babkoff, H., Caspy, T., Mikulincer, M., & Sing, H. C. (1991). Monotonic and rhythmic influences: A challenge for sleep deprivation research. *Psychological Bulletin*, *109*, 411-428.

Baltes, M. M., Wahl, H. W., & Schmid-Furstoss, U. (1990). The daily life of elderly Germans: Activity patterns, personal control, and functional health. *The Journals of Gerontology*, *45*, 173-179.

Bartley, M. (1994). Unemployment and ill health: Understanding the relationship. *Journal of Epidemiology and Community Health*, *48*, 333-337.

Baum, C. M., & Edwards, D. (1993). Cognitive performance in senile dementia of the Alzheimer's type: The kitchen task assessment. *American Journal of Occupational Therapy*, *47*, 431-436.

Bediako, G., & Vanek, J. (1999). Trial international classification of activities for time use statistics. Paper presented at the International Conference on Time-Use (ICTU), University of Luneburg.

Bond, M. J. F. (1988). Some correlates of structure and purpose in the use of time. *Journal of Personality and Social Psychology*, *55*, 321-329.

Camporese, R., Freguja, C., & Sabbadini, L. L. (1998). Time use by gender and quality of life. *Social Indicators Research*, *44*, 119-144.

Carlson, M. (1995). The self-perpetuation of occupations. In R. Zemke & F. Clark (Eds.), *Occupational science: The emerging discipline* (pp. 143-158). Philadelphia, PA: F. A. Davis.

Castles, I. (1994). *How Australians use their time.* Canberra: Australia Bureau of Statistics.

EVIDENCE WORKSHEET

Author(s)	Year	Topic	Method	Conclusion
Camporese et al.	1998	Time use by gender and quality of life	Descriptive study DES	Suggests that a disparity in roles related to time spent in housework between men and women contributes to a difference in perceived quality of life
Monk et al.	1990	The Social Rhythm Metric—An instrument to Quantify the Daily Rhythms of Life	DES	Older adults have distinct rhythms influenced by routines, and disruption in these routines may lead to difficulties that compromise health and well-being
Reich & Williams	2003	Exploring the properties of habits and routines in daily life	DES	Factor analysis of responses from a sample of students suggested that underlying factors of habit pertain to cognition and sensory reactions, habitual behaviors, and motivations of approach and avoidance
Robinson & Bostrom	1994	The overestimated workweek: What time diary measures suggest	DES	Comparisons of estimates and time diaries suggest that people perceive that they are working more than they actually are
Rowles	2000	Habituation and being in place	DES	From an ethnographic study of growing old in an Appalachian community, it was shown that older people make habitual adjustments in the use and the meaning of the spaces and the places of their lives as they accommodate to changing circumstances

Chase, P., & Dibble, H. (1987). Middle Paleolithic symbolism: A review of current evidence and interpretations. *Journal of Anthropological Archaeology*, *6*, 263-296.

Christiansen, C. (1993). Three perspectives on balance in occupation. In F. C. R. Zemke (Ed.), *Occupational science: Selections from the symposia*. Philadelphia, PA: F. A. Davis.

Clark, F. A. (2000). The concepts of habit and routine: A preliminary theoretical synthesis. *The Occupational Therapy Journal of Research*, *20*, 123S-138S.

Corbin, P. K. A. (1999). The incorporation of physical disability into the self (adolescents, adjustment, identity development). *Dissertation Abstracts International: Section B: the Sciences & Engineering*, *60*(4-B), 1884.

Csikszentimihalyi, M. (1978). Intrinsic rewards and emergent motivation. In M. L. D. Green (Ed.), *The hidden costs of rewards*. New York, NY: Lawrence Erlbaum.

Csikszentimihalyi, M. (1990). *Flow—The psychology of optimal experience*. New York, NY: Harper and Row.

Cutchin, M. P. (2000). Retention of rural physicians: Place integration and the triumph of habit. *The Occupational Therapy Journal of Research*, *20*(Supplement 1), 106S-111S.

Cynkin, S. (1979). *Occupational therapy: Toward health through activities* (1st ed.). Boston, MA: Little, Brown & Co.

Dean, K., Colomer, C., & Perez-Hoyos, S. (1995). Research on lifestyles and health: Searching for meaning. *Social Science and Medicine*, *41*(6), 845-855.

Decousus, H. (1994). Chronobiology in hemostasis. In H. E. Touitou (Ed.), *Biologic rhythms in clinical and laboratory medicine* (pp. 555-565). New York, NY: Springer-Verlag.

Dewey, J. (1922). *Human nature and conduct*. New York, NY: Henry Holt.

Dunn, W. W. (2000). Habit: What's the brain got to do with it? *The Occupational Therapy Journal of Research*, *20*(Supplement 1), 2S-5S.

Eisler, A. D., & Eisler, H. (1994). Subjective time scaling: Influence of age, gender, and Type A and Type B behavior. *Chronobiologia*, *21*, 185-200.

Elliott, D. S. (1993). Health enhancing and health compromising lifestyles. In A. C. Millstein (Ed.), *Health enhancing and health compromising lifestyles* (pp. 119-145). New York, NY: Oxford University Press.

Emirbayer, M., & Mische, A. (1998). What is agency? *American Journal of Sociology*, *102*, 962-1023.

Fidler, G. S. (1996). Lifestyle performance: From profile to conceptual model. *American Journal of Occupational Therapy*, *50*(2), 139-147.

Halberg, F. (1960). Temporal coordination of physiologic function. *Cold Spring Harbor Symposia*, *25*, 289-310.

Halberg, F. (1994). *Introduction to chronobiology*. Minneapolis, MN: Medtronic.

Harvey, A. S. (1990). Guidelines for time use data collection. *Social Indicators Research, 30*, 97-228.

Harvey, A. S. (2000). *Use of context in time use research. Paper Given at Expert Group Meeting on Methods for Conducting Time-Use Surveys*. New York, NY: United Nations Secretariat-Statistics Division.

Holmes, T. H. (1967). The social readjustment rating scale. *Journal of Psychosomatic Research, 11*, 213-218.

Holmes, T. H., & Rahe, R. H. (1967). The Social Readjustment Rating Scale (SRRS). *Journal of Psychosomatic Research, 11*, 213-218.

Horne, J. A. (1985). Sleep and sleepiness following a behaviourally "active" day. *Ergonomics, 28*, 567-575.

Ironmonger, D. (1999). *An overview of time use surveys. International Seminar on Time Use Studies*. Ahmedabad, India: Ministry of Statistics and Programme Implementation, Government of India.

James, W. (1890a). The perception of time. In *Principles of psychology* (Vol. 1). New York, NY: Henry Holt.

James, W. (1890b). *Principles of psychology*. New York, NY: Holt.

Little, B. R., Lecci, L., & Watkinson, B. (1992). Personality and personal projects—Linking big 5 and pac units of analysis. *Journal of Personality, 60*, 501-525.

Ludwig, F. M. (1997). How routine facilitates well-being in older women. *Occupational Therapy International, 4*, 213-228.

Ludwig, F. M. (1998). The unpackaging of routine in older women. *American Journal of Occupational Therapy, 52*, 168-174.

McLennan, W. (1997). *How Australians use their time*. Canberra, Australia: Australian Bureau of Statistics.

Mellor, D. H. (1998). *Real time II*. London: Routledge.

Michelson, W. (1985). *From sun to sun: Daily obligations and community structure in the lives of employed women and their families*. Ottawa, Canada: Rowman and Allanheld.

Monk, T. H., Flaherty, J. F., Frank, E., Hoskinson, K., & Kupfer, D. J. (1990). The social rhythm metric—An instrument to quantify the daily rhythms of life. *The Journal of Nervous and Mental Disease, 178*(2), 120-126.

Neville, A. (1980). Temporal adaptation: Application with short-term psychiatric patients. *The American Journal of Occupational Therapy, 34*, 328-331.

Peloquin, S. (1990). Time as a commodity. *American Journal of Occupational Therapy, 43*, 775-782.

Pittendrigh, C. S. (1960). Circadian rhythms and the circadian organization of living systems. *Cold Spring Harbor Symposia, 25*, 159-182.

Rao, S. M., Mayer, A. R., & Harrington, D. L. (2001). The evolution of brain activation during temporal processing. *Nature Neuroscience, 4*, 317-323.

Reich, J. W. (2000). Routinization as a factor in the coping and the mental health of women with fibromyalgia. *The Occupational Therapy Journal of Research, 20*(Supplement 1), 41S-51S.

Reich, J. W., & Williams, J. (2003). Exploring the properties of habit and routine in daily life. *OTJR: Occupation, Participation and Health, 23*(2), 48-56.

Reich, J. W., & Zautra, A. (1991). Analyzing the trait of routinization in older adults. *International Journal of Aging and Human Development, 32*, 161-180.

Robinson, J. P. (1999). The time-diary method. In A. S. Pentland & M. A. M. Lawton (Eds.), *Time use research in the social sciences* (pp. 47-89). New York, NY: Kluwer Academic Plenum Publishers.

Robinson, J. P., & Bostrom, A. (1994). The overestimated workweek: What time diary measures suggest. *Monthly Labor Review, 117*(8), 11-23.

Robinson, J. P., & Nicosia, F. N. (1991). Of time, activity, and consumer behavior: An essay on findings, interpretations, and needed research. *Journal of Business Research, 22*, 171-186.

Rowles, G. (2000). Habituation and being in place. *The Occupational Therapy Journal of Research, 20*(Supplement 1), 52S-67S.

Rubenstein, R. L. (1986). The construction of a day by elderly widowers. *International Journal Aging and Human Development, 23*, 161-193.

Schleidt, M., & Kien, J. (1997). Segmentation in behavior and what it can tell us about brain function. *Human Nature, 8*, 77-111.

Sjoberg, L. M. (1990). Action and emotion in everyday life. *Scandinavian Journal of Psychology, 31*, 9-27.

Smyth, A. H. (Ed.). (1905). *The writings of Benjamin Franklin*. New York, NY: MacMillan.

Sobel, M. E. (1981). *Lifestyles and social structure. Concepts, definitions, analyses*. New York, NY: Academic Press.

Stones, M. J., & Kozma, A. (1989). Happiness and activities in later life: A propensity formulation. *Canadian Psychology, 30*, 526-537.

Szalai, A. (Ed.). (1972). *The use of time*. The Hague, Netherlands: Mouton.

Tsang, A. M., & Klepeis, N. E. (1995). *Descriptive Statistics Tables from a Detailed Analysis of the National Human Activity Pattern Survey (NHAPS) Data (No. U.S. EPA Contract No. 68-W5-0011)*. Las Vegas, NV: U.S. Environmental Protection Agency.

Whiteford, G. (1995). A concrete void: Occupational deprivation and the special needs inmate. *Journal of Occupational Science, 2*, 80-81.

Whiteford, G. (1997). Occupational deprivation and incarceration. *Journal of Occupational Science: Australia, 4*, 126-130.

Whiteford, G. (2000). Occupational deprivation: Global challenge in the new millennium. *British Journal of Occupational Therapy, 64*, 200-210.

Whiteford, G. (2004). When people cannot participate: Occupational deprivation. In C. Christiansen & E. Townsend (Eds.), *Introduction to occupation: The art and science of living* (pp. 221-242). Upper Saddle River, NJ: Prentice-Hall.

Whitrow, G. J. (1989). *Time in history—Views of time from prehistory to the present day*. Oxford: Oxford University Press.

Young, M. (1988). *The metronomic society*. Cambridge, MA: Harvard University Press.

Chapter Four: Time Use and Patterns of Occupations Reflections and Learning Activities

Julie Bass-Haugen, PhD, OTR/L, FAOTA

REFLECTIONS

In this chapter, we learned that time and our daily occupations are interconnected. That is, we really can't understand our occupations unless we consider our use of time. We can't describe our use of time without using a framework of occupations. We also learn that time can be viewed and analyzed in a variety of different ways. Both objective and subjective components of time have been used to explore our occupational patterns.

In elementary school, we began to get a handle on the objective measures of time in our culture. We learned about different measures of time (e.g., seconds, minutes, hours, days, weeks, months, seasons, years, centuries, etc.), how to tell time using a clock and calendar, and events (e.g., holidays, birthdays, the school day, etc.) that occurred at different periods of time. We also started to associate objective periods of time with our occupations. We may remember watching a favorite TV show on a certain day of the week at a certain time. We may have watched the clock in the classroom in eager anticipation of our 30-minute lunch and recess period. As we grew older, the objective components of time likely became even more important as we scheduled the many activities in our life.

The subjective components of time are evident in our varied experiences and perceptions of time. We have all had experiences in which the same period of time, say 10 minutes, feels like it has gone by way too fast (e.g., the last 10 minutes of an exam) or is an eternity (e.g., waiting for someone to pick you up). You might find it interesting that these individual experiences have been investigated to identify the factors that contribute to different experiences. For example, older adults often report that the years are flying by compared with the passage of time during their youth. This difference in the perception of time at different ages has been well documented. What were some of the other factors that contributed to individual differences in perception of time?

The next section of the chapter discussed influences on our use of time. Why is it that I use my time in a certain way and you use your time in a different way? How can we explain the fact that my most productive work time is between 4 and 11 AM and someone else has more energy between 8 PM and 2 AM? One explanation has to do with differences in physiology and physical status. Our energy levels are driven by a number of physiological factors that include hormones and biological clocks. In turn, we know that our physical status is influenced by other factors, including sleep patterns, nutrition, and illness.

The idea that our use of time is influenced by natural rhythms of the human body related to rest and activity explains a lot in terms of occupational engagement. When our body needs a break, it is no wonder that we choose sedentary activities like reading and watching TV. We also know of times when our body just has to do something and during these times, we might feel energized to go for a bike ride or even vacuum the carpet. It may seem common sense that the rest/activity cycle of our body drives the occupations we choose at a given time. It is interesting, however, that the reverse also holds. That is, the occupations we choose as part of our routine influence our rest/activity cycle and help set our biological clock.

Time use is not just a phenomenon of interest to those who study human occupation. It has huge implications for the economy, marketing, public health, and community planning. We saw by the examples of time use studies in this chapter that different investigators have their own twists on the methods for studying time and the classifications of activities. We will explore these methods and classifications in some of the individual and group activities. Studies of time use help us describe averages and variations in patterns of occupations for a 24-hour day for many populations.

Individuals show variation in the duration and frequency of time involved in specific occupations. I remember visiting the Sistine Chapel and gazing in awe at the ceiling done by Michelangelo. How could he possibly have devoted enough hours in one day or in one lifetime to complete such an enormous work of art? One explanation has to do with the concepts, flow, and occupational perseverance discussed in this chapter. I suspect Michelangelo had such a passion for this project that he could "lose himself" in his work. I would guess his level of focus was about 150% all the time, night and day. Flow results from the pure joy of doing something you love. We can see it in the basketball player who shoots baskets for hours on end. We can see it in the scientist who works in his or her lab long into the night. We can see it in a musician or dancer who works toward perfection on one small piece of his or her work.

The terms *habits*, *routines*, *ritual*, and *lifestyle* were used to characterize aspects of time use as it relates to occupational engagement. However, it is clear from the chapter that there are not consistent definitions of these terms. Habits are those patterns of thought and behaviors that are repeated and semi-automatic and they generally support engagement in the more demanding occupations of our lives. They may include very specific behaviors to patterns that represent an overall approach to life. When I look at my own life, I see that many of the things that I do are habitual in nature and make it possible for me to do other things that are more interesting. For example, it is a good thing that I don't have to expend my creative energies on brushing my teeth in the morning or pulling into the same parking space at work. These are habits that perhaps allow me to reserve my creativity for more important things, like preparing for teaching.

Routines are obviously linked to habits, but this chapter indicated that we can't understand a person's routines just by looking at habits. While a habit can be described in terms of a single entity, a routine consists of a number of occupations, the order in which they are done, and the general environmental characteristics that support performance. We use routines to varying degrees in our life. In fact, the people who live and work with us can often describe us in terms of our routines. My children are well aware of my Saturday morning routine that consists of a few occupations (e.g., drinking coffee, reading the newspaper) that are as predictable as clockwork. I don't think this routine would fall in the classification of routinization, but of course my children know not to disrupt it too often.

Rituals are also important in our lives. They are the occupations that have significance on a personal or cultural level. The person who is part of a ritual can often describe the key aspects that make it special. For example, Thanksgiving is a holiday filled with rituals for many families. In my family, eating the pies that my mother makes is the highlight of the day. The ritual includes one piece of each kind of made-from-scratch pie, mounds of homemade whipped cream (and licking the beaters after it is made), and a discussion about how it is the best-ever pie she has made.

Our lifestyles are made up of all our habits, routines, and rituals. Your lifestyle is different from my lifestyle and everyone else for that matter. How you take care of yourself, how you meet your individual needs, how you contribute to society, and how you relate to others is your own style. We are only just beginning to study and understand how different lifestyles relate to the health of an individual and a community.

Any time there is a change or disruption in our occupational patterns and use of time, there is also the possible change in our health and well-being. Many of us have taken "stress" tests in popular magazines that are based on the number of significant changes that have recently occurred in our life. If you look carefully at the test items, you will likely see that they many of them inquire about habits, routines, rituals, and lifestyle. There are also large-scale studies that seek to understand changes in the population and the influence on health. For example, our increasingly sedentary lifestyle is of interest to public health officials who are concerned about heart disease, obesity, and ergonomic problems.

I hope after reading this chapter you have a perception of time and time use that is influenced by your understanding of occupations. Occupations do give us a different lens for how to view our time, habits, routines, rituals, and lifestyle. Well, it is now "time" to get going with some other activities.

Journal Activities

1. Look up and write down a dictionary definition of time, habit, routine, ritual, and lifestyle. Highlight the component of the definitions that are most related to the descriptions of occupation in Chapter Four.
2. Identify the most important new learning for you in this chapter.
3. Identify one question you have about Chapter Four.
4. Reflect on your current use of time.
5. Describe one of your habits.
6. Describe a routine in your life. Is it place-related?
7. Describe a ritual in your family that marks a beginning, end, or transition.
8. Describe your lifestyle.
9. Describe your rest/energy cycle. What factors change your rest/energy cycle?

Technology/Internet Learning Activities

1. Use a discussion database to share specific journal entries or individual activities.
2. Use a good Internet search engine to find one example of a time use survey.
   - Enter the words "time use" in your search line, and enter other words for specific interests.
   - Age: children, adolescent, adult, seniors

- Country: United Kingdom, Canada, American, Australia, international
- What is the source for this survey?
- Evaluate the quality of the Web site.
- Who is the target audience for the survey?
- What is the format or the types of questions? Diary? Forced choice questions?
- Record three interesting categories/questions related to occupation and time use.
- Does the survey include questions related to primary occupations, secondary occupations, context/environment, classifications of occupations, demographic characteristics, habit, routine, ritual, lifestyle?

3. Use a good Internet search engine to find one example of national or international research on time use.
   - Enter the word "time use" or "time use research" in your search line and enter other words for specific interests
   - Age: children, adolescent, adult, seniors
   - Country: United Kingdom, Canada, American, Australia, international
   - What is the source for this research?
   - Evaluate the quality of the Web site.
   - Who is the target audience? Age? Country?
   - How were the data obtained? Diary? Survey? Number of participants?
   - Record three interesting findings related to occupation, time use, and the data supporting these findings.
   - Describe one area of new learning from exploring this research.
4. Use a good Internet search engine to find the Social Readjustment Rating Scale.
   - Enter the words "Social Readjustment Rating Scale" in your search line.
   - Complete the scale according to instructions.
   - Record your score.
   - Interpret your score using the scale below:
     - <100 very low stress
     - 100 to 199 typical stress
     - 200 to 299 moderately high stress
     - >300 very high stress
   - Discuss your score in terms of your habits, routines, rituals, lifestyle.
5. Explore Web sites for the following topics.
   - Enter the following words in your search line: International Association Time Use Research, United Nations Time Use, Time Management Academic.
   - Record Internet sites for future interest.

Applied Learning

Individual Learning Activity #1: Analyzing Your Use of Time

Instructions:

- Pick one week to record your use of time on the time use survey.
- For each primary occupation, record the total amount of time per day spent on that activity. Record totals in 0.25 hour (or 15 minute) units of time. Example: 1 hour 15 minutes = 1.25 hrs. (Note: record total travel time for all obligatory activities—work, school, other).
- Obtain subtotals for each of the main areas of time use.
- Compute your weekly average for each of the main areas of time use. Add the subtotals for all 7 days and divide by 7. Record your results for each area in the average time column.
- Write a summary of your findings by examining your results. How would you interpret your results? Are these typical results for you? Are they ideal results?

- Compare your findings with the research averages for the main areas as discussed in the chapter and presented in the table.
- What happens to your work subtotal if you include the school subtotal as part of your "work"?
- Examine the care of others area. If you had significant time recorded in this area, what other areas would be decreased compared to research averages?
- How would you improve this survey to more accurately obtain time use data?
- How is this time use survey (see p. 88) similar and different from the survey in Chapter One?

ACTIVE LEARNING

Group Activity #1: Sharing Personal Characteristics of Time Use for an Occupation

Preparation: Read Chapter 4
Time: 20 to 30 minutes
Instructions:

- Individually:
  - ✧ Think about the various ways you use your time for the following occupations: reading a textbook, exercising, eating a nutritious meal, going to a party.
- In small groups:
  - ✧ Select one of the following occupations for members of the group to discuss: reading a textbook, exercising, eating a nutritious meal, going to a party.
  - ✧ Briefly discuss your performance of this occupation.

Discussion:

- Discuss the following questions related to your use of time for this occupation:
  - ✧ How does your energy level influence your use of time?
  - ✧ How do expectations (by yourself, others) influence your use of time?
  - ✧ How does the location, place, or environment influence your use of time? Use the chart on p. 88.
  - ✧ How does your daily rhythm influence your use of time?
- Discuss the similarities and differences in time use of group members for this occupation.

Group Activity #2: Learning About Habits, Routines, Rituals, Lifestyles

Preparation: Read Chapter 4
Time: 45 to 60 minutes

Habits

Instructions:

- Individually:
  - ✧ Take a few minutes to think of an example of a habit of action and a habit of thought. For each example, think of what, when, where, why, and how it is done (e.g., signaling a turn in a car; generating a basic, mid-week grocery list).
- In small groups:
  - ✧ Share your examples of habits of action/thought with other members in the group.
  - ✧ Fill in the table on p. 89 for each habit listed.

Discussion:

- Discuss each habit and answer the following questions based on Chapter Four:
  - ✧ Does it increase your skill in action by helping you focus on elaboration of action?

Time Use Survey

Area	*Primary Occupation*	*S*	*M*	*T*	*W*	*T*	*F*	*S*	*Average Time*	*Research*
Self-Care	Eating									
	Dressing									
	Grooming/Bathing									
	Subtotal Self-Care									2.4 hrs
Sleep/Rest	*Subtotal Sleep/Rest*									8.0 hrs
School	Class/Tutor/Lesson									
	Study/Practice									
	Athletics/Clubs/Other									
	Subtotal School									
Work	Paid									
	Volunteer									
	Internship									
	Travel/Commute									
	Subtotal Work									6.0 hrs.
Leisure	Passive—TV, Read, Stereo, Computer									
	Active—Exercise, Recreation, Shop									
	Social—In-person, Internet/E-mail, Phone									
	Cultural—Theatre, Museums, Concerts									
	Spiritual—Church, Personal Growth activity									
	Subtotal Leisure									
Care of Others	Children									
	Parents/Family/Others									
	Subtotal Care of Others									
Household	Homemaking—Cleaning, Laundry									
	Cooking									
	Shopping—Grocery									
	Subtotal Household									2.4 hrs
TOTAL										

Habit	*Thought or Action*	*Increase Skill in Action?*	*Reduce Fatigue?*	*Free Attending?*	*Function Without Attention?*
Signaling turn in car	Action	Yes	Yes	Yes	Yes
Basic grocery list	Thought	Yes?	Yes	Yes	Yes

- ✧ Does it reduce fatigue by requiring an economy of effort?
- ✧ Does it free your attention for unpredictable things and help you detect novel stimuli?
- ✧ Does it help you function without having to recall and attend to specific elements?

Routines

Instructions:

- Individually:
  - ✧ Take a few minutes to think of your morning, studying, and grocery shopping routines.
  - ✧ For each example, think of what, when, where, why, and how it is done.
- In small groups:
  - ✧ Select a routine for the small group to discuss: morning routine, studying routine, grocery shopping routine.
  - ✧ Describe individual steps, sequences, and occupations for the routine.

Discussion:

- Discuss how a specific environment or situation supports the routine.
- Discuss what happens to the routine when the environment or situation is changed.
- Discuss how your routine interconnects you with the routines of others in your life.
- Discuss whether routinization is evident in your routine.

Rituals

Instructions:

- Individually:
  - ✧ Think of examples of rituals associated with beginnings, ends, and transitions. For each example, think of what, when, where, why, and how it is done.

- In small groups:
  - ✧ Select a ritual to discuss what is associated with a beginning, end, or transition event.
  - ✧ Briefly describe the ritual.

Discussion:

- Discuss each ritual in terms of the characteristics of rituals discussed in Chapter Four.
- Fill in the grid below to summarize each ritual.

  Example: My children's birthdays have become quite ritualistic in recent years. We have a family birthday party that includes a made-from-scratch Black Forest cake, the child's choice of a favorite meal at home with the immediate family, a red "you are special" plate for the birthday person, and the "happy birthday" song in our own version. I don't recall any ceremonial dress for the family birthday party.

Ritual	*Example*	*Ritual #1*	*Ritual #2*	*Ritual #3*	*Ritual #4*
Prescribed	Yes				
Intentional	Yes				
Meaningful	Yes				
Special significance	Yes				
Special language	Yes				
Symbolic objects	Yes				
Specific places	Yes				
Ceremonial dress	No				
Special status people	Yes				

Lifestyle

Instructions:

- Individually:
  - ✧ Think how you (or others) would characterize your lifestyle.
  - ✧ What key words come to mind as you think about your lifestyle.

    Example: One person might use the key words of busy, involved, committed, family-centered, spiritual, simple, wholesome, interested, and adventuresome to describe a lifestyle.
- In small groups:
  - ✧ Share the key words that you associate with your lifestyle.

Discussion:

- Discuss how the key words you shared fit/don't fit with the dimensions of lifestyle discussed in Chapter Four.
  - ✧ Self-maintenance
  - ✧ Intrinsic gratification
  - ✧ Social contribution
  - ✧ Interpersonal relatedness
  - ✧ Activity engagement
  - ✧ Nutritional habits
  - ✧ Coping mechanisms

Group Activity #3: Sharing Results of Individual and/or Technology/Internet Learning Activities

Preparation:

- Read Chapter Four.
- Complete assigned Individual and/or Technology/Internet Learning Activities.

Time: 20 to 30 minutes

Materials: Notes from completed assignments

Instructions:

- Individually:
  - ✧ Prepare notes for assigned activities.
- In small groups:
  - ✧ Select an Individual and/or Technology/Internet Learning Activity to discuss.
  - ✧ Share your results from the activity.

Discussion:

- Discuss how your results related to information on occupation and time use in Chapter Four.
- Discuss any personal insights you had about your own occupations and time use.
- Discuss your most interesting/surprising finding.
- Discuss the questions/areas of inquiry you identified after doing this activity.

Chapter Five Objectives

The information in this chapter is intended to help the reader:

1. Define occupational choice.
2. Identify different motivational constructs that inform the concept of occupational choice.
3. Discuss the process by which an individual selects self-directed life activities that support tasks and roles within different environments.
4. Discuss how the environment dictates an individual's occupational choices.
5. Discuss how genetics, culture, and social policy inform complex questions regarding the differential aspects of how people make occupational choices.

Key Words

collective agency: Operates through shared beliefs of efficacy, pooled understandings, group aspirations and incentive systems, and collective action (personal agency beliefs are not independent of, but rather formed through, a broad network of sociostructural influences) (Bandura, 2000).

culture: Provides people with a set of values, assumptive beliefs, and implicit inferences about how the world operates that enable them to find meaning in and make sense of the events in their lives. "Culture provides the cognitive tools through which we understand and regulate behavior" (Cantor & Zirkel, 1990, p. 140).

ego-involved activity: Activity in which a person's self-esteem depends on attaining a specific level of performance (Ryan, 1982).

genotype (i.e., DNA): The genetic constitution of an individual (Jewell & Abate, 2001).

intrinsic motivation: That aspect of motivation that is based in innate, organismic needs for competence and self-determination, even in the face of obstacles offered by the social environment (Deci & Ryan, 1985).

locus of control: Beliefs about the control individuals believe they have over the outcomes of events in their lives (Rotter, 1966).

motivational processes: Mediate the formation of decision; create the impulse or intention to act (Kuhl, 1985, 1986).

nature: Primitive state of existence, untouched and uninfluenced by civilization (Jewell & Abate, 2001).

nurture: The sum of environmental influences acting upon an organism (Jewell & Abate, 2001).

occupation: "The interaction of the person with his or her self-directed life activities" (Baum & Law, 1997, p. 279).

occupational choices: "Deliberate commitments to enter into an occupational role, acquire a new habit, or undertake a personal project" (Kielhofner, 1992, p. 192).

occupational performance or function: "The point when the person, the environment, and the person's occupation intersect to support the tasks, activities, and roles that define that person as an individual" (Baum & Law, 1997, p. 281).

phenotype: Emerges through the process of development and exposure to a variety of experiences; is a set of observable characteristics of an individual or group as determined by its genotype and environment (Jewell & Abate, 2001).

possible selves: "Cognitive manifestations of enduring goals, aspirations, motives, fears, and threats" (Markus & Nurius, 1986, p. 58).

proxy agency: The efforts of intermediaries can contribute to a person's sense of self-efficacy (Bandura, 2000).

role scripts: "Appreciative tendencies that allow one to comprehend social situations and expectations and to construct behavior that enacts a given role" (Kielhofner, 1992, p. 193).

self-efficacy: Judgments as to how well one can perform actions required to deal with a prospective situation (Bandura, 1977, 1982, 1991).

task-involved activity: Activity characterized by engagement because a task is interesting, challenging, or has other inherent qualities (Ryan, 1982).

volitional processes: Control intentions and impulses so that an action is carried out; mediate the enactment of decisions to act and protect them (Kuhl, 1985, 1986).

volitional structure: "A stable pattern of dispositions and self-knowledge generated from and sustained by experience" (Kielhofner, Borell, Helfrich, & Nygard, 1995, p. 41).

volitional subsystem: "A system of dispositions and self-knowledge that predisposes and enables people to anticipate, choose, experience, and interpret occupational behavior" (Kielhofner, 1995, p. 30).

The self is not something ready-made,
but something in continuous formation through choice of action.
John Dewey

Chapter Five

Personal and Environmental Influences on Occupations

Gretchen Van Mater Stone, PhD, OTR/L, FAOTA

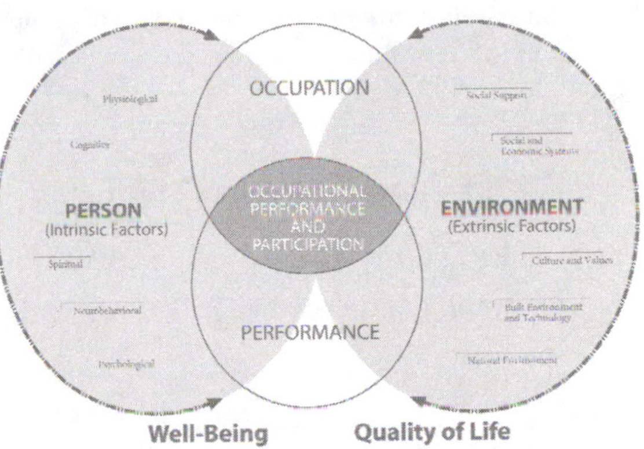

Setting the Stage

In this chapter, the influences of personal and environmental factors on the selection and performance of occupations are explored. First, theories and ideas fundamental to understanding human motivation from an intrinsic perspective are briefly reviewed. In this discussion, concepts such as agency, self-efficacy, and personal goals expressed as possible selves are reviewed. Then, environmental factors, such as culture and social policy, are considered in relation to their influence on occupational choices. Research-based examples are provided that clearly demonstrate that occupations are reciprocal transactions between people and their environments.

Don't miss the companion Web site to *Occupational Therapy: Performance, Participation, and Well-Being, Third Edition.* Please visit us at http://www.cb3e.slackbooks.com.

Stone, G. V. M. (2005). *Personal and environmental influences on occupations.* In C. H. Christiansen, C. M. Baum, and J. Bass-Haugen (Eds.), Occupational therapy: Performance, participation, and well-being (*3rd ed.*). *Thorofare, NJ: SLACK Incorporated.*

Introduction

Occupation is a term that describes "the interaction of the person with his or her self-directed life activities" (Baum & Law, 1997, p. 279). Occupational performance, or function, is "the point when the person, the environment, and the person's occupation intersect to support the tasks, activities, and roles that define that person as an individual" (Baum & Law, 1997, p. 281). Given these definitions, two central questions come to the forefront: What is the process by which an individual selects self-directed life activities that support tasks and roles within different environments? To what extent does the environment dictate an individual's occupational choices? Psychological theories of motivation, genetics, culture, and social policy inform these complex questions regarding the differential aspects of how people make occupational choices. Occupational choices are defined as "deliberate commitments to enter into an occupational role, acquire a new habit, or undertake a personal project" (Kielhofner, 1992, p. 192).

Occupational Choices Within Contexts and Social Environments:

Contributions of Psychological Theories of Motivation

Although there are multiple perspectives on human motivation, widely accepted theories address four common areas: how behavior is energized, sustained, directed, and stopped (Jones, 1955). Early theories of motivation maintained that behavioral responses were the result of drive and habit strength. Drives were thought to be physiologically based, and habits were developed through reinforced practice that resulted in direct pursuit of an end state. Behaviors were thought to be operant in that they were energized, sustained, directed, and stopped in response to environmental stimuli (Hull, 1943; Mook, 1987; Skinner, 1953). Given this view, the environment completely dictates an individual's choices, and no attention is given to self-directed activity such as thoughts and feelings.

Numerous examples can be found to support the supposition that the environment does reinforce certain behaviors; however, operant conditioning falls short of explaining why humans strive to explore new avenues of learning or why primates are curious (Harlow, 1953). Murray (1938) believed that humans have psychological as well as physiological needs and that these needs are triggered by environmental forces called *press*. Thus, the environment arouses human behavior but does not completely dictate an individual's choices. Lewin (1951) and others proposed a more interactive role of the individual with the environment. This view, under the umbrella of expectancy-value theories, suggests that the extent to which individuals engage in specific activities is related to expectations that their actions will lead to valued outcomes offered by the environment. Expectations are largely based on future events rather than past experiences. Individuals set goals and regulate their behavior based on consequences relative to goal attainment. Individuals select activities they find arousing because they strive to extend their capabilities. White (1959) termed this striving to extend one's capabilities as *competence motivation* and proposed that this corresponds to feelings of being efficacious in one's environment. Expectancy-value and attribution theories address self-directed activity, such as thoughts and feelings relative to environmental events. Thus, the individual makes occupational choices based on perceived impact from the environment.

Rotter (1966, 1975) recognized that striving does not always result in success and that individuals develop beliefs about why their efforts meet with success or failure. He introduced the term *locus of control* to suggest that individuals may limit their choices to engage in specific activities based on their beliefs about the control they have over the outcomes of events. Individuals who have an internal locus of control relative to a task are more likely to attribute poor performance to low effort, rather than low ability. That is, if they believe that they are capable of succeeding on a task and an outcome is under their own control, then failure must be due to lack of effort. Attributions such as this help people to continue striving, despite poor performance. Individuals with an external locus of control are more likely to interpret poor performance on uncontrollable events in the environment and may disengage from the activity or devalue the activity.

Currently, social-cognitive approaches to motivation predominate, such as those advanced by Mischel (1973) and Bandura (1977). Bandura suggests that both attributional approaches to motivation and traditional expectancy-value theories are encompassed by self-efficacy. Motivation is affected by attributions that raise or lower self-efficacy, not a person's actual ability. For example, feelings of anxiety are not the result of doubts about being able to accomplish a task, but rather fear of one's ability to develop effective coping strategies to deal with defeat or success (Bandura, 1991). Self-efficacy refers to judgments of how well one can perform actions required to deal with a prospective situation; thus, perceived self-efficacy is situation-specific. Bandura (1977, 1982) believes that the extent to which individuals believe they are capable, or efficacious, is a major contributing factor to goal selection and attainment. Thus, he considered efficacy to be the central self-regulatory mechanism of human agency. Self-regulation of behavior occurs through judgmental processes and through cognitive processing of self-observations (Bandura, 1991). Judgmental processes involve comparing self with others, determining the value of the activity, and establishing beliefs about that which determines a successful performance. According to Bandura, whether a person believes that he or she is capable of producing a desired action influences the individual's choices, aspirations, level of effort and perseverance, resilience to adversity, and vulnerability to stress and depression. Thus, self-efficacy is also a self-persuasion process (Bandura, 1998).

Bandura believes that people exercise personal agency (i.e., they take action that will produce an effect) unless they are constrained by one or more of three factors. They may face environmental constraints, they may not feel capable of achieving a goal, or the expected outcome may change. Studies have documented that self-efficacy belief, independent of actual ability, predicts perseverance, performance, and selection of appropriate strategies. Thus, the greatest constraint to occupational choice may be the belief that one is not capable of performing new and challenging tasks. In addition to believing in the power to make things happen through direct personal agency, Bandura has advanced the idea of "proxy agency" (Bandura, 2000). By this, he means that one can become more efficacious through the efforts of intermediaries. Given this perspective, personal care assistants who enable individuals with severe disabilities to live in their own homes could serve as intermediaries that contribute to perceptions of high self-efficacy among those they serve. Social-cognitive theories frame motivational issues in terms of how the individual perceives him- or herself in relation to specific environmental situations. The extent to which individuals believe themselves to be capable in specific environmental situations influences occupational choice.

The construct of self-efficacy is robust in that it has served as a theoretical basis for multiple studies of health-related concerns. Lorig and colleagues (1999) evaluated the effectiveness of choices made by individuals with a chronic disease following an intervention designed to enhance self-management based on efficacious beliefs. Individuals in the intervention group demonstrated an increase in weekly minutes of exercise and social/role activities. They also had fewer hospitalizations and days in the hospital. Similarly, Conn (1998) studied lifelong leisure exercise among adults 65 to 100 years of age. She found that perceived barriers, age, and self-efficacy expectation had a strong direct effect on exercise, whereas perceptions of the expected outcome had no appreciable effect. Kurlowicz (1998) examined the effects of perceived self-efficacy and functional ability on depressive symptoms in older adults after elective total hip replacement surgery. She found that interventions to enhance older patients' perceived self-efficacy while hospitalized may enhance functional ability, which in turn may decrease the likelihood of depressive symptoms postoperatively. Barriers to health-promoting behaviors for people with disabilities are negatively associated with general self-efficacy, perceived health status, and the likelihood of engaging in health-promoting behaviors (Stuifbergen & Rogers, 1997).

Theorists offer other perspectives as to why individuals choose to engage in some activities and not others. Why do they readily assume some roles and avoid others? Deci and Ryan (1985) coined the term *intrinsic motivation* to capture that aspect of motivation that is based in innate, organismic needs for competence and self-determination, even in the face of obstacles offered by the social environment. They propose that individuals are active agents who seek out opportunities in the environment. Intrinsic motivation includes behaviors in which satisfaction is concurrent with one's involvement in the activity, rather than being linked to some separable effect of the activity (Koestner & McClelland, 1990). Deci and Ryan (1985) propose that personality may play a role in what they term the relative salience of the competence-relevant versus autonomy-relevant aspects of an event in the environment. To one person, social praise may reinforce the belief that one is competent. To another person, social praise may be a threat to self-determination. Interestingly, Deci and Ryan found that men view praise as an affirmation of their competence at the activity whereas women view praise as an attempt at social control, which results in diminished feelings of self-determination, thus undermining their intrinsic motivation.

Ryan (1982) distinguished ego-involved activity and task-involved activity. Ego involvement refers to a condition in which a person's self-esteem depends on attaining a specific level of performance. In contrast, task-involved activity is characterized by engagement because a task is interesting, challenging, or has other inherent qualities. According to Ryan, ego-involvement creates self-imposed pressure to perform, similar to that offered by some form of external evaluation. Nicholls (1984) adds that, in ego-involving situations, a person's goal is to demonstrate high competence relative to others, and mastery of the task is only a means to this end, whereas in the task-involving situation, mastery of the task is an end in itself. Active engagement in task-involving situations may be as much of a contributing factor to health and well-being as mastering a task to meet specified criteria.

Tying level of effort to ego versus task conditions, Jagacinski and Nicholls (1984) found that when people try hard under task-involving conditions, they experience a positive sense of competence, whereas under ego-involving conditions, trying hard results in a lower perception of competence. Koestner and McClelland (1990) conducted a study that has direct implications when some level of mastery is expected. They found that subjects who were task-involved interpreted praise for trying hard as an indication of competence and appeared more intrinsically motivated to continue working. The implication is that if clients complete everyday tasks, such as self-maintenance tasks, under ego-involvement conditions, they could perceive praise for trying hard as decreased competence and thus subsequent performance could also decrease. Task-oriented activities are more prone to increase intrinsic motivation. Dweck and Leggett (1988) found that ego-oriented activities have resulted in avoidance of challenges and impaired performance in the face of obstacles. How is it possible to encourage task-involved conditions versus ego-involved conditions? One way is to carefully monitor the language used when providing feedback to others who are attempting to accomplish a task. An example of task-specific language to an elderly adult who is engaged in self-feeding following a stroke would be, "You scooped four spoons full of mashed potatoes today, and took some peas along, too. You are managing semi-solid foods well." In contrast, language that could precipitate an ego-involved condition would include comments such as, "Soon you'll be able to eat with others in the cafeteria. Your family will be so pleased." Under the ego-involved condition, competence is substantiated through the evaluative comments of others. Under the task-involved condition, competence is substantiated through the use of self-evaluation relative to task completion.

Analysis of conditions under which engagement in tasks is optimized has long been the central focus of practitioners of occupational therapy, a profession devoted to the study of human occupation. As early as 1922, Adolph Meyer proposed that occupation is "any form of helpful enjoyment" and he described occupation as "free, pleasant, and profitable" (Meyer, 1922, p. 2). According to Meyer, occupation used to enhance health does not depend on attaining a specific level of performance. Rather, the simple act of engaging in an activity that is enjoyable promotes well-being. Similarly, Trombly (1995) makes a distinction between occupation-as-end and occupation-as-means. Although purposefulness and meaningfulness are essential components of each of these two views of occupation, Trombly recognizes that the goals and therapeutic processes of these two views are different. Occupation-as-end is focused on levels of activities, tasks, and roles. Occupation-as-means focuses on a therapeutic approach in which engagement in activity is used to bring about changes in performance among people who have impairment, such as strength and range of motion. This is not unlike the distinction made by Dweck and Leggett (1988) who elaborated on the concept of ego- versus task-oriented conditions to goal orientation. According to Dweck and Leggett, performance goals are pursued for the express purpose of seeking positive feedback about competence, whereas learning goals are pursued for the purpose of increasing mastery relative to a task. Koestner and McClelland (1990) simplify this by stating that people can be cued into either proving their ability or improving their ability. Goals that are task-oriented could be categorized as learning goals, whereas goals that are ego-oriented could be categorized as performance goals.

Performance and learning goals need not preclude one another. Rather, occupational choices may include both goal orientations. Again, using the example of an individual who has physical and sensory losses following a stroke, accompanying one's family on a trip to the mall could be approached with an overall learning goal orientation. However, specific aspects of the task, such as drinking coffee at the food court, could be undertaken as a performance goal. Completing a specific task, indicating competence in a specific context, leads to overall increased intrinsic motivation and, subsequently, reinforces occupational choice The concept of self-determination is key. Language such as, "Mr. Smith, I want you to do this for me" or "Mrs. Jones, you can do this if you just try hard enough" reflect an environment that precludes occupational choice. When emphasis on self-determination is minimized, self-directed activity and intrinsic motivation are diminished. The importance of self-determination is emphasized in the definition of occupation offered by Baum and Law at the beginning of this chapter. Occupation is a term that describes "the interaction of the person with his or her *self-directed* (italics added) life activities" (Baum & Law, 1997, p. 279).

Koestner and McClelland (1990) point out that self-regulation is necessary because there are many things people must do that are neither interesting nor challenging. They note that Ryan and colleagues (1985) have extended the theory of intrinsic motivation to include processes by which "extrinsic regulation of behavior can be gradually transformed into internalized forms of self-regulation" (p. 534). This internalization process involves first assimilating the social environment and then accommodating to it. Internalization becomes possible when the environment provides structure but also supports feelings of autonomy and relatedness. Environments that facilitate the process of internalization offer a variety of meaningful tasks from which individuals can choose and offer the opportunity for successful performance. Under the frameworks of both goal orientation and intrinsic motivation, individuals who take an active role in setting goals and who retain ownership of those goals are more likely to select self-directed life activities that support tasks and roles within different environments.

Markus and her colleagues (Markus & Nurius, 1986, 1987; Markus & Sentis, 1982) have advanced an interesting explanation as to why individuals might strive to reach more challenging future goals at the expense of immediate reinforcement. They have coined the term *possible selves* to explain the interface between motivation and self-concept. In essence, they propose that what really motivates us is some sense of what we could be at some point in the future. Possible selves are "cognitive manifestations of enduring goals, aspirations, motives, fears, and threats" (Markus & Nurius, 1986, p. 58). Thus, the process of making occupational choices involves not only having a sense of who you are now, but also being able to accurately represent what it takes to be the person you want to be. This construct is helpful in explaining why students study long hours and work hard to develop professional competencies. They put forth the effort because they envision themselves as successful at some point in the future. Similar to the work of Markus and her colleagues, King (1998) believes that control over one's life and the perception that one has impact on the world is critical to the experience of subjective well-being. He proposes that pursuing daily goals contributes to a sense of being in control of not only the present, but also the future. Setting long-term goals serves as a source of agency and meaning. When life goals appear to be unattainable, a person must disengage, re-evaluate the situation, and establish what he or she terms a new "life dream." Clients who experience cognitive deficits or who have lost their sense of "self" may be unable to actively participate in day-to-day decisions about what they want to do.

Representations of possible selves include visions of both desired and undesired end states. Once again, an example of a person receiving rehabilitation following a stroke will illustrate the point. People who are able to relate the value of taking part in an activity in a clinic setting to some positive outcome after they return home are more likely to participate. Individuals who relate participation to avoidance of a negative outcome are also likely to participate. However, individuals who believe that participating in an activity is so disparate with what they were formally capable of doing and who are unable to visualize themselves in a different but still acceptable way may perceive the activity to be an outward sign of the loss of function rather than a means of regaining function. This helps to explain why the same man who is willing to work long hours on learning to walk again refuses to participate in activities to relearn how to dress himself. When individuals refuse to participate in activities, they are deprived of important information about themselves. Markus believes that self-schemas include information about who you are, largely by observing what you do. In essence, people observe themselves making choices. They watch themselves engaging in activities. This results in procedural knowledge or action-based memories in the form of motor skills, habits, and strategies. Not only do people need to know who they are and where they want to go, they also need to know how to get there. Markus and Nurius (1987) believe individuals include plans and strategies for approaching or avoiding personally significant possibilities. "...It is the possible self that puts the self into action, that outlines the likely course of action" (p. 159). Individuals select self-directed life activities that support tasks and roles within different environments they expect to encounter in the future.

Making plans and developing strategies for skills is difficult for individuals who do not have sufficient information to evaluate how they will function in a specific context. Individuals cannot develop strategies to compensate for a problem if they do not realize that the problem exists. An example from a person with a brain injury will make a point. Acknowledging that individuals with right brain damage and unilateral neglect often lack awareness of their disabilities, Tham and colleagues (2000) examined how individuals with cerebrovascular lesions and neglect experienced, discovered, and handled their disabilities in the context of their everyday lives. Using a phenomenological research method, they found that the individuals they studied came to understand the consequences of unilateral neglect through the performance of everyday tasks. Self-evaluating and self-monitoring one's own performance relative to goal-directed activity enables one to modify strategies for accomplishing a goal. That is, not only do people need to keep focused on the intended outcome, they also need to keep focused on the strategies they use as they work toward their goal. It is the selection and use of strategies that enables one to sustain and direct occupational performance. Individuals select strategies and put the self into action so they can function in specific environmental contexts.

Motivated people can be distracted by task-irrelevant thoughts, and it is volitional processes that guide action under demanding performance circumstances (Kuhl, 1985, 1986). According to Kuhl, the construct of volition refers to action orientation involving overt and covert processes of self-control. Volitional processes are "postdecisional." They come into play after the decision is made to complete a task. Kuhl proposes that motivation creates the impulse or intention to act; volition controls intentions and impulses so the action is carried out. Thus, motivational processes mediate the formation of decisions and promote decisions, whereas volitional processes mediate the enactment of those decisions and protect them. The challenge is to identify mechanisms that control concentration and aid progress in the face of environmental and personal obstacles to performance.

Kielhofner (1995) describes a volitional subsystem within a Model of Human Occupation. He refers to the term *volition* as connoting "will or conscious choice," explaining that this term emphasizes "the deliberate process of willing behavior in contrast to other concepts of motivation which de-emphasize conscious choice" (p. 29). The volitional subsystem is defined as "a system of dispositions and self-knowledge that predisposes and enables persons to anticipate, choose, experience, and interpret occupational behavior" (Kielhofner, 1995, p. 30). Volitional structure and volitional process are distinguished within the volitional subsystem. Volitional structure refers to "a stable pattern of dispositions and self-knowledge generated from and sustained by experience" (Kielhofner et al., 1995, p. 41), whereas volitional process "refers to the actual workings and procedures of anticipating, experiencing, choosing, and interpreting occupational behavior" (Kielhofner et al., 1995, p. 41).

Kielhofner (1992) proposes that "occupational choices ordinarily result from considerable deliberations and may involve an extended process of information-gathering, reflection, and imagination" (p. 192). He believes that people engage in volitional narratives to "integrate past, present, and future into a coherent whole through highly personal life stories" (Kielhofner, 1992, p. 192). According to Kielhofner, these volitional narratives can be powerful motivators in that they can energize or paralyze volitional choices. Perspectives on volition reveal that individuals select valued activities among many offerings in the environment, but they also must remain focused and regulate their behavior in the face of many environmental distractions so that intentions are realized.

According to Zirkel and Cantor (1990), it is the larger sociocultural context that frames personal construct of life events. How individuals decide which tasks are crucial for independent function at a specific time period in their lives helps to clarify occupational choices and affective reactions to daily life activities. For example, some high school-aged students who are members of families with lower socioeconomic status may construe life tasks as preparing to enter the workforce following graduation. Other students in the same age group who are members of families with higher socioeconomic status may construe their current life tasks as preparing to enter college. Cantor and Zirkel's approach model emphasizes sociocultural and "age-graded mandates" (Cantor & Zirkel, 1990, p. 150). However, even striving toward socially valued projects is characterized by "a strongly idiographic flavor because individuals do experiment with these social agendas and frequently find their own tasks and projects from within the broader array of 'choices'" (Cantor & Zirkel, 1990, p. 151). Some adults construe retirement as a time to adopt a calmer lifestyle centered on home and family. Others construe retirement as a time for extended travel and a more active social life. Parameters established by sociocultural environmental context influence the occupational choices of individuals.

Two central questions initially identified in this chapter are informed by examination of psychological theories of motivation. "What is the process by which an individual selects self-directed life activities that support tasks and roles within different environments?" Current approaches to human motivation recognize that this process is largely a cognitive process that occurs within a social environment in that what people know about themselves develops through interactions with others. Cognition contributes to goal-directed behavior in that individuals articulate, represent, and solidify what it is they want to do in particular life settings and life periods. People tend to adopt a temporal perspective when making occupational choices in that they envision their future, possible self, sometimes thinking backward and anticipating alternative futures. They adopt strategies most likely to help them realize the choices they have made, including blocking irrelevant thoughts and actions that could interfere with task engagement.

To what extent does the environment dictate an individual's choices? The environment dictates an individual's choices by offering or failing to offer expected valued outcomes. When there is a match between expectations and values, and when there is a match between environmental challenges and the capabilities of individuals, individuals believe themselves to be efficacious. As a result, they will strive to complete even more challenging tasks and assume multiple roles in familiar and new environments. The environment and events that occur within that environment do not influence occupational choices. Rather, it is the person's interpretation of the environment relative to self.

Contributions of Genetics

What is the process by which an individual selects self-directed life activities that support tasks and roles within different environments? To what extent does the environment dictate an individual's occupational choices? These questions invite consideration of the ongoing tension between the relative influences of nature (primitive state of existence, untouched and uninfluenced by civilization) and nurture (the sum of environmental influences acting upon an organism) on human behavior. As early as 1865, Francis Galton identified a struggle between nature and nurture; however, there is compelling evidence that interaction between genetically determined and environmental factors is continuous. That which is given at birth and that which emerges through interactions with the environment both determine how individuals are characterized. It is commonly accepted that individuals inherit gene combinations from two parents, which form the genotype (i.e., the DNA, or the genetic constitution) of an individual. The individual's phenotype emerges through the process of development and exposure to a variety of experiences. A phenotype is a set of observable characteristics of an individual or group as determined by its genotype and environment. Because of the complex interactions between genes and environment, a given organism's genotype never fully determines its phenotype, the actual living creature that eventually develops. The science of behavioral genetics confirms that there are experiential differences between any two people functioning in the same environment, including children growing up in the same family. Studies of monozygotic twins reared apart and genetically unrelated children adopted together confirm that environmental influences are specific to each individual and may not be generalized across a group of people. Hegman and DeFries (1970) and Loehlin and Nicholls (1976) hypothesize that there may be an underlying physiological structuring that mediates the influence of both genetic and environmental factors.

The science of molecular biology has given birth to the Human Genome Project, whose decoding of the human genome has begun to open up the actual digital code governing biological development. The magnitude of this project serves as an early indication of the limitless possibilities for understanding the genetic contributions to human behavior. The Universal Declaration on the Human Genome and Human Rights (United Nations Educational, Scientific, and Cultural Organizations, n.d.) reads, "The human genome underlies the fundamental unity of all members of the human family, as well as the recognition of their inherent dignity and diversity. In a symbolic sense, it is the heritage of humanity." Ironically, increased understanding of the human genome reveals that although each human is unique, there are more similarities than differences among the human race. Social, cultural, and environmental influences may affect genetic predispositions, and genetic predispositions affect how humans respond to the environment. Evolutionary biologists suggest that the brain is not a blank tablet to be shaped by society, but rather an organ that has adapted over time to deal with its environment and to solve certain key problems of social competition and cooperation. Behavioral geneticists offer new rigorous statistical methods for teasing out the genetic from the environmental components of behavior. Cognitive neuroscience offers discoveries linking behavior to the physiology and biochemistry of the brain.

It supports the conception of the plasticity within the brain and, thus, the organism. Individuals respond to the environment; conversely, exposure to the environment can subsequently impact at the level of the organism. Optimal levels of stimulation and enhancement place demands on the organism that lead to preferred levels of occupational performance. Too little or too much stimulation from the environment is less satisfying and will be less likely to stimulate positive change in the organism. Individuals thrive in environments that give them the opportunity to make choices that result in optimal experiences. The environment can be either enabling or disabling. Individuals who experience physical and/or sensory impairments at the level of the organism are still able to function if the environment is accommodating. At times, it is possible to alter the environment to provide necessary support without changing the person. Some changes in the environment may elicit new responses in the organism, thus expanding options for occupational choice and opening new avenues for occupational performance. At other times, changes in the environment may be sufficient to enable the individual to freely choose those occupations that are personally meaningful. What is the relevance of these findings within the larger conceptualization of interactions among person-environment-occupation in general and occupational choice in particular? One implication is that people functioning in the same environment may not, in fact, experience the same thing. Underlying physiological mechanisms serve to mediate both genetic and environmental factors, thus both the environment and the individual dictate occupational choice.

Contributions of Culture

To what extent does the cultural environment dictate occupational choice? Summarizing current conceptions of culture, Cantor and Zirkel (1990) write:

> A culture provides people with a set of values and assumptive beliefs, and implicit inferences about how the world operates, which enable them to find meaning in and make sense of the events in their lives… A culture helps orient the kinds of personal constructs that are likely to develop; it prescribes the dimensions along which self-schemas are likely to develop, and it provides a set of culturally prescribed goals and tasks from which to choose… Culture provides the cognitive tools through which we understand and regulate behavior. (p. 140)

Thus, occupational choices may be a reflection of socially transmitted behavior patterns and beliefs.

The 1997 Institute of Medicine (IOM), Division of Health Sciences Policy, Committee on Assessing Rehabilitation Science and Engineering defines culture as including "both material culture (things and the rules for producing them) and nonmaterial culture (norms or rules, values, symbols, language, ideational systems such as science or religion, and arts such as dance, crafts and humor)" (Institute of Medicine, 1997, p. 154). The committee makes a distinction between enabling and disabling aspects of culture. Examples of how culture enables individuals with disabilities are, "Expecting people with disabling conditions to be productive" and "Expecting everyone to know sign language." Examples of how culture can be a disabling factor are, "stigmatizing people with disabling conditions" and "valuing physical beauty" (Institute of Medicine, 1997, p. 155).

The IOM report specifically addresses how culture can affect the likelihood that pathology may become impairment or a functional limitation. For example, well-educated Americans may constitute a subculture that values health advice such as breast cancer screening. As a result, women who undergo breast screenings are less likely to develop impairment from a potential pathological condition. The report emphasizes that whether a functional limitation is seen as being disabling will depend on the culture. "The culture defines the roles to be played and the actions and capabilities necessary to satisfy that role. If certain actions are not necessary for a role, then the person who is limited in ability to perform those actions does not have a disability" (Institute of Medicine, 1997, p. 157). As an example, the report contrasts the roles of a college professor and a secretary. Presumably, the college professor could continue to retain his or her role if he or she experienced arthritis in her hands, whereas a secretary who was required to type could not. For the professor, arthritic hands would not be a functional limitation if typing assistance were provided, whereas arthritic hands would pose a functional limitation for the secretary. Culture defines the roles of individuals. As Kielhofner writes, "When people perform role-related behavior, they employ role scripts. These role scripts are appreciative tendencies that allow one to comprehend social situations and expectations and to construct behavior that enacts a given role" (1992, p. 193).

The IOM report points out that a disability can exist without functional limitations given cultural constraints. For example, in the United States, facial disfigurement might not pose a functional limitation per se, and yet a person's access to a position in which he or she must interact with the public, such as the position of salesperson, may be culturally unacceptable. Thus, the person would be excluded from assuming the role. The committee clarifies that "culture affects not just whether there is a disability caused by the functional limitation but also where in the person's life the disability will occur" (Institute of Medicine, 1997, p. 157). People may experience disabilities in family or other personal relationships, not just in the workplace. Leidy and Haase (1999) conducted a naturalistic, qualitative study to describe the meaning of functional performance from the perspective of 12 men and women (aged 50 to 76 years) with a moderate to severe chronic disease. Functional performance was defined as "finding purpose and meaning through activity." Two affective responses were derived as a result of careful observations, having a sense of effectiveness, or "being able," and having a sense of connectedness, or "being with." These findings serve to illuminate a dimension of functional performance that is not often addressed. People with disabling conditions not only want to feel capable; they also want to feel included.

Harwood, Schoelmerich, Ventura-Cook, and Schulze (1996) studied the effects of culture and class influences on Anglo and Puerto Rican mothers' beliefs about desirable and undesirable long-term socialization goals for their children. They found that both culture and socioeconomic status contribute independently to group differences, but that cultural effects appear to be stronger. Of particular interest was how these mothers thought their children should behave in social situations and the extent to which they valued development of the individual to the greatest extent possible. Children who are taught to be reticent in social situations and who are not encouraged to develop challenging life dreams are likely to set less challenging goals in the future.

Gill (1999) examined the value of choice making as it affects economics in the workplace. She suggests that cultural context; social networks; and affiliations with class, ethnicity, and gender affect choices made about work. One prime example of a health-related behavior that has been found to have cultural determinants is that of obesity in the United States. Nies and colleagues (1998) compared lifestyles among obese and nonobese African American and European American women in the community. They found that the prevalence of obesity among African American women is twice that of European America women. More than 60% of the African American female population older than 45 years is obese. The investigators hypothesized that both obesity and race would have independent effects on health-promoting behaviors. Using the Health-Promoting Lifestyle Profile (HPLP), the investigators measured six variables, including self-actualization, health responsibility, adhering to regular exercise patterns, establishing meal patterns and making healthy food choices, interpersonal support, and stress management. These authors found the obese women had significantly lower scores than the nonobese women on all scales. However, the only subscale for which the African American women had significantly lower scores than European American women was nutrition. The authors suggest that this may be because culture is often expressed through food and eating habits.

Similarly, Kim and colleagues (1998) examined racial differences in health status and health behaviors of older adults. They found that, when covaried with education and income, racial differences in self-perceived health were eliminated. Only two health behaviors, physical activity and eating breakfast regularly, showed significant racial differences. Investigating level of functional disability among older inner-city African Americans with few socioeconomic resources, Miller and colleagues (1996) found that, compared with other groups of similar ages and gender, these individuals had diminished lower extremity strength and balance, presumably due to minimal levels of leisure time exercise. They were more dependent in terms of daily living activities and had increased health concerns. Consistently, studies have revealed that occupational choices are influenced by habits and culture that subsequently affect health status. They provide support for the formative role of family, culture, and social organizations. People complete tasks to accomplish their own goals, but these same tasks may also be part of "rituals" reinforced by the larger cultural group.

Kao (2000) examined group and individual images of the future possible self among adolescents. On the basis of interviews with 66 Asian, Black, White, and Hispanic 9th to 12th grade students, she found stereotypes that link ethnic group membership to academic ability as well as other skills. According to these students, Asian youth are gifted in their academic abilities, while Blacks are seen as less successful in academics. Stereotypes about Hispanics focused on occupations that involve manual labor. Of special concern to Kao is that young people form judgments about which ethnic groups will be successful in different areas of their lives based on these stereotypes, and they set goals primarily in terms of stereotypical images attached to their ethnic groups. Kao also found that these stereotypes are reinforced through racially and ethnically segregated extracurricular activities.

Brickman (1999) investigated knowledge upon which plans for the future were based. She included three adolescents from varying ethnic backgrounds in her study via interviews, historical data, autobiographical reports, and surveys tapping students' present classroom goals. She concluded, "knowledge about the future is represented as plans and that much of this knowledge was the result of sociocultural experiences." Additionally, she reports that it is difficult to devise a plan outside of one's own experiences. Present tasks are only instrumental if one has the knowledge of what is expected of one's self in a specific role in the future. In summary, culture provides a frame of reference as individuals make occupational choices. Some choices reinforce roles and activities consistent with group membership. Other choices serve to alienate one's self from others with whom they are the most similar.

Contributions of Social Policy

The preceding section reflects the views of psychologists and their assumptions about how culture contributes to the social construction of self. However, these theories do not address how political forces, class structure, or other socioeconomic factors influence occupation choice and subsequent quality of life. Social policy largely determines the availability of roles in society and social position. Bandura refers to the effects of the social environment as "collective agency." He says that human adaptation and change are rooted in social systems. Personal agency beliefs are not independent of, but rather formed through, a broad network of sociostructural influences. He believes individual and social interactions are bidirectional in that people are producers as well as products of social systems. Explaining this position, he says that collective agency operates through shared beliefs of efficacy, pooled understandings, group aspirations and incentive systems, and collective action. How people view their collective agency to produce desired outcomes may be influenced by socioeconomic status and cultural experiences.

It is obvious that social policy influences the extent to which resources are available to individuals who have diminished productivity and who may need costly services. It may be less obvious that economics contributes to the likelihood that individuals will acquire pathologies that may be disabling. People with fewer economic resources are less likely to receive care for infectious diseases and more chronic conditions. Progressive lack of care can influence whether a pathological condition progresses to impairment and whether impairment then affects the ability of the individual to function with a disabling condition (Institute of Medicine, 1997). For example, an individual with few economic resources may be diagnosed with a pathological condition such as diabetes. Inadequate or delayed medical care may result in impairment, such as amputation of a limb. If resources are not available to purchase a prosthetic device, the individual may not be able to work or fully participate in other aspects of society. Perhaps the individual has a prosthetic device, but needs public transportation. Without transportation the individual may not be able to resume his role as a primary wage earner for a family. Society may value basic health care as well as the right to work, but without a fully operational system that supports employment, this individual who could otherwise fulfill his role would experience a disability.

Current public policy in the United States is moving away from interventions where clients are passive recipients of care and the focus is on impairments. Instead, emphasis is on models of social inclusion where clients develop the resources to fully participate in society (Institute of Medicine, 1997). Two major federal research organizations are concerned with disability: the National Institute of Health's NCMRR and the U.S. Department of Education's NIDRR. Funding from these organizations is sensitive to public policy and supports research efforts that target social inclusion rather than impairment.

A healthy economy supports people with disabilities. People with disabilities are more likely to secure jobs in growing communities. Communities with a strong tax base are more likely to provide accessible public transportation and public building, or support payments for personal assistance benefits. Conversely, "economic factors also can affect disability by creating incentives to define oneself as disabled" (Institute of Medicine, 1997, p. 159). Disability compensation programs have been found to reduce the number of people with impairments who work because they create incentives to leave the labor force.

The 1997 IOM concluded:

> ...the amount of a disability is not determined by levels of pathologies, impairments, or functional limitations, but instead is a function of the kind of services provided to people with disabling conditions and the extent to which the physical, built environment is accommodating or not accommodating to the particular disabling condition. Because societies differ in their willingness to provide the available technology and, indeed, their willingness to provide the research funds to improve that technology, disability ultimately must be seen as a function of society, not of a physical or medical process. (Institute of Medicine, 1997, p. 148)

Acknowledging that public policy affects the objective and subjective experience of disability, the IOM committee formulated four questions that typify known areas of need.

For example, "Has the Americans with Disabilities Act of 1990 (ADA) affected the practices of hiring people with limitations? Has the implementation of architectural guidelines improved accessibility to public and private facilities? Have efforts to include children with and without disabling conditions in the same educational environments decreased discriminatory attitudes and behaviors among those without disabling conditions? How do the different definitions of disability in such federal programs as Social Security, Vocational Rehabilitation, and Individuals with Disabilities Education Act affect the extent to which people with limitations participate in work or school?" If, in fact, occupation meets "the [person's] intrinsic needs for self-maintenance, expression, and fulfillment within the context of personal roles and environment" (Law et al., 1996, p. 16), then engagement in occupation is central to overall health and well-being.

As a result of the growing pressures for accountability in health care, the prevalence of functional outcome studies documenting the benefits of occupational choice is increasing. For example, older adults demonstrate improved process performance when given their choice of tasks even though motor performance per se may not improve (Stauffer, Fisher, & Duran, 2000). Preferred activities, such as leisure activities, have been found to predict vocational choice, and productivity among adolescents is enhanced when work characteristics are similar to leisure activities (Hong, Milgram, & Whiston, 1993).

LaMore and Nelson (1993) examined whether giving adults with mental disabilities options at the beginning of an art activity would motivate them to paint more than when they were not given options. They found that subjects painted significantly more when they had a choice than when they did not have a choice. McColl and colleagues (1986) examined why hospitalized anorexics often do not report feelings of satisfaction or effectiveness in the performance of activities. They concluded that the importance of choice in activity was an important factor. Duncan-Myers and Huebner (2000) tested the association between perceptions of personal control and quality of life among older people as revealed through perception of choice in performance areas, including 29 self-care and leisure activities. Findings revealed a significant positive correlation between the amount of choice residents perceive they have and their quality of life. Residents living in a nursing home repeated arm movements more when given the choice between a simulated game of basketball and rote exercise (Zimmerer-Branum & Nelson, 1995). Similarly, following a cerebrovascular accident, individuals demonstrated increased standing time when they were given the choice to participate in personally meaningful activities (Dolecheck & Schkade, 1999).

Overall, there is compelling evidence that occupational choice enhances occupational performance. Occupational choice is a reflection of how one perceives one's self within the social context of everyday living. Occupational choices are influenced by assumptions about what is expected of one's self in different roles, and they are influenced by the desire to be viewed by self and others as being competent. Individuals use information available from the environment to make judgments about the extent to which their occupational performance is acceptable. These judgments influence subsequent occupational choices. The extent to which occupational choices are challenging and valued by society affects one's sense of personal worth.

Evidence Worksheet

Author(s)	*Year*	*Topic*	*Method*	*Conclusion*
Brickman	1999	How perceptions of the future influence achievement motivation	Descriptive	Knowledge about the future is represented as plans and much of this knowledge was the result of sociocultural experiences. Occupationally embedded exercise versus rote exercise: A choice between occupational forms by elderly nursing home residents, it is difficult to devise a plan outside of one's own experiences. Present tasks are only instrumental if one has the knowledge of what is expected of one's self in a specific role in the future
Conn	1998	Older adults and exercise: self-efficacy related constructs	Path analysis	Perceived barriers, age, and self-efficacy expectation have a strong direct effect on exercise, whereas perceptions of the expected outcome have no appreciable effect
Deci & Ryan	1985		Descriptive	Men view praise as an affirmation of their competence at the activity, whereas women view praise as an attempt at social control, which results in diminished feelings of self-determination, thus undermining their intrinsic motivation
Dolecheck & Schkade	1999	The extent dynamic standing endurance is effected when CVA subjects perform personally meaningful activities rather than nonmeaningful tasks	Descriptive	Following a cerebral vascular accident, individuals demonstrated increased standing time when they were given the choice to participate in personally meaningful activities
Duncan-Myers & Huebner	2000	Relationship between choice and quality of life among residents in long-term care facilities	Descriptive	A positive correlation was found between the amount of choice residents perceive they have and their quality of life

(continued)

Author(s)	*Year*	*Topic*	*Method*	*Conclusion*
Harwood et al.	1996	Culture and class influences on Anglo and Puerto Rican mothers' beliefs regarding long-term socialization goals and child behavior	Descriptive	Both culture and socio-economic status contribute independently to group differences, but cultural effects appear to be stronger; children who are taught to be reticent in social situations and who are not encouraged to develop challenging life dreams are likely to set less challenging goals in the future
Hong et al.	1993	Leisure activities done by adolescents predict occupational choice in young adults	Descriptive, longitudinal study	Preferred activities, such as leisure activities, have been found to predict vocational choice; productivity among adolescents is enhanced when work characteristics are similar to leisure activities
Jagacinski & Nicholls	1984	Conceptions of ability and related affect in task involvement and ego involvement	Descriptive	When people try hard under task-involving conditions, they experience a positive sense of competence, whereas under ego-involving conditions, trying hard results in a lower perceptions of competence
Kao	2000	Group images and possible selves among adolescents: linking stereotypes to expectations by race and ethnicity	Descriptive	Young people form stereotypes that link ethnic group membership to academic ability as well as other skills; they form judgments about which ethnic groups will be successful in different areas of their lives based on these stereotypes, and they set goals primarily in terms of stereotypical images attached to their ethnic groups; these stereotypes are reinforced through racially and ethnically segregated extracurricular activities
Kim et al.	1998	Racial differences in health status and health behaviors of older adults	Descriptive	When covaried with education and income, racial differences in self-perceived health were eliminated. Only two health behaviors, physical activity and eating breakfast regularly, showed significant racial differences

(continued)

Author(s)	*Year*	*Topic*	*Method*	*Conclusion*
Kurlowicz	1998	Perceived self-efficacy, functional ability, and depressive symptoms in older elective surgery patients	Descriptive	Interventions to enhance older patients' perceived self-efficacy while hospitalized may enhance functional ability, which in turn may decrease the likelihood of depressive symptoms postoperatively
LaMore & Nelson	1993	The effects of options on performance of an art project in adults with mental disabilities	Descriptive	Examined whether giving adults with mental disabilities options at the beginning of an art activity would motivate them to paint more than when they were not given options; found that subjects painted significantly more when they had a choice than when they did not have a choice
Leidy & Haase	1999	Functional status from the patient's perspective: The challenge of preserving personal integrity	Naturalistic, qualitative study	People with disabling conditions not only want to feel capable, they also want to feel included
Lorig et al.	1999	Evidence suggesting that a chronic disease self-management program can improve health status while reducing hospitalization	Descriptive	Individuals in a self-efficacy intervention group demonstrated an increase in weekly minutes of exercise and social/role activities. They also had fewer hospitalizations and days in the hospital
McColl et al.	1986	When doing is not enough: the relationship between activity and effectiveness in anorexia nervosa	Descriptive	Importance of choice in activity is an important factor in reports of satisfaction or effectiveness in the performance of activities
Miller et al.	1996	Inner-city older blacks have high levels of functional disability	Descriptive	Occupational choices are influenced by habits and culture that subsequently affect health status. They provide support for the formative role of family, culture, and social organizations. People complete tasks to accomplish their own goals, but these same tasks may also be part of "rituals" reinforced by the larger cultural group

(continued)

Author(s)	*Year*	*Topic*	*Method*	*Conclusion*
Nies et al.	1998	Comparison of lifestyles among obese and non-obese African American and European American women in the community	Descriptive	Obese women score lower than nonobese women on all scales of the Health-Promoting Lifestyle Profile (HPLP). However, the only subscale for which the African American women had significantly lower scores than European American women was nutrition. This may be because culture is often expressed through food and eating habits
Ryan	1982	Control and information in the intrapersonal sphere: an extension of cognitive evaluation theory	Experimental	Distinguished ego-involved activity and task-involved activity. Ego involvement refers to a condition in which a person's self-esteem depends on attaining a specific level of performance. In contrast, task-involved activity is characterized by engagement because a task is interesting, challenging, or has other inherent qualities. According to Ryan, ego-involvement creates self-imposed pressure to perform, similar to that offered by some form of external evaluation
Stauffer et al.	2000	ADL performance of black Americans and white Americans on the assessment of motor and process skills	Descriptive	Older adults demonstrate improved process performance when given their choice of tasks even though motor performance per se may not improve
Tham et al.	2000	The discovery of disability: a phenomenological study of unilateral neglect	Phenomenological	Individuals with CVA came to understand the consequences of unilateral neglect through the performance of everyday tasks. Self-evaluating and self-monitoring one's own performance relative to goal-directed activity enables one to modify strategies for accomplishing a goal
Zimmerer-Branum & Nelson	1995	Occupationally embedded exercise versus rote exercise: a choice between occupational forms by elderly nursing home residents	Descriptive	Positive correlation between the amount of choice residents in a nursing home perceive they have and their quality of life

References

Bandura, A. (1977). Self-efficacy: Toward a unifying theory of behavioral change. *Psychological Review, 84*, 191-215.

Bandura, A. (1982). Self-efficacy mechanism in human agency. *American Psychologist, 37*, 122-147.

Bandura, A. (1991). Self-regulation of motivation through anticipatory and self-reactive mechanisms. In R. Dienstbier (Ed.), *Nebraska Symposium on Motivation, 1990: Perspectives on motivation. Current theory and research in motivation*, Vol. 38 (pp. 69-164). Lincoln, NE: University of Nebraska Press.

Bandura, A. (1998). Personal and collective efficacy in human adaptation and change. In J. Adair & D. Belanger (Eds.), *Advances in psychological science, Vol. 1: Social, personal, and cultural aspects* (pp. 51-71). Hove, England: Psychology Press/Erlbaum.

Bandura, A. (2000). Social cognitive theory: An agentic perspective. *Annual Review of Psychology, 52*, 1-26.

Baum, C. M., & Law, M. (1997). Occupational therapy practice: Focusing on occupational performance. *American Journal of Occupational Therapy, 51*, 277-288.

Brickman, S. (1999). How perceptions of the future influence achievement motivation. Dissertation Abstracts International, A (Humanities and Social Sciences), Vol 59(9-A).

Cantor, N., & Zirkel S. C. (1990). Personality cognition and purposive behavior. In L. A. Pervin (Ed.), *Handbook of personality: Theory and research*. New York, NY: The Guilford Press.

Conn, V. (1998). Older adults and exercise: Path analysis of self-efficacy related constructs. *Nursing Research, 47*, 180-189.

Deci, E. L., & Ryan, R. M. (1985). *Intrinsic motivation and self-determination in human behavior*. New York, NY: Plenum.

Dolecheck, J. R., & Schkade, J. K. (1999). The extent dynamic standing endurance is affected when CVA subjects perform personally meaningful activities rather than nonmeaningful tasks. *Occupational Therapy Journal of Research, 19*, 41-55.

Duncan-Myers, A., & Huebner, R. (2000). Relationship between choice and quality of life among residents in long-term care facilities. *American Journal of Occupational Therapy, 54*, 504-508.

Dweck, C. S., & Leggett, E. L. (1988). A social cognitive approach to motivation and personality. *Psychological Review, 45*, 256-273.

Gill, F. (1999). The meaning of work: Lessons from sociology, psychology and political theory. *Journal of Socio-Economics, 28*, 725-743.

Harlow, H. G. (1953). Mice, monkeys, men and motives. *Psychological Review, 60*, 23-32.

Harwood, R., Schoelmerich, A., Ventura-Cook, E., & Schulze, P. (1996). Culture and class influences on Anglo and Puerto Rican mothers' beliefs regarding long-term socialization goals and child behavior. *Child Development, 67*, 2446-2461.

Hegman, P., & DeFries, C. (1970). Are genetic correlations and environmental correlations correlated? *Nature, 226*, 284-286.

Hong, E., Milgram, R., & Whiston, S. (1993). Leisure activities in adolescents as a predictor of occupational choice in young adults: A longitudinal study. *Journal of Career Development, 119*, 221-229.

Hull, C. L. (1943). *Science and human behavior*. New York, NY: Macmillan.

Institute of Medicine, Committee on Assessing Rehabilitation Science and Engineering, Division of Health Sciences Policy (1997). *Enabling America: Assessing the role of rehabilitation science and engineering*. Washington, DC: National Academy Press.

Jagacinski, C. M., & Nicholls, J. G. (1984). Conceptions of ability and related affect in task involvement and ego involvement. *Journal of Educational Psychology, 76*, 909-919.

Jewell, E. J., & Abate, F. (Eds.). (2001). *New Oxford American dictionary*. New York: Oxford University Press.

Jones, M. R. (Ed.). (1955). *Nebraska symposium on motivation* (Vol. 3). Lincoln, NE: University of Nebraska Press.

Kao, G. (2000). Group images and possible selves among adolescents: Linking stereotypes to expectations by race and ethnicity. *Sociological Forum, 15*, 407-430.

Kielhofner, G. (1992). *Conceptual foundations of occupational therapy* (2nd ed.). Philadelphia, PA: F. A. Davis.

Kielhofner, G. (1995). Internal organization of the human system for occupation. In G. Kielhofner (Ed.), *A model of human occupation: Theory and application* (2nd ed.). Baltimore, MD: Williams and Wilkins.

Kielhofner, G., Borell, L., Helfrich, C., & Nygard, L. (1995). Volitional subsystem. In G. Kielhofner (Ed.), *A model of human occupation: Theory and application* (2nd ed.). Baltimore, MD: Williams and Wilkins.

Kim, J., Bramlett, M., Wright, L., & Poon, L. (1998). Racial differences in health status and health behaviors of older adults. *Nursing Research, 47*, 243-250.

King, L. (1998). Personal goals and personal agency: Linking everyday goals to future images of the self. In M. Kofta & G. Weary (Eds.), *Personal control in action: Cognitive and motivational mechanisms. The Plenum series in social/clinical psychology* (pp. 109-128). New York, NY: Plenum Press.

Koestner, R., & McClelland, D. C. (1990). Perspectives on competence motivation. In L. A. Pervin (Ed.), *Handbook of personality: Theory and research*. New York, NY: The Guilford Press.

Kuhl, J. (1985). From cognition to behavior: Perspectives for future research on action control. In J. Kuhl & J. Beckmann (Eds.), *Action control: From cognition to behavior* (pp. 267-275). New York, NY: Springer-Verlag.

Kuhl, J. (1986). Motivational and information processing: A new look at decision making, dynamic change and action control. In R. M. Sorrentino & E. T. Higgins (Eds.), *Handbook of motivation and cognition* (pp. 404-434). New York, NY: Guilford Press.

Kurlowicz, L. (1998). Perceived self-efficacy, functional ability, and depressive symptoms in older elective surgery patients. *Nursing Research, 47*, 219-226.

LaMore, K., & Nelson, D. (1993). The effects of options on performance of an art project in adults with mental disabilities. *American Journal of Occupational Therapy, 47*, 397-401.

Law, M., Cooper, B., Strong, S., Stewart, S., Rigby, P., & Letts, L. (1996). The person-environment-occupational model: A transactive approach to occupational performance. *Canadian Journal of Occupational Therapy, 63*, 9-23.

Leidy, N., & Haase, J. (1999). Functional status from the patient's perspective: The challenge of preserving personal integrity. *Research in Nursing & Health, 22*, 67-77.

Lewin, K. (1951). Intention, will, and need. In D. Rapaport (Ed.), *Organization and pathology of thought* (pp. 95-153). New York, NY: Columbia University Press.

Loehlin, C., & Nicholls, R. C. (1976). *Heredity, environment and personality*. Austin, TX: University of Texas Press.

Lorig, K., Sobel, D., Stewart, A., Bandura, A., Ritter, P., Gonzalez, V., et al. (1999). Evidence suggesting that a chronic disease self-management program can improve health status while reducing hospitalization. *Medical Care, 37*, 5-14.

Markus, H., & Sentis, K. (1982). The self in social information processing. In J. Suls (Ed.), *Psychological perspectives on the self* (Vol. 1, pp. 41-70). Hillsdale, NJ: Erlbaum.

Markus, H., & Nurius, P. (1986). Possible selves. *American Psychologist, 41*, 954-969.

Markus, H., & Nurius, P. (1987). Possible selves: The interface between motivation and the self-concept. In K. Yardley and T. Honess (Eds.), *Self and identity: Psychosocial perspectives*. New York, NY: John Wiley & Sons.

McColl, M. A., Friedland, J., & Kerr, A. (1986). When doing is not enough: The relationship between activity and effectiveness in anorexia nervosa. *Occupational Therapy in Mental Health*, 6, 137-150.

Meyer, A. (1922). The philosophy of occupational therapy. *Archives of Occupational Therapy, 1*, 1-10.

Miller, D., Carter, M., Miller, J., & Fornoff, J. (1996). Inner-city older Blacks have high levels of functional disability. *Journal of the American Geriatrics Society, 44*, 1166-1173.

Mischel, W. (1973). Toward a cognitive social learning reconceptualization of personality. *Psychological Review, 80*, 252-283.

Mook, D. G. (1987). *Motivation: The organization of action*. New York, NY: Norton.

Murray, H. A. (1938). *Explorations in personality*. New York, NY: Oxford University Press.

Nicholls, J. G. (1984). Achievement motivation: Conceptions of ability, subjective experience, task choice, and performance. *Psychological Review, 91*, 328-346.

Nies, M., Buffington, C., Cowan, G., & Hepworth, J. (1998). Comparison of lifestyles among obese and nonobese African American and European American women in the community. *Nursing Research, 47*, 251-257.

Rotter, J. B. (1966). Generalized expectancies for internal versus external control of reinforcement. *Psychological Monographs, 81* (1, Whole No. 609).

Rotter, J. B. (1975). Some problems and misconceptions related to the construct of internal versus external reinforcement. *Journal of Consulting and Clinical Psychology, 43*, 56-67.

Ryan, R. M. (1982). Control and information in the intrapersonal sphere: An extension of cognitive evaluation theory. *Journal of Personality and Social Psychology, 43*, 450-461.

Ryan, R. M., Connell, J. P., & Deci, E. L. (1985). A motivational analysis of self-determination and self-regulation in education. In C. Ames & R. E. Ames (Eds.), *Research on motivation in education: The classroom milieu* (pp. 13-51). New York, NY: Academic Press.

Skinner, B. F. (1953). *Science and human behavior*. New York, NY: Macmillan.

Stauffer, L., Fisher, A., & Duran, L. (2000). ADL performance of black Americans and white Americans on the assessment of motor and process skills. *American Journal of Occupational Therapy, 54*, 607-613.

Stuifbergen, A. K., & Rogers, S. (1997). Health promotion: An essential component of rehabilitation for persons with chronic disabling conditions. *Advances in Nursing Science, 19*, 1-20.

Tham, K., Borell, L., & Gustavsson, A. (2000). The discovery of disability: A phenomenological study of unilateral neglect. *American Journal of Occupational Therapy, 54*, 398-406.

Trombly, C. (1995). Occupation: Purposefulness and meaningfulness as therapeutic mechanisms. *American Journal of Occupational Therapy, 49*, 960-972.

United Nationals Educational, Scientific, and Cultural Organization. (n.d.). Universal declaration on the human genome and human rights, 1997. Retrieved July 25, 2001, from http://www.unesco.org/shs/human_rights/hrbc.htm.

White, R. W. (1959). Motivation reconsidered: The concept of competence. *Psychological Review, 66*, 297-333.

Zimmerer-Branum, S., & Nelson, D. L. (1995). Occupationally embedded exercise versus rote exercise: A choice between occupational forms by elderly nursing home residents. *American Journal of Occupational Therapy, 49*, 397-403.

Zirkel, S., & Cantor, N. (1990). Personal construct of life tasks: Those who struggle for independence. *Journal of Personality & Social Psychology, 58*, 172-185.

Chapter Five: Personal and Environmental Influences on Occupations Reflections and Learning Activities

Julie Bass-Haugen, PhD, OTR/L, FAOTA

REFLECTIONS

This chapter provided an important overview of current thought regarding how it is that we make choices regarding our occupations. Without this background, it might appear that we have a couple of occupational options floating around in our brains at any given time and one option takes control of the situation—and that is the one that we do. Well, fortunately or unfortunately, the explanations regarding occupational choice are a little more complex than that. One of the key ideas related to occupational choice is that it requires a deliberate commitment—a thoughtful, intentional response.

When we examined choice, we learned about why people do the things they do. Two questions were proposed at the beginning of this chapter: 1) What is the process by which an individual selects self-directed life activities that support tasks and roles within different environments? Another way to state this: How does a person choose occupations? 2) To what extent does the environment dictate an individual's choices? Another way to state this: How do things outside the person (i.e., the environment) influence choice?

Three approaches were used to answer these questions and introduce us to different ideas about choice. First, the discipline of psychology has introduced concepts and theories that explain our motivations. These ideas fall under the umbrella of motivational theories and include behaviorism, expectancy-value, social-cognitive, intrinsic/extrinsic, future orientation, volitional behavior, and sociocultural phenomena. Whew! Second, the field of genetics is now offering us new and rapidly changing insights regarding all aspects of human behavior, including occupational choice. Third, cultural influences on occupational choice are important to understand in our increasingly diverse national and international communities

I'll try to summarize each motivational theory by answering the two questions in a very succinct way. Obviously, to fully understand the answer for each question, some understanding of the underlying theory is important as well. Here is a simplified version of the questions again:

- How does a person choose occupations?
- How do things outside the person (i.e., the environment) influence choice?

I will also use a specific example to examine motivational theories and identify what an explanation might be related to occupational choice. The example I will use is the different occupational choices my brother, Robert, and I make regarding learning a language. Why is it that he chooses to teach himself a language, like Portuguese, and I do not?

Behaviorism

- Physiologically-based drives and habits influence choice and are reinforced through practice. But, and this is a big but, behaviors are only activated in response to something in the environment.
- Environment completely dictates choice.

Behaviorism suggests that innate drives influence our choice to do something, like learn a language, but these innate drives are activated (or not activated) in response to something in our environment. So, in my language example, there is something that occurs in my environment that is different from my brother's environment. Something in Robert's environment reinforces his choice to learn a language. What might it be?

Expectancy-Value

- Our expectations (or attributions) about whether or not our actions will lead to valued outcomes or future goal attainment influence choice. Our belief about the control we have over outcomes (locus of control) influences choice. Our motivation for competence in some area influences choice.
- Environment arouses needs and behavior but doesn't dictate choice.

Expectancy-value suggests that my brother and I have different expectations regarding the effect that learning a language will have on our future personal goals and our ability to achieve them. Robert perhaps believes that his efforts to learn Portuguese will translate to a positive outcome (i.e., mastering the language) and achievement of some personal or professional goal (i.e., working as a translator). When he stumbles in his performance, he attributes it to not enough effort on his part and so he tries harder (i.e., internal locus of control). On the other hand, I can't envision that my efforts to learn a language will be fruitful or relate to any current goals of mine. I also don't stick to it as I never can seem to find the "just right" language learning tools (i.e., external locus of control).

Social-Cognitive

- The extent to which we believe we are capable in a certain situation (i.e., self-efficacy) influences choice. We make judgments about personal capability, the value of activity, our definition of good performance, and sometimes the beliefs of others, and these judgments influence choice.

- Beliefs about capability in certain environmental situations influence choice, not the environment itself.

The social-cognitive perspective suggests my brother and I have very different beliefs about our capability to learn languages. Say we rent a DVD movie that has the option to use Portuguese as the language. I suspect Robert views this option as a wonderful opportunity to advance his Portuguese skills because he can use the general story line, the audio, and the captions to follow 75% of the movie. I, on the other hand, feel like I will be totally lost and not get any benefit from spending 2 hours of my time on the endeavor. You see, I believe Robert is more capable of learning Portuguese. He has already picked up several languages (American Sign Language, Spanish, German). I, on the other hand, once asked an Italian bus driver where the gabinetti stop (i.e., restroom) was instead of the garibaldi stop because of my limited capability for the language.

Intrinsic-Extrinsic

- Our innate (intrinsic) needs for competence and self-determination may influence choice. Our perceptions about the occupation itself and our goals for doing it may also influence choice. Some choices are made because performance of the occupation is tied to our self-esteem, demonstration of competence, and fulfillment of roles (e.g., ego-involved activities, occupations-as-ends, performance goals). Some choices are made because performance of the occupation is interesting, challenging, and tied to our motivation for learning (e.g., task-involved activity, occupations-as-means, learning goals).
- Good environments may provide structure and support feelings of autonomy and relatedness that in turn influence intrinsic motivation and choice.

Intrinsic-extrinsic theories suggest that my brother and I have different innate needs for mastering a language. Robert has gone to Brazil just to have an opportunity to learn more Portuguese. He has Brazilian friends who are obviously thrilled that he is learning the language, and they give him lots of opportunity to practice via e-mail. Robert also chooses to spend much of his free time engaged in tasks that support his learning (e.g., movies, novels, music), and he does this just for the pure enjoyment of it. I have not had any of these experiences or reinforcements. I have spent so much of my life in an academic setting that, unfortunately, I equate learning a language with fulfilling a language requirement in college. Furthermore, when I try to learn a language, I get impatient because it seems to take forever to make any progress, and I can never master the language.

Future Orientation

- Our definition of a "possible self" influences choices. People may choose to do activities that they believe help them become their chosen possible self or avoid becoming a negative possible self.
- Individuals make choices to perform in specific environments that are related to their future possible selves.

My future orientation regarding language is quite different from my brother's. Even if I wasn't an occupational therapist and educator, I don't think I could ever envision a future role for myself with "ability to speak different languages" as a key component of it. Robert, on the other hand, has all kinds of ideas about how he might use this new occupation in the future. In fact, I would guess he would describe language as part of his current and future identity.

Volitional Behavior

- Our motivations help us to formulate choices. Our volition (or will, conscious choice) helps us to implement choices.
- Volitional processes are used to select among many choices, keep focused, and regulate behaviors in an environment with many distractions.

My brother and I have volitional behaviors that reflect our different interests. Given all the occupational options that are available at any given point in time, Robert chooses to do an occupation that is related to language, and he does it! I may choose to do an occupation related to mother-child relationships, and I do it! We make and carry out our choices regardless of the other distractions around us.

Sociocultural Phenomena

- A larger sociocultural context frames life events and influences choice.
- The environment, specifically the sociocultural environment, influences choice.

My brother and I had basically the same sociocultural home environment in our younger years. However, we have had very different sociocultural influences in our adult years. Robert's sociocultural context of an international, cosmopolitan city obviously shaped his life events in a different way from mine, a mid-western metropolitan area. These contexts, in turn, influence the choices we have made about occupations.

Whew! That was a lot of motivational theory and a lot of different ideas. Can we make any summary statements? Let's go back to our original questions.

- How does a person choose occupations? Motivational theories seem to agree that there is an internal process (cognition) that is shaped by the people in our life (social environment). This internal process influences our behavior and links our past, present, and future choices.
- How do things outside the person (i.e., the environment) influence choice? The person interprets the environment as it relates to self. If the person believes there is a match between the environment and self, then occupational choices will reflect that belief. So it is not the environment itself that influences choice, but the person's beliefs about the environment.

Genetics provide us another angle to answer the two questions posed at the beginning of the chapter. The old nature versus nurture question provided scientists some opportunity for lively discussion in the past. Now, we believe that humans develop from the interaction of their genetic code with environmental influences.

- Both the person (i.e., genetic code) and the environment influence occupational choice.
- There is a reciprocal relationship between genetic characteristics and the environment. One influences the other. These two factors in turn influence performance and choice. Optimal environments support optimal performance.

Back to the example. This occupational choice—to learn or not to learn Portuguese—is greatly influenced by both our genetic code and the environment. Aha! There is something that my brother has in his genetic code and in his environment that makes this occupation important and meaningful for him to do. Whatever it is, it is not in my genetic code and environment. Now I don't feel so bad!

Our culture is another potential influence on occupational choice.

- If our culture includes our beliefs, values, and the lens we use for the world, then it makes sense that our culture would shape our choices.
- There is a reciprocal relationship between our cultural environment and occupational choice. Our culture influences the roles we adopt and our behaviors. Our occupational choices in turn either reinforce or weaken our fit with a specific culture.

My brother and I have very similar beliefs and values in a number of areas. We both grew up in the same family that valued life-long learning, curiosity about life, and persistence in our efforts. However, there must be something different in our culture beyond the family. What might it be?

Social policy is also a potential influence on occupational choice.

- Social policy, which includes things like economic resources, public policy, social systems, and public initiatives, influences our ability to make desired occupational choices, especially if we are part of a group that is targeted or neglected by social policy.
- Our social policy is part of our environment. This aspect of environment may either support or limit a person's engagement in certain occupations. This is particularly true for some populations (e.g., people with disabilities) and some occupational choices (e.g., work).

Now, I don't think social policy has influenced my brother's and my occupational choices related to language but I am not entirely sure. I will have to talk with him about this the next time we get together.

Well, you made it through a very challenging chapter. The next time you choose to try a new sport, volunteer at a community agency, or learn Portuguese, it should make you pause and consider all the possible internal and external influences on that choice.

Journal Activities

1. Look up and write down a dictionary definition of choice. Highlight the component of the definition that is most related to the descriptions of occupation in Chapter Five.
2. Identify the most important new learning for you in this chapter.
3. Identify one question you have about Chapter Five.
4. Reflect on an occupation you chose to do in the past.
5. Describe one personal influence and one environmental influence on that choice without referring to the text.
6. Reflect on an occupation you chose NOT to do in the past.
7. Describe one personal influence and one environmental influence on that choice without referring to the text.

Technology/Internet Learning Activities

1. Use a discussion database to share specific journal entries.
2. Use a good search engine to find the Web site for the Human Genome Project.
   - Enter the phrase "Human Genome Project" in the search line.
   - Answer the following questions:
     - ✧ What is a human genome?
     - ✧ What agencies sponsor or coordinate the Human Genome Project?
   - Briefly summarize the main purposes and activities of the Human Genome Project.
   - Describe three ethical, legal, and social issues identified by the Human Genome Project that relate to behavior; choice; and social, cultural, and environmental factors.
3. Use a good search engine to find the Web sites that may address cultural and social policy influences on occupational choice.
   - Enter the phrase "Institute of Medicine" in the search line.
   - Explore the Institute of Medicine Web site for topics related to "culture" using the search line in the site.
   - Answer the following question:
     - ✧ What is the mission of the Institute of Medicine (IOM)?
   - Identify several Programs or Boards of the Institute of Medicine.
   - Identify three interesting topics on culture directly or indirectly related to occupational choice.
   - Skim one topic. Propose one idea on how occupational choice relates to this topic.
   - Enter the phrase "NCMRR" or "NIDRR" in the search line.
   - Explore the National Center for Medical Rehabilitation Research or National Institute on Disability and Rehabilitation Research.
   - Explore the site for topics related to culture, choice, and policy using the search line in the site.
   - Answer the following questions:
     - ✧ What is the mission or purpose of the agency?
     - ✧ Identify three core funding/program/research areas for the agency.
     - ✧ Identify three interesting topics directly or indirectly related to occupational choice.
     - ✧ Skim one topic. Propose one idea on how occupational choice relates to this topic.

Applied Learning

Individual Learning Activity #1: Narrating Your Story About an Occupational Choice

Instructions:

- Identify an occupation (or role) that required you to make a deliberate choice (e.g., playing a musical instrument, competing in a specific sport, working at a particular job).
- Reflect on your choice and answer the two questions in the chapter from at least three different perspectives discussed in the chapter.

	How Did You Choose the Occupation?	*How Did the Environment Influence the Choice?*
Behaviorism		
Expectancy-Value		
Social-Cognitive		
Intrinsic Versus Extrinsic Motivation		
Future Orientation		
Volitional Behavior		
Sociocultural Phenomenon		
Genetics		
Culture		
Social Policy		

Group Learning Activities

Group Activity #1: Discussion of Major Motivational Theories

Preparation:

- Read Chapter Five.
- Complete Individual Learning Activity #1.

Time: 1 to 1.5 hours

Instructions:

- Individually:
  - ✧ Complete Individual Learning Activity #1.

- In the classroom:
  - ✧ List the occupational choices examined in Individual Learning Activity #1.
  - ✧ Identify one occupational choice from the list above or a new choice that is in common for the entire group (e.g., enrolling in your academic program, choosing a specific career).
  - ✧ Use the grid below to answer the two questions from a variety of perspectives.

	How Did You Choose the Occupation?	*How Did the Environment Influence the Choice?*
Behaviorism		
Expectancy-Value		
Social-Cognitive		
Intrinsic Versus Extrinsic Motivation		
Future Orientation		
Volitional Behavior		
Sociocultural Phenomenon		
Genetics		
Culture		
Social Policy		

Discussion:

- What perspectives were difficult to represent for your example of an occupational choice?
- What perspectives made the most sense as they relate to your example of occupational choice? Why? Would this be true with every example?
- What perspectives were the hardest to understand as they relate to your example of occupational choice? Why? Would this be true with every example?

Chapter Six Objectives

The information in this chapter is intended to help the reader:

1. Understand that creating meaning through doing is a key concept that has historical roots in early occupational therapy.
2. Explore meaning as a cultural and socially constructed concept.
3. Describe meta-theories about meaning that focus on how spiritual and existential beliefs connect a person to the world and to the universe.
4. Describe the flow experience.
5. Discuss a model for analysis of experiences in daily occupations.
6. Describe the phenomenological view on meaning as the subjective life-world that humans enter prior to understanding and explanation.
7. Explore the philosophical tradition that emphasizes that humans create meaning through understanding their experiences as parts of stories.
8. Show examples of how narrative perspectives can be used in therapeutic story making through the experience of doing.
9. Explore different ways of how meaning in occupation has been empirically investigated and understood in research.
10. Appreciate the dynamic and complex nature of human understanding that influences the creation of meaning through occupational participation.

Key Words

employment: Choosing a course of action with the context of a personal narrative.
life-world: The subjective experiences of an individual within the context of his or her daily activities and relationships.
narrative: The personal story or account of an experience over time that provides a framework for understanding events.
phenomenology: The study of things as they are perceived.
sociocultural: Involving both social and cultural factors.
spirituality: The quality or condition of being spiritual or concerning one's self with metaphysical meaning.

Words may show a man's wit but actions his meaning.
Benjamin Franklin

Chapter Six

Occupation and Meaning

Hans Jonsson, PhD, OT(Reg) and Staffan Josephsson, PhD, OT(Reg)

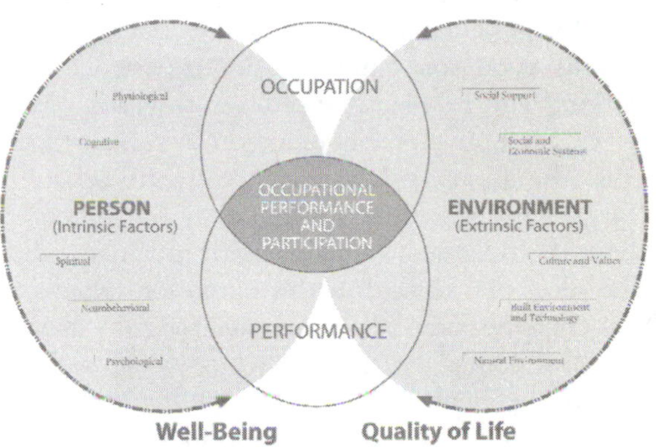

Setting the Stage

In this chapter, the idea of meaning as derived from human occupations is explored. People derive meaning from what they do. Concepts of plasticity, dynamics, and change are seen as guiding perspectives in the particular view of occupation-based meaning expressed here. We propose two general sources of meaning within occupation: a sociocultural perspective and a life-world perspective. The first shows how culture, social interaction, and agreement influence meaning. The second approach suggests that the life story of the individual creates a framework personal meaning.

Don't miss the companion Web site to *Occupational Therapy: Performance, Participation, and Well-Being, Third Edition.* Please visit us at http://www.cb3e.slackbooks.com.

Jonsson, H., & Josephsson, S. (2005). Occupation and meaning. In C. H. Christiansen, C. M. Baum, and J. Bass-Haugen (Eds.), Occupational therapy: Performance, participation, and well-being *(3rd ed.). Thorofare, NJ: SLACK Incorporated.*

Meaning Making Through the Experience of Doing

> When [the patient] gets down to honest work with her hands she makes discoveries. She finds her way along new pathways. She learns something of the dignity and satisfaction of work and gets an altogether simpler and more wholesome notion of living. This in itself is good, but better still, the open mind is apt to see new visions, new hopes and faith. There is something about simple, effective work with the hands that makes (humans)... creators in a very real sense—makes them kin with the great creative force of the world. From such a basis of dignity and simplicity anything is possible. Many a poor starved nature becomes rich and full. All this aside from the actual physical gains that may come from new muscular activities. (Hall & Buck, 1915)

This quotation builds on the experience of people working with people in hospitals in the early 20th century. The authors probably relied on historical experiences from the humanistic moral treatment school (Bing, 1981). This school was inspired by ideas from Europe about the treatment of people with psychiatric disorders. The ideas put forward in this quotation express an idea that could be named "meaning making through the experience of doing." By doing different occupations, people acquire experiences that create meaning in their lives.

Let us tell a story of meaning making from the perspective of a man named Anders (Lundemark, 1996). Anders was in a traffic accident at the age of 52 and was in a coma for 4 weeks before waking up partially paralyzed after a traumatic brain injury. He was transferred to a rehabilitation unit. There, he started to do things with his hands, first making quite simple products. When the experience taught him that he really could make things, he asked his occupational therapist to give him the most difficult thing to do. He then was given a piece of leather and the task of making a wallet out of it. Anders says, "For three weeks I worked with this. During this time, I thought: If I can make this, I can manage everything. And today, this wallet is one of my most important belongings" (Lundemark, 1996, p. 17). The story ends with Anders returning to his former work and being able to find a continuation in his life (Figure 6-1).

Let us now look at the quotation from 1915 and the example of Anders together. Hall and Buck (1915) say that humans make discoveries and find new pathways by doing (or working as the quotation says). Anders describes this process in working with his wallet in therapy. This is, of course, good, say Hall and Buck, but, better still, it is additive. It's not only good for the moment, but it also opens minds and gives new visions, new hopes, and faith. In other words, it gives new meaning. Anders describes this process as a conviction that, from his experience working with the wallet, he could manage anything. The quotation continues to say that the experience from doing gives you a belonging to the creative forces of the world and a dignity where anything is possible. The photo of Anders showing the wallet shows he's belonging to the forces that he values in his professional life and he has attained dignity in his way back to life. Today, this wallet is a symbol for Anders. In rehabilitation, it was a significant occupation that gave new meaning.

Occupations, of course, are not only crafts as in this example, but can be reading a book, learning a new language, or playing on the computer. Doing occupations creates meaning in our lives. Consequently, meaning is an essential part of an occupational perspective of the human being. The above story gives one example of the centrality of meaning in human occupation. The question remaining is how this concept can be explored and understood.

Introduction to Meaning and Occupation

In this chapter, we will explore meaning from aspects that are relevant for an occupational perspective. First, philosophical and theoretical thinking about meaning and occupation will be reviewed. Second, we will discuss and review empirical studies regarding human occupation. Finally, a synthesis regarding occupation and meaning will be discussed in terms of the character of plasticity in meaning and occupation.

Theories on Meaning

Meaning can be understood from several different theoretical and philosophical traditions. One key distinction that can be made among theories of meaning is to distinguish between theories relating to social and cultural perspectives of meaning and theories relating to the consciousness and experiences of the individual. This distinction might simplify reasoning about meaning, and it suffices as a point of departure in exploring these perspectives.

Social and Cultural Perspectives on Meaning

Culture is a word often used in everyday language. It has been defined as "the beliefs and perceptions, values and norms, and customs and behaviors that are shared by a group or society and passed from one generation to the next through both formal and informal education" (Barris,

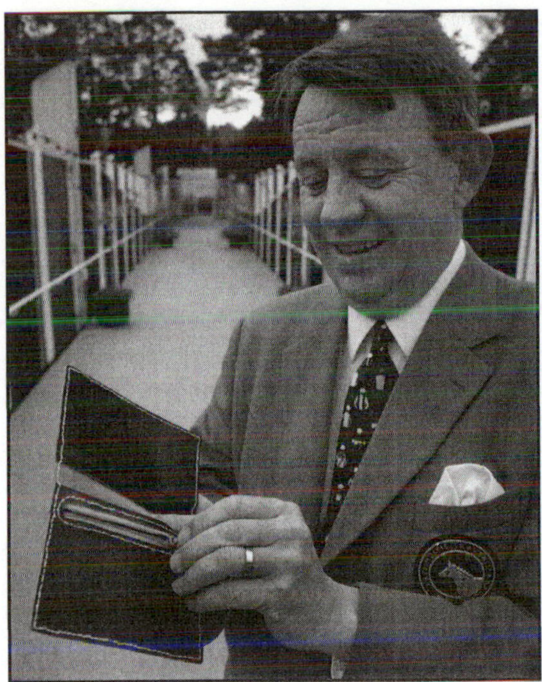

Figure 6-1. Anders with the "work of his hands."

Kielhofner, Levine, & Neville, 1985, p. 55). Simply stated, culture is systems of socially shared meanings. The meaning we attach to everyday occupation is closely connected and interwoven with our culture. Meaning is given to life and its features through language. Thus, culture relies on language and our ability to think symbolically (Bruner, 1986, 1990).

Culture is not a socially shared system of meaning; it is also often understood as socially constructed. Berger and Luckman (1966) in their influential book, *The Social Construction of Reality*, address how cultures are living systems made and reshaped in everyday life through social encounters with other human beings. The concept of independence can serve as an example. Independence is a core value in western culture and includes dimensions such as individualism, initiative, and self-reliance. Such independence is valued as good and desirable. Interest-ingly, in other cultures, independence is not always seen as a goal. Rather, interdependence is valued and promoted (Brown & Gillespie, 1992). In line with the reasoning of Berger and Luckman (1966), dependence as well as independence could be seen as a result of the needs of the everyday culture reflecting the social life developed in various societies. In other words, independence is not a personality trait among western citizens. It is interesting to reflect on how the growing mobility of human beings in our world will affect western cultural beliefs such as independence (Figure 6-2).

> *Different Tools for Eating as Reflection of Culture*
>
> The different procedures and occupational patterns used when eating everyday food can serve as an illustrative example of human culture. Few of us think of our own way of eating as a reflection of our culture. However, when encountering people from other cultural groups, it suddenly becomes apparent that we eat differently. For example, the habit to basically eat with a fork and use a knife occasionally is common and proper in America. In Europe, a proper way to eat is to use both fork and knife all the time. However, most habitants of this earth would find both of these ways of eating improper and hard to understand.

The French sociologist Pierre Bordieu (Bordieu & Passeron, 1977; Calhoun, LiPuma, & Potone, 1993) created a concept called *habitus regarding the cultural and political frames* (or *fields* as Bordieu calls them) in which an individual is located. The habitus creates a field that shapes one's attitudes about what is possible and preferable as well as the experience of meaning. This theory suggests that to understand the individual experience of meaning, you need to know the habitus. The theory rejects cultural determinism (i.e., the individual's will has no importance) as well as individualism (i.e., the individual's will is the only thing that matters). The habitus creates a field that outlines the frames into which an individual navigates.

Spirituality and Meaning

In the discussion of meaning, the concept of spirituality has been put forward as a fundamental concept of meaning addressing the existential questions of humankind: Why do we exist? What is the meaning of life? Spirituality has been closely connected to religious beliefs. However, as Christiansen (1997) points out, rather the opposite connection could be made: "Religions are organized traditions of rules and orthodoxy that attempt to serve spiritual needs of their followers" (p. 170). Spirituality has been defined as "a higher self, a spiritual direction or greater purpose, which nurtures people through life events and choices" (CAOT, 1997, p. 42). In this view, spirituality has a meta-meaning that guides humans both in their choices of occupations and in how they interpret the meaning of their experience of doing.

Connected to spirituality is also the concept of "being" as proposed by Rowles (1991) and later Wilcock (1998a, 1998b). Being is the enjoyment of inner life, to reflect and to simply exist (Wilcock, 1998b). Being is one part of

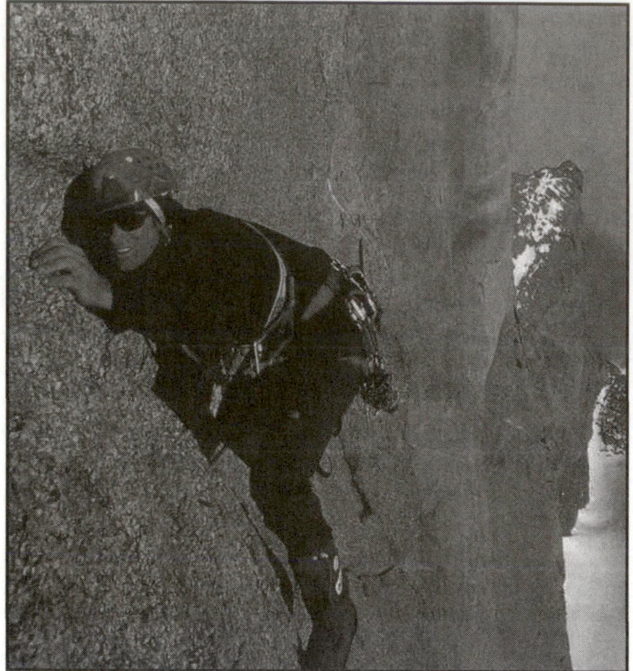
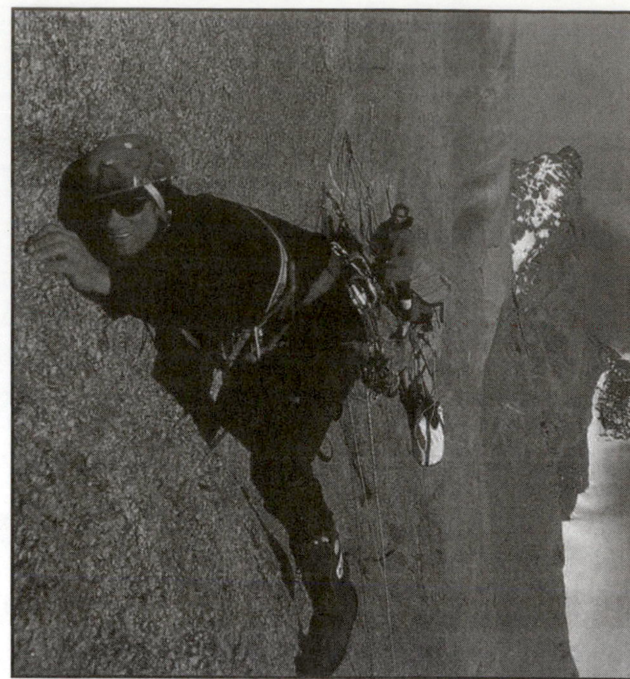

Figure 6-2. Is independence always better than interdependence?

what Wilcock describes as an interrelated wholeness of doing, being, and becoming. Experiences of meaning in occupation are, from that perspective, connected to both the direct experiences (doing) and to how we are situated in the world (being), as well as to the competence and identity to which this leads (becoming).

Another theory that connects to spirituality and meaning is the salutogenetic orientation regarding health and life satisfaction developed by the Israeli sociologist Antonovsky (1979, 1987). In this theory, Antonovsky developed the concept named sense of coherence that has a close relationship to health. The experience of meaningfulness, comprehensibility, and manageability are the three constituents in the sense of coherence. Meaning is experienced when the daily experiences of the world are comprehensible and when a person recognizes that he or she has the resources available to meet demands that are seen as worth investment and engagement. The concept of sense of coherence has been used in studies of the quality of experience in daily living (Brännholm, Fugl-Meyer, & Frölunde, 1998; Persson, Eklund, & Isacsson, 1999).

Spirituality is one important element in the complex arena of human meaning making. Awareness of the spiritual needs of the client's everyday occupation might be crucial for the individual's ability to find meaning in new circumstances caused by disease or handicap. However, spirituality also comprises elements in human existence that are difficult to verbalize or capture behind the barriers of theoretical language. This state of affairs might make spirituality even more important to be considered when a person is in vulnerable life circumstances.

The Flow Experience as Meaning in Occupation

Csikszentmihalyi developed a sociopsychological theory called flow theory (1975, 1998). He has studied the experience of meaning that occurs in the direct interaction between the person and his or her everyday activities. When the challenge of the activity matches the skills of the individual, a certain state of mind occurs—a flow experience—with total involvement in which the individual feels joy, excitement, and happiness. This state of doing creates not only meaning in the direct experience but also meaning in life as a whole. Csikszentmihalyi states:

> ...the way to improve the quality of life is not primarily through thinking, but through doing. The issue is not to figure out how to be happy, satisfied, or contented; but to act in ways that will bring about those states of experiences directly. (1993, p. 38)

Research has pointed out that experiences of high quality in life go together with the experiences of flow in daily life (Csikszentmihalyi & Csikszentmihalyi, 1992; DeVries, 1992; Gerhardsson & Jonsson, 1996; Persson, 1996). A methodology called the *experience sampling method* (ESM) has been developed to collect data about

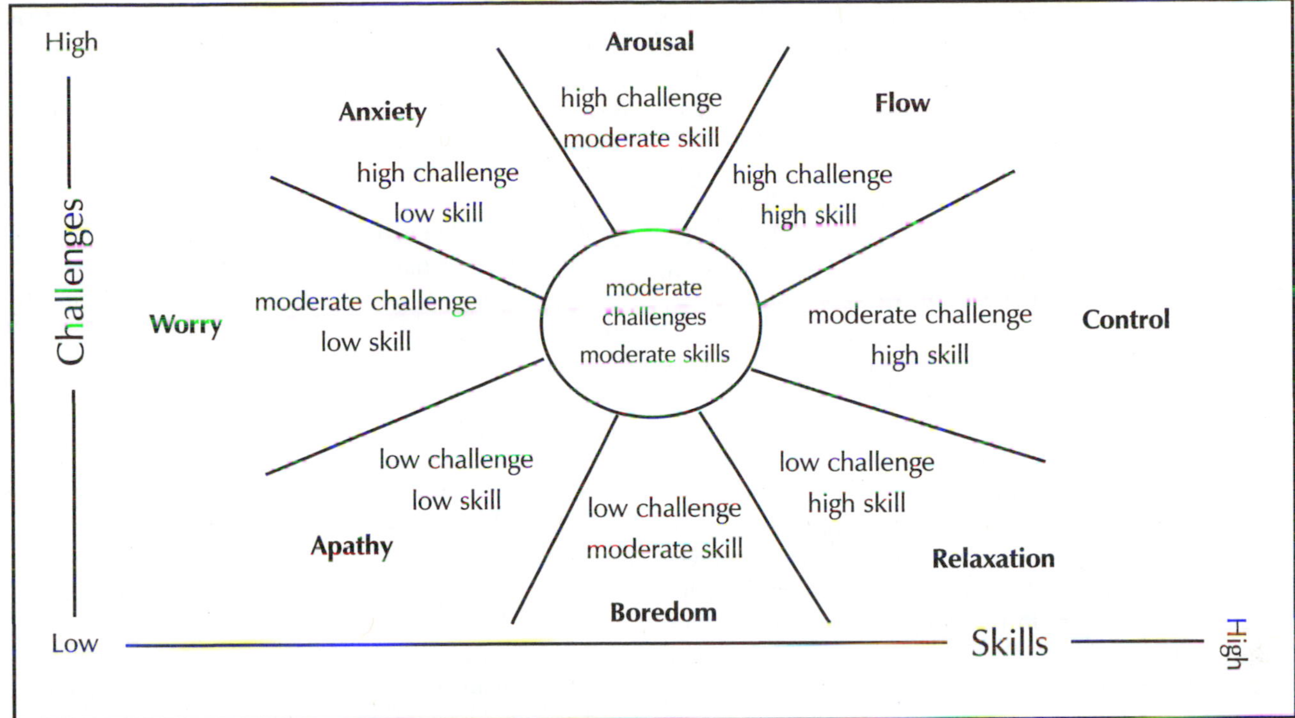

Figure 6-3. Eight-channel model for analysis of experiences in daily occupations. (Adapted from Massimini, F., & Carli, M. (1988). The systematic assessment of flow in daily experience. In M. Csikszentmihalyi & I. Csikszentmihalyi (Eds.), *Optimal experience: Psychological studies of flow in consciousness* (pp. 266-287). New York, NY: Cambridge University Press and Csikszentmihalyi, M. (1990). *Flow: The psychology of optimal experience.* New York, NY: Harper & Row.)

individuals' subjective experiences of what they do (Csikszentmihalyi, 1990; Massimini & Carli, 1988). Research using the ESM methodology has developed a taxonomy (Figure 6-3) of eight qualities of experiences of daily activities as depending on the experienced relationship between challenges and skills in the activity. An example of research using these methods is a study where individual experience quality profiles were developed, based on the eight-channel flow model (Persson et al., 1999) (see Figure 6-3).

As can be seen in the above review of social and cultural perspectives on meaning, the theories and reasoning often interweave with a more individual focus. For example, in Rowles' concept of being in place and in flow theory, the individuals are in focus. In the next section, we discuss theories in which experiences are in focus.

A Life-World Perspective: Phenomenology and Narrative

The Phenomenological Approach

Phenomenology is based on the German philosopher Edmund Husserl's writings from the late 19th and the early 20th century (Karlsson, 1993; Kvale, 1996). This philosophy is focused on the individual's perspective of his or her world and approaches the consciousness and experiences of everyday life. Husserls argued that this philosophy should be the starting point for all studies on human life given that the only access we have to the world is through the individual's perception and experience of it (Giorgi, 1985; Karlsson, 1993). A central term in this way of approaching meaning is the life-world. Life-world could be presented as the world the individual encounters in everyday life, a direct experience prior to any explanation or theory. Consequently, the life-world is lived experiences. Phenomenology has influenced in various ways the present understanding of meaning in relation to occupation. The growing interest in exploring human occupation based on individuals' experiences is an example of the influence of phenomenology. Several studies have researched life-world experiences in relation to occupation (Andersson & Borell, 1998; Nygård & Borell, 1998).

The Narrative Turn

Stories have an important position in everyday human life. We tell stories, we read stories, and we talk about stories. Stories and other narrative material are often seen as cornerstones in human cultural and artistic life. However, in the past decades, stories have taken an important position also in theory on human occupation (Barrett, Beer, & Kielhofner, 1999; Clark, Larson Ennevor, & Richardson, 1996; Clark, Carlson, & Richardson, 1997; Helfrich & Kielhofner, 1994; Helfrich, Kielhofner, & Mattingly, 1994; Jonsson, Borell, & Sadlo, 2000a; Jonsson, Josephsson, & Kielhofner, 2001; Jonsson, Kielhofner, & Borell, 1997; Kirsh, 1996; Mallinson, Kielhofner, & Mattingly, 1996; Mattingly, 1998).

A narrative view says that humans' understanding of life shares features from understanding a story or a novel. Humans construct their understanding of reality using similar mechanisms as those used when they read and understand a story. In other words, human understanding is narratively constructed. This notion had such a great impact on the way meaning was described and theoretically understood that it justifies the claim that there has been a narrative turn in the human sciences (Mattingly, 1998; Polkinghorn, 1988). The narrative turn here stands for a shift from a biomedical and behaviorist understanding of human motivation to an understanding where fiction, stories, and narrative play an important role.

However, the idea that stories play an important part in human meaning making is not new in human history. For example, when Aristotle wrote his *Poetics* more than 2,300 years ago, he took part in an intensive discourse about the role of stories and fiction in human life (Aristotle, 1970). Why are stories so central in human life? Should stories imitate life, or is it even true that stories take part in shaping life?

> A narrative view on time can be illustrated with this quotation:
>
> [Time is] "measured not by minutes or hours, but by intensity, so that when we look at our past it does not stretch back evenly but piles up into a few notable pinnacles, and when we look at the future it seems sometimes a wall, sometimes a cloud, sometimes a sun, but never a chronological chart" (Forster, 1927, p. 28).

One contemporary philosopher contributing to this discussion about stories is Paul Ricoeur (1984). In the early 1980s, he presented his thesis about time as narratively constructed rather than understood in hours and minutes. Humans cannot process all information they receive through perception. Rather, a selection must be made, and from that selection, the individual formulates a meaning. The term Ricoeur used for this process was *emplotment*. By linking single events together in a meaningful plot, life becomes understandable. Such a plot is by necessity one possible meaning from thousands of others that could be constructed. When an individual engages in the process of finding a new occupational life after disease or trauma, he or she is establishing new possible emplotments of life.

Occupation as Ongoing Stories

When an individual enters into the middle of another person's life that has a history as well as a prospective future, the meaning of the situation is not given just by the situation itself. Rather, the meaning results from the placement of the situation in a larger configuration, plot of events, historical events, and possible futures (Mattingly, 1998).

Depending on how the situation is placed in these larger plots, different stories can be created. The following story illustrates this quality of everyday life (Josephsson, Backman, Nygard, & Bor, 2000):

> Eva is spending a lot of time trying to assist her mother. Eva is a woman in her 30s, and her mother Anna is in her 70s. Anna has been a capable woman managing, as a single mother, to raise her daughter. However, now, things have changed. For two years, Anna has had the diagnosis of Alzheimer's disease, and now her life gives proof of very typical features of dementia. She has difficulty in remembering, and, consequently, her occupational life is ruined. She also shows very strong emotions when approached by others about her situation or when others try to intervene in her daily life. When visiting the day care center Anna attends every week, Eva understands that her mother's place at the center is questioned because of her neglect of personal care. Other visitors become annoyed, and the staff has difficulties in handling the situation. In Eva's words, when a friend approaches her on the subject, "they need me to assist in caring for my mother." Eva engages in long sentences about the disease and her mother's need for her assistance.
>
> But then Eva pauses for a while. Her words go in another direction. She tells about her teens and how she had been in constant conflict with her mother. She smiles a little when she admits that she saw the home that she then shared with her mother as merely a food and laundry depot. But I am back now she says. I have things to share, and I want to learn from my mother. It is just that the possibility does not seem to be there anymore. "My big sorrow is that I don't have a good meeting place with my mother."

This story illustrates how the meaning of a problem is shifting by how the situation is placed within a larger emplotment of events. The plot changed from being about a mother with a challenging disease to being centered on Eva's need for establishing a new form of fellowship with her mother. As exemplified by Eva's words in the story, this quality is often visible in everyday conversation.

Meaning in this tradition is largely narratively constructed and is in contrast to physical traits. Stories can change, and plots can take other directions as illustrated in the story of Anna and Eva where the meaning of the problem shifted. Such meaning revisions often result from collaborating with other human beings in everyday life. The use of metaphor in narratives has been found to be key to understanding the experiences of clients (Mallinson et al., 1996). Metaphors are something familiar that stand in place of a non-understood situation. Metaphors of entrapment and of losing momentum in life are especially common. In the example of Anna and Eva, the metaphor could be the idea of a meeting place.

Studies of Meaning in Connection to Occupation

As has been seen in earlier sections, there are several theories and perspectives in which the concept of meaning can be understood. In the following section, we will connect these theories to the everyday world of occupation. We will then see how the perspectives identified earlier—the social, the cultural, and the life-world perspectives—will interweave.

The Variety of Meanings in Occupation

The notion that meanings are shared and constructed in cultures and in social contexts does not imply that meanings of occupations are the same among different people. What one person experiences as challenging and exciting, others can experience as boring and destructive.

It is important to consider the variety of meanings that can be experienced in the same occupation, even in the most common everyday activity. One example of research that highlights this variety is an interview and observation study about the meaning of meals for seniors in Denmark (Bundgaard, Christiansen, & Schultz, 1999). The study showed the following variety of meanings, where several of the seniors expressed more than one meaning:

- Filling time and giving variety of the day
- Expressing and maintaining identity
- Making one's self useful
- Creating and keeping up social contacts
- Keeping up self-determination and independence
- Maintaining physical and mental well-being
- Giving the possibility of creativity and development
- Giving the joy of experience

All these factors were seen as contributing to these seniors' well-being by keeping up lifestyles, social contacts, experiences, and action.

A similar type of study researched the meaning of making and drinking a cup of tea for five British women (Hannam, 1997). The authors found six shared categories through which significant meanings were experienced. One of the categories was meaning through objects. This category referred to the importance of using special objects, like an Indian tea service, with both aesthetic and family traditional meanings. While this is an example of individual variations in the same shared culture, another study looked at 15 people from a variety of cultures in the activity of making a cup of tea (Fair & Barnitt, 1999). In this study, both cultural and individual preferences were found, like religious importance and individual relaxation. The authors' conclusion was that the way an occupation like tea making was conducted must be seen both in the context of culture and from the perspective of individual preferences.

Let us now turn to the experience of a larger area of occupation: work. In a study of the meaning of work, as experienced a few years before retirement in Sweden (Jonsson et al., 1997), a number of positive and negative values of work were found (Table 6-1).

The same aspect of work could assume both a negative and a positive meaning for the individual. For example, in the category external structure, the alarm clock was taken as an illustration with both a negative meaning ("I really long for the time when I can get rid of this terror in the morning"), as well as a positive meaning ("I really think I need this clock to get me up in the morning.")

The varieties of meaning in an occupation, as well as how individual preferences can result in very different types of experiences, stress the importance of grasping the individual experience of meaning. Furthermore, this individual experience of meaning has to be understood in relation to other occupations and their meanings. In the study regarding the meaning of work before retirement (Jonsson, et al., 1997), a positive aspect of work like "using one's knowledge and capacities" could be of very critical importance for one person who did not find that he or she could experience this aspect of meaning in other occupations. Another person had types of leisure engagements where this aspect of occupational meaning also was fulfilled. Consequently, leaving work was not such a big step for this person as for the former one. This example highlights the relative aspect of meaning in occupation.

Table 6-1 Positive and Negative Values of Work as Expressed by a Group of People Aged 63 Years

Positive	*Negative*
Social contacts and fellowship	Undesired social contacts
Using one's knowledge and capacities	Uninteresting work and boring routines
Being a part of a larger whole	Structural changes of workplace and staff
Having something to do	Diversion of energy from preferred occupations
Being productive	Stress and the burden of responsibility
Having an external structure	Rigidity of external structure
Earning one's income	

Meaninglessness and Occupational Deprivation

So far, this chapter has been concerned about meaning. However, what is the opposite of meaning? People sometimes express a lack of meaning in their everyday occupational lives. What is meaningless occupation? When and how is occupation experienced as meaningless? A few studies have been conducted regarding boredom and occupational deprivation as two expressions of not experiencing meaning in occupation. One study was about occupational deprivation among inmates in a security prison (Whiteford, 1997). Lack of engagement in meaningful occupation was the basis of this deprivation. The prison environment did not offer possibilities for engaging in meaningful occupations with one small exception: a fish tank. This fish tank was highly appreciated as a meaningful oasis in an occupational desert. Tending to the fish tank led to self-discipline and organized constructive performance in an environment where the opposite was the most common way to react. In a study of young offenders (Farnsworth, 1998), boredom was experienced half of the time and seemed closely connected to lack of engagement in productive occupations such as education and work. Lack of meaning in occupations was also present in some narratives of Swedish retirees that contained only a flat chronological description of one occupation after another (Jonsson, Borell, et al., 2000; Jonsson et al., 1997). In contrast to this type of report, there were narratives loaded with meaning in occupation that were told with enthusiasm and passion. Some occupations stood out from others and were narrated with great emphasis. This type of occupation, named *engaging occupation*, was closely tied to the experience of meaning and engagement in a person's occupational life (Jonsson, 2000; Jonsson et al., 2001). Interestingly, engaging occupation could be found in all areas of human occupation: in home and family as well as in work or in leisure.

Before leaving the concept of meaninglessness, let us raise some signs of caution. Following earlier arguments on how meaning is constructed, meaninglessness could be viewed also as a form of meaning. In fact, by definition, meaninglessness is a form of meaning. Let us also relate this idea of meaninglessness to the earlier discussion about meaning as a constantly reformulative phenomenon. An occupation that in the direct experience can be seen as meaningless, such as a part of an educational program, can later in a professional situation turn out to be of great significance. From the narrative thinking presented earlier, it was not possible at first to emplot this experience into a present narrative, but later, the experience was reformulated and thus became a meaningful part of one's present narrative.

Meaning in Occupation as Relationship

In the literature, meaning in occupation has mainly been understood as being either internal to the individual or in the interaction between the individual and the occupation. Recent studies of occupational transitions, however (Jonsson, Borell, et al., 2000; Jonsson, Josephson, & Kielfhofner, 2000), suggest an additional aspect of meaning and occupation, namely that occupations also get part of their meaning in rela-

> Balance between occupations has a relationship to meaning as has been expressed in this quotation: "If all the year were playing holidays, To sport would be as tedious as to work; But when they seldom come, they wish'd for come." (Shakespeare, 1598, Henrik IV 1.2)

tionship to other occupations. Under stable conditions, it might be difficult to see this type of meaning, but in a process of change, it becomes more obvious. An example of this aspect of meaning is shown in how a summer cottage changed meaning for a person before and after retirement. Before retirement, the cottage provided an oasis of 3 days of well-deserved rest and relaxation after a long working week. After retirement, this meaning, to the person's own surprise, had changed as there was no work from which to relax, and the three days could be 33 or more. "It's not the same any longer, I don't have the feeling for it any longer" was the comment regarding this change of meaning. In a narrative way of looking at this example, one could say that this person developed difficulties emplotting this experience when the overall organization of the plot had changed.

It is important to understand the difficulties a person may experience in foreseeing the consequences that big occupational transitions have on the experience of meaning in different occupations. Occupational transitions may upset the dynamic balance that is between different occupations, a balance that has a direct influence on the experience of meaning in an occupation.

Summary—The Plasticity of Meaning in Occupation

In this chapter, we have outlined a perspective where meaning is expressed as a central issue for an occupational perspective of human beings: meaning making through the experience of doing. Plasticity, dynamics, and change have been guiding perspectives in this view of meaning. It is certainly not the only perspective for understanding the concept of meaning. Other perspectives, such as personality psychology (Friedman & Schustack, 1999), address the rigidity of perception and view experiences of meaning as emerging from relatively stable traits in a stable personality. Although relevant as a perspective, it is out of the scope of this chapter to further address these types of perspectives.

To better grasp the concept of meaning, we proposed two general categories regarding theories on meaning and occupation: a sociocultural perspective and a life-world perspective. To the former, we linked theories addressing culture and social construction of meaning. To the latter, we linked phenomenology and its focus on the life-world of the individual and meaning in occupation as narratively constructed.

A narrative approach has been stressed as a way to understand how humans make meaning out of different occupational experiences. The concept of emplotment expresses this meaning making process. The narrative is not only shaped by the process of emplotment, it is also constantly reshaped in a process of interaction with the narrative and the living world with a character of plasticity.

Let us return to the story of Anders with which we began this chapter. The way Anders originally emplotted his experiences of rehabilitation might have changed as his life progressed. It does not make his experiences at that time less relevant. However, when Anders now tells his story from the perspective of new experiences in his life story, he might give another meaning to the experiences than those he gave in the quoted example.

References

Andersson, G., & Borell, L. (1998). Experience of being occupied: Some elderly people's positive experiences of occupations at community-based activity centers. *Scandinavian Journal of Occupational Therapy, 5*, 133-139.

Antonovsky, A. (1979). *Health, stress and coping: New perspectives on mental and physical well-being*. San Francisco, CA: Jossey-Bass.

Antonovsky, A. (1987) *Unraveling the mysteries of health*. San Francisco, CA: Jossey-Bass.

Aristotle (1970). *Poetics* (G. Else, Trans.). Ann Arbor, MI: University of Michigan Press.

Barrett, L., Beer, D., & Kielhofner, G. (1999). The importance of volitional narrative in treatment: An ethnographic case study in a work program. *Work, 12*, 79-92.

Barris, R., Kielhofner, G., Levine, R., & Neville, A. (1985). Occupation as interaction with the environment. In G. Kielhofner (Ed.), *A model of human occupation: Theory and application* (pp. 42-62). Baltimore, MD: Williams & Wilkins.

Berger, P. L., & Luckman, T. (1966). *The social construction of reality*. New York, NY: Doubleday.

Bing, R. K. (1981). Eleanor Clark Slagle lectureship 1981: Occupational therapy revisited: A paraphrastic journey. *American Journal of Occupational Therapy, 35*, 499-518.

Bordieu, P., & Passeron, J. C. (1977). *Reproduction in education, society and culture*. London: Sage.

Brännholm, I. B., Fugl-Meyer, A. R., & Frölunde, A. (1998). Life satisfaction, sense of coherence and locus of control in occupational therapy students. *Scandinavian Journal of Occupational Therapy, 5*, 39-44.

Brown, K., & Gillespie, D. (1992). Recovering relationships: A feminist analysis of recovery models. *American Journal of Occupational Therapy, 46*, 1001-1005.

Bruner, J. (1986). *Actual minds, possible worlds*. Cambridge, MA: Harvard University Press.

Bruner, J. (1990). *Acts of meaning*. Cambridge, MA: Harvard University Press.

Bundgaard, K. M., Christensen, B., & Schultz, T. (1999). *En bid af ældres hverdagsliv* (A part of elderly everyday living). Odense.

Evidence Worksheet

Author(s)	*Year*	*Topic*	*Method*	*Conclusion*
Fair & Barnitt	1999	The meaning of making a cup of tea for people with a variety of cultural backgrounds	Descriptive	Meaning in occupation has to be understood from cultural, personal, and lifespan perspectives
Farnsworth	1998	The subjective experiences in occupation for young offenders	Descriptive statistics using a pager	High degree of boredom seems to be connected to lack of engagement in productive occupations like work or education
Helfrich & Kielhofner	1994	The experience of meaning of therapy	Narrative	Meaning of therapy was assigned in how this episode was emplotted into a larger volitional narrative
Jonsson et al.	2001	The experience of meaning in occupation through the transition from worker to retiree	Narrative analysis Longitudinal studies	Occupations that had significant meanings for the participants had a number of certain characteristics and was named *engaging occupation*
Nygård & Borell	1998	Life-world from a phenomenological perspective of two women with early dementia	Phenomenological, case studies over time	The experiences of the life-world as taken for granted gradually decreased, and objects and tasks of everyday life increasingly had an existential meaning as they threatened order and control in the participant's life
Whiteford	1997	The occupational world of inmates in a security prison	Descriptive, participant observation	Lack of meaning for the inmates contributed to disorientation and psychotic episodes

Calhoun, C., LiPuma, E., & Postone, M. (Eds.). (1993). *Bourdieu: Critical perspectives*. Chicago, IL: University of Chicago Press.

Canadian Association of Occupational Therapists. (1997). *Enabling occupation: An occupational therapy perspective*. Ottawa: CAOT Publications ACE.

Christiansen, C. (1997). Acknowledging a spiritual dimension in occupational therapy practice. *American Journal of Occupational Therapy, 51*, 169-172.

Clark, F., Carlson, M., & Polkinghorne, D. (1997). The legitimacy of life history and narrative approaches in the study of occupation. *American Journal of Occupational Therapy, 51*, 313-317.

Clark, F., Larson Ennevor, B., & Richardson, P. L. (1996). A grounded theory of techniques for occupational storytelling and occupational story making. In R. Zemke & F. Clark (Eds.), *Occupational science: The evolving discipline* (pp. 373-392). Philadelphia, PA: F. A. Davis Company.

Csikszentmihalyi, M. (1975). Play and intrinsic rewards. *Journal of Humanistic Psychology, 15*, 41-63.

Csikszentmihalyi, M. (1990). *Flow—The psychology of optimal experience*. New York, NY: Harper & Row.

Csikszentmihalyi, M. (1993). Activity and happiness: Towards a science of occupation. *Journal of Occupational Science, 1*, 38-42.

Csikszentmihalyi, M. (1998). *Finding flow: The psychology of engagement with everyday life*. New York, NY: BasicBooks.

Csikszentmihalyi, M., & Csikszentmihalyi, I. (Eds.). (1992). *Optimal experience: Psychological studies of flow in consciousness*. New York, NY: Cambridge University Press.

DeVries, M. (Ed.). (1992). *The experience of psychopathology: Investigating mental disorders in their natural settings*. New York, NY: Cambridge University Press.

Fair, A., & Barnitt, R. (1999). Making a cup of tea as part of a culturally sensitive service. *British Journal of Occupational Therapy, 62*, 199-205.

Farnsworth, L. (1998). Doing, being, and boredom. *Journal of Occupational Science, 5*, 140-146.

Forster, E. M. (1927). *Aspects of the novel*. New York, NY: Harcourt Brace Jovanovich.

Friedman, H. S., & Schustack, M. W. (1999). *Personality—Classic theories and modern research*. Boston, MA: Allyn & Bacon.

Gerhardsson, C., & Jonsson, H. (1996). Experience of therapeutic occupations in schizophrenic subjects: Clinical observations organized in terms of the flow theory. *Scandinavian Journal of Occupational Therapy, 3*, 149-155.

Giorgi, A. (1985). *Phenomenology and psychological research*. Pittsburgh, PA: Duquesne University Press.

Hall, H. J., & Buck, M. M. C. (1915). *The work of our hands: A study of occupations for invalids*. New York, NY: Moffat, Yard & Company.

Hannam, D. (1997). More than a cup of tea: Meaning construction in an everyday occupation. *Journal of Occupational Science, 4*, 69-74.

Helfrich, C., & Kielhofner, G. (1994). Volitional narratives and the meaning of therapy. *American Journal of Occupational Therapy, 48*, 318-326.

Helfrich, C., Kielhofner, G., & Mattingly, C. (1994). Volition as narrative: Understanding motivation in chronic illness. *American Journal of Occupational Therapy, 48*, 311-317.

Jonsson, H. (2000). Anticipating, experiencing and valuing the transition from worker to retiree: A longitudinal study of retirement as an occupational transition. Doctoral dissertation, Department of clinical neuroscience, occupational therapy and elderly care research, Division of occupational therapy, Karolinska Institutet, Sweden.

Jonsson, H., Borell, L., & Sadlo, G. (2000). Retirement: An occupational transition with consequences on temporality, rhythm and balance. *Journal of Occupational Science, 7*, 5-13.

Jonsson, H., Josephsson, S., & Kielhofner, G. (2000). Evolving narratives in the course of retirement. *American Journal of Occupational Therapy, 54*, 463-476.

Jonsson, H., Josephsson, S., & Kielhofner, G. (2001). Narratives and experience in an occupational transition: A longitudinal study of the retirement process. *American Journal of Occupational Therapy, 55*, 424-432.

Jonsson, H., Kielhofner, G., & Borell, B. (1997). Anticipating retirement: The formation of narratives concerning an occupational transition. *American Journal of Occupational Therapy, 51*, 49-56.

Josephsson, S., Bäckman, L., Nygård, L., & Borell, L. (2000). Nonprofessional caregivers' experience of occupational performance on the part of relatives with dementia: Implications for caregiver program in occupational therapy. *Scandinavian Journal of Occupational Therapy, 7*, 61-66.

Karlsson, G. (1993). *Psychological qualitative research from a phenomenological perspective*. Stockholm: Amqvist & Wiksell.

Kirsh, B. (1996). A narrative approach to addressing spirituality in occupational therapy: Exploring personal meaning and purpose. *Canadian Journal of Occupational Therapy, 63*, 55-61.

Kvale, S. (1996). *Interviews: An introduction to qualitative research interviewing*. London: Sage Publications.

Lundemark, T. (1996). Arbetsterapeuter hjälpte Anders vinna sitt livs lopp (Occupational therapists helped Anders to win the race of his life). *Arbetsterapeuten, 12*, 16-18.

Mallinson, T., Kielhofner, G., & Mattingly, C. (1996). Metaphor and meaning in a clinical interview. *American Journal of Occupational Therapy, 50*, 338-346.

Massimini F., & Carli, M. (1988). The systematic assessment of flow in daily experience. In M. Csikszentmihalyi & I. Csikszentmihalyi (Eds.), *Optimal experience: Psychological studies of flow in consciousness* (pp. 266-287). New York, NY: Cambridge University Press.

Mattingly, C. (1998). *Healing dramas and clinical plots: The narrative structure of experience*. Cambridge, MA: Cambridge University Press.

Nygård, L., & Borell, L. (1998). A life-world of altering meaning: Expressions of the illness experience of dementia in everyday life over three years. *Occupational Therapy Journal of Research, 18*, 109-136.

Persson, D. (1996). Play and flow in an activity group—A case study of creative occupations with chronic pain patients. *Scandinavian Journal of Occupational Therapy, 3*, 33-42.

Persson, D., Eklund, M., & Isacsson, Å. (1999). The experience of everyday occupations and its relation to sense of coherence—A methodological study. *Journal of Occupational Science, 6*, 13-26.

Polkinghorn, D. E. (1988). *Narrative knowing and the human sciences*. Albany, NY: State University of New York Press.

Ricoeur, P. (1984). *Time and narrative*. Chicago, IL: University of Chicago Press.

Rowles, G. D. (1991). Beyond performance: Being in place as a component of occupational therapy. *American Journal of Occupational Therapy, 45*, 265-272.

Shakespeare, W. (1598). Henrik IV 1.2. Retrieved February 17, 2002, from http://www.shakespeare.com/FirstFolio/1_KING_HENRY_IV/1.2.html

Wilcock, A. A. (1998a). *An occupational perspective on health*. Thorofare, NJ: SLACK Incorporated

Wilcock, A. A. (1998b). Reflections on doing, being, and becoming. *Canadian Journal of Occupational Therapy, 65*, 248-256.

Whiteford, G. (1997). Occupational deprivation and incarceration. *Journal of Occupational Science, 4*, 126-130.

Chapter Six: Occupation and Meaning Reflections and Learning Activities

Julie Bass-Haugen, PhD, OTR/L, FAOTA

Reflections

In Chapter One, we saw that occupations are exceedingly complex and can be described in many ways. In Chapter Six, we learned that occupations help us to find meaning in our lives.

The chapter began by telling a very moving story about a seemingly simple project that Anders did while he was recovering from a traumatic brain injury. Anders saved a wallet he made because it so beautifully represented his life at one period of time and was a reminder of the goals he achieved on the road to recovery. With a little imagination, we can almost see the wallet—perhaps with some errors in construction or a pattern that seems rather simple for a man of his age. Certainly, the wallet would not be anything that would win a creative arts award. Yet, this object was symbolic of an important occupation in Anders' life. Why?

The remainder of the chapter provided some hints on what we know about the meaning of occupation. Culture and spirituality were discussed as important contributions to the development of meaning. However, if you have ever tried to describe your culture or spirituality, you realize they are very complex dimensions because they are either too familiar to appreciate or too foreign to understand. This perspective on meaning comes from a socio-cultural perspective. The other approach to meaning introduced in this chapter is the life-world perspective. The life-world perspective is based on phenomenology and narrative.

It was only recently that I was able to convey the meaning of one of my occupations, canoeing, and the connections of these meanings to my culture and my sense of spirituality. For years, I assumed anyone who tried canoeing would immediately understand my meaning of this occupation.

It never crossed my mind that my meaning of canoeing was tied to the culture of a specific group of people. As I have talked with different people over the years, it is clear that I have a canoeing connection with people from similar cultures, and then there are other people who "just don't get it" from my perspective. My meaning of canoeing is associated with the beliefs, values, customs, and behaviors of my community. Let me give you a little background. I grew up in Minnesota, the Land of 10,000 Lakes, an area of the country that has used canoes for hundreds of years. Canoeing is used to introduce children to nature and is regarded as a safe, coming-of-age experience for adolescents. Canoeing is a common occupation of vacationing friends and families and is part of the routines and lifestyles of many people in my community. Canoeing is also a priority in the broader community, with evidence of this in the products sold by area businesses, activities of local associations, and the resources available for canoeing. Even those individuals who do not canoe understand the importance of this occupation to our community.

My meaning of canoeing is also tied to the types of experiences that give me a heightened awareness of my spirituality. The rhythm inherent in paddling, the expansiveness of the wilderness in comparison to me, and the renewal of my senses are all part of the meaning I have for this occupation. My engagement in canoeing over the years has nurtured the development of my identity and inner self, my relationship with a higher being, and my connection with the natural environment.

This chapter proposed that our most meaningful occupations are often those same occupations from which we experience a state of flow. It has certainly been true for me. I can get totally lost in a state of reverie while canoeing. I remember paddling hour after hour against the wind on big lakes despite a lot of aches and pains while we made our way to the target stopping point at the end of a long day. There was no need to check the time or ask how long we had been on the water. We simply continued until we had met our goal for the day.

Now, let's look at canoeing from a life-world perspective. From the chapter, we see that phenomenology and narratives are two approaches for this perspective. Let's look first at the word *phenomenology*. Do you remember what the suffix "-ology" means, as in psychology or sociology? Of course, it is "the study of." Now look at the rest of the word, phenomenon. When I looked up the definition of phenomenon in several dictionaries, I found four words routinely used in part of the definition—fact, event, object, experience. So without even looking up a formal definition of phenomenology, I would guess that it might involve studying facts, events, objects, and experiences related to my occupation of canoeing. Of course, there is more to phenomenology than this but it is a good beginning.

The other approach to getting a life-world perspective is narrative or stories. The meaning of an occupation is often not realized without the stories that come from our experiences. Stories help us construct the meaning of an occupation and keep an occupation in the foreground of our life even when we are unable to do the occupation. I could fill this chapter with stories of canoeing. My stories would indirectly convey my meaning for this occupation and keep alive special experiences I have had. If you had a whole day to listen to my canoeing stories, you would see a thread that links the individual stories I selected. My selection of stories, the way I order them, and the way I have them unfold is part of the meaning making or emplotment process.

This chapter ended with discussions of the many different meanings a single occupation can have, meaningless occupations, occupational deprivation, and the meaning that is derived from occupations when they are connected to other occupations. Now, when you hear someone ask, "What is the meaning of life?" I hope you will look to your occupations as one way of answering this important question.

Journaling Activities

1. Look up and write down a dictionary definition of meaning, culture, and spirituality. Highlight the component of the definition that is most related to the descriptions of these terms in Chapter Six.
2. Identify the most important new learning for you in this chapter.
3. Identify one question you have about Chapter Six.
4. Reflect on the meaning of an occupation in your life using a process similar to the one discussed in the chapter and in the reflection section. This occupation may be a past or current occupation. Discuss the following in your journal entry for Chapter Six.
   - Describe an occupation that has meaning to you.
   - Describe the meanings of this occupation to you in terms of the following:
     - Culture
     - Spirituality
     - Flow
     - Storying
   - How has this occupation changed over time?
   - How is this occupation embedded in other aspects of your life?
   - How does this occupation relate to your habits, routines, or lifestyles?

Technology/Internet Learning Activities

1. Use a discussion database to share specific journal entries or individual learning activities.
2. Use an online library or a good Internet search engine to review information on one of the following topics:
   - Flow Csikszentmihalyi or Flow Massimini
   - Emplotment
   - Phenomenology
   - Coherence or sense of coherence
   - Constructivism activity or activity theory or socio-cultural theory
3. Select three sources of information for the topic that are related to Chapter Six.
   - Document the source, the type of source (e.g., research study, theoretical paper, instructional site, etc.), the quality of the source, and your process for finding the source.
   - Conduct an informational scan of each source.
   - Document three key ideas from each source that are related to Chapter Six.
   - Summarize how each key idea contributes to your learning about the meaning of occupations (what questions do you have, what light bulbs went on, what things do you wonder about).

Applied Learning

Individual Learning Activity #1: Exploring the Meaning of Work

Investigate the meaning of work for individuals.
Instructions:

- Ask three people to participate in a brief interview about their work (Note: If at all possible, select people of different ages/backgrounds and who have different types of work).
- Document the job title for their work.
- Document the top five responsibilities they have as part of their work.
- Document the positive aspects or meanings of work from their perspective.
- Document the negative aspects or meanings of work from their perspective.
- Summarize the similarities and differences in meaning of work for these three individuals.

Individual Learning Activity #2: Examining the Meaning and Meta-Meaning of an Occupation

Investigate the meaning of an occupation from the perspective of another person.
Instructions:

- Select an occupation that you would not like doing (e.g., marathon running, watching wrestling, ironing).
- Find a person who does like the occupation and performs it regularly.
- Interview the person regarding the meaning of the occupation and a story (or two) about the occupation in his or her life.
- Document the meaning of the occupation for this person.
- Describe how this meaning is different from your own for this occupation.

Individual Learning Activity #3: Emplotment of an Occupation or Experience

Analyze the meaning and plot of an occupation at two different points in time.
Instructions:

- Select an occupation or experience that had one meaning at one point in time and can be re-evaluated now (e.g., a school experience, a family ritual, a coming-of-age event).
- Describe the occupation or experience from your perspective at that point in time—details, meaning, feelings, perceptions, attitudes, etc.
- Describe the occupation or experience from your perspective now—details, meaning, feelings, perceptions, attitudes, etc.

  (Note: It was hard for me to identify an occupation or experience that would work for this activity until I started thinking about it. Maybe a couple of examples will help you get started. When I was an adolescent, I remember numerous family or community events in which my parents said, "you have to go." You can imagine my perspective as a 16-year-old, I'm sure. Now, I look back at some of those experiences quite differently. I also remember some experiences in my youth that seemed like total failures. Now, I can look at those same experiences as a personal growth opportunity.)

Active Learning

Group Learning Activity #1: Jigsaw Learning of Key Topics in Chapter Six

Preparation:

- Read Chapter 6.

- Review instructions for Technology/Internet Learning Activity #2.
- Assign one topic from the list to each individual in a group.

Time: 45 minutes to 1 hour
Materials: Flip chart, chalk board, white board, or virtual discussion space
Instructions:

- Individually (use instructions from Technology/Internet Learning Activity #2):
  - ✧ Research your assigned topic.
  - ✧ Prepare a summary on your assigned topic.
- In small groups:
  - ✧ Teach the topic to the rest of the group members.
- In a large group:
  - ✧ If there is more than one group, the groups may share summaries of each topic with other groups.

Small or Large Group Discussion:

- Was the "meaning of occupation" a key idea or just one component of each topic?
- What other words were used to describe occupations?
- How might this topic help us in our understanding of the meaning of occupations?
- What questions did you have as you learned more about each topic?

Group Learning Activity #2: A Historical and Futuristic View of the Meaning of Occupation

Preparation: Read Chapter Six
Time: 30 to 45 minutes
Materials: Flip chart, chalk board, white board, or virtual discussion space
Instructions:

- Select an occupation that was popular in past history.
  - ✧ Describe the characteristics of the occupation then and now.
  - ✧ Describe the likely meanings of the occupation in past history (say, early 1900s).
  - ✧ Describe the meanings of this occupation today (e.g., quilting, wood-working, horse-back riding, travel, family reunions, political debates, care of pets, ironing, writing letters, listening to the radio).
- Select an occupation that is popular today.
  - ✧ Describe the characteristics of the occupation now and possibly in the future.
  - ✧ Describe the meanings of the occupation today.
  - ✧ Describe the likely meanings of the occupation in the future (say, 2050) (e.g., talking on a cell phone, visiting the library, commuting to work/school, watching a football game, space exploration, going to a movie).

Occupation:	*Past:*	*Current:*
Meanings:		
Occupation:	*Current:*	*Future:*
Meanings:		

Small or Large Group Discussion:

- Describe the characteristics of the occupations for the two time periods.
- How were the "meanings of occupation" similar and different for the two time periods?
- How did the "lived experience" for different periods of time influence the meanings?
- What types of stories did you imagine as being associated with the meanings of these occupations at different points in time?
- What other occupations have had (or will have) changes in their meanings over time?

Chapter Seven Objectives

The information in this chapter is intended to help the reader:

1. Compare and contrast various approaches for defining health.
2. Understand the relationship between health and occupational needs.
3. Understand the relationship between well-being and occupational needs.
4. Review the World Health Organization definition of health.
5. Understand the significance of the Ottawa Charter for Health Promotion.

Key Words

health: According to the World Health Organization, a state of complete physical, mental, and social well-being, not merely the absence of disease or infirmity; defined in terms: negatively (absence of illness), positively (wellness of the organism), or having a constitutional or temperamental reserve of health or energy.

mediate, enable, advocate: Roles that health professionals need to play to build healthy public policy, create supportive environments, strengthen community action, develop personal skills, and reorient health services.

mental well-being: A feeling of contentment associated with emotional, intellectual, and spiritual satisfaction enabling effective interaction with others and peace with self.

occupation: In the context of this chapter, an agent of health that is a means of developing well-being according to individual capacities in conjunction with environmental demands.

occupational balance: A regular mix of physical, mental, social, spiritual, and rest occupations that provide an overall feeling of well-being.

occupational justice: The just and equitable distribution of power, resources, and opportunity so that all people are able to meet the needs of their occupational natures without compromising the common good.

physical well-being: A feeling of bodily health and wellness.

social well-being: A feeling of contentment and freedom in interpersonal relationships enabling the development of ideas and action deemed of benefit to society. Also applicable to communities and societies at large.

well-being: An individual perception of a state of happiness, physical and mental health, peace, confidence, and self-esteem that for many is associated with occupations, relationships, and environments.

Our greatest happiness does not depend on the condition
of life in which chance has placed us,
but is always the result of a good conscience, good health,
occupation, and freedom in all just pursuits.
Thomas Jefferson

Chapter Seven

Relationship of Occupations to Health and Well-Being

Ann A. Wilcock, PhD, RegOT(SA)

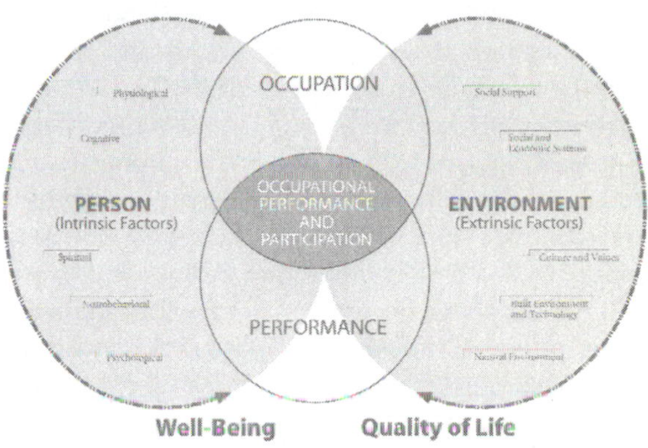

Setting the Stage

In this chapter, the relationship of occupation to health and well-being is explored. The discussion begins by contrasting definitions of health as well-being with those centered on health as absence of disease. It is argued that occupation is a natural human need that must be met for physiological, developmental, psychological, and sociocultural reasons. The chapter then explores how environmental contexts create differing definitions of health and well-being across individuals and communities and concludes with a discussion of how occupation influences happiness and well-being.

Wilcock, A. A. (2005). Relationship of occupations to health and well-being. In C. H. Christiansen, C. M. Baum, and J. Bass-Haugen (Eds.), Occupational therapy: Performance, participation, and well-being *(3rd ed.). Thorofare, NJ: SLACK Incorporated.*

INTRODUCTION

In this chapter, the relationship of occupation to health and well-being will be explored. The discussion picks up on the call for the reorientation of all health professionals toward the pursuit of health as well as the absence of illness made by the World Health Organization (WHO) nearly three decades ago, which has still to be taken seriously. That call provides authority to claim good health and well-being as laudable and desirable objectives in their own right. However, as Rene Dubos maintained in the 1950s:

> Solving problems of disease is not the same thing as creating health and happiness. This task demands a kind of wisdom and vision which transcends specialized knowledge of remedies and treatments and which apprehends in all their complexities and subtleties the relation between living things and the total environment. (Dubos, 1959)

Occupation as an agent of health and well-being is very much needed in the 21st century. The idea of it as an agent of health and well-being has a solid foundation that is at least 2,400 or so years old. So, it is not a new thought, but those of earlier ages are hidden in unfamiliar words and contexts and often were addressed not as central issues but as a part of different concepts. Indeed, thought and action about occupation for health and well-being cross cultural boundaries, disciplines, thought, and time.

In seeking to clarify people's ideas about the relationships between health, well-being, and occupation, it is important to recall that, in present times, in postindustrialized societies, the ideas held and practices followed are dominated by medical science, which limits the acceptability or even the possibility of considering the subject from another perspective. This is not suggesting that the medical science approach is necessarily incorrect, but that it can be added to from other knowledge bases to improve future attempts to enhance health and well-being. Additionally, and in part because of acceptance of a medical science view, current social and political thinking fails to fully acknowledge people's need for a range of meaningful occupation for their health's sake, recognizing it principally as an economic requirement.

Because of the limited appreciation of occupation as an agent of health and well-being, it is necessary to consider each separately and as a part of that fundamental relationship. The discussion in this chapter will start and finish with that task. It will also discuss the WHO's holistic view of health and well-being. WHO's view includes appreciation that there is an association between positive health and what people do. That will be followed by considering occupation mainly as a physiological mechanism for health, as a means of enabling individual capacities for well-being, and as a sociopolitical determinant of health and well-being.

HEALTH IN RELATION TO OCCUPATION

In seeking to understand health from an occupational perspective, it is helpful to begin before the relationship became complicated by modern medical ideas, which is one reason to take an historical approach as a foundation to consider the present. The notions that emerge from that exploration provide questions for modern research, which is still in its infancy. In each section, an attempt will be made to define or describe essential concepts.

Health as a Physiological State

Researchers in different countries and from a range of disciplines recognize that ideas, definitions, and descriptions of health differ. Herzlich, for example, studied a mainly middle class group of "lay" individuals from Paris and Normandy and found that people described health according to three main dimensions: negatively as the absence of illness, positively as a state of "equilibrium" or wellness, and thirdly as having a constitutional or temperamental "reserve of health," which could be drawn upon (Herzlich, 1973). A more recent exploration of views about health and lifestyles, sampling 9,000 adults in the United Kingdom, is helpful with regard to how widespread such ideas might be among the population (Blaxter, 1990). Mildred Blaxter's survey revealed that people describe health variously, principally elicited from two questions:

> (1) Think of someone you know who is very healthy. Who are you thinking of? How old are they? What makes you call them healthy? (2) At times people are healthier than at other times. What is it like when you are healthy? (Blaxter, 1990, p. 16)

How those questions were answered will be discussed throughout the chapter where most appropriate.

Despite many attempts, it appears that health is a concept that many find difficult to define in a positive sense because it is often not thought about seriously until someone experiences a state of illness. Definitions and descriptions from a negative absence of illness or a positive wellness stance will be discussed in this section of the chapter.

Health Defined Negatively

It certainly appears easier to define health by default; that is, by reflecting on ill-health and its consequences to understand health in a functional or positive sense. Yet, concepts of ill health differ between societies and individuals. There are those who regard illness as the consequence of evil or due to the wrath of the gods. There are some who suggest it is a direct consequence of social disadvantage and others who regard it as a mechanistic breakdown due to congenital or environmental causes. Some regard people with physical disability as ill, or certainly not healthy, and others hold that psychosocial illness has no similarity with illness manifesting physical symptoms.

Doyal and Gough provide an absence of illness description with a combined physiological and occupational message in their award winning book, *A Theory of Human Need:*

> Physical health can be thought of transculturally in a negative way. If you wish to lead an active and successful life in your own terms, it is in your own objective interest to satisfy your basic need to optimize your life expectancy and to avoid serious physical disease and illness conceptualized in biomedical terms. This applies to everyone, everywhere. (Doyal & Gough, 1991, p. 59)

Blaxter (1990) found, among her respondents, that about 15% of the people surveyed couldn't think of anyone who was healthy, and about 10% couldn't describe how it felt, or didn't think about health. Some who couldn't describe it seemed to imply that "health" felt ordinary. It was the "norm" and therefore without qualities that could be described. As one 28-year-old office worker said, "I don't think I know when I'm healthy; I only know if I'm ill" (p. 20). This group tended to be people who did not value health highly and elderly respondents who often saw their own health as poor.

Another group described health as "not suffering any symptoms, never having anything more serious than a cold, never seeing the doctor, having no aches and pains" or really serious illnesses and "never having had to go to hospital." This "not-ill" description of health was given in relation to others by about 37% of the respondents, but only by about 13% in response to their own health. It was "markedly associated with the [respondent's] own state of health" and surprisingly more often by those who were not suffering illness. Additionally, despite the idea being previously thought more characteristic of the socially disadvantaged, in this case, the response was "more frequently used by the better educated and those with higher incomes" (Blaxter, 1990, pp. 20-21).

Health Defined Positively

In considering the other extreme, Kass (1981), who offers his own positive description, explains that it is not possible to define health precisely. In 1981, though, he provided the following simple attempt, which is particularly useful. Health, he said, is "the well-working of the organism as a whole."

He added a more complex rider, which is similar to the idea of health as feeling ordinary suggested earlier, but also links it with "doing" so giving that idea a more positive slant. It is, he said:

> A natural standard or norm—not a moral norm, not a value as opposed to a fact, not an obligation, but a state of being that reveals itself in activity as a standard of bodily exercise or fitness, relative to each species and to some extent to individuals, recognizable if not definable and to some extent attainable.

Kass' linkage of a "state of being" with "activity" also anticipates the notion of people as "occupational beings."

In Blaxter's study, positive descriptions included ideas about health, most of which had occupational implications, such as physical fitness, energy, being functionally able, being psychosocially fit, and healthy behavior. Respondents who defined health as healthy behavior were mainly young people or those with less education. They "stressed the role of 'bad habits' in the causation of disease and the importance of self-responsibility" by associating health with not drinking or smoking, "virtuous" eating patterns, and exercise. It was also among younger people that physical fitness was strongly identified with health. While young men "stressed strength, athletic prowess, [and] the ability to play sports," young women frequently defined "physical fitness in terms of its outward appearance," commonly mentioning body size and the condition of complexion, eyes, and hair (Blaxter, 1990, pp. 20-23).

Many would resist the idea that people with disabilities are labeled as sick. It is, therefore, gratifying to learn that in Blaxter's study, "many disabled and/or elderly people insisted on calling their health 'excellent.'" Additionally, in describing health for others, some people with disability or "suffering from serious conditions" were called "healthy because they coped so well" (Blaxter, 1990, pp. 22-32).

Energy was "the word most frequently used by all women and older men to describe health, and for younger men it came a close second to fitness." Respondents referred to either physical energy or psychosocial vitality or combined them. They used words such as being "lively, alert, full of get up and go, full of life, not tired, not listless." For many young men, "not staying in bed appeared to mark really positive healthiness," while for older men, the "concept of energy and vitality was most often expressed as enthusiasm about work" as it was for women of any age. Women also "defined health as '...doing everything easily, feeling like conquering the world, being keen and interested, lots of get up and go,' ... [and] 'having the energy to be with other people.'" Indeed, women were considerably more likely to define health, especially for themselves, in terms of their relationships with other people. Those ideas overlap with the notion of health as function, which will be discussed later (Blaxter, 1990, pp. 25-27).

In beginning to build up a preliminary working definition of health in relation to occupation from a physiological point of view, Kass' notion that it is "the well-work-

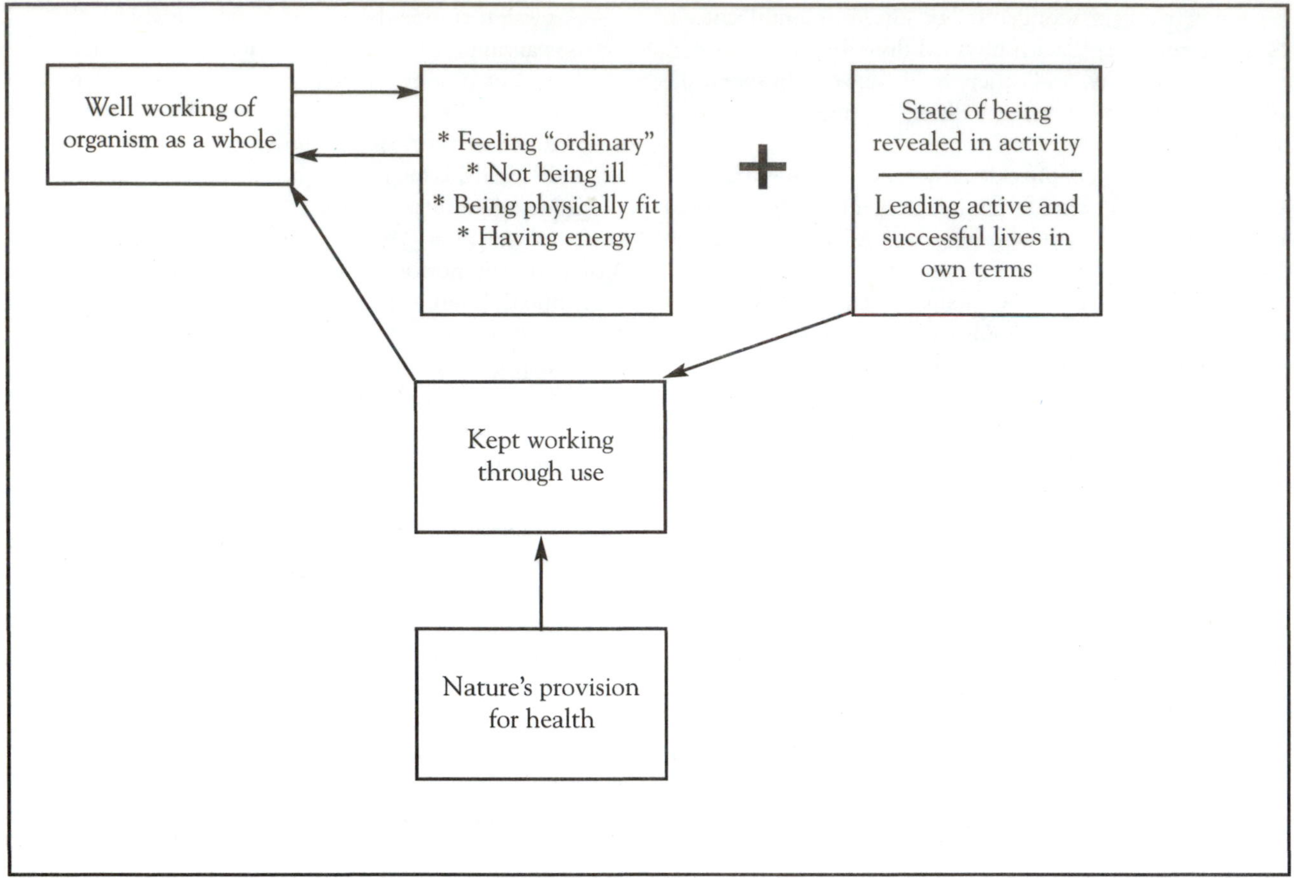

Figure 7-1. Preliminary working definition of health in relation to occupation from a physiological point of view.

ing of the organism as a whole" appears to be a useful foundation. It sits well with the array of Blaxter's findings already discussed—feeling "ordinary," not being ill, being physically fit, and having energy. It requires a closer tie with occupation such as Doyal and Gough's phrase about individuals leading active and successful lives in their own terms and Kass' other term that health was a "state of being that reveals itself in activity." Both of those are profoundly important because it is through actively and regularly engaging in a well-balanced range of occupations that the organism as a whole works well. Feeling "ordinary," being physically fit and having energy, and even not being ill depends to a great extent on keeping all parts of the body, brain, and mind working well through use. As the medical historian Sigerist (1955) commented, "Work is essential to the maintenance of health because it not only determines the chief rhythm of our life, balances it, and gives meaning and significance" but also because "an organ that does not work atrophies and the mind that does not work becomes dumb" (p. 254-255). That is one of nature's major provisions for health (Figure 7-1).

Nature's Occupational Provision for Health

That occupation is one of nature's major provisions for health may be easier to appreciate if it is first considered in respect to animals other than human beings. Animals who lead a natural life within their ecological niche, if it is not affected by environmental degradation, tend to be healthy and to exhibit the appearance of well-being and satisfaction. This doesn't mean that all live a long life or that high infant mortality is not the norm, but that those who survive are more than able to resist disease and infection because they are adapted to the resident pathogens, risks, and predators that are constituents of their ecosystems. As a part of their natural lifestyle, the animals engage in occupations to meet their needs and requirements for survival. For example, they find food and water, often picking out specific herbage if they feel unwell, select or make shelter, interact with others, educate their young, explore, play, and observe their world. It is through such occupations that the animals maintain and enhance physical fitness, stimulate their mental capacities toward future challenges, and build a supportive community that will be protective in times of need. They keep in "good shape" and they keep healthy through their ongoing interaction with the environment, through what they do, and through being true to their species' nature (Wilcock, 1998a).

It was the same for early humans. They, too, kept in "good shape" and healthy through their ongoing interaction with the environment, through what they did, and through being true to their species' nature (McNeill, 1979; Stephenson, 1972). Dunton was quite correct when he suggested in his credo "that occupation is as necessary to life as food and drink" (Reed & Sanderson, 1980). Our species' nature was, and still is, decidedly occupational. Archeological and anthropological opinion suggests that, throughout their existence, humans have engaged in occupation in a more complex manner than other animals, often in response to sociocultural factors (Bronowski, 1973; Campbell, 1988; Jones, Martin, & Pilbeam, 1992). Such interaction supports Ornstein and Sobel's (1988) claim that "the major role of the brain is to mind the body and maintain health" through making "countless adjustments," which preserves stability between "social worlds, our mental and emotional lives, and our internal physiology" (pp. 11-12). With that in mind, it becomes clear that the need to engage in occupation is fundamental when considering health from a physiological point of view.

Since time immemorial, people have proclaimed that living a "natural life" is health giving. Many early civilizations held legends of a long past Golden Age central within their communal beliefs in which people were not at odds with nature and that they were, as a consequence, happy, healthy, and long lived. The Greeks placed theirs in distant places and the Chinese, the remote past. In civilized societies, similar beliefs are rationalized as philosophical theories particularly concerned with harmonizing life with the ways of nature. That is as true today, with increasing interest being shown in "natural remedies" and the proliferation of alternative therapies, as it was in the 18th century when Jean-Jacques Rousseau maintained "that man in his original state was good, healthy and happy and that all his troubles came from the fact that civilization had spoiled him physically and corrupted him mentally" (Dubos, 1959, pp. 7-8).

Apart from such legends, early in the history of humankind, it is known that people lived a very different kind of life from the present, fitting into a self-balancing, self-regulating ecological system. They preyed on other life forms and were prey to them. Health care as we know it did not exist, and yet medical archeologists have gathered a substantial amount of evidence to convince them that people living in those times experienced very little infection (Dobson, 1992). Within a natural environment, the major morbidity and mortality concerns had to do with accidents; predators; adequate nutrition; and occasional disturbances such as drought, fire, and floods. As the population of people began to increase, dominate the food chain, and to adapt, as well as adapt to, different habitats, they transformed the balance of nature through engagement in different occupations. At the same time, they altered patterns of disease. It is obvious in those early days that it was through their occupations that they met the other requirements of life, kept bodies and minds fit, and skills honed through using them in the ordinary course of life.

That natural process has not changed despite its being obscured by the processes of civilization. In 1931, John Maynard Keynes, the economist, observed that "the struggle for subsistence always has been hitherto the primary, most pressing problem of the human race... Thus we have been expressly evolved by nature" (Keynes, 1931). If this need is removed:

> Mankind will be deprived of its traditional purpose... Thus for the first time since his creation man will be faced with his real, his permanent problem—how to use his freedom... how to occupy the leisure, to live wisely and agreeably and well... It is a fearful problem for the ordinary person, with no special talents, to occupy himself, especially if he no longer has roots in the soil or in the custom or in the beloved conventions of a traditional society. (Keynes, 1931)

Some 70 years later, without fully understanding the fundamental health purposes of occupation, humankind is indeed faced with a fearful problem. In part, this is due to the fact that health-maintaining needs and functions, rather like the autonomic nervous system, are built into the organism to just go on working. In part, it is due to little being written in mainstream health care about the benefits of a natural lifestyle or of the need for a balance of ongoing physical, mental, and social occupations as integral aspects of health. There is equally scant information about people as occupational beings and the inbuilt consequences of that.

Health and Occupational Needs

It is possible to state, quite categorically, that people have "occupational needs" that are related to health. They prompt "the doing of 'something'" to overcome physiological, psychological, or social discomfort to maintain the well-working of the organism. For example, they prompt the gathering, preparing, or eating of food. They prompt the sharing of tasks or the need to find an antidote for pain. They can be considered the species' primary health mechanism because the occupations they prompt are the means of providing the other basic requirements of life. They predate and, in a way, led to the development of medical science, which in those terms can be regarded as "the doing of something" to alter the experience of illness (Wilcock, 1998a).

Doyal and Gough (1991) remind us that:

> Our mammalian constitution shapes our needs for such things as warmth and food in order to survive and maintain health. Our cognitive aptitudes and the bases of our emotionality in childhood (due to human children's relatively early birth because of brain size, and subsequent dependence) shape many other needs—for supportive and close relationships with others, for example. (p. 37)

"Need" is defined as a "human requirement" (Norton, 1980). Doyal and Gough (1991) recognize need has a "biological background." It is not, as they write:

> Disconnected from 'human nature,' or to the physiological and psychological make-up of homo sapiens. To argue for such disconnection would be to identify humanity with no more than human reason and to bifurcate human existence from that of the rest of the animal world. (pp. 35-36)

Other useful "occupationally focused" definitions of need date from the 1970s, such as that it is "the condition of lacking, wanting, or requiring something which if present would benefit the organism by facilitating behavior or satisfying a tension," and also "a construct representing a force in the brain which directs and organizes the individual's perception, thinking and action, so as to change an existing, unsatisfying situation" (Wolman, 1973, p. 250). In that way, "needs" relate to facilitating what is required for living organisms to maintain health and to experience well-being (Watts, 1985). To do that, "needs" serve to overcome physiological, psychological, or social discomfort such as pain, boredom, or loneliness, which demand some kind of action; to protect and prevent potential disorder, needs stimulate and motivate the exercise of capacities; and to reward use, so that the organism will continue to work well, the needs for purpose, satisfaction, fulfillment, and pleasure are common experiences. Such physiological needs are structured to interact and provide feedback (Wilcock, 1993a).

To ensure the well-working of the organism as a whole, occupational needs that stimulate and motivate the exercise of capacities are associated with people's physical make-up such as their bipedal gait, unique hand structure, and highly developed brain. The latter is evolved to such an extent that, for example, it enables language; creativity; adaptation to different environments or the ability to change them; fulfillment of needs for belonging; exercise of biological capacities for scholarship, exploration, and adventure; and development of potential, to maintain the well-working of the organism (Wilcock, 1998b).

Occupational needs are therefore inborn health agents integral to the collaboration between biological rhythms and homeostasis (Campbell, 1998), which link the organism with the environment as part of an "open system," relating structures and function and not differentiating between the physical, mental, or social (Bertalanffy, 1968). That is a simplification of many complex systems, but it is useful if it enables an appreciation of occupations' fundamental purposes, which can easily be overlooked in the detail of complexity.

Health as a Concept Dependent on Environmental and Sociocultural Context

The idea of what health is depends to a great extent upon environmental and sociocultural contexts. That becomes very apparent when immersed in data from periods other than the present. Two examples of health beliefs that differ from the present will be briefly described to clarify the effects of context on fundamental concepts, such as the relationship between health and occupation.

The first to be discussed is the classical period in Greece, when modern medicine is said to have had its genesis. During that time, the use of specific occupations as part of health care formed part of the daily lives of most citizens. Indeed, physical occupations for strength and beauty were seen as important enough to warrant state intervention, and their use is reflected in the tales and poetry of master story-tellers, in the myths of the gods and religious medicine, in philosopher's views as they queried the essence of all things, as well as in the recommendations of physicians who are immortalized in today's culture. By the 18th century, Fuller was still advising people of the use of occupations as advocated by Herodicus, Hippocrates, Mercurialis, and Galen (Wilcock, 2001).

Although a variety of occupations were recognized as health giving, it was hardly surprising in a world in which wars and conquest were commonplace that youth and occupations deemed to promote strength and physical beauty were considered of more value than others. Not dissimilar in some ways to today when, driven by marketplace agendas, youth and physical beauty are once more ascendant, gymnasia and physical exercise reigned supreme as healthful occupation. The idea of wisdom and of music, however, was also linked with the older gymnasia, which, in ancient Greece, were general places of learning. Mental and physical exercises were carried out alongside each other, in part, because there was a strong belief in mind and body interaction and in the notion of "balance." It was believed that illness resulted from imbalance of the four humors and that a physician's job was to advise on due proportion, to "restore a healthy balance" to aid "the natural healing powers believed to exist in every human being" (Wilcock, 1998b, p. 137).

One aspect of classical health beliefs that differs most from those highly regarded by occupational therapists was the difference made between the health needs of slaves and of citizens. That was founded on, what would be now, a totally unacceptable notion that the mundane activities of daily life concerned with people's "physiological" requirements were inhuman, unhealthy, and brutalizing. Indeed, that notion resulted in the citizens needing to invent the gymnasia to replace the health giving effects of daily occupation, which they attempted to eradicate from their lives. Some insightful writers of the times did allude to the fact that slaves were generally healthy because they engaged in a variety of occupations (Wilcock, 2001).

The second period to be discussed in relation to a difference in views about health is the Middle Ages. Health care during that period was dominated by monasticism, so it follows that the mainstream approach was spiritual. The view held at the time was that life on earth was merely to provide the gateway to everlasting happiness or purgatory and that it was more important to maintain and develop spiritual health than that of the body. With that belief, the occupations that were chosen were different, overwhelmingly emphasizing the spirit rather than the corporeal. They were used as a medium of spiritual health and recovery, the obvious choice being prayer. Participation in crusades met the needs of some, and pilgrimages to holy places, shrines, and relics, which were popular with rich and poor alike, became the precursor of the health enhancing "holidays" of modern times. In addition to that, labor was seen as an essential component of spiritual wellness while good or moral occupation led to good health or the opposite to sickness.

Monastic medicine played a large part in transmitting the medical ideas of the classical world into the future and was instrumental in the development of the growth of secular, university-based medicine. Within that context, occupation, as physical exercise, was one important principle to maintain and promote health based on Galen's understanding of that process. Indeed, the growth of medicine, which promulgated old medical knowledge, was underpinned by a preventive approach within which occupation, while not playing the most important role—which was given to food—was integral to more than one of the six rules of a regimen based on the humoral view of physiology. That view of health and the health message of the regimen was to last until the 19th century and was broadcast to rich and poor alike, as well as medical men, through professional and lay texts and popular verses (Wilcock, 2001).

Health as Differing According to Individuals and Communities

Notions of health not only differ according to environmental or sociocultural context, but also among individuals and between communities within the same time span. For individuals, those different notions are part of their uniqueness. Despite obvious species, ethnic, and family characteristics that are similar, every individual differs somewhat. Not even identical twins have "the exact pattern of nerve cells... at the same time and place" (Edelman, 1992, p. 64). Nor have they exactly corresponding numbers of branches of any one neuron because of developmental "cellular processes such as cell division, movement and death" (Edelman, 1992, p. 25). Indeed, "the kinds of unique individuality in our brain networks makes that of fingerprints or facial features appear gross and simple by comparison" (Sperry, 1982, pp. 209-219). In the cerebral cortex alone, it has been estimated that there are between 20 and 100 billion neurons, and about one million billion connections, all of which are capable of many combinations so that "the sheer number and density of neuronal networks in the brain" reaches "hyperastronomical" figures and "the brain might be said to be in touch more with itself than with anything else" (Ornstein & Sobel, 1988, p. 39). In addition to that, as geneticists and biologists come closer to understanding the structure and function of genes by using biochemical technology, "they have uncovered inherited variation at almost every level of organization" to the extent that "it is certain that every human being who has lived or ever will live is genetically unique" (Jones, 1992, pp. 264-267). This suggests that, despite commonalities of family, community, and experience, individuals could be more likely than not to hold different concepts to each other.

Having said that, it is important to bear in mind that, because of our genetic make-up, nurture also plays a part in how people think. Csikszentmihalyi and Csikszentmihalyi (1988) remind us that:

> ...at a certain point in ontogenesis, each individual begins to realize his or her own powers to direct attention, to think, to feel, to will, and to remember. At that point, a new agency develops within awareness. This is the self. ()

With knowledge of the self comes an increased need to conform with others of the species (Csikszentmihalyi & Csikszentmihalyi, 1988). That reminder provides explanation for the communal similarities in the ways we think.

In terms of health concepts, the individuality of people makes sense of Blaxter's array of findings, as well as her conclusions that views of health differ over the life course, have clear gender differences, and are, for most, a multidimensional concept. She found that there were other ways than those mentioned above of what health is to different people. About 14% of respondents chose the notion of "health as function" to describe health for someone else, particularly when talking about men or about the elderly, and more than 30% defined health for themselves in functional terms. Although important for all age groups, it was more frequently mentioned by middle-aged to older people and incorporated ideas about being able to perform physically demanding work, "social, family, and community activity," to "work despite an advanced age," to do "extra work," or "being fit to work," as well as "being mobile or self-sufficient." Some, including the young, saw health as "being able to do what you want to when you want to," and a few said, "simply and explicitly that 'health is freedom.'" Another way, often associated with health as energy, as social relationships, or as function was the description of health as psychosocial well-being. For some, it was a separate concept used to describe spirituality, mental alertness, happiness, enjoyment, and a relaxed attitude. For those in "the middle years, [this] was the most popular concept" for describing self-health particularly for women and by those with more education (Blaxter, 1990, pp. 28-29).

It is obvious that individuals, more often than not, adopt major concepts that are common among the population into which they were born or in which they live, as is the case in postindustrial societies, which, largely, accept a medical science view of health. The differences are often variations of a general community understanding or are the result of personal experiences that made a lasting impression.

Within postindustrial capitalist communities, it is easy to disregard broader concepts of health that relate to families, communities, and to the ecology in favor of an individualistic medical science view. Some other societies, often living a more natural life, such as Australian aboriginals, place as much, if not more, value on kin and community than individuality. It is not surprising, therefore, to find that the Australian Aboriginal Health Organization defines health as "the social, emotional, spiritual, and cultural well-being of the whole community." They recommend that "health services should strive to achieve that state where every individual can achieve [his or her] full potential as a human being and thus bring about total well-being of [his or her] community as a whole" (Agius, 1993, p. 23).

Communities were and still are a fundamental source of protection and succor to many peoples, where the good of "tribe" is appreciated to be at least as important as individual survival. Indeed, such people often have difficulty in understanding why those living in postindustrial societies "have become alienated from the most fundamental truth of our nature, our spiritual oneness with the living universe," and our dependence on maintaining it's physical health, as well as our own (The Asian NGO Coalition, 1993) (Figure 7-2).

Well-Being in Relation to Occupation

Defining well-being is a start to the process of relating it to occupation and health, but as could be expected, it also varies. For example, in *Roget's New Thesaurus of Synonyms and Antonyms* (Roget, 1972), it stands with words like *happiness* and *prosperity* as well as *health*. In an 80s Resource Center for Health and Well-being brochure, it is defined as "a state that transcends the limitations of body, space, time, and circumstances, and reflects the fact that one is at peace with one's self and with others" (Johnson & Schmit, 1986, pp. 753-758); within the health promotion fraternity as "a subjective assessment of health [that] is less concerned with biological function than with feelings such as self-esteem and a sense of belonging through social integration" (Nutbeam, 1986, p. 126); and within an earlier edition of this textbook as "one's sense of contentment and order," and finding meaning, acceptance, and belonging in one's life (Depoy & Kolodner, 1991, p. 312-313). In the Ottawa Charter for Health Promotion, well-being is linked with everyday life, with opportunity for personal development, and with caring communities (WHO, 1986).

Psychologists have long been interested in trying to understand, describe, and measure well-being in various aspects of life, such as Bradburn who considered its structure (Bradburn, 1969), Andrews and Withey (1976) who explored social indicators, and Diener (1984) who looked at it as a subjective phenomenon. In related studies, it has been linked with income, employment, social supports, community adhesion, perceived status and marital state, education, religious attitudes, beliefs and activities, the quality of the environment, and quality of life generally (Argyle, 1987; Burckardt, Woods, Schultz, & Ziebarth, 1989; Cohen et al., 1982; Homel & Burns, 1989; Isaksson, 1990; Koeing, Kvale, & Ferrel, 1988; McConatha & McConatha, 1985; Ullah, 1990; Warr, 1990). In some instances, it is used interchangeably with "wellness." That term, which has become increasingly popular, embraces a range of notions about what are deemed to be healthy behaviors, such as physical fitness; not smoking; not overeating or drinking excessively; adequate and regular sleep and meals; meaningful and productive work; and loving, caring relationships (Gross, 1980), all of which link well-being firmly with holistic notions of health (Figure 7-3).

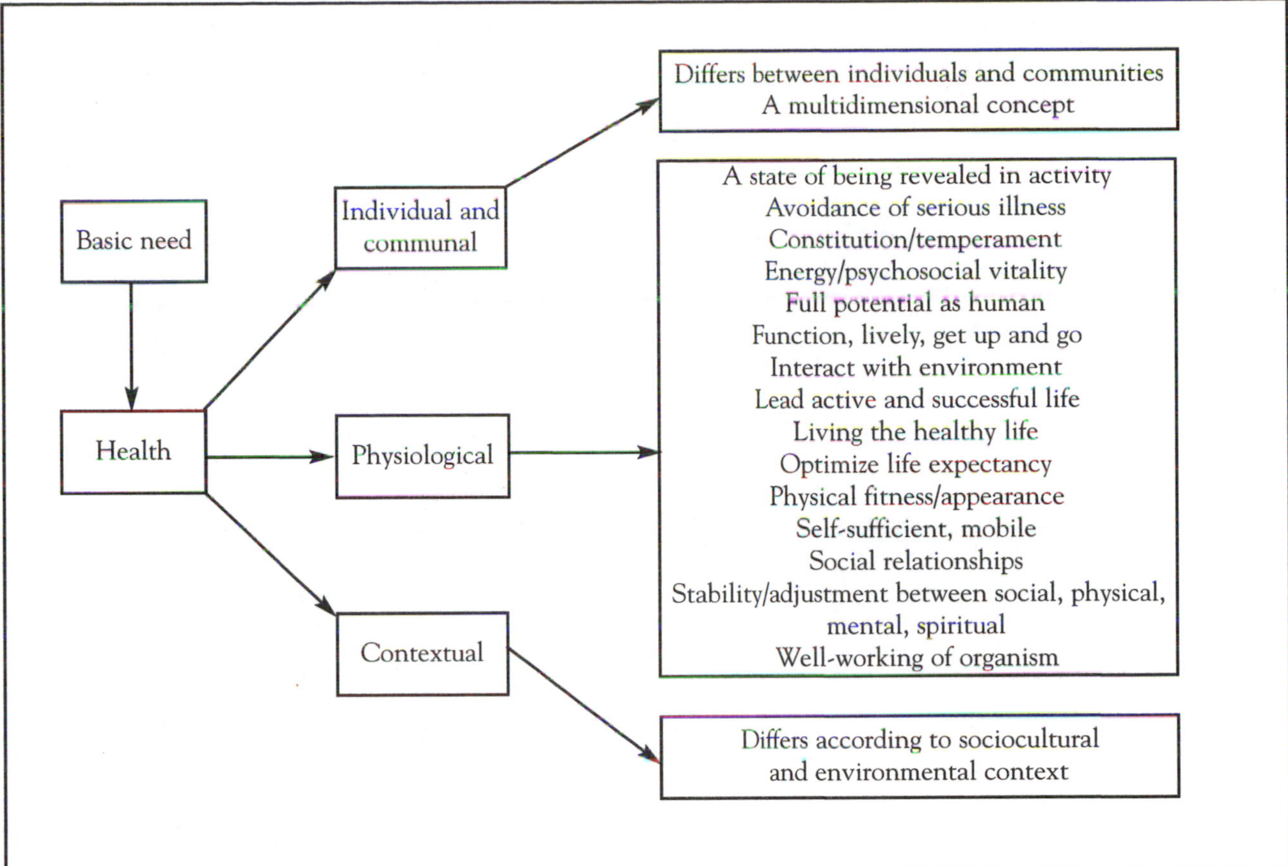

Figure 7-2. Health defined.

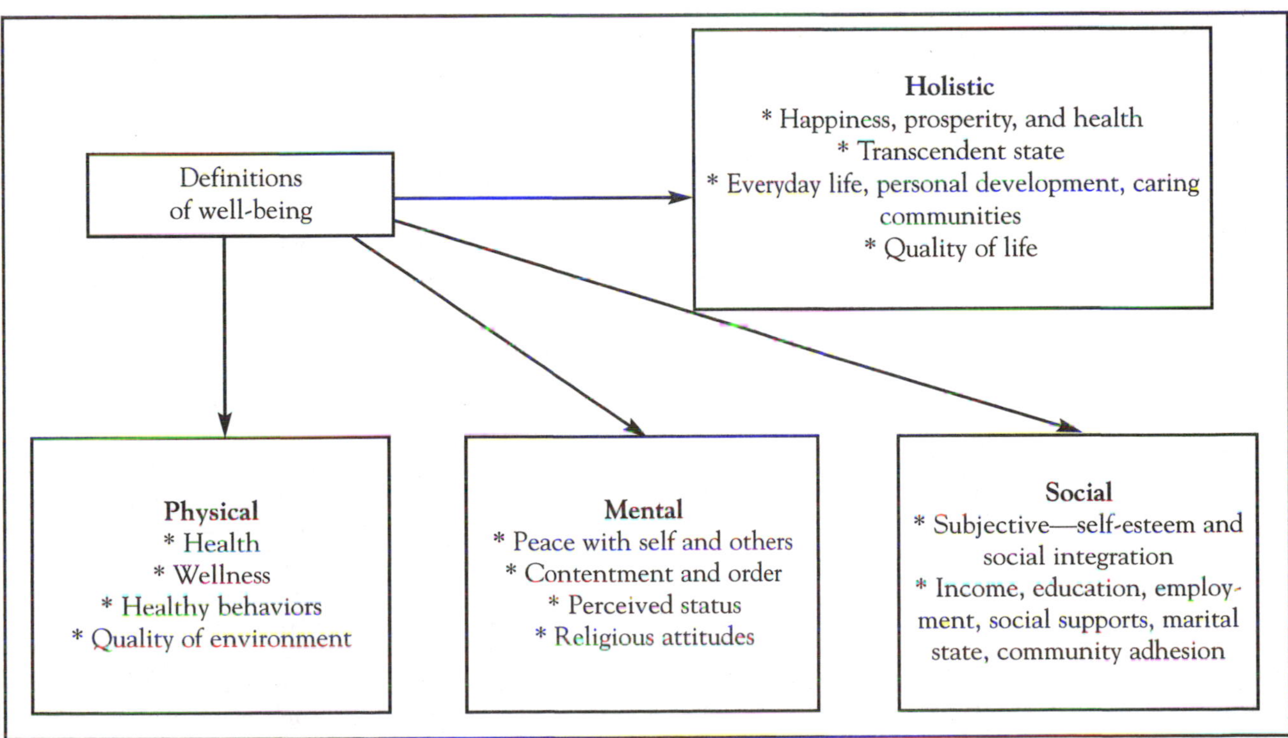

Figure 7-3. Definitions of well-being.

Well-Being as Related to Health

Well-being has long been associated with concepts about health. Athenian statesman Pericles, sometime between 490 to 429 BC, is reputed to have defined health as the "state of moral, mental, and physical well-being [that] enables a (person) to face any crisis in life with the utmost facility and grace" (Moss, 1989, personal communication). However, in the present day, the place to start any discussion of well-being, when among health professionals, is with the WHO's definition of health coined as early as 1946. It is one of the most important definitions ever created but is referred to so often that people fail to appreciate its significance. Its description of health "as a state of complete physical, mental, and social well-being not merely the absence of disease or infirmity" has stood the test of more than 50 years of enormous strides in medical science as well as rapid social change (WHO, 1946).

Most health professionals have read it or heard it said many times. It is a definition that a significant body of health writers have kept in mind, despite some criticism about it from medical scientists that it is not only difficult to measure, but "idealistic, unattainable, and largely irrelevant" (Caplan, Englehart, & McCartney, 1981; Nutbeam, 1986, p. 113). This criticism is not surprising in view of the medicalization of health, which is apparent in countries where people have been socialized to think in terms of ill-health as a physical phenomenon for which there is a medical cure and not seriously about health relating to well-being in everyday life (Newman, 1986).

If the WHO definition is considered really seriously, it does more than suggest that health professionals cannot afford to be reductionistic. It demands exploration to find out how to achieve a state of complete physical, mental, and social well-being because there is precious little work done on it yet, which makes it difficult to take appropriate action. The WHO calls for all health professionals to reorient their practice toward positive health. Thus, it becomes important not only to understand just what is well-being, but also how it relates to engagement in occupation, for practice to be guided by more than intuitive insights.

Achieving physical, mental, and social well-being appears to call for a variety of skills and abilities, which, while they may not amount to overall "well-being" in themselves, can be viewed as prerequisites (Kanner, Coyne, Schaefer, & Lazarus, 1981). Physical well-being is, perhaps, the aspect of health that has received the most attention and is the easiest to understand. When people are able to experience well-being in a physical sense they will be able to carry out occupations they need or wish to do without undue consideration of body functioning. The experience often follows exercise, as many runners and gymnasia devotees attest. It is also well accepted that well-being achieved through use of physical capacities has an effect on overall well-being, through, for example, increased blood and oxygen supply to the brain (Kirchman, 1983; Sydney & Sheppard, 1977). Such acceptance is supported by studies such as Folkins' and Syme's (1981), which found evidence of a positive relationship between exercise, well-being, self-concept, and work ability; Chamove's (1986), which found that moderate physical exercise by people with psychiatric disorders decreased their depression, anxiety, and disruptive and psychotic behavior; increased self-concept and social well-being; and aided sleep and relaxation; and Oliver's (1972), which found that improved play and social interaction are benefits of physical education as well as growth, fitness, agility, and coordination.

Mental well-being is described in many popular texts that address healthy living, such as the *The Good Health Guide* (The Open University, 1980), *Health Through Discovery* (Dintiman & Greenberg, 1986, and *Understanding Your Health* (Payne & Hahn, 1995). Popular texts like those encompass ideas about the development of emotional, intellectual, and spiritual capacities, which, in combination, enable people to interact effectively with others, be reflective, problem solve, make decisions, cope with stress, clarify values and beliefs, be flexible, and find meaning in their lives. In similar vein, the National Mental Health Association of America describes mentally well people as those who are at ease with themselves, are not overcome or incapacitated by their own feelings despite experiencing all types of emotions, like fear, anger, love, jealousy, guilt, or joy, and are accepting of many of life's disappointments; as those who are at ease with others and are concerned about their interests, able to give and receive love, and have relationships that are satisfying and lasting; as those who are able to meet life's demands, deal with its problems, accept responsibility, and plan and establish realistic goals (Payne & Hahn, 1995).

Social well-being is dependent on satisfying interpersonal relationships within "just" cultural and social parameters that permit or encourage people to develop ideas deemed of benefit to society or to challenge injustice.

Happiness

Associated with the notion of well-being and health is that of happiness in which interest has been displayed for centuries. More recently, Argyle's personal study of the psychology of happiness found that relationships, such as marriage and other close, confiding, and supportive relationships, enhance health by both preserving the immune system and encouraging good health habits (Argyle, 1987). He also reports that socially valued activities, including religious beliefs and paid employment if it is satisfying, appear to have a positive correlation with both health and happiness. During the past decade with other social psy-

Table 7-1

Frequency of Respondents' Awareness of Well-Being

Occurrence	*Frequency*	*Percentage*
Never	1	0.75%
Rarely	17	12.3%
Occasionally	26	18.8%
Frequently	70	50.7%
Always	12	8.7%
Other	4	2.9%

(n=131; 1 missing value)

chologists, Strack, Argyle, and Schwartz (1991) also found a goodness of fit between well-being and happiness.

Well-Being as Reported by Individuals

It is important to understand what well-being means to people generally as well as to "experts." To that end, a study exploring individuals' perception and experiences of well-being was undertaken in Adelaide, South Australia (Wilcock et al., 1998). It was predicted that what constitutes well-being for different people would vary, not only because of the uniqueness of human beings, but because of the potential for variation in the physical, mental, and social dimensions frequently used to describe well-being, and because individuals may assign different levels of significance and meaning to those dimensions. That notion is supported by the many theories about well-being and by its apparent relationship with health, which is a far from static concept, but one that reflects how individuals see themselves as growing, changing people, the meaning of which alters with age.

In a survey of 138 subjects, participants were asked to define their concept of well-being, how it felt to them, and how often they experienced the feeling. The sample was made up of seven "cluster" samples from high schools, an elderly citizen's village, families, a suburban neighborhood, the city shopping center, churchgoers, and fourth-year students. Despite the mix, many of the subjects were female, single, Caucasian, and young, so similar studies need to be carried out with different sample groups.

Ninety-five percent of the sample had experienced a feeling they described as well-being, with half of them (50.7%) professing that they experienced the feeling frequently. That category included responses such as 2 to 3 times a week, 75% of the time, daily, more often than not, and most of the time. Twelve participants experienced well-being all the time, 26 occasionally, 17 rarely, and only one participant had never experienced it (Table 7-1).

The four most common responses to the question asking them to briefly describe well-being appear to support the relationship between health and well-being and between them and happiness. Forty-two percent related it to having a sound mind, 41.3% to a healthy body, 38.4% to being happy, and 31.9% to being "healthy." The next most popular response concerned concepts such as self-esteem, self-confidence, and feeling good about one's self, which make up the category "self" (29.7%) and appear to give authority to occupational therapists' concern with enabling such feelings through appropriate occupations with meaning to an individual (Table 7-2).

In describing the sorts of feeling they associated with the experience of well-being, the outstanding response was happiness (52.9%). Other feelings reported frequently were peace (35.5%) and confidence (22.5%) (Table 7-3).

In answer to a question that asked what situation or environment they associated with a feeling of well-being, the most common response related to occupations. Included within that were leisure (19.6%), achievement (15.2%), work (9.4%), rest (7.2%), selfless activity (5.1%), self-care (2.2%), and religious practices (1.4%), which when added together totaled 60% of the responses. That total does not take into account any occupations carried out in conjunction with social relationship or spiritual (as opposed to religious) situations, so it could well be that most of the sample identified some form of occupational experience as one of the circumstances associated with well-being. Of the other two most common responses, 56% concerned relationships and 37% surroundings. It appears that what people do, whom they do it with, and where they do it were deemed to be very important (Table 7-4). The key words used by participants coded in the most frequently given categories are shown in Table 7-5.

Table 7-2

Respondents' Descriptions of Well-Being

Description	*Frequency*	*Percentage*
Mind	58	42%
Body	57	41.3%
Happiness	53	38.4%
Healthy	44	31.9%
Self	41	29.7%
Relationships	21	15.2%
Occupation	11	8%
Spiritual	9	6.5%
Materialistic	5	3.6%
Other	16	11.6%

n is greater than number of respondents as some gave more than one answer.

Table 7-3

Frequency of Respondents' Descriptions of Feelings Associated With Well-Being

Feelings	*Frequency*	*Percentage*
Happiness	73	52.9%
Peace	49	35.5%
Confidence	31	22.5%
Energy	25	18.1%
Belonging	22	15.9%
Fulfillment	20	14.5%
Loving	18	13%
Control	10	7.2%
Health	8	5.8%
Freedom	8	5.8%
Relationships	7	5.1%
Fortunate	4	2.9%
Sadness	2	1.4%
Other	8	5.8%

n is greater than number of respondents as some gave more than one answer.

Table 7-4

The Situations or Environments Associated With Well-Being

Situation	*Occupation*	*Relationships*	*Surroundings*	*Health*	*Other*
	60.1%	56.5%	37%	5.8%	5.1%

These total more than 100% because some respondents gave more than one answer.

Table 7-5

Key Words in Occupation, Relationships, and Surroundings Categories

Category	*Other Key Words Included in Category*
Occupation	Work, leisure, recreation, exercise, going out, travelling, rest, relaxation, sleep, religious practices, selfless and familial activity, self-care, grooming, hairdressing, dressing up, indulgence, achievement, learning, education, personal goals
Relationships	Personal relationships, social, friends, family, partnerships, neighbors, strangers
Surroundings	Accommodation, home, school, physical, environments, weather, country, church, peace

As a result of that survey, it is possible to argue that what constitutes well-being for different people does vary and that occupation is, indeed, an important element within well-being that is closely associated with both health and happiness. From this sample, well-being might be defined as an individual perception of a state of happiness, physical and mental health, peace, confidence, and self-esteem [that] for many is associated with occupations, relationships, and environment.

Antonovsky (1990) adds yet another notion to the complexity of individual differences in well-being, which he describes as a "sense of coherence." He defines that as:

> A global orientation that expresses the extent to which one has a pervasive, enduring though dynamic feeling of confidence that (1) the stimuli deriving from one's internal and external environments in the course of living are structured, predictable, and explicit; (2) the resources are available to meet the demands posed by these stimuli; and (3) these demands are challenges, worthy of investment and engagement. (Antonovsky, 1990, p. 117)

His theory, which addresses an individual's level of coping within his or her "own boundaries," proposes that the difference between who stays well and who does not is related to his or her sense of coherence. Those with a strong sense will be better able to cope and to experience well-being. Any person's boundaries, he argues, enclose what is important to him or her and may be broad for some and narrow for others. To have a strong sense of coherence, "one need not necessarily feel that all of life is highly comprehensible, manageable, and meaningful" (Antonovsky, 1990, pp. 117-119).

Well-Being as Related to Communities and Environments

Nutbeam (1986) suggests that well-being in its entirety belongs within the broad context of a social model of health, and Doyal and Gough (1991) go so far as to suggest that "to be denied the capacity for potentially successful social participation is to be denied one's humanity" (p. 184). Notions such as those reflect the fact that, of all animals, humans have created the largest and most complex societies (Dunbar, 1992). Throughout human history, the majority of people have lived in social collectives, conforming, more or less, to the behavioral expectations and rules set by their collective, whether formally or informally. Williams (1979) argued that there are four fundamental rules of such collectives concerned with how individuals order their everyday lives to enable group goals essential for the continuance of mutual support. They cover, first, the satisfaction of basic needs for health and survival; second, adequate biological reproduction and structure for child socialization; third, transmission and understanding of necessary skills and values throughout the group; and fourth, a system of authority to ensure the rules are kept. With those rules in place, it is possible for individual action to meet social preconditions, even if meeting them is largely unconscious. Doyal and Gough (1991) reason that such collectives of individuals are a societal precondition for the satisfaction of basic needs, such as health and well-being. Giddens (1984) reasons that the processes between individual action and social structure are two-way.

If collective living is a precondition of basic needs, then it is hardly surprising that community well-being is so important or that ideas about what well-being is differs according to a community's cultural and spiritual philosophies, socially dominant views, and type of economy. One difficulty, though, in postindustrial societies is that because of the individualistic and material values that are sustained by market forces, community well-being is often not at the forefront of effort. Individuals in large urban communities can be particularly at risk of having a paucity of social contacts and, as a result, may be susceptible to stress and illness. That is, perhaps, particularly true for some people with disability, whose occupational deprivation, among other factors, leads to few personal contacts. Blaxter found that "those who had the fewest family, friendship, working, and community roles had the lowest psychosocial well-being," and "for all age/gender groups except the young men, it is obvious that low income and lack of social support are each associated with high illness" (Blaxter, 1990). Low income made no difference for men under 40 as long as there was adequate social support. She found that "not only socioeconomic circumstances and the external environment, but also the individual's psychosocial environment, carry rather more weight, as determinants of health, than healthy or unhealthy behaviors" (Blaxter, 1990, pp. 105-109, 223, 233).

Cultural forces and values add a social dimension to the relationship between occupation and well-being, which was recognized in earlier times, perhaps more so than today. For example, in the 16th century, the young king, Edward VI, son of Henry VIII, agreed that one of his royal palaces, Bridewell, should become one of only five royal hospitals within London. This he called the House of Occupations, as it was for the training and rehabilitation of the occupationally deprived and depraved, rather than for those with illness of a medical kind. Occupational health and well-being were recognized as a social and community need to prevent avoidable poverty and vice. Other examples of programs aimed at community well-being include Scottish physician W.A.F. Browne's early 19th century notion that the basis of community life in asylums for the mentally ill should be "Justice, Benevolence and Occupation" and Welsh-born Robert Owen's (1771-1858) drive toward establishing communal living and working conditions to act as a force for social change. His vision of a reformed society can be traced forward to Elizabeth Casson, the founder of the first occupational therapy school in England, through the community work of Octavia Hill in housing management, the open space movement and the establishment of the National Trust (Wilcock, 2001).

That latter example reminds us of the link between well-being and environment, which is true not only of the social environment but of the natural world. The *Ottawa Charter for Health Promotion*, which will be considered in more depth in the next section of the chapter, recognizes "the inextricable links between people and their environment [which] constitute the basis for a socio-ecological approach to health" (WHO, 1986). The *Charter* argues for:

> The conservation of natural resources throughout the world, and... the need to encourage reciprocal maintenance, to take care of each other, our communities and our natural environment... [so] that the society one lives in creates conditions that allow the attainment of health by all its members. (p. 3)

It also calls for a commitment to "address the overall ecological issue of our way of living" and to "counteract the pressures towards harmful products, resource depletion, unhealthy living conditions, and environments." In acknowledging that urgent consideration needs to be given to factors detrimental to the natural and social environment, the *Charter* can be seen to recognize the adverse results of many current occupational structures and technology, and the place of environment in health and well-being (Wilcock, 2000) (Figure 7-4).

World Health Organization's Holistic View of Health, Well-Being, and What People Do

It has already been noted that the WHO definition of health is of great importance. Another that is equally significant is the *Ottawa Charter for Health Promotion* mentioned above (WHO, 1986). It is a central document in world health policy that resulted from the combined wisdom of 212 delegates from 38 countries when they met in Ottawa at the first WHO Health Promotion Conference in 1986. It has provided the guiding principles of three further meetings in other parts of the world. It is so occupationally framed that it could have been written by an occupational therapist.

The document stresses that the favored roles of health professionals should be those of advocate, enabler, and mediator. Future directions could aim at advocating occupation for health or mediating in cases of occupational injustice. That last suggestion might prompt the question, "What is occupational justice?" Just briefly, it is a term that has made its debut during the past few years. It was featured in *An Occupational Perspective of Health*

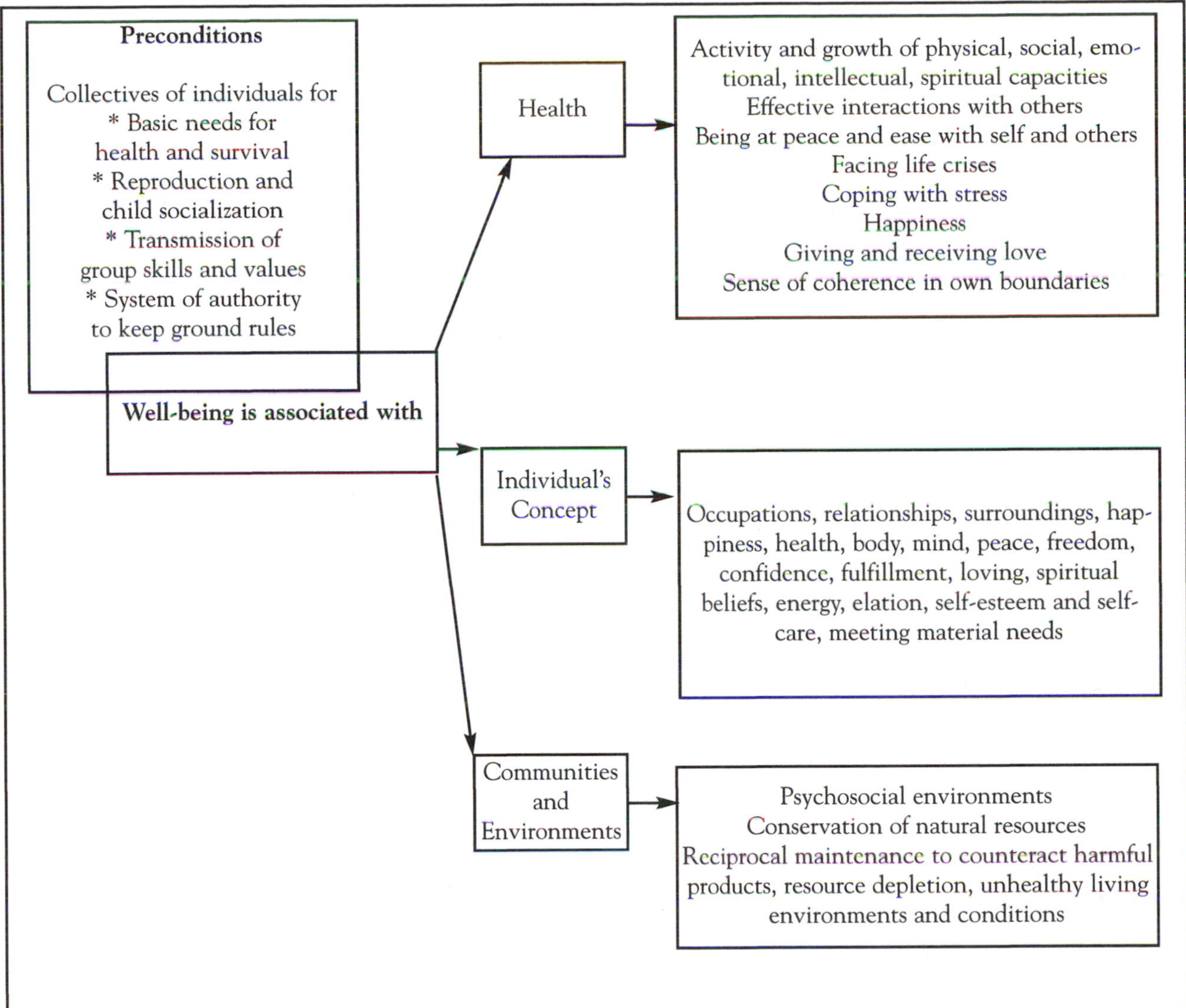

Figure 7-4. Well-being's association with health, individuals, communities, and environments.

(Wilcock, 1998b), the concept having drawn heavily upon earlier work done by Townsend (1993). In broad terms, it is about the just and equitable distribution of power, resources, and opportunity so that all people are able to meet the needs of their occupational natures and so experience health and well-being. Justice is just one of the prerequisites for health mentioned in the *Ottawa Charter*.

The *Ottawa Charter's* concern for justice is apparent in the view that "To reach a state of complete physical, mental, and social well-being, an individual or group must be able to identify and to realize aspirations, to satisfy needs, and to change or cope with the environment" (WHO, 1986, p. 2). That suggests how the WHO's definitive vision of health can be achieved. As occupation is the fundamental mechanism by which people "realize aspirations, satisfy needs, and cope with the environment," this provides a clear mandate for the further development of services to that end (Wilcock, 1993b).

The *Charter* advocates five major strategies. They are that all health professionals need to:

1. Build healthy public policy.
2. Create supportive environments.
3. Strengthen community action.
4. Develop personal skills.
5. Reorient health services toward the pursuit of health.

In support of those strategies, it goes on to argue that the promotion of health goes beyond health care, putting it on the agenda of policymakers in all sectors. It is important for everyone to build healthy public policy, not just those who are classified as needing intervention for medically diagnosed mental or physical problems. Almost a century ago, an interesting text about the history of English philanthropy said:

> Legislation is in some sense an expression of a social ideal; it is also, and perhaps more commonly, a recognition of forces already become actual. Sometimes a point of departure for major advance, it is often merely a summary of actual conditions. (Kirkman Gray, 1905, p. 35).

What are our social ideals in terms of the relationship between occupation and health? If we can articulate what they are at present and consider them of importance to all individuals, then they are of national importance, too, and need to be included in policy documents. We could ask, for example, if policies about redundancies for the sake of productivity also address the costs of unemployment, which include rises in sickness rates. In community health terms, those personal/social health costs make a mockery of reduced costs in production. Another example concerns education policies being geared more and more toward high achievers in intellectual terms. The cost of those initiatives in health terms, without opportunities also being put into place for young people with different occupational aptitudes and potentials, could be surmised as increased rates of dropouts from school, youth suicide, and substance abuse. The list of possibilities is endless, but it would be most useful if any recognition of the link used the terminology of *occupation for health* (Wilcock, 2000).

To create supportive environments, the *Ottawa Charter* advocates the generation of living and working conditions that are safe, stimulating, satisfying, and enjoyable in the knowledge that "health cannot be separated from other goals" and that "changing patterns of life, work, and leisure have a significant impact on health" (WHO, 1986, p. 3). Such living and working conditions are not created by ergonomic considerations, safe practice, performance factors, or economics alone, which tends to be the emphasis of many organizations and professionals. They are also about being stimulating, satisfying, and enjoyable from the participant's own perspective.

The *Ottawa Charter* suggests that at the heart of health promotion is the empowerment of communities, their ownership, and control of their own endeavors and destinies. Alongside that strategy, health professionals are exhorted to support personal and social development through providing information, education for health, and enhancing life skills.

In the fifth and last strategy concerned with the reorientation of health services, it is argued that the role of the health sector, as well as refocusing on the total needs of the individual as a whole person, must do the following:

- Move increasingly in a health promotion direction beyond its responsibility for providing clinical and curative services
- Give stronger attention to health research as well as make changes in professional education and training
- Change the attitude and organization of health services

People in general do not adequately understand the central place of occupation in health and well-being, and such understanding is of primary and general importance. If health practitioners move increasing in a health promotion direction, they must do the following:

- Give stronger attention to occupation for health research and make changes in professional education and training to help them enable all people to better understand occupation for health
- Work toward changing attitudes and the organization of health services to increase their understanding and inclusion of occupation for health concepts
- Refocus on the total needs of individuals as whole people including their occupational personae

Occupation for Health and Well-Being

As this textbook substantiates, there are many definitions of occupation, some narrower than others, but together they encompass the whole range of human activity whether physical, mental or social, obligatory or chosen, biological or sociocultural in origin, or, according to cultural mores, described as either work, play, or rest. Whatever definition is chosen as the guide to practice, occupation is, without doubt, a central aspect of the human experience and so much a part of everyday life and health that it is taken for granted.

Occupation: A Physiological Mechanism for Health; a Means of Developing Well-Being According to Individual Capacities; a Sociopolitical Determinant of Health and Well-Being

Despite occupation being the major natural mechanism to meet basic needs and maintain health, in the million or so years that humans have lived on earth, their everyday lives have changed almost beyond recognition. On the whole, individuals are no longer required to undertake either sustained or substantial physical occupations. They undertake them at will rather than for necessity. On the whole, they regularly experience a very different form of mental stress, for necessity rather than will, and, for most, sociocultural demands are constantly changing. So, although affluent societies appear to have an abundance of occupational choices to meet occupational health needs, the values placed upon different aspects of occupation, as well as other constraints, affect access and efficacy. Additionally, the cultural dividing of occupation into work, leisure, and sleep impedes the conscious awareness of the need to balance energy expenditure and rest, obligatory with self-chosen occupations, and social activity and solitude.

Effects such as those from continuous cultural evolution, the development of occupational technology, and the accompanying changes to social structures and values have resulted in the factors and feelings associated with people's occupations becoming extremely complex. To increase the complexities, the meaning of occupations differ for each individual according to age; gender; innate capacities and interests; experience; and particular cultural, societal, communal, and family circumstances. Over and above those factors, teasing out the relationship between it and health (which is equally complex) is a difficult task because the wide ranging health benefits of occupation have been largely ignored by mainstream medicine.

One study that began the process was an enquiry based on the provision of wide-ranging occupational intervention. It was a randomized controlled trial to evaluate the effectiveness of preventive occupational therapy for older adults living independently in government-subsidized apartment blocks in Los Angeles. The study demonstrated significant benefits across health, function, and quality of life domains for its 361 subjects (Clark et al., 1997). Upholding those findings was another population-based study of social and productive activities with a random sample of 2,761 male and female elderly Americans. Reported in the *British Medical Journal*, the investigation found that:

> Social and productive activities (occupations) that involve little or no enhancement of fitness lower the risk of all cause mortality as much as fitness activities do. This suggests that in addition to increased cardiopulmonary fitness, activity may confer survival benefits through psychosocial pathways. Social and productive activities that require less physical exertion may complement exercise programmes and may constitute alternative interventions for frail elderly people. (Glass, deLeon, Marottolil, & Berkman, 1999)

More studies like those and that of Blaxter and her associates discussed earlier would be invaluable to substantiate the interaction between occupation, health, and well-being.

To further substantiate the work toward occupation for health, major components that surfaced in the previous sections associated with health and well-being are selected for comment from an occupational perspective. That approach will suggest what aspects of occupation might be most useful to address in research, practice, and education if future directions aim at positive health in response to the WHO's recommendation (Figure 7-5).

Two of the notions that emerged from earlier in the chapter are those of prerequisites or preconditions for states of health or well-being. The notions are so fundamental that they must be the first issues to be addressed. In his analysis of preconditions for well-being, Williams, and an array of others after him, argued that people need to live in mutually supportive social collectives. The fundamental rules of such collectives are concerned with material production, reproduction, the transmission of skills and values, and rules for the community (Braybrooke, 1987; Doyal & Gough, 1984, 1991; Williams, 1979). As occupation at various levels of society is fundamental in all four conditions, the question is prompted as to whether or not practitioners of occupation for health and well-being should get involved in concerns such as those and try to improve them so that population well-being is enhanced overall. Such involvement would demand a proactive political stance rather than a reactive conservative one.

If involvement became the case, questions would need to be asked and answered about whether contemporary occupational structures, the social environment, and political agendas that support them enable the maximum number of people to experience adequate health and well-being or if there are major groups who are disadvantaged. Instead of accepting the present sociopolitical situation, health practitioners with an interest in occupation, health, and well-being would need to be investigating effects and possibilities of major and minor changes, which could provide more people with occupationally satisfying and fulfilling lives. Such practitioners must also have strong ideas about what to aim for and must be prepared to at least comment on policies and current practices. Exploration of the idea of occupational justice, which was mentioned earlier, is one way of becoming more aware of such issues and of eventually being in a situation to address them more effectively. Addressing them should lead to societal and individual well-being as well as improved health status.

More research on the physical, mental, and social factors integral to occupation, health, and well-being is called for. The results of one such study suggest that it would be worthwhile. The study of 146 respondents in South Australia explored perceptions of occupational balance and its relationship to health (Wilcock et al., 1997). The notion of balance was central to the philosophy propounded by Adolf Meyer (1922). Others followed, such as Rogers (1984) who spoke passionately to the belief that a

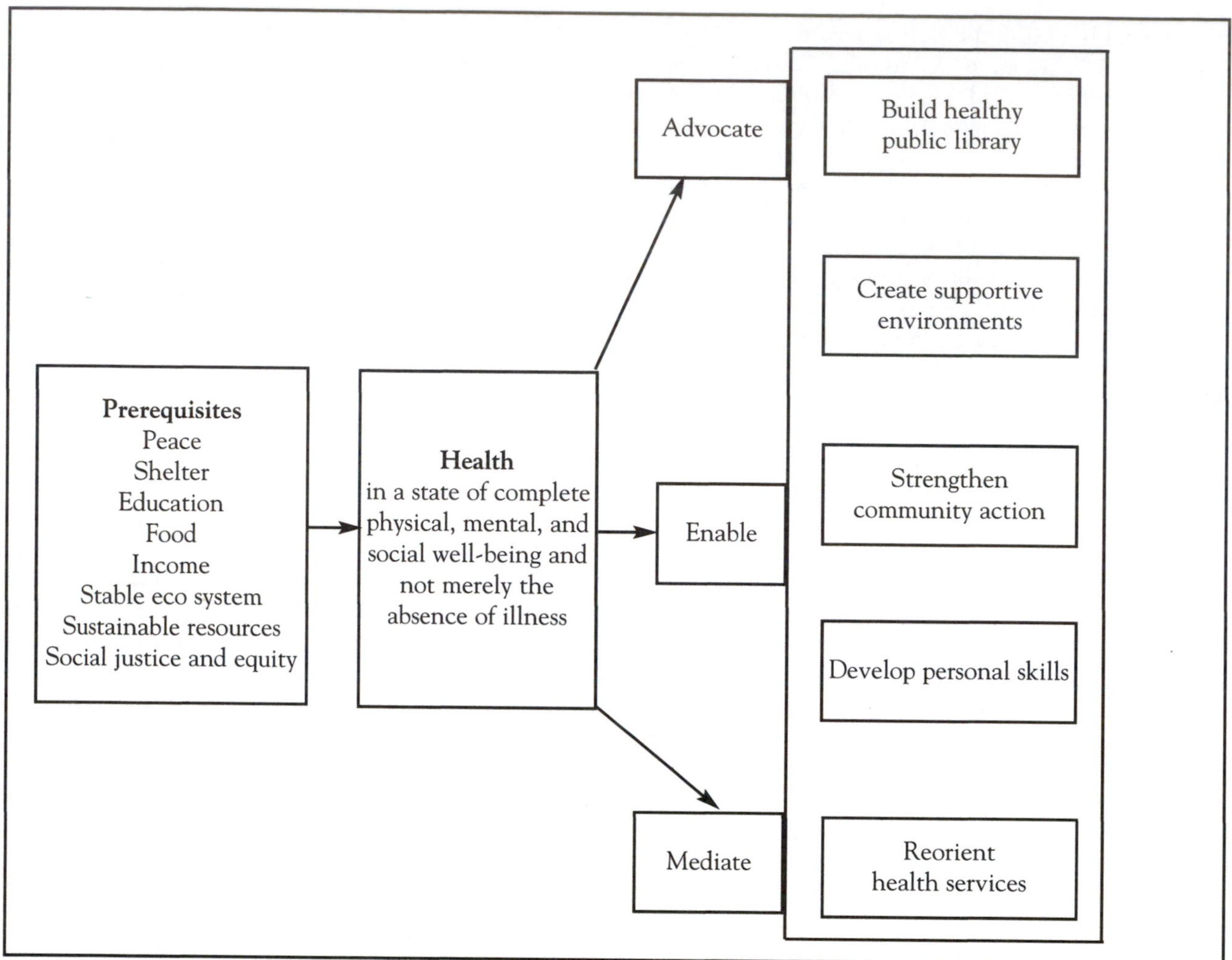

Figure 7-5. WHO's holistic view of health and well-being.

balance of self-care, play, work, and rest are essential for healthy living, and that occupation is the means by which balance is achieved and physical and mental well-being attained. However, a limited understanding of occupational balance suggests that it is chance, rather than design, which leads to health and well-being. When the natural balance between active and rest occupations is considered from studies of more primitive cultures, it would seem that artificial constructs such as a 5-day week or an 8-hour day have little to recommend them in terms of biologically-based temporal rhythms and how they impact on health. Such disregard continues despite studies such as those by Monk (1988), Rosa and Colligan (1988), and Dinges and colleagues (1988), which have found that irritability, malaise, fatigue, stomach complaints, diminished concentration, diminished functional capabilities, mood changes, and increased susceptibility to accidents can result when sleep-wake patterns are disrupted by shift work. That is a far cry from health and well-being.

In the South Australian study of occupational balance and health, the researchers chose to consider it in terms of physical, mental, social, and rest occupations, more or less in line with the WHO's definition of health. In seeking to discover individuals' perceptions of their own occupational balance and health status, participants were selected from different living situations and ages ranged between 13 to 85 years. The sampling closely mirrored gender and urban/rural distributions in South Australia. Participants were asked to rate both their current and their perceived ideal involvement in physical, mental, social, and rest occupations and their health from poor to excellent. The patterns of current balance showed wide variation among respondents with 55 different patterns being chosen, with only two picked more than eight times. The patterns of ideal balance showed less variation. Thirty-nine different patterns were chosen, with four patterns picked more than eight times. The most frequently chosen pattern of ideal occupational balance was moderate involvement in all four categories. Occupational balance, measured in that way, varied between people, as one would expect and, for almost 90% of the participants, current occupational balance was different than how ideal occupational balance was perceived. A significant relationship was found between reported good health and the closeness of current occupational patterns and those perceived by the respondent to be ideal. Despite differences, a picture of healthful occupational balance began to emerge of moderate to high involvement in all physical, mental, social, and rest occupations.

More exploration is needed to focus on other occupational issues that are connected with the physical, mental, social, and rest mix, such as how, through what they do, people attain happiness—a feeling that is obviously central to both health and well-being. Similarly, questions need to be constantly borne in mind and explored about occupation's interaction with other feelings associated with health and well-being, such as about self, or problem solving, or experiencing the whole range of emotions. In terms of mental well-being and social well-being, programs need to ensure they encompass the enabling of emotional, intellectual, and spiritual capacities through use of occupations, which include factors such as those described by the National Mental Health Association of America, for example, as characteristics of mentally well people (Payne & Hahn, 1995). They also need to ensure that practice and research follow occupationally just cultural and social parameters, which permit or encourage people to engage in everyday lives that benefit their communities or to challenge injustice should they become aware of it.

Reaching toward potential has been recognized as relating to health and well-being. In 1935, for example, Nobel prize-winning physiologist Alexis Carrel (1935), described how each human being must actualize all of his or her potentialities to reach an optimum state. In thinking about that concept, it is helpful to consider occupation as a means of developing individual capacities as steps on the way. Following consultation of dictionaries and thesauri, capacity in that context means "the innate and perhaps undeveloped potential, aptitude, ability, talent, trait or power with which each individual is endowed" (Wilcock et al., 1998, p. 253). Capacities vary between individuals according to their genetic make-up, can become apparent long after birth, improve with use, and are the building blocks of unique occupational natures and personalities. Maslow claimed capacities are needs and observed that they "clamor to be used." If not, he said, they "become a disease centre or else atrophy or disappear" (Maslow, 1968, p. 201).

It seems clear that people who regard health as function, for example, will probably be most comfortable if they are enabled to continue with the tasks or work they enjoy and at the level that they feel meets their need for competence or satisfaction. In the well-being study described earlier, the following types of occupation were mentioned as leading to the experience: work, leisure, recreation, exercise, going out, traveling, rest, relaxation, sleep, religious practices, self-less and familial activity, self-care, grooming, hairdressing, dressing up, indulgence, achievement, learning, education, and personal goals. A question that must be asked is whether or not occupational therapists would be able to offer or to tap into a sufficient range of options in terms of occupations to meet their potential clients' health and well-being requirements?

Programs that provide intervention for individual, group, or community well-being need to be the subject of continual appraisal and investigation as well as being openly addressed in public forums to raise population awareness and understanding of the profession's role (Figure 7-6).

CONCLUSION

Bearing in mind the ideas articulated throughout the centuries, as well as findings from more recent studies, well-being from an occupation and health perspective needs to embrace the notions of happiness, personal potential, community action, and be people driven. It requires recommendation, facilitation, and utilization of a range of physical, social, and emotional experiences as people go about meeting their basic needs, so that engagement in occupation provides physical exercise, motivation, socialization, opportunities to develop self-esteem, meaning, and purpose, as well as intellectual challenge (Foster, 1983; Lilley & Jackson, 1990). Additionally, there is evidence for a balance of physical and intellectual capacities, spiritual experiences, emotional highs and lows, satisfying and stimulating social relationships, relaxation, and time for self. This does not imply constant high-powered mental, physical, or social "doing" or "feeling," rather that those should be interwoven with timelessness and higher-order meaning (Rappaport, 1979) and simply being or becoming happy with self according to individual nature and need (do Rozario, 1994). Occupations that will have most obvious effects on well-being are those that are socially sanctioned and valued and that enable people freedom to effectively use physical and mental capacities in combination with social activity. Physical, mental, and social well-being cannot easily be separated. They are part of an integrated system that warns, maintains, and rewards through people's awareness of their needs and how they feel.

Through ongoing use of their capacities by engagement in a range of purposeful, fulfilling, balanced, motivating physical, mental, and social occupations, people can maintain homeostasis, keep body parts, neuronal physiology, and mental capacities functioning at peak effi-

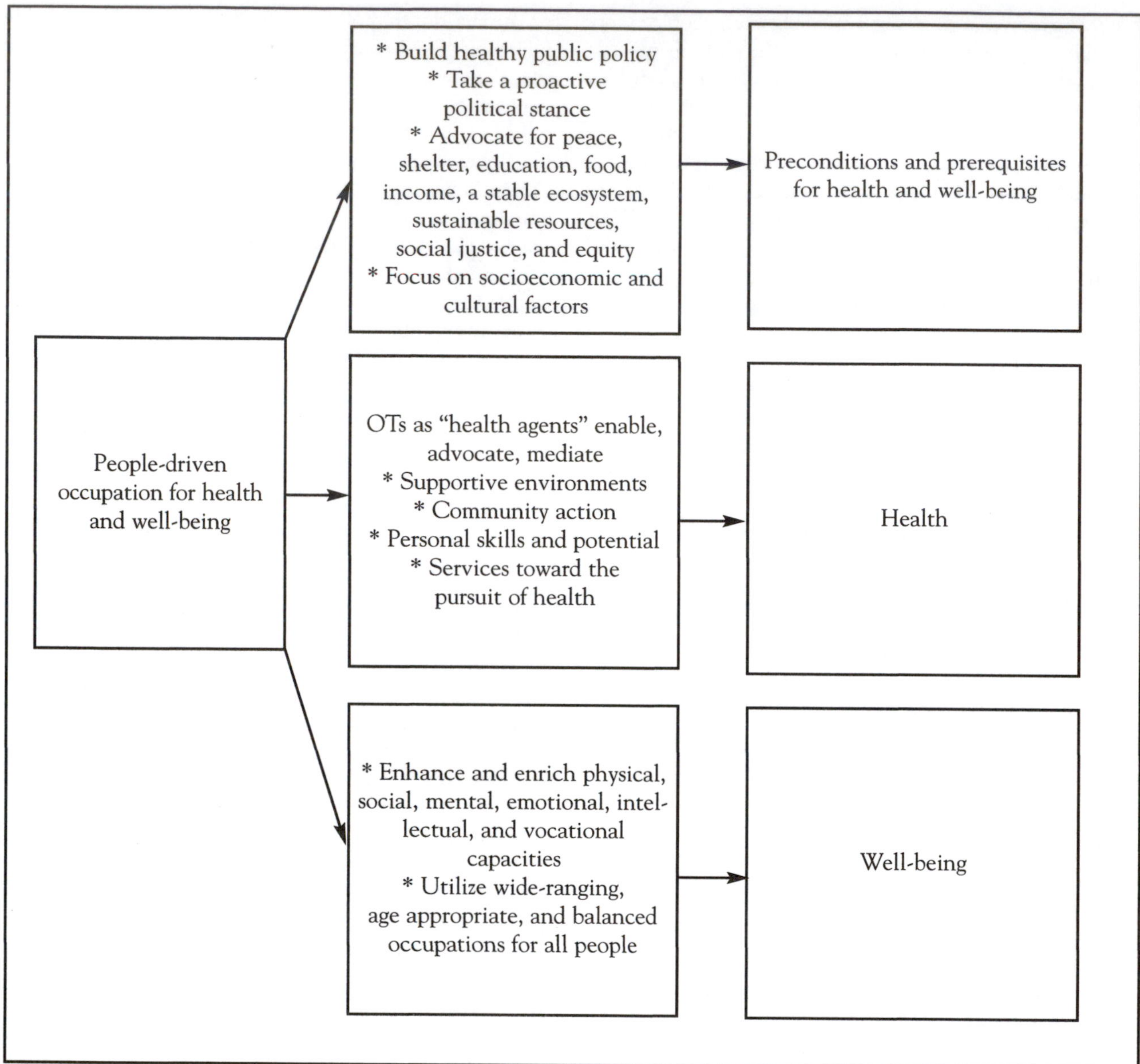

Figure 7-6. Occupational approaches to meet people's health and well-being requirements.

ciency and maintain and develop satisfying and stimulating social relationships. As society comes to understand this, medicine's view of health will begin to shift. Already the mandate from the WHO places emphasis on health as a resource for living, not merely an absence of disease.

REFERENCES

Agius, T. (1993). Aboriginal health in Aboriginal hands. In J. Fuller, J. Barclay, & J. Zollo (Eds.), *Multicultural health care in South Australia. Conference proceedings*. Adelaide: Painters Prints.

Andrews, F. M., & Withey, S. B. (1976). *Social indicators of well-being*. New York, NY: Plenum Press.

Antonovsky, A. (1990). The sense of coherence as a determinant of health. In J. D. Matarazzo, S. M. Weiss, J. A. Herd, N. E. Miller, & S. M. Weiss (Eds.), *Behavioral health. A handbook of health enhancement and disease prevention*. New York, NY: John Wiley and Sons.

Argyle, M. (1987). *The psychology of happiness*. New York, NY: Methuen & Co.

Bertalanffy, L. (1968). *General systems theory*. New York, NY: George Baziller.

Blaxter, M. (1990). *Health and lifestyles*. New York, NY: Tavistock/Routledge.

Evidence Worksheet

Authors	Year	Topic	Method	Conclusion
Blaxter	1990	Views of health and lifestyles	Quantitative and qualitative population survey	There are clear gender differences as well as at different stages of life in how people describe health for themselves and others
Clark et al.	1997	Preventative occupational therapy for older adults in the community	Experimental: Randomized controlled trial	All participants showed benefits across health, function, and quality of life domains
Csikszentmihalyi & Csikszentmihalyi	1988	Optimal experience: Studies of changes in consciousness of time during enjoyable occupations	Time use study: Experience sampling	During occupations which meet "a just right" challenge for individuals time appears to pass more quickly
Glass et al.	1999	The role of social and productive activities in older adults	Experimental: Randomized controlled trial	Social and productive activities as well as fitness activities play an important role in decreasing mortality in individuals
Kanner et al.	1981	Stress management for life events	Qualitative	A variety of skills and abilities are prerequisite to overall well-being
Wilcock	1998b	The relationship between occupation and health	History of ideas	Occupation is a major biological mechanism for health
Wilcock et al.	1998	Individual's perception and experiences of well-being	Questionnaire: Trial using cluster sampling	Occupation plays an important role within health and well-being. The view of well-being varies between people

Bradburn, N. M. (1969). *The structure of psychological well-being*. Chicago, IL: Aldine.

Braybrooke, D. (1987). *Meeting needs*. Princeton, NJ: Princeton University Press.

Bronowski, J. (1973). *The ascent of man*. London: British Broadcasting Corp.

Burckardt, C., Woods, S., Schultz, A., & Ziebarth, D. (1989). Quality of life of adults with chronic illness: A psychometric study. *Research in Nursing and Health, 12*, 347-354.

Campbell, B. G. (1988). *Humankind emerging* (5th ed.). New York, NY: Harper Collins Publishers.

Campbell, J. (1998). *Winston Churchill's afternoon nap*. London: Paladin.

Caplan, A. L., Englehart, H. T., & McCartney, J. J. (1981). *Concepts of health and disease*. Reading, MA: Addison-Wesley.

Carrel, A. (1935). *Man the unknown*. London: Burns and Oates.

Chamove, A. (1986). Exercise improves behaviour: A rationale for occupational therapy. *British Journal of Occupational Therapy, 49*, 83-86.

Clark, F., Azen, S. P., Zemke, R., Jackson, J., Carlson, M., Mandel, D., et al. (1997). Occupational therapy for independent-living older adults: A randomized control trial. *Journal of the American Medical Association, 278*, 1321-1326.

Cohen, P., Struening, E. L., Genevie, L. E., Kaplan, S. R., Muhlin, G. L., & Peck, H. B. (1982). Community stressors, mediating conditions and well-being in urban neighborhoods. *Journal of Community Psychology, 10*, 377-390.

Csikszentmihalyi, M., & Csikszentmihalyi, I. S. (Eds.). (1988). *Optimal experience: Psychological studies of flow in consciousness*. Cambridge: Cambridge University Press.

Depoy, E., & Kolodner, E. L. (1991). Psychological performance factors. In C. Christiansen & C. Baum (Eds.), *Occupational therapy: Overcoming human performance deficits*. Thorofare, NJ: SLACK Incorporated.

Diener, E. (1984). Subjective well-being. *Psychological Bulletin, 95*, 542-575.

Dinges, D., Whitehouse, W., Carota-Orne, E., & Orne, M. (1988). The benefits of a nap during prolonged work and wakefulness. *Work and Stress, 2*, 139-153.

Dintiman, G. B., & Greenberg, J. S. (1986). *Health through discovery* (3rd ed.). New York, NY: Random House.

do Rozario, L. (1994). Ritual, meaning and transcendence: The role of occupation in modern life. *Journal of Occupational Science: Australia, 1*(3), 46-53.

Dobson, A. (1992). People and diseases. In S. Jones, R. Martin, & D. Pilbeam (Eds.), *The Cambridge encyclopedia of human evolution*. Cambridge: Cambridge University Press.

Doyal, L., & Gough, I. (1984). A theory of human need. *Critical Social Policy, 4*, 1.

Doyal, L., & Gough, I. (1991). *A theory of human need*. London: Macmillan.

Dubos, R. (1959). *Mirage of health*. New York, NY: Harper and Row Publishers Inc.

Dunbar, R. (1992). Why gossip is good for you. *New Scientist, 136*(1848), 28-31.

Edelman, G. (1992). *Bright air, brilliant fire: On the matter of the mind*. London: Penguin Books.

Folkins, C. H., & Syme, W. E. (1981). Physical fitness training and mental health. *American Psychologist, 36*, 373-389.

Foster, P. (1983). Activities: A necessity for total health care of the long-term care resident. *Activities, Adaptation and Ageing, 3*, 17-23.

Giddens, A. (1984). *Profiles and critiques in social theory*. New York, NY: Macmillan.

Glass, T. A., de Leon, C. M., Marottoli, R. A., & Berkman, L. F. (1999). Population based study of social and productive activities as predictors of survival among elderly Americans. *British Medical Journal, 319*, 478-483.

Gross, S. (1980). The holistic health movement. *The Personnel and Guidance Journal, 59*(2), 96-100.

Herzlich, C. (1973). *Health and illness: A social psychological analysis*. London: Academic Press.

Homel, R., & Burns, A. (1989). Environmental quality and the well-being of children. *Social Indicators Research, 21*, 133-158.

Isaksson, K. (1990). A longitudinal study of the relationship between frequent job change and psychological well-being. *Journal of Occupational Psychology, 63*, 297-308.

Johnson, J., & Schmit, H. Resource Center for Health and Well-being, Inc. Unpublished brochure, 1983. In Johnson, J. A. (1986). Wellness and occupational therapy. *American Journal of Occupational Therapy, 40*(11), 753-758.

Jones, S. (1992). Genetic diversity in humans. In S. Jones, R. Martin, & D. Pilbeam (Eds.), *The Cambridge encyclopedia of human evolution*. Cambridge: Cambridge University Press.

Jones, S., Martin, R., & Pilbeam, D. (Eds.). (1992). *The Cambridge encyclopedia of human evolution*. Cambridge: Cambridge University Press.

Kanner, A. D., Coyne, J. C., Schaefer, C., & Lazarus, R. S. (1981). Comparison of two modes of stress management: Daily hassles and uplifts versus life events. *Journal of Behavioral Medicine, 4*, 1-39.

Kass, L. R. (1981). Regarding the end of medicine and the pursuit of health. In A. R. Caplan, H. T. Engelhart, & J. J. McCartney (Eds.), *Concepts of health and disease: Interdisciplinary perspectives*. MA: Addison Wesley Publishing Co.

Keynes, J. M. (1931). Economic possibilities for our grandchildren. In *Essays in persuasion*. London: MacMillan.

Kirchman, M. M. (1983). The preventive role of activity: Myth or reality—A review of the literature. *Physical and Occupational Therapy in Geriatrics, 2*(4), 39-47.

Kirkman Gray, B. (1905). *A history of English philanthropy*. London: P. S. King & Son.

Koeing, H., Kvale, J., & Ferrel, C. (1988). Religion and well-being in later life. *The Gerontologist, 28*(1), 19-27.

Lilley, J., & Jackson, L. (1990). The value of activities: Establishing a foundation for cost effectiveness. A review of the literature. *Activities, Adaptation and Ageing, 14*(4), 12-13.

Maslow, A. H. (1968). *Toward a psychology of being* (2nd ed.). New York, NY: D. Van Nostrand Co.

Maslow, A. H. (1970). *Motivation and personality* (2nd ed.). New York, NY: Harper and Row.

McConatha, J. T., & McConatha, D. (1985). An instrument to measure self-responsibility for wellness in older adults. *Educational Gerontology, 11*, 295-308.

McNeill, W. H. (1979). *Plagues and people*. London: Penguin Books.

Meyer, A. (1922). The philosophy of occupational therapy. *Archives of Occupational Therapy, 1*, 1-10.

Monk, T. (1988). Coping with the stress of shift work. *Work and Stress, 2*, 169-172.

Moss, J. (1989). Personal communication. Department of Public Health, University of Adelaide.

Newman, M. A. (1986). *Health as expanding consciousness*. St Louis, MO: The C. V. Mosby Company.

Norton, A.L. (Ed). (1980). *Concepts of occupational therapy* (pp. 203-204). Baltimore: Williams and Wilkins.

Nutbeam, D. (1986). Health promotion glossary. *Health Promotion, 1*, 113.

Oliver, J. (1972). Physical activity and the psychological development of the handicapped. In J. Kane (Ed.), *Psychological aspects of physical education and sport*. London: Routledge & Kegan Paul.

Ornstein, R., & Sobel, D. (1988). *The healing brain: A radical new approach to health care*. London: MacMillan.

Payne, W. A. & Hahn, D. B. (1995). *Understanding your health*. (4th ed.). St Louis, MO: Mosby.

Rappaport, R. (1979). *Ecology, meaning, and religion*. Richmond: North Atlantic Books.

Reed, K. L., & Sanderson, R. S. (1980). *Concepts of occupational therapy* (pp. 203-204). Baltimore: Williams and Wilkins.

Rogers, J. C. (1984). Why study human occupation? *American Journal of Occupational Therapy, 38*, 47-49.

Roget, P. M. (1972). *Roget's New Thesaurus of Synonyms and Antonyms*. London: The Number Nine Publishing Company.

Rosa, R., & Colligan, M. (1988). Long workdays versus rest days: Assessing fatigue and alertness with a portable performance battery. *Human Factors, 5*, 87-98.

Sigerist, H. E. (1955). *A history of medicine, Vol. 1, Primitive and archaic medicine*. New York, NY: Oxford University Press.

Sperry, R. (1982). Some effects of disconnecting the cerebral hemispheres. *Les Prix Nobel*, 1981.

Stephenson, W. (1972). *The ecological development of man*. Sydney: Angus and Robertson.

Strack, F., Argyle, M., & Schwartz, N. (Eds.). (1991). *Subjective well-being: An interdisciplinary perspective*. Oxford: Pergamon Press.

Sydney, K. H., & Sheppard, R. J. (1977). Activity patterns of elderly men and women. *Journal of Gerontology, 32*, 25-32.

The Asian NGO Coalition, IRED Asia. (1993). *Economy, ecology and spirituality: Toward a theory and practice of sustainability*. IRED, Asia: The People Centered Development Forum.

The Open University in association with the Health Education Council and the Scottish Health Education Unit. (1980). *The good health guide*. London: Pan Books.

Townsend, E. (1993). Muriel Driver Memorial Lecture. Occupational therapy's social vision. *Canadian Journal of Occupational Therapy*, 60, 174-183.

Ullah, P. (1990). *The association between income, financial strain and psychological well-being among unemployed youths*. London: The British Psychological Society.

Warr, P. (1990). The measurement of well-being and other aspects of mental health. *Journal of Occupational Psychology, 63*, 193-210.

Watts, E. D. (1985). Human needs. In A. Kuper & J. Kuper (Eds.), *The social science encyclopedia*. London: Routledge.

Wilcock, A. A. (1993a). A theory of the human need for occupation. *Journal of Occupational Science: Australia, 1*, 17-24.

Wilcock, A. A. (1993b). Biological and sociocultural aspects of occupation, health and health promotion. *British Journal of Occupational Therapy, 56*, 200-203.

Wilcock, A. A. (1998a). Occupation for health. *British Journal of Occupational Therapy, 61*, 340-345.

Wilcock, A. A. (1998b). *An occupational perspective of health*. Thorofare, NJ: SLACK Incorporated.

Wilcock, A. A. (2000). *The Thelma Cardwell Lecture: Occupation for Health: Re-activating the Regimina Sanitatis*. Toronto: University of Toronto.

Wilcock, A. A. (2001). *Occupation for health: Volume 1: A journey from self-health to prescription*. London: British College of Occupational Therapists.

Wilcock, A. A., Chelin, M., Hall, M., Hamley, N., Morrison, B., Scrivener, L., et al. (1997). The relationship between occupational balance and health: A pilot study. *Occupational Therapy International, 4*, 17-30.

Wilcock, A. A., van d'Arend, H., Darling, K., Scholz, J., Siddall, R., Snigg, C., et al. (1998). An exploratory study of people's perception and experiences of well-being. *British Journal of Occupational Therapy, 61*, 75-82.

Williams, R. (1979). *Politics and letters*. London: Verso.

Wolman, B. (Ed.). (1973). *Dictionary of behavioral science*. New York, NY: Van Nostrand, Reinhold Co.

World Health Organization. (1946). *Constitution of the World Health Organization*. International Health Conference, New York.

World Health Organization, Health and Welfare Canada, Canadian Public Health Association. (1986). *Ottawa charter for health promotion*. Ottawa, Canada: Authors.

Chapter Seven: Relationship of Occupations to Health and Well-Being
Reflections and Learning Activities

Julie Bass-Haugen, PhD, OTR/L, FAOTA

REFLECTIONS

In this chapter, we examined the relationships between occupation, health, and well-being. You might ask, was it necessary? Isn't it enough just to understand occupation? Here, we learned occupations are an integral part of the human experience and influence our quality of life at any given point in time. Health and well-being were the key concepts used to describe quality of life in this chapter.

Think for a moment about the terms *health* and *well-being*. Are your definitions of these terms exactly the same as mine? Not likely. What influences my definitions of these words? What influences yours? You might guess that the things we read shape our definitions as well as our personal experience, our outlook on life, and the perspective of people in our circle of influence. Do my personal definitions of health and well-being influence my life in any significant ways? Do your personal definitions of health and well-being influence your life in a different way? Yes, to both questions!

The first section of this chapter discussed health and its relationship to occupation. There are many different ways to think about health. Figure 7-2 depicted health as a basic need that can be studied from individual/communal, physiological, and contextual perspectives. The physiological perspective provides us with a variety of definitions to consider.

In western culture, our medical systems greatly influence our ideas about health. From this perspective, it is far easier to think about health by first thinking about not having health. If someone we know has landed in the hospital because of an accident, a major illness, or a disease, our image of that person at that particular time is likely one of ill health. It is easy to take the next step then and infer that anyone who does not have ill health must be healthy. This definition of health was introduced as "health defined negatively" and is similar to the feelings we might have after recovering from a bad cold or the flu. When we no longer have those terrible symptoms of the cold or flu, it is enough to make us feel healthy again regardless of our overall health status.

Now let's look at health from the opposite angle, "health defined positively." Think of all the people you know and select two who you regard as the healthiest. What makes them stand out as healthy? When I did this little exercise, I was surprised how my images matched the positive perceptions of health discussed in the chapter. The people I thought of always seem to have lots of energy, lead a good life, and are physically fit. Note that these are all positive attributes, and, thus, they agree with "health defined positively."

These definitions of health defined negatively or positively had not mentioned anything about occupations. We might ask, "Are occupations necessary for life?" and "Are occupations necessary for health?" It might be hard to answer these questions with a resounding "yes!" if we have never had to think much about the basic necessities of life and health. Pause for a minute and think of stories you know about people who have struggled at some point in their life. People living in refugee camps have been known to develop specific routines for their day (e.g., cleaning the tent or latrine, teaching the children, playing games) as a way to hold on to some meaning and purpose (i.e., occupations for life). Many people who lived during the Great Depression needed to plant, tend, and harvest gardens to have adequate nutrition (i.e., occupations for health). These examples emphasize the natural, basic relationships that exist between health and occupation and life itself.

Food, warmth, and relationships with others were identified as basic necessities of life and health. We can easily identify occupations that support these necessities of life. Eating, for example, is a necessary occupation to fulfill our requirements for food intake. Occupations may also serve to meet our innate needs related to physiological, psychological, and social comfort. Exercise, for example, is a good occupation to meet our body's physiological needs. We could argue (along with many famous scholars) that occupations are the vehicles by which we meet our health-related needs. Throughout the ages, specific occupations have been identified by a culture as health-giving or health-restoring (e.g., exercise, prayer, work).

Our perspective on health is also influenced by unique characteristics of individuals and communities and contextual factors. Some of these characteristics might include gender, age, genetics, social-cultural factors, environment, and even views on health itself. Let me ask a couple of questions to illustrate this idea. Are there unique characteristics of health for children who have asthma as compared with children who do not have this condition? Are there unique characteristics of health for people who work in a coal mine as compared to those who work in an office? Are there unique characteristics of health for people who live near a toxic waste area as compared to those who live near a pristine wilderness area? Are there unique characteristics of health for citizens of an industrialized, wealthy country as compared to citizens of an impoverished, developing country? What are the possible images of health that came to your mind in each of these examples? Our ideas about health are shaped by both individuals and the larger environment.

Well-being was the other term explored in this chapter. The WHO acknowledged the importance of well-being in its 1946 definition of health. Unfortunately, many people only remember the "absence of disease" phrase in this definition and not the "state of complete physical, mental, and social well-being" phrase. What is well-being? We all have a sense of what it means intuitively, but it presents a real challenge when we try to identify a unifying definition. Why is this the case? Well-being is a holistic concept that addresses several personal dimensions (e.g., physical, mental, social), includes a strong subjective component (e.g., peace, happiness), and is associated with many situations (e.g., occupations, relationships).

Despite the challenge of defining well-being, there is increased interest in studying well-being from both an individual and community perspective. There is alot of recent evidence of strong links between health, well-being, and occupation. The chapter outlined some of these important studies.

We have established that well-being is a worthy individual state, but how is it related to the needs and occupations of populations? Well, like it or not, we are generally part of a community or a society or a population of people. And if the community, society, or population is going to thrive, certain needs have to be met: basic health and survival; reproductive and developmental; skills and values; and law and order. All of these needs require occupational engagement and performance. For example, one component of survival—food—would require engagement in several occupations. In my community, the occupations related to food include buying food, cleaning food, preparing food, storing food, and, last, but not least, eating food.

My community meets most of these needs related to health and well-being. However, I know of communities, societies, and populations that do not thrive. In fact, their health and well-being is at risk. Recent research is suggesting that an occupational framework is a good way to look at the health and well-being of people and solve the problems of at-risk populations. For example, if I was concerned about mortality rates of older adults in my community, I might examine the social, productive, and fitness activities of these adults after reading the chapter. If I found that older adults in my community had limited opportunity for occupational engagement in these areas, I could advocate for formal and informal community interventions that would change this situation. I could befriend my older neighbors who have become isolated in recent years. I could petition the city council to address transportation issues that limit occupations. I could support community-based organizations that provide occupational opportunities for older adults. These are examples of sociopolitical approaches that address occupational health and well-being.

The well-being of a people or community is the goal of many health professionals in the world. There is concern not only for the individual but also for the broader community in which that person lives. This focus on well-being suggests that all people have the right to live life to its fullest potential (i.e., to achieve personal goals, fulfill needs, and cope with the environment) not just have basic health. These are obviously lofty goals. However, groups like the *Ottawa Charter for Health Promotion* of the World Health Organization feel these goals are achievable with careful planning and deliberate efforts. This chapter outlined strategies for improving the well-being of all people.

After reading this chapter, I suspect you have some new insights on health and well-being. And perhaps you have developed some interest in addressing health and well-being issues from an occupational perspective!

Journal Activities

1. Look up and write down dictionary definitions of health and well-being. Highlight the components of the definitions that are most related to their descriptions in Chapter Seven.
2. Identify the most important new learning for you in this chapter.
3. Identify one question you have about Chapter Seven.
4. Examine your own health and well-being.
   - Develop your personal definition of health.
   - Develop your personal definition of well-being.
   - Identify three occupations that positively influence your health and well-being.
   - Identify three occupations that negatively influence your health and well-being.
   - Identify three personal goals for optimal health.
   - Identify three personal goals for optimal well-being.
   - Identify three occupational goals as they relate to health and well-being.

Technology/Internet Learning Activities

1. Use a discussion database to share specific journal entries.
2. Use a good Internet search engine to scan resources and organizations for health and well-being.
   - Enter the phrase "health organization" in your search line.
   - Add other words to your search line for any specific interests.
     - ✧ Age: children, adolescent, adult, seniors
     - ✧ Country: United Kingdom, Canada, American, Australia, international
   - Scan the first 30 to 50 sites.
   - Look at the Web sites for three to five interesting health organizations.
   - Evaluate the quality of the Web site.
   - Document the organization and its Web site.
   - What is the primary mission and objectives of each organization?
   - Summarize the activities of the organization that are related to health and occupation.
   - Enter the phrase "well-being organization" in your search line.
   - Add other words to your search line for any specific interests.
     - ✧ Age: children, adolescent, adult, seniors
     - ✧ Country: United Kingdom, Canada, American, Australia, international
   - Scan the first 30 to 50 sites.
   - Look at the Web sites for three to five interesting well-being organizations.
   - Evaluate the quality of the Web site.
   - Document the organization and its Web site.
   - What is the primary mission and objectives of each organization?
   - Summarize the activities of the organization that are related to well-being and occupation.
3. Use a good Internet search engine to find the Web site of the World Health Organization.
   - Enter the word "World Health Organization" in your search line.
   - What is the address of this Web site?
   - Evaluate the quality of the Web site.
   - What is the primary objective or mission of the WHO?
   - What is the WHO's current definition of health? What year was this definition proposed?
   - Describe the current strategic goals and activities of WHO.
   - Summarize how these goals and activities relate to occupation.
   - Examine information on the *Ottawa Charter* in the Web site.
4. Use a good Internet search engine to find the Web site of the World Health Organization.
   - Enter the word "World Health Organization" in your search line.
   - Explore two to three health topics on the WHO Web site (e.g., child development, child health, disabled people, health promotion, human rights, mental health, occupational health, violence).
   - Identify the health topic you are exploring and its location on the WHO Web site.
   - Describe the health topic and the primary WHO objectives related to this topic.
   - Summarize one example of the relationship between occupation and health for this topic.
   - Identify one question you have about occupation as it relates to this topic.

Applied Learning

Individual Learning Activity #1: Investigating the Occupations, Health, and Well-Being of a Community

Instructions:

- Select a population that you can study by making observations in a public location (e.g., adolescents at recreation center, college students in a dormitory, elders in a senior citizen center, young adults in a shopping mall). Document the population, the location, and the time of the observation.
- Observe this population in a public location for approximately 1 hour.
- Describe the occupations you observe during this time period.
- Describe observable characteristics and behaviors of this population.
- Describe notable individual differences in occupations, characteristics, and behaviors.
- What conclusions do you make about the health and well-being of this population? (Use definitions of health and well-being from the chapter as a guide.)
- What conclusions do you make about the relationship between occupations and health and well-being for this population?

Individual Learning Activity #2: Exploring Individual Views on Health (Blaxter, 1990)

Instructions:

- Identify five people who you can interview regarding their views on health.
- For each person, record the gender and age.
- Ask each person questions based on the Blaxter (1990) study as summarized in the chapter.
  - ✧ Think of someone you know who is very healthy. Who are you thinking of? How old are they? What makes you call them healthy?
  - ✧ At times, people are healthier than at other times. What is it like when you are healthy?
- Record all answers for each question (Note: A person may give several answers to each question).
- Classify the answers for the two primary questions in the tables below.
- Write a brief conclusion of your findings.
- Discuss how your findings are similar and different from results presented in the chapter.

What Makes You Call [a person you are thinking of] Healthy?

Person	*Age*	*Gender*	*Health Defined Negatively*	*Health Defined Positively*	*Health Defined in Occupational Terms*
#1					
#2					
#3					
#4					
#5					

What is it Like When You Are Healthy?

Person	Age	Gender	Health Defined Negatively	Health Defined Positively	Health Defined in Occupational Terms
#1					
#2					
#3					
#4					
#5					

Individual Learning Activity #3: Exploring Individual Views on Well-Being (Wilcock, 1998b)

Instructions:

- Identify five people who you can interview regarding their views on well-being.
- For each person, record the gender and age.
- Ask each person questions based on the Wilcock (1998) study as summarized in the chapter.
  - ✧ How would you describe well-being?
  - ✧ What situations or environments do you associate with a feeling of well-being?
  - ✧ Describe the sorts of feelings that you associate with well-being.
- Record the specific answers for each question (Note: A person may give several answers to each question).
- Classify the answers for the primary questions in the table below.
- Write a brief conclusion of your findings.

Person	Age	Gender	Description of Well-Being	Situations or Environments	Feelings Associated With Well-Being
#1					
#2					
#3					
#4					
#5					

Active Learning

Group Activity #1: Analyzing Views on Well-Being (Wilcock, 1998b)

Preparation:

- Read Chapter 7.
- Complete Applied Learning Activity #3.

Time: 45 minutes to 1 hour

Materials:

- Completed tables from Applied Learning Activity #3
- Flip chart, chalkboard, white board, or virtual board

- Make a master copy of the following tables.

Instructions:

- Individually:
  - ✧ Review the individual responses you were given for each question.
  - ✧ Classify the individual responses for each question in the following tables.
  - ✧ Tally the number of responses for each item in the following tables.
- In small groups:
  - ✧ Record the tallies for each group member in the following tables.
  - ✧ Add up the tallies to obtain a frequency for each item.
  - ✧ Record the frequency for each item in the master copy of the tables.
  - ✧ Obtain the total frequency for each table by adding up the item frequencies.
  - ✧ Obtain a percentage for each item by dividing the item frequency by the total frequency.

Description of Well-being	*Tally/Frequency*	*Percentage*
Materialistic		
Spiritual		
Occupation		
Relationships		
Self		
Healthy		
Happiness		
Body		
Mind		
Other		
Total		

Situations Associated With Well-being	*Tally/Frequency*	*Percentage*
Occupation		
Relationships		
Surroundings		
Health		
Other		
Total		

Feelings Associated With Well-being	*Tally/Frequency*	*Percentage*
Sadness		
Fortunate		
Elation		
Freedom		
Health		
Control		
Loving		
Fulfillment		
Belonging		
Energy		
Confidence		
Peace		
Happiness		
Other		
Total		

Discussion:

- Summarize your findings for each question. Discuss the highlights. Discuss any surprises.
- Compare your findings for each question to the results from the Wilcock (1998b) study as presented in the chapter.
- Discuss similarities and differences in your findings to the results from the Wilcock (1998b) study.
- What questions do you now have that might be a foundation for a new study on well-being?

Group Activity #2: Getting Involved in Issues of Health and Well-Being

Preparation:

- Read Chapter 7 and Figure 7-5.
- Collect and review news articles of health concerns in specific populations.

Time: 30 to 60 minutes

Materials: Recent news articles of health concerns in specific populations

Instructions:

- Individually:
  - ✧ Share news articles with your group.
- In small groups:
  - ✧ Select a current health issue of interest to explore in more detail.
  - ✧ Identify the prerequisites for improved health in this area.
  - ✧ What are the occupations of importance for this area of health?
  - ✧ Identify the actions you could take to advocate, enable, or mediate improved health in this area.
  - ✧ Provide examples of specific activities that you could do to build public policy, create supportive environments, strengthen community action, develop personal skills, and reorient health services.

Discussion:

- Discuss the impact of this health problem on your community.
- Discuss whether the prerequisites seem reasonable to achieve for this area of health.
- Discuss your personal readiness to take action on this health issue.
- Discuss the steps your group could take to become change agents for this health concern.

Chapter Eight Objectives

The information in this chapter is intended to help the reader:

1. Define occupational issues of concern, including delay, deprivation, disparities, interruption, and imbalance.
2. Appreciate the relationship of occupational issues to major health, education, and community concerns.
3. Identify past and current populations at risk for having occupational issues.
4. Describe factors used to describe populations at risk for occupational issues.
5. Discuss the relationships among specific occupational issues, personal factors, and environmental characteristics.
6. Discuss the characteristics of and occupational goals for several at-risk populations.

Key Words

occupational delay: Atypical schedule of occupational development generally associated with developmental disabilities or at-risk populations.

occupational deprivation: Lack of occupational opportunities due to certain personal or environmental characteristics.

occupational disparities: Inequalities in occupational patterns due to different choices/values or unequal opportunities.

occupational imbalance: Patterns of occupations that do not meet unique needs, interests, and commitments (Wilcock, 1998).

occupational interruption: A change in occupational engagement or performance due to changes in personal or environmental factors.

population at risk: Groups of individuals who are vulnerable to a disease or condition (McKenzie, Pinger, & Kotecki, 1999).

Human progress is neither automatic nor inevitable...
Every step toward the goal of justice requires sacrifice, suffering, and struggle;
the tireless exertions and passionate concern of dedicated individuals.
Martin Luther King Jr.

Chapter Eight

Occupational Issues of Concern in Populations

Julie Bass-Haugen, PhD, OTR/L, FAOTA; Mary Lou Henderson, MS, OTR/L; Barbara A. Larson, MS, OTR/L, FAOTA; and Kathleen Matuska, MPH, OTR/L

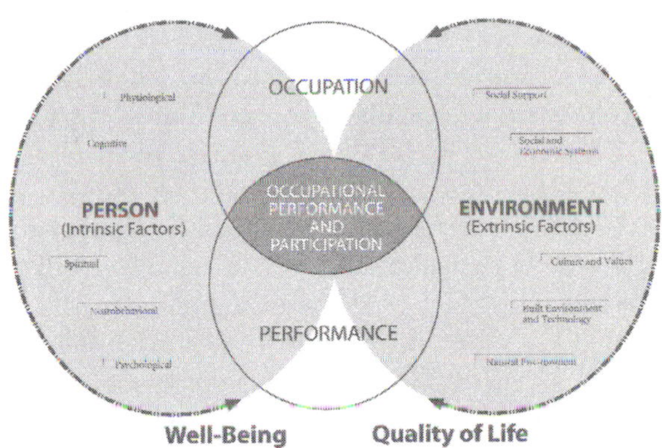

Setting the Stage

Occupational performance is influenced by many personal and environmental factors. Sometimes, personal and environmental factors contribute to enhanced performance or exploration of new occupations. At other times, personal and environmental factors can delay, deprive, or interrupt occupational performance or contribute to occupational imbalance or disparities. This chapter is about those patterns of occupations that are not optimal. Individuals and populations may experience occupational delay, deprivation, disparities, interruption, or imbalance at any time and may be faced with numerous occupational issues during the lifespan. Occupational issues of concern may negatively influence the health, well-being, and quality of life of both individuals and populations. Interventions may be needed to improve occupational performance in these situations.

When occupational issues occur, limitations in activities and restrictions in participation are likely and may directly contribute to problems in human functioning and disability. Furthermore, these occupational issues may influence personal and environmental dimensions. For example, when a person cannot engage in active, physical occupations, muscle strength or cognitive function may decline. Also, when a population does not have sufficient employment opportunities, the economic condition of the community may deteriorate. The purpose of this chapter is to introduce occupational issues of concern in various populations.

Bass-Haugen, J., Henderson, M. L., Larson, B. A., & Matuska, K. (2005). Occupational issues of concern in populations. In C. H. Christiansen, C. M. Baum, and J. Bass-Haugen (Eds.), Occupational therapy: Performance, participation, and well-being *(3rd ed.). Thorofare, NJ: SLACK Incorporated.*

Defining Occupational Issues of Concern

The occupational issues of concern at any given time are complex and varied. A number of terms have been proposed to characterize the nature of occupational issues for a given population. Terms like *delay*, *deprivation*, *disparities*, *interruption*, and *imbalance* may help us to understand the underlying cause of the concern and explore remedies that will improve occupational performance.

Occupational delay is evident when occupational development occurs on a schedule that is not typical. Delay is found in situations that "put off to a later time; defer; postpone" or "impede the process or progress of; retard; hinder" (Flexner, 1987, p. 526) opportunities for occupational performance. Occupational delay is generally associated with the lifespan period from infancy to young adulthood and is evident in children with developmental disabilities or from at-risk populations.

There are an estimated 4 million individuals with developmental disabilities in the United States (U.S. Department of Health and Human Services [DHHS] Administration on Developmental Disabilities, 2002). The global incidence of developmental disabilities is believed to be enormous, but no reliable estimates are available (Institute of Medicine, Committee on Nervous System Disorders in Developing Countries and Board of Global Health, 2001). The Developmental Disabilities Act and the DHHS Administration on Developmental Disabilities define developmental disability as:

> ...severe chronic, disabilities that are due to mental and/or physical impairment, which manifest before age 22 and are likely to continue indefinitely. They result in substantial limitations in [three] or more areas: self-care, receptive and expressive language, learning, mobility, self-direction, capacity for independent living, and economic self-sufficiency, as well as the continuous need for individually planned and coordinated services. (U.S. DHHS Administration on Developmental Disabilities, 2002)

Children with developmental disabilities may have a diagnosis of mental retardation, cerebral palsy, genetic and chromosomal anomalies, autism, learning disabilities, severe orthopedic impairments, visual and hearing impairments, serious emotional disturbances, and traumatic brain injury (Liptak, 1995).

Populations at risk for occupational delay include those groups of individuals who have a possible or probable risk of developing an undesirable trait or outcome. Examples of at-risk populations include runaway and homeless youth, children living in poverty, adolescents engaging in unhealthy behaviors, and children in foster care (U.S. DHHS Administration of Children and Families, 2001a). These at-risk populations are usually identified and described by regional, national, or international organizations as they develop projections and goals for various populations.

Occupational deprivation occurs when "an external agency or circumstance keeps a person from 'acquiring, using, or enjoying something.'" (Wilcock, 1998, p. 145). External agencies and circumstances may include personal characteristics (e.g., disease, body structure/function) and environmental characteristics (e.g., finances, social network). Deprivation may be defined as an act or instance of taking something away from or withholding—especially the necessities of life or of healthful environmental influences (Mish, 1988)—or "to remove or withhold something from the enjoyment or possession of (a person or persons)" (Flexner, 1987, p. 535). Deprivation may occur in preschool children living in poverty who do not have access to safe playgrounds and in adults with mental illness who are unable to maintain a job because of medication problems.

Occupational disparities are evident when occupational patterns differ for different populations. A disparity is a "lack of similarity or equality; inequality; difference" (Flexner, 1987, p. 567). Occupational disparities are often associated with complex factors that may include behavioral, economic, cultural, and political influences. Some disparities occur due to the different values and choices made by people. Other disparities occur due to unequal opportunities available for different populations.

When the disparities are attributed to equity issues, occupational injustice claims may be made. Occupational justice was defined by Wilcock in this text as a fairly recent term that refers to the "just and equitable distribution of power, resources, and opportunity so that all people are able to meet the needs of their occupational natures, and so experience health and well-being;" thus, injustice is the lack of this characteristic. Injustice is also defined as a "violation of the rights of others, unjust or unfair action or treatment" (Flexner, 1987, p. 983). Injustice issues are identified and addressed by many national and international groups concerned with human rights issues. Some recent issues of concern are poverty in developing countries, refugee camps, and racism/classism in the United States.

Occupational interruption occurs when occupational engagement or performance is temporarily affected by a change in personal or environmental factors. When patterns of occupations are interrupted, there is a "... break in the continuity or uniformity of (a course, process, condition, etc.)..." (Flexner, 1987, p. 998). Interruption may influence occupational performance on a temporary or long-term basis and may occur in an individual or population. Examples may include medical conditions (e.g., cancer, orthopedic injuries), personal life stresses (e.g., death in the family, divorce, bankruptcy), natural disasters (e.g., floods, tornadoes), and societal conditions (e.g., economic recession, housing shortages).

Wilcock (1998) writes that *occupational imbalance*:

> ...involves a state that occurs because people's engagement in occupation fails to meet their unique physical, social, mental, or rest needs and allows insufficient time for their own occupational interests and growth as well as for the occupations each feels obliged to undertake in order to meet family, social, and community commitments. (p. 138)

Imbalance is unique to the individual because "capacities, interests, and responsibilities differ." Imbalance may occur in children who have too many commitments and, thus, little unstructured play time; women who are trying to meet the needs of both their young children and their elderly parents (i.e., the sandwich generation) (Brody, 1981); workers who have jobs that require excessive repetition of the same tasks (Centers for Disease Control [CDC] National Institute for Occupational Safety and Health, 1997); and individuals in the early stage of retirement (Jonsson, Staffan, & Kielhofner, 2000).

These definitions of occupational delay, deprivation, disparities, interruption, and imbalance provide an introduction to occupational issues of concern. It should be obvious that there is overlap in the definitions themselves and in their occurrence in specific populations. Examples of these occupational issues will be presented with specific cases that cross the lifespan.

Populations at Risk for Occupational Issues

Occupational issues of concern often occur in at-risk populations (Table 8-1). A population at risk is defined as "those in the population who are susceptible to a particular disease or condition" (McKenzie et al., 1999, p. 66).

In a changing world, the populations at risk for occupational issues change over time. In the past century, interventions were targeted to specific populations to address their occupational needs. During the settlement movement of the early 1900s, creative occupations were used with various populations-at-risk, especially immigrants, to address individual and societal problems associated with poverty and industrialization (Addams, 1961). During the first half of the 20th century, the mental hygiene movement, the philosophy of pragmatism, and the arts and crafts movement also supported the use of occupations with individuals having various maladies (e.g., psychiatric illnesses and tuberculosis) (Clark, Wood, & Larson, 1998).

Occupations in the 20th century were also a primary means of restoring health and functional ability to individuals with disabilities secondary to medical conditions. Improvement in occupational performance was a primary goal in rehabilitation programs and special education programs. Specific populations having occupational interventions included veterans returning from wars with injuries or posttraumatic stress; individuals with medical conditions like stroke, spinal cord injury, or psychiatric diagnoses; and children with developmental disabilities. Many of these interventions were provided by occupational therapy practitioners. The education and practice of these professionals focused on occupational interventions and the supporting components of occupation. These populations are examples of past populations at risk for occupational issues. A discussion of several current populations-at-risk follows. By the time this text is published, other populations will surface that have occupational issues of concern.

The International Classification of Function (ICF) framework of the World Health Organization (World Health Organization [WHO], 2001) provides us with an important tool for describing individuals and populations-at-risk for occupational issues. The ICF dimensions of body structure, body function, and environment can help us understand the specific personal and environmental characteristics that support and limit occupational performance. The ICF framework also includes activity and participation dimensions that enable us to examine the complete constellation of occupations for an individual.

In community health, we must identify the general characteristics of the population at risk; examine the incidence, significance, and importance of the issue in the population; determine population factors that relate to the issue; and consider the issue in terms of human policies and the current political climate. Several dimensions are often used to characterize at-risk populations: gender, age, health status, ethnic background, socioeconomic levels, education, and geographic residence. These dimensions are examined because we find that occupational issues are often found in specific populations.

Community health initiatives emphasize the importance of describing at-risk populations because of disparities in health status for different groups. *Healthy People 2010* (U.S. DHHS, 2000) has a primary goal to eliminate health disparities for different populations. There are still substantial differences in mortality and morbidity rates for different populations associated with race, income, and gender. Disparities are also found in populations having different educational levels, disabilities, geographic residences, and sexual orientations. Many of these health disparities are related to occupational issues and are believed to result from variations in personal characteristics, environmental factors, and health behaviors.

Table 8-1

Sample of Occupational Issues of Concern in Populations

Target Area	*Possible Occupational Issues*	*General Population*	*Specific Populations of Concern*	*Incidence*	*Health Issues*	*Source*
Physical activity	Imbalance	Adolescents and adults	Women; individuals with disabilities, lower incomes, less education; African Americans and Hispanics; older adults; people in northeastern and southern parts of U.S.	40% of adults don't engage in any physical activity	Bones, muscle; weight control; psychological well-being and risk of depression/anxiety	*Healthy People 2010* (U.S. DHHS, 2000)
Substance abuse	Delay, deprivation, interruption, and imbalance	Adolescents and adults	Alcohol use in adolescents ages 12 to 17	23% of adolescents age 12 to 17 used alcohol/drugs, 16% of adults engaged in binge drinking, and 6% of adults used illicit drugs during the past month	Child/spousal abuse, sexually transmitted disease, unintended pregnancy, school failure; motor vehicle accidents, drownings, suicide, homicides; increased health costs, low worker productivity, and substantial disruptions in family, work, and personal life; heart disease, cancer, liver disease, fetal alcohol syndrome	*Healthy People 2010* (U.S. DHHS, 2000)

(continued)

Table 8-1

Target Area	*Possible Occupational Issues*	*General Population*	*Specific Populations of Concern*	*Incidence*	*Health Issues*	*Source*
Mental health	Interruption, imbalance, and disparities	Adults and older adults	Older people on medications and with coexisting medical conditions; rates among nursing home residents is estimated as 15% to 25%. Incidence is also higher in women especially among those who are poor, on welfare, less educated, unemployed, and specific minority populations	20% of the U.S. population has mental illness during a given year with depression being the most common disorder; >19 million adults suffer from depression—the leading cause of disability and more than two-thirds of suicides each year Only 23% of adults diagnosed with depression received treatment	Associated with other medical conditions. Mental health is essential to personal well-being, family, and interpersonal relationships and health of a society	*Healthy People 2010* (U.S. DHHS, 2000)
Injury and violence	Disparities, deprivation, and imbalance	All populations	Males, especially African American males; adolescents in the 15 to 24 age group	There are 15.8 deaths per 100,000 persons from motor vehicle accidents with 15% of them being in the 15 to 24 age group. Nearly 40% of traffic fatalities in 1997 were alcohol related. In 1997, more than 32,000 people died from firearm injuries and 42% were victims of homicide;	Significant mortality rates. Permanent health conditions associated with injury. Mental health issues	*Healthy People 2010* (U.S. DHHS, 2000)

(continued)

Table 8-1

Target Area	*Possible Occupational Issues*	*General Population*	*Specific Populations of Concern*	*Incidence*	*Health Issues*	*Source*
				African American men are seven times more likely to be victims		
Runaway and homeless youth	Delay, interruption, and imbalance	Adolescents	Half are 15 to 16 years old; 66% of the youth seek shelter assistance because of problems with parental relationships	500,000 to 1.5 million young people run away or are forced out of their homes every year; 200,000 are estimated to be homeless and living on the streets	Long-term dependence on social services; related problems of street youth	U.S. DHHS Administration for Children and Families (2001a, 2001b)
Domestic violence	Interruption and imbalance	Women	Not specific to any group of women	Approximately 4 million annual occurrences of domestic abuse against U.S. women; 2.4 million children are abused by parents each year	Injuries, mental health issues	
Refugees	Interruption, disparities, and deprivation	Families	Targeted groups are often local and regional	Since 1975, approximately 2,325,000 refugees have been resettled in the U.S. In fiscal year 1998, over 90,000 refugees were admitted for resettlement	Health issues associated with limited economic self-sufficiency and delayed social adjustment	*Healthy People 2010* (U.S. DHHS, 2000)

At-risk populations may be identified by different governmental agencies. At a regional level, states or provinces often establish goals or priorities for populations with certain characteristics living in specific geographic, economic, and political environments. For example, one state might have a particularly large immigrant population that is adjusting to different social and cultural norms. At a national level, countries usually establish priorities for funding and programs that are linked with specific populations. For example, the U.S. welfare to work program has represented a major shift in the lives of people who previously had limited requirements for employment.

Populations with disease or pathology are often identified as those at greatest risk for occupational issues. However, there has been growing interest in the occupational issues of populations that are typically described as healthy. These issues may be initially targeted in public health and education prevention programs as a means of decreasing the incidence of major health problems and then popularized in magazines and talk shows. Some recent issues of discussion have included the neck and back problems of children carrying heavy backpacks (Guyer, 2001), the changing face of rural communities (HHS Rural Task Force, 2002), the shortage of affordable housing (U.S. Department of Housing and Urban Development [HUD], 2002), and isolation of some elders in their communities (Chop, 1999).

A description of at-risk populations may begin with an awareness of people in our own community and the occupational issues they have. The next step, however, requires a review of sources of information about the population and issue and the projections and goals proposed by community organizations.

Sources of Information

There are numerous community organizations that serve as valuable sources of information and provide projections and goals for populations at risk. These community organizations may be part of health, education, or social service arenas and classified as governmental, quasi-governmental, and nongovernmental (McKenzie et al., 1999). Governmental organizations are defined as those international and national agencies that are funded by taxes and managed by the government. Governmental organizations may be at the federal, regional, state, or local level. Quasi-governmental organizations are defined as those agencies that receive some governmental funding but otherwise operate independently from governmental agencies (e.g., Red Cross). Other funds are received from a variety of private sources. Nongovernmental organizations are defined as those agencies that are funded by private sources for a specific mission and include voluntary health agencies; professional associations; foundations; and other service, social, religious, and corporate organizations.

Healthy People 2010 (U.S. DHHS, 2000) is a specific source of information that summarizes the national health priorities for the United States as established by the DHHS. *Healthy People 2010* seeks to increase quality and years of life and eliminate health disparities. If you read the objectives for *Healthy People 2010*, you will not find specific mention of occupational issues. However, it is clear that many of the goals are directly related to habits, routines, and lifestyles or the patterns of occupations that contribute to good or ill health.

Introduction to Six Populations at Risk for Occupational Issues

In this chapter, we will examine six at-risk populations. Two primary assumptions were used to select the six populations discussed here. First, the populations represent the entire lifespan and have a variety of occupational issues of concern. Second, the goals for these populations emphasize different dimensions and may be addressed by several types of intervention strategies. The goals may be realized through different human service systems (e.g., health, education, community) and models of intervention (e.g., direct, consultation, education).

Each population is examined using a standard process. First, the age group is described, and a brief summary of general issues and goals is provided. This discussion includes background information on the incidence, urgency, and importance of issues for this age group. Then, two subpopulations for each age group are examined for specific occupational issues of concern. The dimensions supporting and limiting occupational performance are reviewed, and occupational goals are proposed.

Infants, Children, and Adolescents

There are approximately 70.4 million infants, children, and adolescents (birth to 18) in the United States (Federal Interagency Forum on Child and Family Statistics, 2001), representing approximately 26% of the population. The number of children is approximately equal in three age groups: birth to 5, 6 to 11, and 12 to 18.

The years from birth through age 5 represent a time of incredible physical growth. During this time, the development of most personal factors required for occupational performance occur, including neurobehavioral, physiological, psychological, and cognitive aspects. Development in these areas is necessary for performance of activities and participation in broader environments during the elementary school years, ages 6 to 11 years. Adolescence, the period from puberty to maturity, is often a turbulent period with hormonal changes, maturation of body structures and functions, and increasing independence. These years are a time of exploration, idealism, and cynicism and offer an opportunity to begin planning for the future; adopt healthy attitudes about life choices; and develop meaningful roles with families, friends, and communities. This is also a period when young people may engage in a variety of risky behaviors.

One of the most important areas of development for the child is the social-emotional aspect of occupational performance. The child needs to develop trust of self and others, regulate emotions and behaviors, cope and adapt to changing environments and contexts, and eventually to function as a contributing member of his or her society. Occupational opportunities are important for developing these abilities. Initially, the family has the greatest influence on this process, with the immediate neighborhood and community supporting the efforts of the family. Gradually, these socializing influences expand to include school, peers, and community.

There are many factors that threaten the development of infants, children, and adolescents. Homelessness and substance abuse are two of the current factors that put young people at great risk for participation in society and pose significant occupational threats (U.S. DHHS, 2000). The overall goals for this age group are to improve overall quality of life, promote healthy social-emotional development, develop occupational potential, and prepare them to deal with the many risks encountered during these years.

Homeless Families

The Stewart B. McKinney Homeless Assistance Act of 1987 defines homelessness as people who:

> ...lack a regular and adequate night time residence; have a night time residence that is supervised public or private shelter; sleep in an institution that provides temporary residence; or sleep in a public or private place not ordinarily used as sleeping accommodations for humans". (Yamaguchi & Strawser, 1997, p. 91)

Currently, there are an estimated 3 to 4 million people in the United States who are homeless, including approximately 400,000 families with 1.1 million homeless children. National data show that families with children are the fastest growing group of homeless people in the United States. The "typical" homeless family consists of a single mother who is about 30 years old with three children averaging 5 years of age (Nunez & Fox, 1999).

There are many occupational issues of concern for children who are homeless, including *delay, deprivation, interruption, and disparities*. These occupational issues are related to health problems, instability in the home environment, limited social support systems, poor access to educational and community resources, and mental health issues. The lack of routine health care frequently may lead to increased rates of chronic health problems such as poor nutrition, chronic ear and respiratory infections, and skin diseases, which in turn put children at increased risk for occupational delay. Occupational deprivation and interruption occur when there is no stability in the home environment and when a family is housed in less than ideal living conditions or has to relocate frequently. A family that has to move frequently may not be able to maintain an assortment of toys and books that promote occupational engagement. Families who are homeless also have poor access to schools, limited and unsafe places to play, and few adult role models and playmates. The occupational disparities evident in people who are homeless may be related to social justice issues—poverty, racism, and classism—with African Americans being heavily overrepresented and whites significantly underrepresented in most regions of the United States (Nunez & Fox, 1999).

Homelessness can affect all levels of health in the ICF framework, including body structure, body function, activity, and participation. Children who are homeless experience more frequent developmental, psychological, and behavioral problems, including short attention span, separation anxiety, withdrawal, aggression, sleep disorders, poor social interaction, and delays in motor and language skills (Yamaguchi & Strawser, 1997). Homelessness leads to more frequent activity problems in learning, language and communication, movement, care of self and others, social interactions, coping, and adaptation. These problems at the person, environment, and activity level lead to limitations in the ability of homeless children and adolescents to fully participate in society.

Homelessness is greatly affected by numerous national, state, and local policies. Frequently, families' problems are so complex and the policies are so numerous that it is difficult to access and provide needed services. Health policies such as Medicaid, welfare policies such as Welfare to Work, and educational policies such as Individuals with Disabilities Education Act (IDEA) all influence the provision of services. Of particular importance for children and adolescents is their right to a free and appropriate education, as guaranteed by IDEA. Subtitle VII-B of the 1987 McKinney Act, Education for Homeless Children and Youth, ensures all children who are homeless the same right to a free and appropriate education as children whose families have permanent housing (Stronge & Hudson, 1999).

The occupational goals for homeless families are to engage in occupations that promote development, coping, and adaptation and to achieve the stability and safety in their home and school environments necessary for optimal occupational performance.

Substance Abuse in Children and Adolescents

America and many other countries have been waging a war on drugs for the past 20 to 30 years. Unfortunately, the war shows no signs of being won. Recent surveys have shown a sharp resurgence in adolescent substance use starting in the early 1990s with the rates for several drugs being higher than at any time since the mid-1980s. One source (Centers for Disease Control [CDC] National Center for Health Statistics [NCHS], 2000) indicated that in 1999 about 50% of all high school students (48% female/52% male) reported alcohol use in the previous 30 days, with binge drinking (five or more drinks on one occasion) reported by 28% of girls and 35% of boys during same 30-day period. This source also indicated that marijuana is the most commonly used illicit drug with 47% of high school students indicating they had ever used it and more than 25% indicating that they had used it one or more times in the past 30 days. Approximately 30% of students indicated that they had their first experience with alcohol and 11% had their first experience with marijuana prior to age 13 (Grant & Dawson, 1998). Research has shown that the younger a person is when he or she begins to use tobacco, alcohol, and drugs, the more likely he or she is to develop addiction and the multiple behavior and social problems that go along with it.

The occupational issues of concern in adolescents who use alcohol and drugs include *delay*, *deprivation*, *interruption*, and *imbalance*. Alcohol and illicit drug use contribute to substantial disruptions and changes in personal, family, and community life (DHHS, 2000). Substance abuse is associated with many serious societal problems including relational and predatory violence, sexually transmitted diseases, unwanted pregnancy and sexual abuse, chronic unemployment and low worker productivity, school failure, injuries and deaths related to motor vehicle and other types of accidents, escalation of health care costs, and homelessness. Long-term heavy abuse can lead to a variety of chronic health problems, including heart disease, cancer, and alcohol-related liver and pancreatic disease. Alcohol use during pregnancy is known to cause fetal alcohol syndrome, a leading cause of preventable mental retardation.

Cigarettes and alcohol are the substances most commonly used by adolescents and frequently are gateways to illicit drugs such as marijuana, cocaine, crack, heroin, acid, inhalants, and methamphetamines, or to the misuse of legally prescribed drugs. Although most adolescents who experiment with these substances do not progress to chronic abuse or dependence (Weinberg, Rahdert, Colliver, & Glantz, 1998), there are still many problems that go along with such use. Even small amounts of use in middle school can have a detrimental impact on academic performance. As substance use becomes more frequent and serious, so do the associated problems that were listed above. Alcohol abuse alone is highly associated with accidents and violence, which are the leading causes of injury and death among young people.

The reasons why adolescents begin to use tobacco, alcohol, and illicit drugs are varied and not fully understood. Common contributing factors are described as the portrayal of these substances in the media, inadequate supervision of children by parents, and poor role modeling by parents related to their own use of a variety of substances. Some people blame adolescent peer pressure to take risks, while others feel many young people are bored, hurt, stressed, insecure, or lonely (Packer, 2000). Young people may start to use as a way to have fun, but over time begin to use as a means to deal with the negative results of their acquired habits. Some adolescents may have an attitude favoring antisocial behavior and a lack of opportunities for positive involvement in school and community activities ("Study Links," 2000).

Multiple factors put adolescents at increased risk for substance abuse and addiction, including family history of addiction; temperament and personality characteristics; and concomitant emotional and mental health issues that involve disorders of behavioral self-regulation such as attention deficit-hyperactive disorder (ADHD), obsessive compulsive disorder (OCD), bipolar disorder, anxiety, or depression. Typically, adolescents at high risk are those who have problems with behavioral self-regulation and difficulties with planning, organizing, attending, abstract reasoning, foresight, judgment, self-monitoring, and motor control (Weinberg et al., 1998).

More resources need to be aimed at the primary and secondary prevention efforts to prevent, delay, and decrease substance use by youth. According to a 3-year study by the National Center on Addiction and Substance Abuse (CASA) at Columbia University, total U.S. state spending to deal with the results of illegal drugs, alcohol, and tobacco use is approximately $78 billion, while only about $3 billion was spent on prevention programs (Parker, 2001). To help prevent substance use, children and adolescents need to engage in a variety of occupations that provide healthy, stimulating, and expanding adventures to increase self-esteem, promote problem solving, and help them learn to regulate behaviors and emotions. Packer (2000) tells teens to say "yes" to getting high, but on their own terms. He writes that we need to offer teens tools and strategies they can use to lead healthy, rewarding lives full of passion, growth, and highs gained through experiences far more intense, rewarding, and long lasting than those achieved through drugs.

The occupational goal for adolescents at risk for substance abuse is to promote engagement in healthy occupations that promote self-regulation, self-esteem, and emotional growth.

Adulthood: Young and Midlife

Adulthood includes the ages between 18 and 65 years old. It is a very important and busy time in the human lifespan. It includes the period of life when people complete their formal education, work to develop financial independence and security, develop significant relationships, reproduce and form families, and make contributions through their vocations to broader society. During this period of life, people also develop and maintain multiple roles (e.g., child, parent, caregiver, citizen, worker, community, volunteer). During the last half of adulthood, many people begin to experience effects of aging and health conditions that influence activity and participation.

The characteristics of current and future adult populations are important to note. In the United States, there have been gradual and multiple changes in the profiles of some individuals in this age group (e.g., higher educational levels, longer hours at work), their families (e.g., delayed reproduction, nontraditional families, increased geographic distances among members, two-worker families), and their communities (e.g., diversity in race, culture, language, disability, aging work force, increased disparities, global influences, labor opportunities). All of these changes in turn influence changes in occupational performance.

Public policy initiatives in the United States will influence many aspects of life for the adult population of the future. Social security benefits will likely be lower. There have been proposed changes in U.S. immigration policy. People will live longer and healthier lives because of advances in and access to medical technology. The makeup of the workforce will include an increased mix of cultures, ages, genders, and races. Industry will continue moving from mass-production occupations to office-worker, service-provider occupations. Increased global competition, due in part to advances in communication, will continue to increase the demand for new technologies (U.S. Department of Labor, 1999).

The fastest population growth is estimated to be in the 45-and-older age groups. This growth reflects the aging of the large baby boom population, those born between 1946 and 1964. With most of this group still a decade or more from retirement, the proportion of the population that is economically active will remain at a record high. Even with this growth in the age 45-and-over population, statistics show there will be a slowing of labor force growth in the coming decades (Minnesota Department of Human Services [MDHS], 1998). The estimated number of workers age 16 and older is expected to fall short of demand (MDHS, 1999).

According to the U.S. Bureau of Labor Statistics, white, non-Hispanics was the largest group in the labor force in 1988, accounting for 79% of the total population. However, from 1988 to 1998, this group had the lowest growth rate, 0.06% a year, among the groups analyzed. The smallest group, Asians, showed the fastest growth rate (Fullerton, 1999). The number of men in the labor force is projected to grow, but at a slower rate than in the past. The labor force participation rate for men is projected to continue declining (Fullerton, 1999). Labor force participation rates of women have been increasing across age groups. The group of women who increased their participation the most during the 1978 to 1988 period was those aged 35 to 44 years (U.S. DHHS, 2000). In contrast to the general pattern, labor force participation rates of women 16 to 24 years of age dropped over the 1998 to 1999 period (Fullerton, 1999). The rate of growth for women in the labor force is expected to slow, but it will still increase at a faster rate than that of men. As a result, the share of women in the labor force is projected to increase from 46% in 1998 to 48% in 2008 (Fullerton, 1999). Immigration will continue to impact the growth of the U.S. labor force. The Hispanic labor force will expand nearly four times faster than the rest of the labor force, accounting for 12.7% of the labor force by 2008, compared with 10.4% in 1998 (MDHS, 1998).

Work is the framework around which economic stability, affordable health care, and personal prosperity depend (U.S. Department of Labor, 1999). America's workforce of the future will include more people of color, older Americans, women, and people with disabilities. The availability of larger pools of workers creates the opportunity to maintain economic growth by tapping new human capital resources (U.S. Department of Labor, 1999). While adults will enjoy longer, healthier lives, they will also remain in the workforce longer before retirement. The percentage of adults who care for dependents other than children, such as aging parents, will continue to rise (Czaja, 1999). There will be a need to understand and interact with individuals from other cultures and areas of the world. Industry shifts will require additional learning to keep up with the changes in technology. While advances in medical technology and public health policy have increased the health and well-being of the population, inequalities in income and education will continue to underlie many health disparities in the United States (U.S. DHHS, 2000). Goals of the adult population are based on the need to provide for themselves, their families, and their future, and include having a sustained income; having access to affordable, quality health care; and securing their retirement income (Fullerton, 1999; U.S. Department of Labor, 1999). Depending on the age and life circumstances of the adult, these goals may have more or less significance or priority at any given time.

Adults in the Sandwich Generation

The sandwich generation (Brody, 1981) has been defined as adults who have significant involvement in occupations that involve care of both young people and adults. During young and middle adulthood, care of children has always been a primary role in many people's lives. However, an increasing number of adults in this age group also have responsibilities of caring for other adults, especially elders.

Caregiving responsibilities may contribute to a risk of *occupational interruption* and *occupational imbalance* for the sandwich generation population. Caregiving can interrupt performance of all other occupations and result in imbalance in some occupations, notably work and leisure. The stresses and tensions that occur from balancing family and work are increasing as these responsibilities of childcare and elder care overlap (U.S. Department of Labor, 1999). Many caregivers are under increased personal stress due to caring for an adult relative or friend at the same time they are raising and caring for young children. These responsibilities make it difficult to maintain a balance in physical, social, mental health, and rest needs. More than half of adult workers providing care have had to make changes at work, such as leaving early, going in late, changing to part time, or taking time off during the day to accommodate caregiving. Six percent of workers providing care report having to give up work entirely as a result of caregiving responsibilities (U.S. DHHS, 2000).

There has been a noted increase in the number of adults/elders who have difficulty performing some occupations. About 7.3 million Americans age 15 and over, or 4% of the population residing in households, have difficulty performing one or more or the following activities: bathing, dressing, eating, using the toilet, and getting into or out of a bed or chair (U.S. Department of Labor, 1999). According to the Bureau of Labor Statistics, the growth rate of this noninstitutionalized population will continue to increase. While the growth rate of people 64 to 75 years old is projected to decrease, the rate of people 75 and older is expected to increase in the next 5 to 6 years (U.S. DHHS, 2000).

More than half of this population requires the assistance of another person to perform activities of daily living. Family members are the primary source of such assistance. Spouses provide 38% of assistance, followed by daughters (19%), other relatives (12%), and sons (8%). Only 9% of those needing assistance use paid providers (U.S. Department of Labor, 1999). In 1996, 22.4 million U.S. households (almost 20%) provided informal care to a relative or friend age 50 or older or had done so in the previous year. During this same year, more than 4 million households spent at least 40 hours a week in caregiving for the elderly, and 1.6 million spent 20 to 40 hours a week. Nearly two out of three family caregivers are working either full- or part-time (U.S. Department of Labor, 1999), and almost three-quarters of current caregivers are women (MDHS, 1999).

Caregiving has an enormous impact on the work life of the caregiver and the work environment. Employers report an increase in the number of requests for time off to care for aging parents. According to the Families and Work Institute, 42% of all workers were projected to be providing some form of elder care in the year 2002 (Galinski & Bond, 1998). In 1998 at Bank Boston, 50% of extended family leave involved care of elderly residents (U.S. Department of Labor, 1999). At State Street Corporation in Boston, unpaid time off for elder care accounted for 15% of all leave requests, up from 8% in the 2 previous years. A 1997 study estimated the aggregate cost of caregiving in lost production to U.S. businesses at $11.4 billion per year (U.S. DHHS, 2000). Those costs were attributed to absenteeism, hiring replacements for those forced to leave because of caregiving responsibilities, workday interruptions, and employee physical and mental health care. It is estimated that future increases in need for family caregiving will have their greatest impact on women in the workforce (MDHS, 1999).

Occupational goals for the sandwich generation address balance in caregiving, work, social, and personal responsibilities; work conditions that facilitate productivity and offer flexibility; support and assistance for caregiving; financial and health care resources; and opportunities for occupations that enrich life.

Midlife Workers

By 2008, the median age of the labor force will approach 41 years (MDHS, 1999). The proportion of people working past age 55 will increase from 45% in 1990 to 65% in 2020. Almost all of this increase will be attributable to people between ages 55 and 64 (MDHS, 1999). Supporting these projections is evidence that two-thirds of baby boomers expect to continue working past age 65, some out of economic necessity and some by choice (American Association of Retired Persons [AARP] Public Policy Institute, 1998).

Many individuals over the age of 50, who are not working, do not define themselves as retired, and most want to continue working full-time. Only 25% of people in this category consider themselves as fully retired, while almost 50% define themselves as temporarily unemployed and 30% as partially retired. However, once unemployed, individuals 55 to 64 years old are more likely to become discouraged workers. They have either stopped looking for work because they either believe no work is available or do not know where to look (MDHS, 1998). In a 1998 study, the AARP indicated that age, physically demanding work, early retirement plans offered by employers, and three or more functional limitations were among the factors that have the most significant impact on retirement for both men and women (MDHS, 1998).

The midlife worker is at risk for *occupational deprivation* and *occupational disparities*. Balancing household, family, work, and community activities provides increased challenges. The number of families with both parents in the workplace had risen to two-thirds by 1998, and the number of single-parent families doubled over the past 30 years (U.S. Department of Labor, 1999). More women in the workplace have forced families to find alternative ways to do the work traditionally done by stay-at-home moms. Some of those include sharing household responsibilities among family members, contracting out such traditional tasks as day care and housekeeping, and eating in restaurants or purchasing take out. Children are participating in more organized activities that often require transportation and participation by one or more parents. Families are dealing with increased time constraints as well as increased financial constraints (U.S. Department of Labor, 1999).

Disability rates among midlife workers, those ages 45 and older, are relatively stable. Challenges for people with disabilities, however, have not significantly changed. Medically, people with disabilities experience more anxiety, pain, sleeplessness, and days of depression than those without activity limitations (U.S. DHHS, 2000). People with disabilities also have other disparities, such as lower rates of physical activity and higher rates of obesity. Many lack access to health services and medical care. The percentage of adults with disabilities who have not completed high school is more than double that of adults with no disabilities. Fewer than 10% of adults with disabilities have graduated from college (U.S. DHHS, 2000). Attention from both policymakers and the private sector has begun to focus on increasing job opportunities for disabled workers. Laws and policies requiring equal access for people with disabilities, coupled with advances in assistive technologies, are estimated to result in rising rates of education attainment for people with disabilities (U.S. DHHS, 2000).

While the vast majority of workers are in good health and do not have any functional limitations or conditions that limit work, it is important to consider the physiological and functional effects of aging on work performance (MDHS, 1998). With the aging process, individuals generally experience a gradual decline in acuity in all five senses (touch, taste, smell, sight, and hearing). Many of these changes can be addressed by modifying individual behaviors and introducing environmental (workplace) modifications (Czaja, 1999). Many midlife workers are seasoned employees and as a result may have more training and safety awareness than younger workers. Younger workers whose bodies are not accustomed to the physical stresses of heavy industry may not be prepared for physically demanding jobs. The midlife worker may be more skilled in the techniques required to do certain jobs (Czaja, 1999).

Occupational goals of midlife workers may address adaptation to continue job performance with changing levels of ability, environmental modification or accommodations to support work performance, balance in worker and other personal roles, and security of financial and benefit resources.

Older Adults

The growth of the population age 65 and older will significantly affect almost all aspects of our society, from individuals and families to policymakers and communities. In 30 years, 20% of the population will be older than 65 years old, and the proportion of old-old adults (older than 85 years) will triple in size (Chop, 1999). The cultural and ethnic backgrounds of older adults in the United States is projected to be very diverse, with minority groups representing 25% of the population by 2030 (U.S. Bureau of the Census, 1990). The majority of the old-old adults are women, and three out of every five of them in 1997, for example, lived alone (AARP, 1998).

Advances in medical care have reduced the morbidity and mortality rates of older adults who are living with chronic health conditions. Currently, 85% of older adults live with a chronic health condition, yet overall disability rates are declining (Manton, Corder, & Stallard, 1997). However, given the advances in health care, more than half of the older population reported having at least one disability, and the percentage of those living with disabilities increases sharply with age. Although chronic health conditions do not necessarily lead to disability, there is some correlation between chronic health conditions and increased rates of depression. More than 85% of depressed older adults have significant health problems, and as many as one in five community-dwelling older adults show signs of clinical depression (Riley, 2001). Currently, the U.S. suicide rate is highest for those older than 65, indicating the significance of this problem (Chop, 1999).

The challenge for this century will be to make the additional years of life as healthy and productive as possible. This is reflected in the goals of *Healthy People 2010* and the National Institute on Aging (NIA). The primary NIA overall goals are to improve the health and quality of life of older people (NIA, 2002). Research and intervention efforts focus on preventing or reducing age-related diseases or disabilities, maintaining physical health and function, enhancing older adults' societal roles and interpersonal support, and reducing social isolation (NIA, 2002).

Older Adults/Retirees

The population projections indicate that there will be significant increases in the number of older adults entering retirement in the near future. This is going to change communities in significant ways, yet the impact is somewhat difficult to predict because it is unknown how the baby boomer generation will adapt to retirement. In 1990, individuals who retired at 65 years spent an average of 3% of their lives in retirement or only a few years. Today, the average retiree spends 25% to 30% of his or her life in retirement or approximately 20 to 35 years (Chop & Robnet, 1999). The transition from work to retirement is also no longer clear cut. It is becoming more of a process than a single event, with an estimated one-third of retirees reentering the work force (Sterns, Junkins, & Bayer, 1999). Most baby boomers believe they will still be working at least part time, doing community service, and devoting more time to hobbies during their retirement years.

Retirement is an occupational transition. It represents a change in usual occupational roles, patterns, and routines that provided some rewards and predictability. Loss of that role can result in an *occupational interruption* and *imbalance*, even if retirement is welcomed and anticipated. Jonsson and colleagues (2000) followed 12 older adults for 7 years through their retirement in Sweden and found that, for most participants, retirement was full of surprises and temporary periods of turbulence. Some participants managed a transition into a satisfying retirement, and others found it an ongoing process of frustration and dissatisfaction. One of their findings was that "the presence or absence of engaging occupations appeared to be the main determinant of whether participants were able to achieve positive life experiences as retirees" (p. 428).

Careful planning is necessary to fill the void with other meaningful occupations to maintain balance between work, rest, and play. Maintaining this important balance has been correlated with higher morale and lifestyle satisfaction among retirees (Jonsson, 1993). The types of occupations that are linked to retirement satisfaction are those that provide regular challenge and engagement with other people and continuity with patterns that proved satisfying earlier in their lives (Osgood, 1993). Most retirees do not start totally new types of activities, but increase the time spent on previously meaningful activities (Jonsson, 1993). Therefore, pre-retirees should take an inventory of the meaningful occupations in their lives and develop a plan to reintroduce or increase time engaged in them. Many older adults will need assistance long before retiring, especially those who have few, if any, meaningful occupations outside of employment. Others will benefit from the planning of a new routine that includes a balance of meaningful occupations with emphasis on those most related to life satisfaction.

Other areas linked to retirement satisfaction include good health, positive attitudes, adequate income, and preparedness for retirement (Christianson & Hammecker, 2001). Financial preparedness is often stressed at the workplace, but most companies do not help their employees with the personal and social planning necessary for successful retirement. There are three primary challenges for older adults entering retirement: the thoughtful preparation for retirement, the act of retirement itself, and the continual adjustment to retirement.

The occupational goals for this population promote smooth transitions into retirement and good quality of life throughout their retirement years.

Old-Old Adults

The old-old (elders older than 85 years) represented just more than 1% of the U.S population in 1994. By 2020, the size of the oldest-old population is expected to double to approximately 7 million and double again by 2040 to 14 million (U.S. Bureau of the Census, 1990). Because the oldest-old have the highest number of chronic health problems and disabilities, the rapid growth of this population has significant implications for families and communities.

Old-old adults are most at risk for occupational *deprivation*, *disparities*, and *imbalance*. One-third of the 70 to 74 age group reported attending movies, sports events, clubs, or other group events, while less than 14% of those older than 85 years reported attending those events (U.S. Bureau of the Census, 1990). Rogers and colleagues (1998) found that many older adults stopped doing certain activities such as shopping, dining out, volunteering, using the library, traveling, and visiting friends or relatives when they experienced difficulties. They also have lower levels of exercise, travel, cultural activities, and outdoors or sports activities than younger adults do, particularly for adults older than 75 years (Kelly, Steinkamp, & Kelly, 1986).

Dependency and disability rates increase significantly for the old-old adults. The percentage of adults older than age 85 having difficulty with activities of daily living such as dressing, preparing meals, and managing money is more than twice that of the 75- to 84-year-olds (U.S. Bureau of the Census, 1990). There is a high correlation between the number of dependencies in activities of daily living and the risk for institutionalization with one in four of those older than 85 placed in a nursing home (Chop, 1999). Increased frailty contributes to higher rates of falls, one of the biggest threats to the independence of older adults, particularly those older than 75 years. Falls are a leading cause of injury and death, and 75% of seniors older than 75 who fracture a hip die within a year of the incident (Christianson & Hammecker, 2001). Obviously, older adults have a lot at stake in preventing a fall. The fear of falling can result in some useful adaptations, such as slowing down or holding onto supports, but can potentially impact participation in meaningful occupations if individuals limit their activities unnecessarily.

For old-old adults, transportation availability has the greatest impact on occupational opportunities and greatly affects their quality of life. According to a 1997 AARP study, one-fourth of the 75-plus age group do not drive, and this number is expected to rise (Straight, 1997). Those with higher incomes are more likely to drive, and older drivers in general limit their options by avoiding night driving, certain routes, or rush hour. Older adults who no longer drive are at a higher risk for social isolation as they take an average of three times fewer trips per week than older drivers do. Fifty percent of these nondrivers take fewer than two trips per week (Straight, 1997). Physical impairments are the primary reason older adults stop diving, but others stop driving because they no longer need to drive, can't afford a car, feel they are too old, or get rides from a spouse. Current public transportation does not seem to be a useful substitute because 86% of the older non-drivers do not use it, citing reasons such as lack of availability, inconvenience, being unable to walk to a bus stop, or other physical limitations (Straight, 1997).

When faced with chronic health conditions, increasing disability, lack of transportation, and fear of falling, old-old adults are forced to make choices and adaptations to activities and social patterns that have proven satisfying in the past to create a satisfying life. According to Atchley's continuity theory (1997), older adults are happiest if they can achieve a sense of stability of activity over time and across different contexts. When they are unable to continue previously meaningful activities, older adults are at risk for isolation and increased dependence leading to depression and deteriorating physical health (Ostir, Markides, Black, & Goodwin, 2000).

One of the major challenges in our aging society is to help older adults cope with and adapt to their activity limitations by helping them find ways to continue participation in meaningful occupations. The occupational goals for old-old adults promote opportunities for participation in meaningful occupations given their increasing frailty.

Future Needs and Directions

There are obviously countless other populations at risk for occupational issues, and by the time this book is published, other at-risk populations will emerge as well. It may seem like an impossible task to accurately identify at-risk populations. What are some strategies for identifying and tracking populations? One important strategy is to constantly engage in environmental scanning at local, national, and international levels. Scanning at different levels is important because the populations of concern at one level may not necessarily be the populations of concern at another level. Environmental scanning can include formal strategies (e.g., review of literature, Internet search) and informal strategies (e.g., community activism, newspapers). A second strategy is to establish a site where you track occupational issues of at-risk populations. This site may include Internet links to governmental, quasi-governmental, and nongovernmental Web sites that routinely study specific populations. How do you identify populations with occupational issues if they are not explicitly named as occupational? Investigate the possible relationships between occupational issues and health issues by examining studies that use related terminology (e.g., activity, lifestyle, and quality of life). You can also raise awareness of possible occupational issues when discussing at-risk populations with colleagues, peers, policy-makers, and community members.

This chapter has introduced terminology related to occupational issues of concern in populations and has described six populations at risk for occupational delay, deprivation, disparities, interruption, or imbalance. The reader is invited to continue learning about at-risk populations and advocate for their needs as they relate to occupational performance.

References

American Association of Retired Persons Public Policy Institute. (1998). *Factors influencing retirement: Their implications for raising retirement age*. Washington, DC: AARP.

Addams, J. (1961). *Twenty years at Hull-House: With autobiographical notes*. New York, NY: Signet.

Atchley, R. C. (1997). *Social forces and aging: An introduction to social gerontology* (8th ed.). Belmont, CA: Wadsworth Publishing Co.

Brody, E. (1981). "Women in the middle" and family help to older people. *Gerontologist, 21*, 471-479.

Centers for Disease Control, National Center for Health Statistics. (2000). Health, United States, 2000, with adolescent health chartbook. Retrieved on October 3, 2002, from http://www.cdc.gov/nchs/hus.htm.

Centers for Disease Control, National Institute for Occupational Safety and Health. (1997). Work-related musculoskeletal disorders (CDC Document #705005). Retrieved September 29, 2002 from http://www.cdc.gov/niosh/muskdsfs.html.

Chop, W. C. (1999). Demographic trends of an aging society. In W. C. Chop & R. H. Robnet (Eds.), *Gerontology for the health care professional* (pp. 1-16). Philadelphia, PA: F. A. Davis.

Chop, W. C., & Robnet, R. H. (1999). *Gerontology for the health care professional*. Philadelphia, PA: F. A Davis.

Christianson, C., & Hammecker, C. (2001). Self-care. In B. Bonder & M. Wagner, (Eds.), *Functional performance in older adults* (2nd ed., pp. 155-178). Philadelphia, PA: F. A. Davis.

Clark, F., Wood, W., & Larson, E. (1998). Occupational science: Occupational therapy's legacy for the 21st century. In M. Neistadt & E. B. Crepeau (Eds.), *Willard and Spackman's occupational therapy* (9th ed., pp. 13-21). Philadelphia, PA: Lippincott.

Czaja, S. J. (1999). Promoting employment opportunities for older adults. Paper presented at the International Conference on Aging, Washington, DC.

Federal Interagency Forum on Child and Family Statistics. (2001). America's children: Key national indicators of well-being. Retrieved October 3, 2002, from http://childstats.gov/ac2001/ac01.asp.

Flexner, S. B. (Ed.). (1987). *Random House dictionary of the English language* (2nd ed.). New York, NY: Random House.

Fullerton, H. N. (1999). Labor force projections to 2008: Steady growth and changing composition. *Monthly Labor Review, 122*, 19-32.

Galinski, E., & Bond J. T. (1998). *The 1998 business worklife study: A sourcebook*. New York, NY: Families and Work Institute.

Grant, B. R., & Dawson, D. A. (1998). Age of onset of alcohol use and its association with DSM IV alcohol abuse and dependence: Results form the National Longitudinal Alcohol Epidemiologic Survey. *Journal of Substance Abuse*, 9, 103-110.

Guyer, R. L. (2001). Backpack=back pain. *American Journal of Public Health, 91*, 16-19.

HHS Rural Task Force. (2002). One department serving rural America: HHS Rural Task Force report to the Secretary. Retrieved October 2, 2002, from http://ruralhealth.hrsa.gov/PublicReport.htm.

Institute of Medicine, Committee on Nervous System Disorders in Developing Countries and Board of Global Health. (2001). Neurological, psychiatric, and developmental disorders. Washington, DC: National Academy Press. Retrieved September 29, 2002, from http://books.nap.edu/books/0309071925/html.

Jonsson, H. (1993). The retirement process in an occupational perspective: A review of literature and theories. *Physical and Occupational Therapy in Geriatrics, 11*, 49-56.

Jonsson, H., Staffan, J., & Kielhofner, G. (2000). Narratives and experience in an occupational transition: A longitudinal study of the retirement process. *The American Journal of Occupational Therapy, 55*, 424-432.

Kelly, J. R., Steinkamp, M. W., & Kelly, J. R. (1986). Later life leisure: How they play in Peoria. *The Gerontologist, 26*, 531-537.

Liptak, G. (1995). The role of the pediatrician in caring for children with developmental disabilities: Overview. *Pediatric Annals, 24*, 232-237.

Manton, K. G., Corder, L., & Stallard, E. (1997). Chronic disability trends in elderly United States populations: 1982-1994. *Proceedings of the National Academy of Sciences of the United States of America, 94*, 2593-2598.

McKenzie, J., Pinger, R., & Kotecki, J. (1999). *An introduction to community health* (3rd ed.). Boston, MA: Jones and Bartlett.

Minnesota Department of Human Services. (1998). *Aging initiatives: Project 2030 final report*. St. Paul, MN: Author.

Minnesota Department of Human Services. (1999). *Workforce and economic vitality issue paper. Aging Initiative: Project 2030*. St. Paul, MN: Author.

Mish, F. (Ed.). (1988). *Webster's ninth new collegiate dictionary*. Springfield, MA: Merriam-Webster Inc.

National Institute on Aging. (2002). Strategic plan to address health disparities. Retrieved May 8, 2002, from http://www.nia.nih.gov/strat-planhd/2000-2005/3.htm.

Nunez, R., & Fox, C. (1999). A snapshot of family homelessness across America. *Political Science Quarterly, 114*, 289-298.

Osgood, N. (1993). Creative activity and the arts. In J. R. Kelly (Ed.), *Activity and aging, staying involved in later life* (pp. 174-186). Newbury Park, CA: Sage Publications.

Ostir, G., Markides, K., Black, S., & Goodwin, J. (2000). Emotional well-being predicts subsequent functional independence and survival. *Journal of the American Geriatric Society, 48*, 473-478.

Packer, A. (2000). Interview on 'Highs! Over 150 ways to feel really, really good... without alcohol or other drugs.' *Curriculum Review, 40*, 15.

Parker, C. (2001). Columbia report: Substance abuse costing states $81 billion per year. *American Hospital Association News, 37*, 5.

Riley, K. (2001). Depression. In B. Bonder & M. Wagner (Eds.), *Functional performance in older adults* (2nd ed., pp. 305-318). Philadelphia, PA: F. A. Davis.

Rogers, W., Meyer, B., Walker, N., & Fisk, A. (1998). Functional limitations to daily living tasks in the aged: A focus group analysis. *Human Factors, 40*, 111-125.

Sterns, H., Junkins, M. P., & Bayer, J. (1999). Work and retirement. In B. Bonder & M. Wagner (Eds.), *Functional performance in older adults* (2nd ed., pp. 179-195). Philadelphia, PA: F. A. Davis.

Straight, A. (1997). Community transportation survey. Washington, DC: AARP. Retrieved February 6, 2001, from http://research.aarp.org/il/d16603_commtran_1.html.

Stronge, J. H., & Hudson, K. S. (1999). Educating homeless children and youth with dignity and care. *Journal for a Just and Caring Education, 5*, 7-19.

Study links peer substance use, school performance. (2000). *Alcoholism & Drug Abuse Weekly, 12*, 6-7.

U.S. Bureau of the Census. (1990). *U.S. population estimates, by age, sex, race, and Hispanic origin: 1989 (current population reports series, p-25, no.1057)*. Washington, D.C.

U.S. Department of Health and Human Services. (2000). *Healthy People 2010* (2nd ed.). Washington, D.C.: U.S. Government Printing Office.

U.S. Department of Health and Human Services, Administration of Children and Families. (2001a). The Administration for Children and Families (ACF) programs. Retrieved May 21, 2001, from http://acf.dhhs.gov/programs.

U.S. Department of Health and Human Services, Administration for Children and Families. (2001b). Fact sheets. Retrieved May 21, 2001, from http://www.acf.dhhs.gov/programs/opa/facts.

U.S. Department of Health and Human Services, Administration on Developmental Disabilities. (2002). ADD Fact Sheet. Retrieved September 29, 2002, from http://www.acf.dhhs.gov/programs/add/Factsheet.htm.

U.S. Department of Housing and Urban Development. (2002). Affordable housing: Who needs affordable housing? Retrieved October 2, 2002, from http://www.hud.gov/offices/cpd/affordablehousing/index.cfm.

U.S. Department of Labor. (1999). *Futurework: Trend and challenges for work in the 21st century, Executive summary.* Washington, DC: Author.

Weinberg, N. Z., Rahdert, E., Colliver, J. D., & Glantz, M. D. (1998). Adolescent substance abuse: A review of the past 10 years. *Journal of the American Academy of Child and Adolescent Psychiatry, 37,* 252-262.

Wilcock, A. (1998). *An occupational perspective on health.* Thorofare, NJ: SLACK Incorporated.

World Health Organization. (2001). *ICF international classification of functioning, disability, and health.* Geneva: World Health Organization.

Yamaguchi, B. J., & Strawser, S. (1997). Children who are homeless: Implications for educators. *Intervention in School and Clinic, 33,* 90-98.

Chapter Eight: Occupational Issues of Concern in Populations Reflections and Learning Activities

Julie Bass-Haugen, PhD, OTR/L, FAOTA

REFLECTIONS

This chapter was a natural next-step in our look at human occupation. We have seen that occupations evolve from one generation to the next, bring meaning to our life, shape our use of time, guide our development, inspire choices, and influence our health and well-being. Ah, the power of occupation! It is natural, then, that we are concerned about people who are not able to realize the full potential of occupation in their lives.

We don't need to look far to find people who have occupational issues of concern. They exist in our community and in every corner of the world. They come in all shapes and sizes—young people, old people, poor people, wealthy people, "healthy" people, and "sick" people. All populations are potentially at-risk for occupational issues.

This chapter could have taken any number of approaches to explore occupational issues of concern in populations. A lifespan approach for populations in the United States was adopted as the framework for this chapter. What other approaches could have been used? A global approach examining populations on each continent? A medical approach examining populations with certain health conditions? A disability approach examining populations with specific disabilities? A social welfare approach examining populations of different economic and social statuses? All of these strategies would have been effective in identifying at-risk populations.

In this chapter, certain terms were introduced as a way to get a handle on occupational issues of concern. *Delay*, *deprivation*, *disparities*, *interruption*, and *imbalance* were the words chosen to represent the array of occupational issues in populations. Some of these words are seen routinely in the health literature. We have all heard of developmental delays and health disparities. However, other words, like *interruption*, were chosen as the best words to convey certain kinds of issues even if they are not prevalent in the literature. What other words could have been used to represent occupational issues of concern?

Now, let's take a look at how the chapter discussed each age group and each population. First, an overall picture of the age group was presented. Who are they? What are they doing at this point in their lives? How many people are there in this age group? What's important at this point in time? What are the challenges and risks associated with this age? What are the occupational goals for this group? Second, a specific concern for this age group was identified. What is the concern? What specific people in this age group are at risk? What is the incidence of this concern? What are the health implications? What are the occupational issues? Finally, the occupational goals for this particular issue were proposed.

Infants, children, and adolescents have many occupational issues of concern. This chapter discussed homelessness and substance abuse as two important issues. During the past few years, many issues have surfaced for this age group, including runaway youth, obesity, physical or sexual abuse, teenage pregnancy, illiteracy, violence, poverty, and dysfunctional families. Even though children have a fair amount of resilience, we have to wonder how children with issues like these can maneuver around all the obstacles in their way and still become successful, productive members of society. Take an issue like literacy. What happens to children who have no support or encouragement for the occupation of reading in their home or community? Children who do not develop the skills and passion for reading are unable to enjoy many of the childhood occupations that require reading and are later limited in their future academic and vocational options. This is clearly an occupational issue of concern!

Young and middle adulthood also present many occupational issues of concern. This chapter discussed adults in the "sandwich" generation and midlife workers as two important issues. During the past few years, many issues have been identified for this age group, including financial debt, sexually transmitted diseases, anxiety and stress, eating disorders, parenting, affordable housing, unemployment, cancer, welfare to work, caregiving, refugee settlement, displaced workers, and divorce. Most of the readers of this text are in this age group. I am sure you can appreciate the occupational challenges you have and those of your peers. Take an issue like financial debt. What happens to young adults who have no training or discipline in occupations related to financial management (e.g., budgeting, balancing checking account)? We hear stories about foreclosures and bankruptcy quite frequently in the news and probably know of people who are completely stressed out because they live beyond their means or need to watch every penny. This is clearly an occupational issue of concern!

Older adults have occupational issues of concern as well. This chapter focused on early retirement years and physical frailty. During the past few years, the news has been filled with other issues of older adults, including medication management, falls, dementia, home management, finances, support systems, health care costs, sensory changes, depression, isolation, grandparent roles, assisted living or accessible housing, long-term care, and living wills. Take an issue like medication management. What happens to older adults who are unable to handle the occupation of medication management? We know of out-of-control health conditions, hospitalizations, injuries, overdoses, and medication psychoses, all resulting from poor medication management. This is clearly an occupational issue of concern!

In these examples and others, occupations are critical factors to consider if we are to fully understand and address the areas of concern. Through your study of human occupation, you are uniquely prepared to present this perspective. Many health, education, and social problems require creative solutions, and so I encourage you to become an activist for the occupational health and well-being of populations.

Journal Activities

1. Look up and write down dictionary definitions of population, delay, deprivation, disparity, interruption, imbalance, and injustice. Highlight the component of the definitions that is most related to their descriptions in Chapter Eight.
2. Identify the most important new learning for you in this chapter.
3. Identify one question you have about Chapter Eight.
4. Reflect on the three age groups discussed in this chapter. Think of one person you know from each age group who likely has occupational issues of concern. For each person, answer the following questions:
   - What are the general characteristics of the person (e.g., gender, age, etc.)?
   - What are the specific occupational issues of concern?
   - What are some specific examples that support your areas of concern.
   - What personal or environmental factors contribute to these occupational issues of concern?
   - Are these occupational issues of concern prevalent in the broader population?
   - What occupational goals would you identify for this person?

Technology/Internet Learning Activities

1. Use a discussion database to share specific journal entries.
2. Use a good Internet search engine to find the Web site for *Healthy People 2010*.
   - Enter the phrase "*Healthy People 2010*" in your search line.
   - Scan the main Web site for *Healthy People 2010*.
   - Describe *Healthy People 2010* and its primary goals.
   - Describe the leading health indicators identified by *Healthy People 2010*.
   - Describe five online resources available for individuals related to "occupations."
   - Describe five resources available for communities related to "occupations."
   - Describe two to three specific objectives and their relevance to occupational issues of concern.
3. Use a good Internet search engine to conduct an environmental scan of one population at risk for occupational issues of concern.
   - Enter search words in your search line to find general statistics on one population issue of interest. Try some of the following phrases in your search line:
     - "fastats" provides information from the U.S. National Center for Health Statistics.
     - "fedstats" provides information from more than 100 U.S. federal agencies.
     - "WHO Statistical Information System" provides information from the WHO.
     - "United Nations Statistics" provides international information from the United Nations.
     - "statistics Canada" provides information on Canada.
     - "state health facts" provides state level data from the Kaiser Family Foundation.

- Scan the site to find a population of interest that may have occupational issues of concern
- Summarize general characteristics of and statistics on the population of interest
- Describe general issues of concern for this population

4. Use a good Internet search engine to conduct an environmental scan of one population at risk for occupational issues of concern and two to three organizations that are concerned with the population.
   - Enter several search words in your search line:
     - ✧ By country: United States, Canada, United Kingdom, etc.
     - ✧ By state or province: Colorado, Minnesota, Virginia, British Columbia, Manitoba, etc.
     - ✧ By type of organization: government, government agency, organization, agency, etc.
     - ✧ By population: children, seniors, adults, etc.
     - ✧ By general or specific issue: health, education, social, aging, disabilities, etc.
   - Document the organization and the Web site.
   - Evaluate the quality of the Web site.
     - ✧ What is the primary objective or mission of this organization?
     - ✧ What specific information does this organization provide on your population of interest?
   - Describe general issues of concern for this population.
   - Propose occupational issues of concern for this population.
   - What are the current goals and objectives of this organization?
   - Describe the current programs and activities of this organization.
   - Summarize how these goals and activities relate to occupation.

Applied Learning

Individual Learning Activity #1: Conducting an Environmental Scan of Occupational Issues of Concern in Your Community

Instructions:

- Conduct an environmental scan of population issues in your community. For example, skim local newspapers or listen to local news for several days.
- Identify five populations that have specific areas of concern or needs. Try to select populations from a variety of age groups.
- Document the specific area of concern or needs for each population.
- Document your original source of information for each population.
- Identify other specific sources of information for this population (e.g., organizations, governmental agencies, Web sites, etc.).
- Propose occupational issues for each population.

Individual Learning Activity #2: Investigating One Occupational Issue of Concern in Your Community

Instructions:

- Select one population and area of concern to study in more detail from your environmental scan.
- Contact an organization for basic information on this population.
  - ✧ Identify specific characteristics of the population that are important to note. Who is at risk for this area of concern?
  - ✧ Identify specific health issues of concern and needs for this population. What specifically is going on with this population?

  - ✧ Describe the incidence and prevalence of this area of concern. How big of an issue is this?
  - ✧ Identify other organizations that address this area of concern. What other organizations are trying to address the same population and concerns?
  - ✧ Inquire whether a contact person from the organization would be willing to meet with a group of students for further information. Explain that you are doing this activity to learn more about populations with health issues and the organizations that serve these populations. Explain that such a meeting is tentative, depending on the next steps in the assignments.
  - ✧ Thank the person from the organization for his or her time.
- Propose occupational issues related to this area of concern.
- Propose occupational goals related to this area of concern.
- Summarize your conclusions about this population as it relates to occupational issues of concern discussed in the chapter.

Active Learning

Group Activity: Exploring the Occupational Issues of Concern in One Population and an Organization That Addresses These Issues

Preparation:

- Read Chapter Eight.
- Complete Applied Learning Activities #1 and #2.

Time: 45 minutes to 1 hour (at least two class sessions)

Materials:

- Information from Applied Learning Activities #1 and #2
- Flip chart, chalkboard, white board, or virtual board

Instructions:

- Individually:
  - ✧ Review your findings from Applied Learning Activity #2.
  - ✧ Evaluate the appropriateness of this population and organization for further study.
- In small groups (two to three people):
  - ✧ Share the results of Applied Learning Activities #1 and #2.
  - ✧ Select a specific population, area of concern, and a related organization for further study.
  - ✧ Review all information collected in the individual learning activity.
  - ✧ Obtain and review any written materials on the related organization.
  - ✧ Set up an informational interview with a contact person in the organization.
  - ✧ Explain that you are trying to understand the needs of this particular population and the ways in which one organization addresses these needs.
  - ✧ Obtain personal perspectives on the organization from the contact person on the mission and objectives, target populations, funding, programs, and services.
  - ✧ Obtain personal perspectives of the contact person on the greatest needs of the population and the organization.
  - ✧ Share information that you have collected on the population and questions you have.
  - ✧ Explore these population concerns and needs from an occupational perspective with the contact person.
  - ✧ Obtain information on ways that individuals can support the needs of the population and the organization.
  - ✧ Send a thank-you note to the contact person after the interview.

Discussion:

- Write a brief summary of your findings from all information collected on the population and the organization and your ideas related to the occupational issues of concern in this population.
- Share the results of your small group work with the class.
- Discuss the implications of looking at the needs of populations from an occupational perspective.

Chapter Nine Objectives

The information in this chapter is intended to help the reader:

1. Be aware of the various methods of inquiry to guide the understanding of human occupation.
2. Formulate a research question appropriate to the study of occupation.
3. Identify existing knowledge relevant to the study of occupation from a variety of literature sources.
4. Be familiar with the Occupational Competency Framework (OCF).
5. Use the OCF to understand the literature from other disciplines from an occupational perspective.
6. Use a variety of methods to gain an understanding of human occupation.
7. Generate new knowledge about the who, what, when, where, how, and why of occupation.

Key Words

case study: A design from the qualitative paradigm consisting of a systematic description and analysis of a particular case or situation.

descriptive study: The collection and measurement of data to describe the characteristics of a variable of interest.

design: The particular approach used by a researcher to answer a question.

ethnography: An approach to studying groups that involves gathering subjective information through interaction, observation, and direct participation with subjects.

experimental study: A research design involving the random assignment of subjects to at least one group that receives an experimental intervention and one group, serving as a control, that does not, with the intention of comparing the results of the two groups to determine differences.

grounded theory: A qualitative design involving multiple stages of data collection, where the researcher collects, codes, and analyzes observational and interview data until the data, being collected, become redundant and relevant categories and relationships are discovered.

method: Processes through which data are collected and measured in a study.

occupationologist: The person who studies occupation.

phenomenology: The study of events that happen as they are perceived.

quantitative paradigm: A tradition in research that emphasizes the collection, measurement, and objective analysis of observable phenomena.

Research is formalized curiosity. It is poking and prying with a purpose.
Zora Neale Hurston

Chapter Nine

Methods of Inquiry: The Study of Human Occupation

Helene J. Polatajko, PhD, OTReg(Ont), OT(C), FCAOT and
Jane A. Davis, PhD (Candidate), MSc, OTReg(Ont), OT(C), OTR

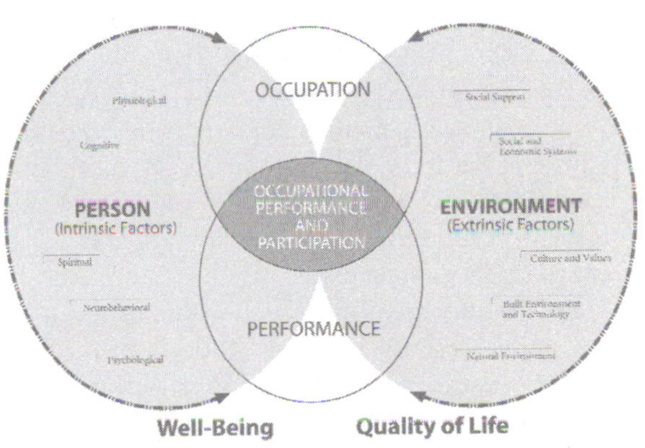

Setting the Stage

This chapter provides you with a guide on how to begin your inquiry into understanding human occupation. In Part One, the focus is on uncovering what is already known. You are given a process to follow to identify all the existing knowledge on the phenomenon of occupation. The process includes identifying the relevant literature, identifying a search strategy, retrieving the information, and determining the relevance of the information to your occupational question. You are also introduced to the Occupational Competency Framework (OCF), which you can use as a tool to help you organize the literature and identify the gaps.

In Part Two, the focus is on generating new knowledge, filling in the gaps. You are provided with the basic knowledge required to begin to answer occupational questions, using who, what, where, when, how, and why as a framework. Finally, you are introduced to the basic paradigms of inquiry along with various designs and methods that you can use to address your occupational questions and begin to fill in the gaps in understanding the occupational human.

Polatajko, H. J., & Davis, J. A. (2005). Methods of inquiry: The study of human occupation. In C. H. Christiansen, C. M. Baum, and J. Bass-Haugen (Eds.), Occupational therapy: Performance, participation, and well-being *(3rd ed.). Thorofare, NJ: SLACK Incorporated.*

INTRODUCTION

Humans of all ages are essentially occupational beings, spending most of their time engaged in doing. Many social interactions also center on what we do or on doing things together. When we first meet someone, we frequently start off by asking, "What do you do?" At the dinner table, parents find out about their children's day by asking, "What did you do today?" When coworkers return from the weekend, they typically ask "What did you do this weekend?" Indeed, what humans do is central to their very being. In many cultures, humans define themselves by what they do (e.g., I am a bus driver, I am a student, I am a teacher). Given the centrality of occupation to our very nature, it is important that we have a good understanding of the occupational human.

The study and understanding of occupation is approached in much the same way as the understanding of any phenomenon. First, you formulate a question, and then you seek to find the answer. Typically, you presume that the answer already exists and all you need to do is look it up. This is generally done by going to the existing literature, be it in books, journals, or on the Internet. On occasion, you discover the answer does not exist, and then you need to carry out your own investigation or experiment to discover the answer.

The specific literature on the human as an occupational being is relatively sparse.[1] Indeed, the express study of human occupation is in its infancy, with the discipline dedicated to this study having its beginnings in the latter part of the last century. At first glance, it would seem that the student interested in understanding human occupation has very little existing knowledge to draw on and must be content with generating new knowledge. However, this is not the case. There is an abundance of information available in a variety of places that provides an understanding of human occupation. The student interested in understanding human occupation must, therefore, become an expert in seeking out this information and interpreting it from an occupational perspective. As well, the student must be able to identify gaps in our understanding and be able to formulate and answer questions designed to fill those gaps.

The purpose of this chapter is to introduce the student to methods for answering occupational questions (i.e., methods to guide the understanding of human occupation). The chapter is organized into two parts: Part 1 describes how you identify existing knowledge (i.e., how to conduct a literature search and, if necessary, interpret it from an occupational perspective), and Part 2 describes how to generate new knowledge (i.e., methods of inquiry).

PART 1: IDENTIFYING EXISTING KNOWLEDGE

The specific study of occupation by the discipline is relatively new. Thus, it can be inferred that the knowledge base on occupation is sparse. This is only partly true. The discipline-specific knowledge base is sparse; however, considerable information on various aspects of human occupation exists. This information can be found in the literatures of various other disciplines. As Neutens and Rubinson (1997) state, the use of documents, knowledge, and research from various disciplines allows for a broader understanding of concepts under study. Part 1 focuses on searching for information to answer an occupational question. The OCF is presented as a means of organizing literature that may hold answers to the occupational question. Examples are given to help the student learn how to approach the literature.

The Occupational Competency Framework

The OCF[2] (Figure 9-1) is a three dimensional model. Based on the notion of Rubik's cube, the model represents the interactional nature of the three dimensions of occupational competency: person, occupation, and environment. The OCF is an adaptation of the Occupational Competency Model (Polatajko, 1992), which, as Rubik's cube, is a 3x3x3 model depicting each of person, occupation, and environment with three components. Consistent with the PEOP Model, the OCF is 5x5x5 cube; each dimension having five components that interact one with the other. The person dimension is comprised of cognitive, affective, physical, neurobehavioral, and physiological components; the occupation dimension: self-care, productivity, leisure, roles, and activities components; and the environment dimension: physical (including tools), social, cultural, natural environment, and economic conditions/resources components.

[1] Yerxa and her colleagues (1990) have called the new science *occupational science*. Polatajko (1992) has suggested that the study of occupation ought to be referred to as *occupationology*.

[2] The Occupational Competence Framework is adapted from Polatajko, H. (1992). Naming and framing occupational therapy: A lecture dedicated to the life of Nancy B. *Canadian Journal of Occupational Therapy*, 59, 189-199.

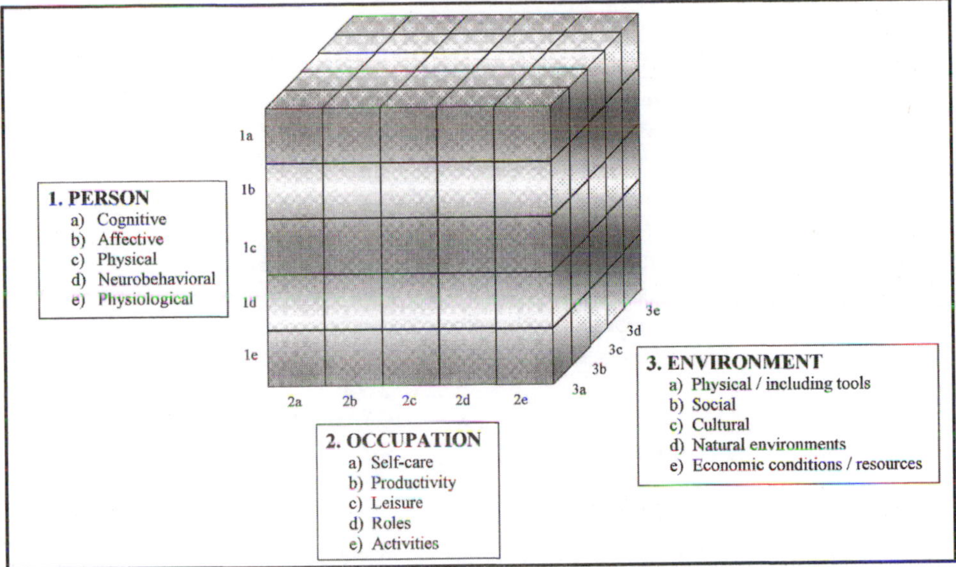

Figure 9-1. The OCF.[2]

The OCF provides the structure to organize the literature for clinical and research use. Specifically, it can be used by students, practitioners, and researchers to identify knowledge generated by other disciplines that provides insights into the occupational human, identify knowledge gaps within our discipline, and organize the literature so it can be easily used.

Application of the Occupational Competency Framework

The first step used in exploring the literature is to choose a phenomenon of interest and to examine the literature for what is already known about that phenomenon. Searching for what is already known requires identifying the relevant literature to search, identifying a search strategy, retrieving the information, and determining the relevance of the information to an occupational question.

Identifying the Relevant Literature to Search

What is known can inform your question. The student of human occupation is interested in person, occupation, and environment in interaction. Many disciplines or fields of study hold information that can inform the topic of human occupation. In Figure 9-2, the major relevant disciplines are mapped onto the OCF. Disciplines fall into place in different positions on the framework. For example, the environment can be understood from the studies of many disciplines, including architecture, forestry, ecology, geography, sociology, political science, and economics. These disciplines can provide information pertaining to various aspects of the environment, including natural and built physical, social, and societal environments. The person, occupation, and environment dimensions intersect with one another, forming further areas in which knowledge exists that could have potential to inform the study of occupation. A number of disciplines examine how people shape and are shaped by their environments (i.e., they investigate the person/environment interaction) (see Figure 9-2).

There are also a number of disciplines that, albeit indirectly, examine self-care, productive and leisure activities and tasks. Many references can be found that discuss theory and provide research into an individual's engagement in occupations (i.e., the interaction of person and occupation). For example, if the student has a question relating to the impact of culture (environment) on occupational choice of the older adult (person), a good starting place would be the literature from the discipline of cultural anthropology, due to its focus on the person and the cultural environment. It is always a good idea to find several articles that address the topic in which you are interested. By reading in the area of study, you will discover a more specific strategy to guide your search. Sometimes, you will find a review article that will identify key words and questions that are yet to be addressed.

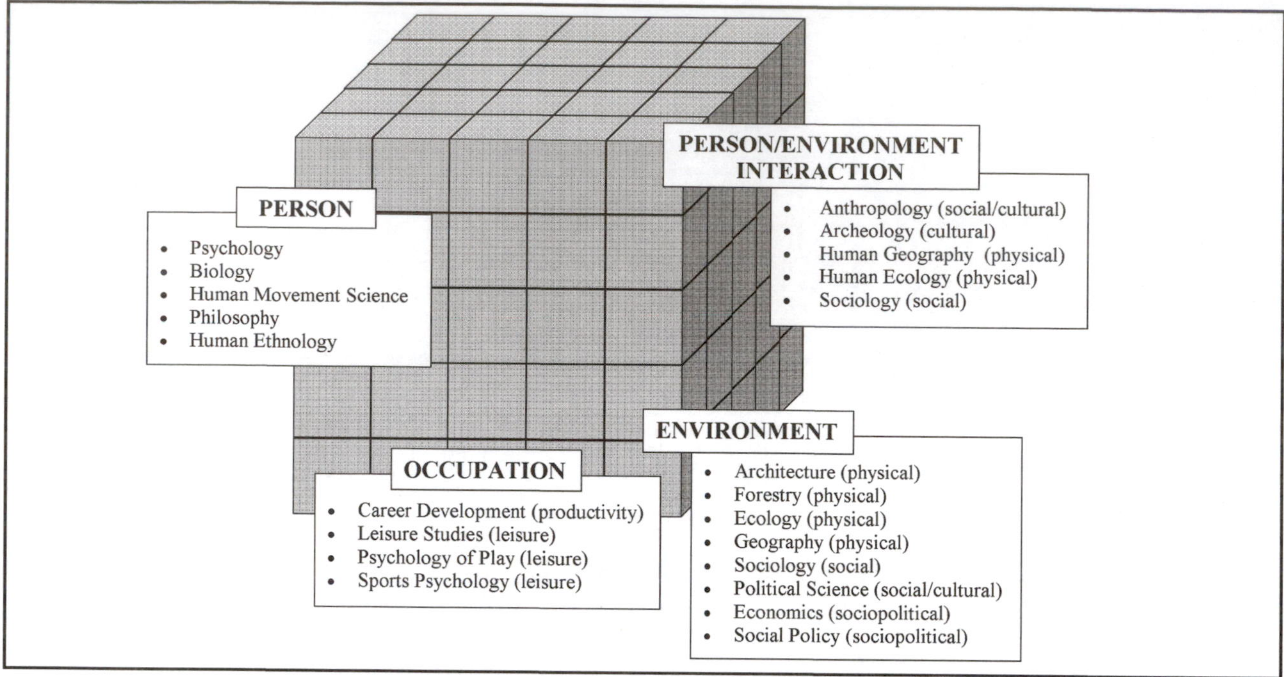

Figure 9-2. A mapping of disciplines on the OCF.[2]

Identifying a Search Strategy

Once relevant disciplines have been identified, your question can lead to a database to search. The best way to start the literature search is to use the current technology (i.e., bibliographic and full text databases, the World Wide Web, and library catalogues) to search for books; journals; magazines; and other video, audio, or written documentation.

To gain access to relevant information, key words have to be determined that are relevant both to the study of occupation and to the disciplines being searched (e.g., human activity, work, play, cultural activities, physical performance, chores). Thesauri and dictionaries can help you to generate an initial list of key words. If your knowledge of the discipline is limited, a good place to start is with a general textbook in the area. To find general textbooks, use the name of the discipline to search titles, and limit the search to the past 3 or 4 years to get the most current textbooks available. Reviewing the textbook by hand will help identify the key words, authors, theories, and concepts to use in subsequent searches. Establishing limits on searches (e.g., publication dates, languages, type of publication) can also help narrow down your search.

Once the databases, keywords, and limits are chosen, you are ready to search for information. This initial search for both journals and books will provide a general listing containing references to theories and ideas from a number of disciplines that could be beneficial to the study of occupation.

Libraries use various search interfaces or software (e.g., Ovid, WebSPIRS, Cambridge Scientific Abstracts), and each search interface uses a different set of commands and a different format to search the literature. The reference librarian can be of help in enabling you to uncover new ways of using the search interfaces more effectively. Your library may even offer classes in how to use the interfaces to explore the corresponding databases. You can become acquainted with many databases that are discipline specific (e.g., ERIC [education], sociofile [sociology], psycINFO [psychology], biological abstracts [biology]) or multidisciplinary (e.g., medline [medicine], cinahl [nursing and allied health], social science abstracts [social sciences], j-stor[3] [social sciences and humanities]). Some databases are available directly through the Internet (e.g., pubmed [medline's internet access], NLM gateway [National Library of Medicine], ingenta [social science], ERIC, j-stor). Different journals are indexed (i.e., available to be searched) through different databases. Some journals of a certain discipline may not necessarily be indexed through its corresponding discipline specific database, and others may be indexed by multiple databases.

[3] j-stor (with over 150 journal titles) requires membership for access but once a member most articles are available in the full format through the Internet. Some institutions have memberships with j-stor as well.

Information can also be found on the World Wide Web using various search engines (e.g., google, dogpile, mamma, yahoo, excite). Most publishers now offer direct online access to at least some of their more recent journal article abstracts (e.g., Psychological Review, Age and Aging). Summaries or abstracts are typically available for free, however, most full text articles require membership or a per article fee. Other online information, such as that found on various Web sites, requires closer scrutiny, as it can be posted by anyone with no verification of accuracy, and there is rarely any type of peer review process of the materials.

Book searches can be done at all libraries, most of which are online and available to all users through library catalogues. Many book searches will provide the table of contents for books from the 1990s to the present, allowing a more in-depth search of the content contained within edited books, in particular, when using "keyword" searches.

Retrieving the Information

Once you have located relevant journal article and book references, you need to determine where you can access them—whether through libraries, hospitals, or associations. If you have been unable to find a journal, you can access interlibrary loans, obtain a reprint directly from the author, or purchase a back issue from the publisher either through online services or by phone.

While searching the library shelves, it is important to examine the shelves surrounding the area where each listed book is located to make sure that an important source didn't get missed. To determine the usefulness of the book, you need to scan the table of contents, the index, and the references and/or bibliography using the key words that you had previously selected. Sometimes, journal articles are published in special theme editions, so always glance at the table of contents of each journal volume you use. The books and journal articles that you accumulate provide additional sources for searching, (e.g., theories, references, keywords).

Determining the Relevance of the Information to an Occupational Question

To benefit from potentially rich sources of information, the relevance of the information from an occupational perspective must be ascertained. Using the OCF as a guide, you can determine if information addresses the dimension of occupation (or one of its components) or if it addresses the person or environment dimension (or one of their components) in interaction with the occupation dimension. For example, searching for information on occupational change with age, you found the chapter by Woodruff-Pak and Papka (1999) on "Theories of Neuropsychology and Aging." This chapter provides a detailed discussion about the physical and cognitive aspects of the person with Alzheimer's disease. In other words, it addresses the person dimension on the OCF. There is minimal discussion of the impact on performance, so it has minimal relevance for an occupational question. Figure 9-3 provides examples of works identified as part of a general search using the OCF (i.e., works that address the occupational dimension or the occupational dimension in interaction with other dimensions of the OCF). Each of the works appearing in Figure 9-3 offers significant discussion of the occupational dimension. It is provided here to serve as a model of how literature from other fields of study can inform occupational practice and set the stage for research.

One work from Figure 9-3, Bandura's notion of self-efficacy, has been chosen to be reframed to answer an occupational question.

- Person: Bandura's Model of Perceived Self-Efficacy

The disciplines or fields of study examining the components of the person (i.e., physical, affective, and cognitive) offer many theories and ideas that can answer occupational questions (see Figure 9-3 for examples).

- Example Occupational Question: What is the role of cognition in occupational competency?

This broad question can be approached by researching different disciplines, including developmental and cognitive psychology and motor learning, and by using various keywords including motivation, physical abilities, self-esteem, self-efficacy, self-perception, self-determination, innate skills, cognitive skills, play, leisure, work, and career choice. One of the concepts that a search using these keywords would uncover is Albert Bandura's Model of Perceived Self-Efficacy, which refers to "beliefs in one's capabilities to organize and execute the courses of action required to manage prospective situations" (Bandura, 1995, p. 2).

Bandura believes that self-efficacy, or an individual's belief in his or her abilities to master performance of an activity, is cognitively regulated and is a determinant of whether a person will choose one activity or another. Although Bandura applies his model mainly to work, this model offers an understanding of activity that can be reframed from the broad perspective of occupation used within this text. Hence, an individual's occupational choice is determined partly by that same individual's belief or perceived self-efficacy in his or her skills and abilities to demonstrate mastery of the chosen occupation.

Bandura believes that perceived self-efficacy is a crucial aspect of "occupational development and pursuits" (Bandura, 1995, p. 23). As an individual is exposed to more occupations across his or her lifespan—whether an infant's self-feeding, a child's reading, an adult's bowling, or an older adult's second career—and is able to engage

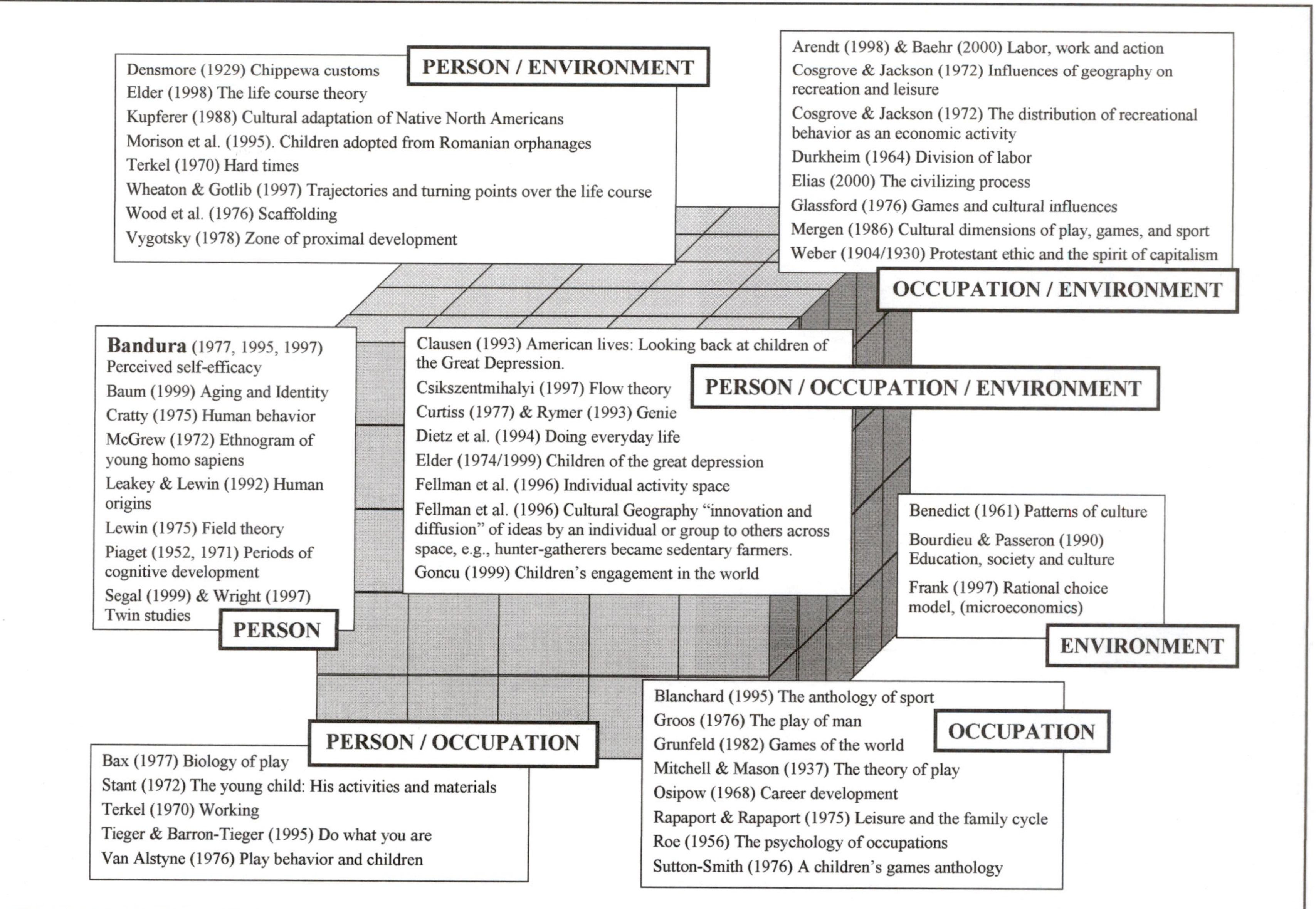

Figure 9-3. Examples of theories, research, and ideas with occupational relevancy as organized within the OCF.[2]

successfully in occupations of his or her choice, the individual will develop perceived self-efficacy in those areas, fostering further occupational development. Bandura (1995) summarizes the interaction of learning new skills and self-efficacy by stating, "...occupational development is a matter of acquiring not only new skills and knowledge but also the sense of efficacy through which innovativeness and productivity are realized" (p. 24).

Bandura (1995) lists four main forms of influence on the development of an individual's beliefs that he or she possesses what is needed for success or, in occupational terms, to achieve occupational competency: mastery experiences, vicarious experiences, social persuasion, and physiological and emotional states. Mastery experiences involve not only the easy successes, but also mastery of the difficult struggles, which require creativity and perseverance. "Some difficulties and setbacks in human pursuits serve a useful purpose in teaching that success usually requires sustained effort" (Bandura, 1995, p. 3). This process allows for the acquisition of "the cognitive, behavioral, and self-regulatory tools for creating and executing appropriate courses of action to manage ever-changing life circumstances" (Bandura, 1995, p. 3). Therefore, from an occupational perspective, mastery experiences help to develop the cognitive components of the person, allowing for the development of occupational competency, such as a child getting his or her first basket in basketball or an insurance salesperson making his or her first sale, and occupational mastery, such as the child growing up to play in the NBA or the insurance salesperson winning national employee of the year for outstanding sales. Vicarious experiences are those provided through watching others who are perceived to be similar to us and/or are engaged in activities that are comparable to ours. Hence, the effect on an individual's self-efficacy will be determined by whether the occupational engagement is successful or not and whether the occupation and person resemble the individual who is observing (Bandura, 1995).

Social persuasion involves an individual's reaction to the verbal persuasion of others. If others can persuade an individual that he or she possesses the abilities to engage in an occupation, that individual is more likely to continue his or her effort toward developing occupational competency and mastery. "Self-affirming beliefs promote development of skills and a sense of personal efficacy" (Bandura, 1995, p. 4); however, confirming results are also required to build efficacy. If an individual is told that he or she sings well by many friends but is then booed off the stage, he or she will doubt that original persuasion and will avoid this occupation in the future, limiting potential occupational development. An individual's physiological and emotional states are the fourth influence on the development of an individual's perceived self-efficacy, as Bandura (1995) believes that a person's judgment of his or her personal efficacy is affected by mood and physical status. If a person's mood is positive and he or she feels physically and mentally relaxed (i.e., the physical and affective components of the person), he or she will possess higher perceived self-efficacy in the successful performance of occupations.

Although Bandura's model mainly examines the person, it also incorporates many interactional aspects that are relevant to the understanding of human occupation. Bandura (1997) believes that many factors play a significant role in the interpretation of experiences, which may foster an individual's self-efficacy, including those of the person, the social environment, and the situation itself. In occupational terms, this refers to the extent to which mastery of occupations influences individuals' beliefs in their abilities, perceived difficulty of the occupation or its component tasks, the amount of cognitive, physical, and/or affective effort they have to expend, their physical and affective states at the time, the amount of help they are given by others within the social environment, and the occupational properties of the situation.

PART 2: METHODS OF INQUIRY

This section, in large part, is drawn from Polatajko (2004) and reprinted with permission from Pearson Education, Inc.

In Part 1 of this chapter, a framework was provided for searching out and using existing knowledge from the literature of other fields. Examples of reframing information from an occupational perspective and thereby enhancing our knowledge of occupation were provided. In Part 2, an overview of methods of inquiry is presented. Examples of a variety of studies using different methods are provided to show how various methods can contribute to our understanding of human occupation.

Part 2 is organized around the six basic questions of inquiry (Ferguson & Patten, 1979): who, what, when, where, how, and why. These six questions have been chosen because they fit well with both of the major paradigms of inquiry, the qualitative and the quantitative.[4] Each question is examined in turn, the question is elaborated

[4] Methods of inquiry emanate from one of two major epistemological perspectives: the naturalistic (also referred to as qualitative) and the positivistic (also referred to as quantitative, experimental-type, or reductionistic) (Jackson, 1999; Lincoln & Guba, 1985). The naturalistic paradigm is based on the assumption that the world is made up of multiple, overlapping realities, which are socially constructed, complex, and constantly changing. The role of the qualitative researcher is to come to an in-depth understanding of these realities and how they are constructed. In contrast, the positivistic paradigm is based on the assumption that the world is made up of observable, measurable facts. The ultimate goal of quantitative research is to explain and predict and to this end, research is expected to be objective, unbiased, and logical (Banister, Burman, Parker, Taylor, & Tindall, 1994; Clark-Carter, 1997; Creswell, 1994; DePoy & Gitlin, 1994; Drew, Hardman, & Weaver Hart, 1996; Glesne & Peshkin, 1992; Lincoln & Guba, 1985; Neutens & Rubinson, 1997).

on, and a number of methods appropriate to the question are identified. The spectrum of possible methods appropriate to the six basic questions of inquiry is broad. It is well beyond the scope of this chapter to present all available designs and methods, let alone describe them in any detail. The intent here is not to be comprehensive, but rather to provide an overview of the more common methods of inquiry for each of the six basic questions. The purpose is to enable the student to identify methods of interest and search out specific sources on those methods.

Gaining an Understanding

Our understanding of occupation can come from three sources: personal experience, existing data sources, and new investigations. Each of us has a great deal of personal experience with our own occupations and those of others. Our experience with occupation, direct or indirect, is very important in helping us develop a basic, informal, understanding of occupation, but it is insufficient. Constructing an understanding of occupation requires careful examination of the phenomenon in its entirety, including the context of the doing, the perspective of the doer, and the framework of the knower. This examination must be built not only on personal experiences but also formal methods of systematic inquiry.

What follows is a description of formal methods of inquiry for the study of occupation. The methods presented are those that are consistent with meeting the aims of any program of disciplinary inquiry (i.e., to describe and explain). The methods identified are by no means novel. They have been drawn from the literature of a number of disciplines concerned with the study of the human. Richards' (1926) observations about his own work apply aptly to these methods: "Few of the separate items are original. One does not expect novel cards when playing a traditional game; it is the hand which matters" (Pedhazur & Schmelkin, 1991, p. xiii).

In this section, care has been taken to identify common methods from both the naturalistic and the positivistic paradigms. This has been achieved by surveying recent methods texts addressing both perspectives from related disciplines—in particular education, social and behavioral sciences (Creswell, 1994; Drew et al., 1996; Glaser & Strauss, 1968; Glesne & Peshkin, 1992; Jackson, 1999; Lincoln & Guba, 1985; Pedhazur & Schmelkin, 1991), health sciences (DePoy & Gitlin, 1994; Neutens & Rubinson, 1997; Portney & Watkins, 1993), and psychology (Banister et al., 1994; Breakwell, Hammond, & Fife-Schaw, 1995; Clark-Carter, 1997; Haworth, 1996; Hayes, 1997).

Inquiry into the phenomenon of occupation should have the same basic structure as inquiry into any other phenomenon: question, design and methods (including methods of data collection, analysis, and interpretation), findings, and conclusion. Only the first few of these will be discussed here as these are the ones that take most careful consideration in determining how to go about studying occupation. The rest follow as a consequence of the decisions made about the first few.

The Question

The first step of any process of inquiry is the formulation of a question. While this is approached somewhat differently within a qualitative framework than within a quantitative framework (see DePoy & Gitlin, 1994 for a good discussion of this), our understanding of occupation is so rudimentary that all the questions of basic inquiry are appropriate to ask (both the descriptive questions: who, what, when, and where; and the explanatory questions: how and why). The specific question will depend on the aspect of occupation that is of interest to the knower and the paradigm of inquiry. In Table 9-1, there are some examples of specific questions that could (and should) be asked about occupation.

Design and Methods

The design and methods[5] to be used to address the questions of scientists studying occupation, as discussed, are those that are appropriate to description and explanation, emanating from the two major paradigms of inquiry. These are the basis for formal inquiry into a phenomenon.

Once a question has been formulated, the next step is to carry out a literature review to determine if the question has already been answered or to refine the question. Then, a design that is consistent with the question and the paradigm of inquiry and corresponding methods are chosen.

Many designs and methods are available to answer occupational questions. The more common ones are summarized in Table 9-2. The classification appearing in Table 9-2 is an amalgam of a number of different classifications,[6] not that of any particular author, although the

[5] There is some confusion in the literature about the use of the terms *method* and *design*. As used here, the term *method*, used in conjunction with the phrase of inquiry (i.e., method of inquiry), refers to all aspects of a study including the paradigm to be used, the design, and the specific methods and procedures used for data collection, analysis, and interpretation. The term *design* refers to the overall structure and plan of a study that emanates from the paradigm of inquiry and the question and determines the specific procedures and methods to be adhered to in conducting the study. The term *method*, used either alone or in conjunction with the phrases of *data collection*, *analysis*, and *interpretation*, refers to the specifics of data collection, analysis, and interpretation, respectively.

[6] There are a number of ways of classifying designs; some are based on purpose, while others are based on data collection strategies or analytical strategies; many are based on a mixed model of naming (Breakwell et al., 1995; Clark-Carter, 1997). There is no agreement on the best classification, nor is there any agreement on the terminology used to name what are essentially the same designs (e.g., the terms *nonexperimental*, *correlational*, *survey*, and *(passive) observational* have all been used to refer to the same designs) (Pedhazur & Schmelkin, 1991).

Table 9-1 The Six Questions of Basic Inquiry and Possible Subquestions Applied to Human Occupation

Purpose	*Question*	*Subquestions*
Describe	**Who** engages in occupations?	Do all people engage in occupations? Does all age, gender, race, religion, ethnicity, ability, health, or socioeconomic status affect occupational engagement? Did early humans engage in occupations?
	What occupations are there?	Are there patterns of occupations (i.e., are there occupational profiles)? Do occupational profiles differ among individuals, groups—systematically? Do the differences in occupational profiles reflect individual or group differences?
	When do people engage in occupation?	Are occupations engaged in at any time of day, week, year, life? Are there daily, weekly, seasonally, yearly, or life patterns of occupational engagement? Have the occupational profiles of humans changed over time?
	Where do people engage in occupations?	Are all/any occupations universal, or are they environmentally specific? Are some environments more conducive to occupational engagement than others? Are specific occupations done in specific places?
Explain	**How** are occupations performed?	How are occupations created/learned? How does the process of occupational engagement happen? What skills are required to perform occupations? How do personal or environmental resources impact occupational performance?
	Why do people engage in occupations?	What meanings are ascribed to occupations? Do people ascribe the same meanings to all occupations? Why do people choose particular occupations and not others? Why do some people seem to need to be occupied all the time while others don't?

classification for the quantitative designs is essentially that presented by Pedhazur and Schmelkin (1991) and Portney and Watkins (1993), and the classification for qualitative designs is that presented by Creswell (1994). The particular design elements that appear in Table 9-2 were chosen not only because they are commonly used but also because they fit well with the constructs: description and explanation; they eliminate like terms having different meanings; or their meaning is logically intuitive.

Table 9-2 also provides a listing of the more common methods of data collection for both paradigms. Design and methods of data collection have been distinguished for the following two reasons:

1. Clarity: Frequently, there is no distinction made between design and methods of data collection, resulting in confusion in the meaning of terms (e.g., an observational study versus observation as a means of data collection).
2. To make it obvious that some methods of data collection (i.e., observation and interview) span the quantitative/qualitative divide (Clark-Carter, 1997).

The more common designs for the quantitative paradigm are descriptive and experimental (Pedhazur & Schmelkin, 1991; Portney & Watkins, 1993). In descriptive studies, information is gathered about the phenomenon of interest for the purpose of documenting the nature

Table 9-2

Common Research Methods[1] in the Quantitative and Qualitative Paradigms

Quantitative	*Qualitative*
Study Designs	**Study Designs**
Descriptive studies (aka correlational, observational, survey)	Ethnography (observational)
Experimental studies (aka quasi-experimental, true experimental)	Case study
	Phenomenology
	Grounded theory
Methods of Data Collection	**Methods of Data Collection**
(Passive) observation	(Participant) observation
Interview	Interview
Questionnaire	Document and record collection
Measurement	Audiovisual materials
Instrumentation	
Document and record collection	
Audiovisual materials	

[1] This classification is an amalgam of classifications presented by Banister et al. (1994), Breakwell et al. (1995), Clark-Carter (1997), Creswell (1994), DePoy & Gitlin (1994), Glaser & Strauss (1968), Glesne & Peshkin (1992), Lincoln & Guba (1985), and Pedhauzer & Shmelkin (1991).

and meaning of the phenomenon at a specific point in time, describing how it changes over time, and exploring relationships among phenomena. In descriptive studies, there is no assignment of subjects or control of variables. In experimental studies, hypotheses regarding cause and effect are tested by the manipulation of certain variables and the control of others. In true experimental studies, assignment of subjects is random. In quasi-experimental studies, it is not.

The more common designs for the qualitative paradigm are ethnography, case study, phenomenology, and grounded theory (Creswell, 1994; Glesne & Peshkin, 1992). In ethnographic studies, through a process of long-term immersion, a researcher gathers information, primarily by participant observation and interview, about the attitudes, beliefs, and behaviors of a group of people or a culture for the purpose of understanding the forces that shape those behaviors and feelings. In case studies, the researcher uses a variety of data collection methods over a sustained period of time for the purposes of understanding a particular activity or phenomenon. In phenomenological studies, through a process of extensive and prolonged engagement, using observations and interviews, the experience and meaning of the individual's lived realities are examined. In grounded theory studies, the researcher, using multiple stages of data collection, collects, codes, and analyzes observational and interview data until the data being collected become redundant. Through a process of constant comparison of data, relevant categories and their relationships are identified and theoretical constructs are formulated.

Several designs can be used to answer any particular question. As well, the same design can be used to answer a number of the questions. The designs corresponding to the basic questions for occupationologists are discussed next, together with exemplars.

Understanding *Who*

It hardly seems necessary to ask the question, "Who engages in occupations?" Experience tells us that everyone—at least everyone we know, everyone we see around us, everyone we see in the media, everyone we hear about, and everyone we read about, be it in the present or in the past—engages in occupations. Further, the answer to this question seems to be well established in the historical, anthropological, social, and psychological literature (i.e., all people, regardless of the variables that typically distinguish groups, engage in occupation).

Yet, there are individuals who don't engage in occupations (Figure 9-4) or who do so very sparingly. Indeed, there likely have been times, perhaps brief, when you

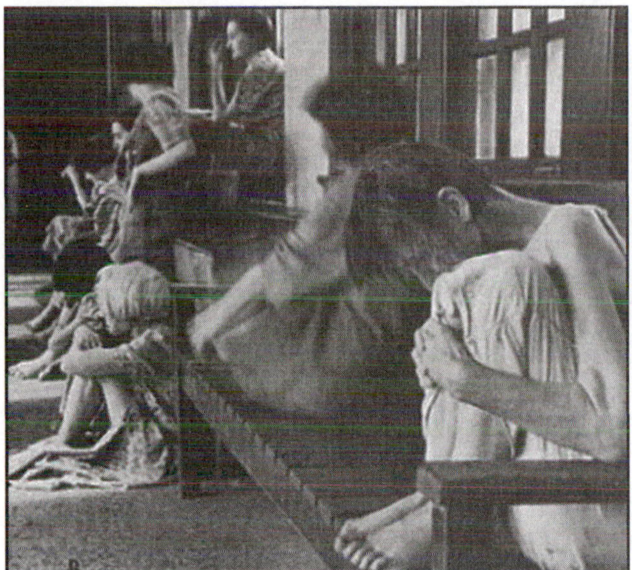

Figure 9-4. Lack of occupational engagement.

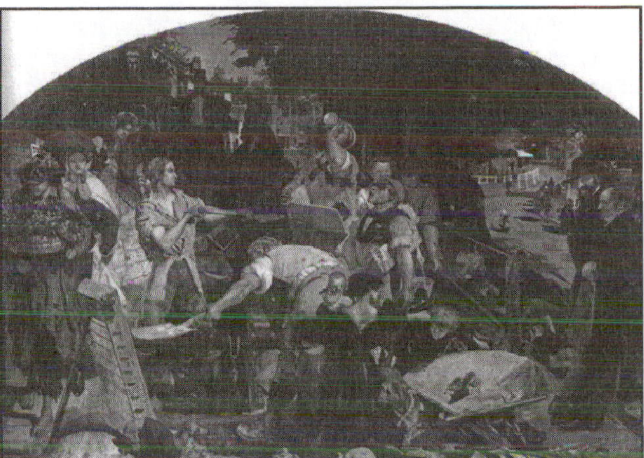

Figure 9-5. Accounts of occupations found in the arts.

yourself did not engage in occupation. Nevertheless, it is self-evident that most humans engage in occupations.

What warrants investigation then, is the exception, "Who does not engage in occupation?" In general, qualitative methods, such as ethnographies, are more likely to lend themselves to finding the exception, although quantitative methods, if used somewhat unorthodoxly (e.g., noting both the rule and the exceptions) may also be useful. Examination of existing data may also be very informative (e.g., documents or records describing individuals or groups of individuals, biographies, and autobiographies).

A good example of an autobiographical account detailing an individual's nonengagement in occupation is *Terry Waite: Taken on Trust* (1993). Terry was held in solitary confinement in Beirut by terrorists for 1,763 days. During most of that time, he was left with nothing to do. With his environment affording him nothing to do for the greater part of most days, Terry created his own, albeit unorthodox, occupations (e.g., he wrote his autobiography entirely in his head throughout the duration of his captivity). What becomes blatantly evident from this book is that nonengagement in occupation is difficult to induce. Further, nonengagement, or more precisely, severely limited engagement, is so difficult to bear that the individual creates whatever occupations can be supported by the environment and resumes a broad range of occupations as soon as the environment will allow. In other words, when considering the who of occupation, the what, when, and where of occupation must also be considered.

Understanding *What*

The question, "What occupations are there?"[7] seems almost as unwieldy a question to ask as the question, "Who engages in occupations?" seems unnecessary. Personal experience tells us that there are a tremendous number of occupations—possibly too many to count. One just needs to look in the do-it-yourself sections of bookstores or in the hobbies or careers section to make this obvious. As well, there are numerous sources, be it in the popular literature; the arts (Figure 9-5); or the historical, anthropological, social, and psychological literature, that give accounts of the various occupations of various people.

It is evident from all of these sources that there are a tremendous number of occupations that different people do at different times and that, therefore, it is less important to have a comprehensive listing of occupations than it is to understand the occupational repertoires and profiles of people. Attempting to understand which people do which occupations (i.e., attempting to establish occupational repertoires and profiles) can be dealt with in a number of ways, including case studies or descriptive studies, to get detailed profiles of individuals; ethnographies, to get detailed profiles of individuals or communities; and surveys, to get profiles of large groups.

Excellent sources for survey data on large groups are national census data. Virtually every country has a national agency that routinely collects demographic, socioeconomic, and social information about the population. The U.S. Census Bureau (United States Department of Commerce, U.S. Census Bureau, n.d.) provides statistics on a large variety of topics that include information

[7] Of course, the question of what occupations there are begs the question: What qualifies as an occupation and what does not? It is not in the scope of this chapter to deal with this question, other than to note that the study of occupation is in desperate need of a taxonomy to guide the work. The author and a group of colleagues are in the process of creating a taxonomy of human occupational activity.

on what people do. In the area of labor and employment alone, it provides information on the demographics of the labor force, commuting to work, occupation, industry, and class of worker. It also provides links to statistics from more than 100 U.S. federal agencies.

Under the Statistics Act, Statistics Canada (2002) is required to collect and publish statistical information on virtually every aspect of the nation's society and economy. Originally, the census was just a simple population count, but today Statistics Canada collects and distributes information from a variety of surveys, offering a rich source of information on the occupations of Canadians. Two types of surveys are routinely used: population surveys, or censuses, in which every possible respondent is approached, or sample surveys based on representative samples of the population. A number of survey designs are employed. These include one-time cross-sectional surveys, repeated surveys that consist of a series of separate cross-sectional surveys and longitudinal or panel surveys that collect information on the same individuals at different points in time. This census is a repeated survey that employs both census taking and sampling techniques.

Although the censuses provide a good overview of the activities of Canadians, they do not provide a detailed breakdown on activity patterns. There are, however, a number of other population surveys available that provide detailed information about activity patterns. The American (University of California, San Diego, Social Sciences and Humanities Library, n.d.) and the Canadian General Social Survey (GSS) (Carleton University Library, Ottawa, Data Centre, 2002) monitor changes in the health and activity of Americans and Canadians, respectively. These surveys provide rich data on what people do.

The Canadian survey is a repeated telephone survey conducted approximately every 5 years and includes questions on educational activity, paid work, unpaid work, personal care activities, physical activities, socializing, passive leisure activities such as watching television and reading, sports and other entertainment activities, and activity limitations. The Canadian GSS is collected from a representative sample of residents 15 years of age and older residing in Canada. Findings indicate that, aside from personal care, the most common activities are tasks around the home, with 90% of the people participating in household work and related activities for an average of 3.6 hours a day. Women spend an average of 1.5 hours more each day on housework than do men. Seventy-seven percent of the population older than the age of 15 watches television for an average of 3 hours a day ranging from a low of 2.3 hours per day for women 25 to 34 years of age to a high of 4.3 hours per day for men older than 65 (Statistics Canada, 1999).

What becomes evident from existing sources documenting human occupation is that there is, and has been, a tremendous variety of occupations that people engage in and that these occupations differ among people, although occupational repertoires and profiles can be discerned. Furthermore, it seems clear that understanding what occupations there are requires putting the question into the context of who, when, and where. In other words, when considering the what of occupation, the who, when, and where of occupation must also be considered.

Understanding *When*

Clearly, our personal experience would suggest that the answer to the question, "When do people engage in occupation?" is always (or, all their waking hours, depending, of course, on whether sleep is considered an occupation or not). Indeed, it is clear to all, in particular to those with children in the back seat of a long car ride, that people always want to be doing something. More interesting questions are, "When do people not engage in occupation?" and "When do which people engage in which occupations, and for how long?" In other words, the occupational patterns of people across the day, week, month, year, and life and across history need to be understood.

Again, there are existing sources that can help with the answer to this question in the popular literature, arts, and the historical, anthropological, social, health, and psychological literature. The work on circadian rhythms can be considered to offer insight into the daily pattern of human occupation. The author suggests that the expression of the circadian rhythm through activity (Fincher, 1984) can be the typical pattern of daily occupations (Figure 9-6). The life course literature on human development and aging can offer insights into the patternicity (i.e., the pattern of human occupation across the life course) (Elder, 1998). Historical analyses of activity patterns provide glimpses into how people's occupations have changed throughout history (Davis, Polatajko, & Ruud, 2002; Wilcock, 1998).

A number of approaches can be used to examine patterns of occupational engagement. Virtually all the qualitative designs could be used to establish occupational patterns. Within the quantitative armament, of particular use, is time in motion studies, either based on self-report data or observational data.

A good example of a study using a self-report time log is the study by Herrmann (1990). Working with a group of 20 single adolescent mothers, Herrmann attempted to describe their daily activities to discern if they were related to the subjects' maternal role or their adolescent role in order to determine the relationship between activities and perceived role conflict among adolescent mothers. She had the young women keep a time log on which they

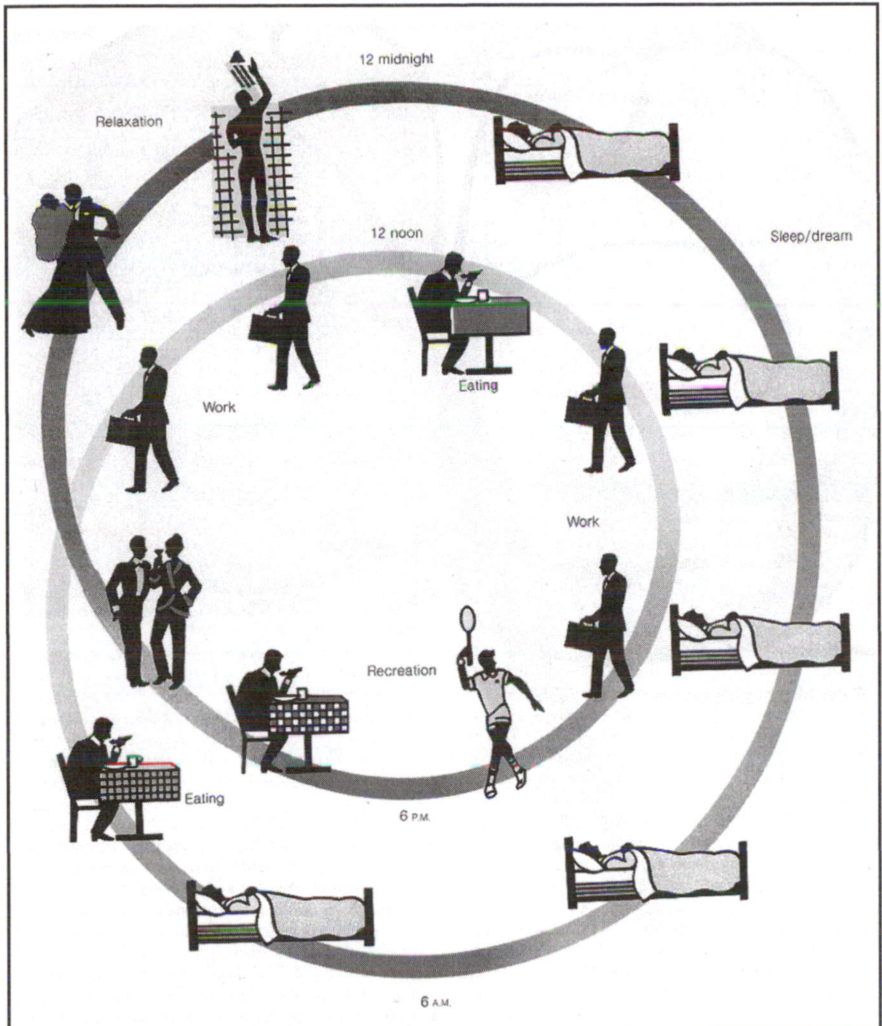

Figure 9-6. Circadian rhythm: typical pattern of daily occupations.

chronicled all their activities over a period of 4 days, ascribing them to either the mothering role or the adolescent role and noting their level of satisfaction with the particular activity. The data from the time log showed that these young women spent the majority of their time (78%) doing adolescent activities, leaving much of the childcare to others. Herrmann points out that, unexpectedly, this pattern was not different on weekdays, when the women were in school, and on weekends.

Herrmann's findings show that occupational patterns are not determined solely by the individual but also by the environment. In particular, her remarking on the lack of change in occupational patterns from weekday to weekend emphasizes the extent to which it is generally held that occupational patterns are not only affected by time but also by the environment in which they are performed. In other words, the who, what, and when of occupation must be considered with respect to where.

Understanding *Where*

As with the previous questions, the answer to the question of where people engage in occupations is also obvious. Personal experience, particularly among those who travel, the popular literature, and the arts all suggest that occupations happen everywhere—even in those environments where there are attempts to prevent occupational engagement (e.g., the story of Terry Waite). What is a more interesting question, therefore, is "What impact does location or geography have on occupational engagement?"

There are several ways of understanding the impact of location or geography on occupations. Again, all the qualitative methods and the descriptive quantitative methods would allow for such an investigation. As well, experimental methods would work well in determining the impact of location on occupation. The literature in such diverse fields as social and human geography, industrial psychology, architecture, sociology of community, urban planning, and community development all provide information on the interaction between occupations and environments.

A rich and colorful source of data on the effects of location and geography on occupations, now and in the past, is *National Geographic*. A browse through issues of *National Geographic* shows that occupations occur everywhere, including under the ocean and on the moon, and that some occupations occur all around the world (e.g., infant care), but are done differently in different places, while others only occur in specific places (e.g., surfing).

Interested in examining the impact of environmental change on occupational engagement, Connor Schisler and Polatajko (2002) carried out an ethnographic study of Burundian refugees in Southwestern Ontario, Canada. Connor Schisler spent more than a year interacting with and participating in the Burundian refugee community. She spent 17 months as an informal participant observer in this community and one academic term conducting formal participant observations. As well, she carried out in-depth interviews with eight of 18 adult members of this community and did individualized member checks with six of these individuals. Using the constant comparison method of data analysis, Connor Schisler found that all participants experienced dramatic changes in their occupations as a result of the physical, social, cultural, and economic differences between Burundi and Southwestern Ontario. Of particular interest was the finding that the changes in occupation resulting from the environmental changes affected the people themselves and that they, too, changed. In other words, where people engage in occupations affects when and what they do, which in turn affects who they are. How does this happen?

Understanding *How*

Whereas the who, what, when, and where of occupation are relatively well understood, relatively little is known about how people perform occupations. Personal experience can only inform us very superficially about the how of occupations. Much of the process of occupational performance is not readily observable or knowable (e.g., only relatively gross movements involved in the performance of a particular occupation can be observed and only the cognitive process available at a meta-cognitive level can be reported). A more in-depth understanding of how occupations are performed requires careful examination of the components of the person and the environment that are involved. Quantitative methods, often involving specialized instrumentations, in an experimental design, are best for an in-depth understanding of the process involved in occupational performance. There are many examples of such studies, especially in the ergonomic, medical, movement science, psychology, and social science literature.

Smyth and Mason (1998) carried out an experimental study to investigate differences in the role of vision and proprioception in a positional aiming task, between normal children and children with a developmental coordination disorder (DCD). The two groups of right-handed children (73 with DCD and 73 control children, matched on age, gender, and verbal ability) were asked to move their hand under a tabletop into alignment with a target on top of the table. The position of the target was made known to the children by vision, proprioception, or both. Accuracy of performance over 24 trials was measured in millimeters along the x and y axes. Results indicated that with proprioception alone, errors were made to the outside of the target; the control children tended to favor proprioceptive input while children with DCD tended to favor visual input, but only with their left hands. The authors concluded that detailed error analysis in aiming tasks provided information about target representation that could not be gleaned from less specific measurement strategies. This study provides experimental evidence of the impact of person and occupational factors on performance and demonstrates the usefulness of controlled studies in determining how occupations are performed. Many more studies of this type, investigating all aspects of performance, are necessary before it can be truly understood how occupations are performed.

Understanding *Why*

The final, and perhaps most important, question to be asked about occupations is "Why?" Of all the questions discussed here, it is the most difficult to answer. There is a general belief, supported by the media, that the basic reason for occupational engagement is survival. In other words, we work because we have to (i.e., we do what we do because it, directly or indirectly, provides us with food and shelter).

Personal experience tells us that there are endless examples of occupational engagement that negate, or at least bring into serious question, this basic survival premise. For example, the survival premise does not explain why people who do not have to work do so, why very young children engage in occupational activity, or why people do the specific things they do. In particular, the basic survival premise does not explain why people do things that put them at serious risk of survival.

All available methods of inquiry need to be used to uncover the why of occupation, and new methods need to be developed. The American GSS (National Research Council, 1999) provides an example of how survey methods can be used to look at work values and the meaning of work. Specifically, in the GSS covering 1973 to 1996, a question asked was, "If you were to get enough money to live as comfortably as you would like for the rest of your life, would you continue to work or would you stop working?"[8] Works by Studs Terkel and Patrick Joyce offer evidence that a phenomenological approach, designed specifically to uncover the meanings people ascribe to their experiences, is particularly useful in learning to understand why people do the occupations they do. *Working*, the 1975 documentary masterpiece by Terkel (1975), and *The Historical Meanings of Work*, a collection of scholarly essays edited by Joyce (1989), provide stories and experiences of individuals in the working world, demonstrating possibilities for how to expand the understanding of the why of occupation.

A study similar to that of Terkel's, but on a much smaller scale, was carried out by Rudman, Cook, and Polatajko (1997). In-depth interviews were carried out with 12 community-dwelling well elderly to discover their perspectives on the role and importance of occupations in their lives. The informants were chosen to allow for maximum variation. After an initial analysis of transcripts using a constant comparative method, two member checking group sessions were held. The results of these discussions were incorporated into the analyses, again using the constant comparative method. The emergent themes indicated that occupations were a means of expressing and managing personal identity, of staying connected to people, of understanding the past and the future, and of organizing time. More importantly, occupations contributed to the sense of well-being of the seniors, to their continued existence, and to the quality of that existence. As one informant put it:

> Most people have a job and that's the only thing, one job all their lives. And the trouble with them is that when they retire, they don't know what the hell to do with themselves. In 2 years, they usually get sick and die. (Rudman, et al., 1997, p. 643)

Conclusion

This chapter has provided the student with an initial understanding of the methods of inquiry used for the study of occupation. Part 1 provided a stepwise method for searching for relevant information in the many literatures that hold potential to offer an understanding of the occupational human. The process was brought together by the introduction of an occupational competency framework that can be used as a tool to organize the literature. In Part 2, the student was provided with methods for finding new knowledge related to the discipline of occupationology or occupational science. The application of the methods discussed in this chapter will allow the student of occupation to begin his or her journey into the world of the occupational human.

References

Arendt, H. (1998). *The human condition* (2nd ed.). Chicago, IL: The University of Chicago Press.

Baehr, P. (Ed.). (2000). *The portable Hannah Arendt*. New York, NY: Penguin Books.

Bandura, A. (1977). *Social learning theory*. Englewood Cliffs, NJ: Prentice Hall, Inc.

Bandura, A. (1995). *Self-efficacy in changing societies*. Cambridge, UK: Cambridge University Press.

Bandura, A. (1997). *Self-efficacy: The exercise of control*. New York, NY: Freeman.

Banister, P., Burman, E., Parker, I., Taylor, M., & Tindall, C. (1994). *Qualitative methods in psychology: A research guide*. Philadelphia, PA: Open University Press.

Baum, R. M. (1999). Work, contentment, and identity in aging women in literature. In S. M. Deats & L. T. Lenker (Eds.), *Aging and identity: A humanities perspective* (pp. 89-101). Westport, CT: Praeger.

Bax, M. (1977). Man the player. In B. Tizard & D. Harvey (Eds.), *Biology of play* (pp. 1-6). London, UK: William Heinemann Medical Books Ltd.

Benedict, R. (1961). *Patterns of culture*. Cambridge, MA: The Riverside Press.

Blanchard, K. (1995). *The anthropology of sport: An introduction*. Westport, CT: Bergin & Garvery.

Bourdieu, P., & Passeron, J. C. (1990). *Reproduction in education, society and culture*. Thousand Oaks, CA: Sage.

Breakwell, G. M., Hammond, S., & Fife-Schaw, C. (Eds.). (1995). *Research methods in psychology*. Thousand Oaks, CA: Sage.

Carleton University Library, Ottawa, Data Centre. (2002). Canadian General Social Surveys (GSS). Retrieved April 4, 2002, from http://www.carleton.ca/~ssdata/gss.html.

Clark-Carter, D. (1997). *Doing quantitative psychological research: From design to report*. Hove, UK: Psychology Press.

Clausen, J. A. (1993). *American lives: Looking back at the children of the great depression*. Toronto, ON: Maxwell Macmillan Canada.

Connor Schisler, A. M., & Polatajko, H. J. (2002). The individual as mediator of the person-occupation-environment interaction: Learning from the experience of refugees. *Journal of Occupational Science*, 9(2), 82-92.

Cosgrove, I., & Jackson, R. (1972). *The geography of recreation of leisure*. London, UK: Hutchinson and Company.

Cratty, B. J. (1975). *Learning about human behavior*. Englewood Cliffs, NJ: Prentice-Hall, Inc.

[8] Most Americans indicated that they would continue to work. The numbers ranged from a low of 65% in 1974 and a high of 77% in 1980. The most recent results (1996) indicate that 68% would continue to work.

Evidence Worksheet

Author	*Year*	*Idea*	*Occupational Evidence*
Occupational reframing: How would this be understood from an occupational perspective?			
Neutens & Rubinson	1997	Using knowledge and research from other disciplines allows for a broader understanding	Supports the notion that ideas about occupation can and should be gleaned from other disciplines to increase the knowledge base of occupation studies
Polatajko	1992	The OCF illustrates the interaction of person, environment, and occupation and provides a structure to organize literature	The OCF can be used as an organizational tool to help understand what occupational knowledge exists, what research has been done, and how these sources of knowledge may be able to inform occupational studies of person, environment, and occupation
Bandura	1995	Perceived self-efficacy is "beliefs in one's capabilities to organize and execute the courses of action required to manage prospective situations" (Bandura, 1995, p. 2). Bandura believes that self-efficacy... is cognitively regulated and is a determinant of whether a person will choose one activity or another	Occupationally reframed, Bandura's notion of perceived self-efficacy can show that mastery experiences help to develop the cognitive components of the person, allowing for the development of occupational competence such as a child getting his/her first basket in basketball, or an insurance salesperson making his/her first sale, and occupational mastery such as the child growing up to play in the NBA, or the insurance salesperson winning national employee of the year for outstanding sales
Who: Who engages in occupation? Who doesn't engage in occupation?			
Waite	1993	In his autobiography, Terry Waite provides a rich, descriptive account of life as a captive in solitary confinement for 1,763 days	This autobiography demonstrates the need for engagement in occupation, which led Terry Waite to find things to do within his environment (e.g., writing his autobiography in his head)
What: What occupations are there?			
Statistics Canada	1999	The Canadian General Social Survey, a repeated telephone survey conducted about every 5 years, includes questions on educational activity, paid and unpaid work, personal care activities, physical activities, socializing, passive leisure activities (e.g., watching television and reading) and entertainment activities (e.g., sports, and activity limitations)	Findings indicate that, aside from personal care, the most common activities are tasks around the home, with 90% of the people participating in household work and related activities for an average of 3.6 hours a day. Above 15 years of age 77% of the population watches television for an average of 3 hours a day
When: When do people engage in occupation? When do people engage in which occupations?			
Herrmann	1990	Herrmann used a self-report time log with 20 single adolescent mothers to attempt to describe their daily activities, to discern if they were related to the	The data showed that these young women spent the majority of their time (78%) doing adolescent activities, leaving much of the childcare to others

(continued)

Author	*Year*	*Idea*	*Occupational Evidence*
		subject's maternal role or their adolescent role to determine the relationship between activities and perceived role conflict among adolescent mothers. The young women kept a time log chronicling all their activities over a period of 4 days, ascribing them to either the mothering role or the adolescent role and noting their level of satisfaction with the particular activity	Herrmann points out that, unexpectedly, this pattern was not different on weekdays, when the women were in school, and on weekends. Herrmann's findings show that occupational patterns are not determined solely by the individual but also by the environment. Her remarking on the lack of change in occupational patterns from weekday to weekend emphasizes the extent to which it is generally held that occupational patterns are not only affected by time but also by the environment in which they are performed
Where: Where do occupations occur? What impact does the where of occupation have on its engagement?			
Connor Schisler & Polatajko	2002	Interested in examining the impact of environmental change on daily occupational engagement, Connor Schisler carried out an ethnographic study of Burundian refugees in Southwestern Ontario, Canada	Connor Schisler found that all participants experienced dramatic changes in their occupations as a result of the physical, social, cultural, and economic environmental differerences between Burundi and Southwestern Ontario. Of particular interest was the finding that environmental changes affected not only the occupations but the people themselves and they too changed
How: How do people engage in occupations?			
Smyth & Mason	1998	Smyth and Mason carried out an experimental study to investigate differences in the role of vision and proprioception in a positional aiming task, between normal children and children with a DCD	Results indicated that with proprioception alone, errors were made to the outside of the target; the control children tended to favor proprioceptive input while children with DCD tended to favor visual input, but only with their left hands. This study provides experimental evidence of the impact of person and occupational factors on performance and demonstrates the usefulness of controlled studies in determining how occupations are performed
Why: Why do people engage in occupation?			
National Research Council	1999	The American GSS provides an example of how survey methods can be used to look at work values and the meaning of work. The GSS asked, "If you were to get enough money to live as comfortably as you would like for the rest of your life, would you continue to work or would you stop working?"	Most Americans indicated that they would continue to work. The numbers ranged from a low of 65% in 1974 to a high of 77% in 1980. The most recent results (1996) indicate that 68% would continue to work. Asking these people why they would continue working would provide a considerable amount of understanding toward the understanding of the why of occupation

(continued)

Author	Year	Idea	Occupational Evidence
Terkel	1975	Studs Terkel, an American journalist, used a phenomenological approach to uncover the meanings people ascribe to their working experiences	These stories are particularly useful in learning to understand why people do the occupations they do
Rudman, Cook, & Polatajko	1997	In-depth interviews were carried out with 12 community-dwelling well elderly to discover their perspectives on the role and importance of occupations in their lives	The themes indicated that occupations were a means of expressing and managing personal identity; of staying connected to people, the past, and the future; and of organizing time. Occupations contributed to the sense of well-being of the seniors, to their continued existence and its quality

Creswell, J. W. (1994). *Research design: Qualitative and quantitative approaches*. Thousand Oaks, CA: Sage.

Csikszentmihalyi, M. (1997). *Finding flow: The psychology of engagement with everyday life*. New York, NY: Basic Books.

Curtiss, S. (1977). *Genie: A psycholinguistic study of a modern day "wild child."* New York, NY: Academic Press.

Davis, J. A., Polatajko, H. J., & Ruud, C. (2002). Occupations in context: Influence of history on the development of the predominant occupations of children. *Journal of Occupational Science*, 9(2), 54-64.

Densmore, F. (1929). *Chippewa customs*. Washington, DC: Government Printing Office.

DePoy, E., & Gitlin, L. N. (1994). *Introduction to research: Multiple strategies for health and human services*. St. Louis, MO: Mosby-Year Book.

Dietz, M. L., Prus, R., & Shaffir, W. (1994). *Doing everyday life: Ethnography as human lived experience*. Mississauga, ON: Copp Clark Longman, Ltd.

Drew, C. J., Hardman, M. L., & Weaver Hart, A. (1996). *Designing and conducting research: Inquiry in education and social science* (2nd ed.). Toronto, ON: Allyn and Bacon.

Durkheim, E. (1964). *The division of labor in society*. Glencoe, IL: Free Press.

Elias, N. (2000). *The civilizing process: Sociogenetic and psychogenetic investigations* (Rev. ed.). Malden, MA: Blackwell Publishers.

Elder, G. H. (1974/1999). *Children of the great depression: Social change in life experience*. Chicago, IL: The University of Chicago Press.

Elder, G. (1998). The life course as developmental theory. *Child Development*, 69(1), 1-12.

Fellman, J., Getis, A., & Getis, J. (1996). *Human geography: Landscapes of human activities*. New York, NY: McGraw-Hill Companies.

Ferguson, D. L., & Patten, J. (1979). *Journalism today: An introduction*. Skokie, IL: National Textbook.

Fincher, J. (1984). *The brain: Mystery of mind and matter*. Toronto, ON: Torstar Books.

Frank, R. H. (1997). *Microeconomics and behavior* (3rd ed.). Toronto, Ontario: McGraw-Hill Companies, Inc.

Glaser, B. G., & Strauss, A. L. (1968). *The discovery of grounded theory: Strategies for qualitative research*. Chicago, IL: Aline.

Glassford, R. G. (1976). *Application of a theory of games to the transitional Eskimo culture*. New York, NY: Arno Press.

Glesne, C., & Peshkin, A. (1992). *Becoming qualitative researchers: An introduction*. White Plains, NY: Longan.

Goncu, A. (Ed.). (1999). *Children's engagement in the world: Sociocultural perspectives*. Cambridge, UK: Cambridge University Press.

Groos, K. (1976). *The play of man*. New York, NY: Arno Press.

Grunfeld, F. V. (1982). *Games of the world: How to make them, how to play them, how they came to be*. Special English edition for the National Committees for UNICEF in Australia, Canada, Ireland, and Switzerland: Swiss Committee for UNICEF.

Haworth, J. (Ed.). (1996). *Psychological research: Innovative methods and strategies*. New York, NY: Routledge.

Hayes, N. (Ed.). (1997). *Doing qualitative analysis in psychology*. Hove, England: Psychology Press.

Herrmann, C. (1990). A descriptive study of daily activities and role conflict in single adolescent mothers. In J. A. Johnson, & E. J. Yerxa (Eds.), *Occupational science: The foundation for new models of practice* (pp. 53-68). New York, NY: The Haworth Press.

Itard, J. M. G. (1962). *Wild boy of Aveyron*. New York, NY: Meredith Publishing Co.

Jackson, W. (1999). *Methods: Doing social research* (2nd ed.). Scarborough, Ontario: Prentice-Hall Allyn Bacon Canada.

Joyce, P. (Ed.). (1989). *The historical meanings of work*. New York, NY: Cambridge University Press.

Kupferer, H. J. (1988). *Ancient drums, other moccasins: Native North American cultural adaptation*. Englewood Cliffs, NJ: Prentice Hall, Inc.

Leakey, R., & Lewin, R. (1992). *Origins reconsidered: In search of what makes us human*. Toronto, Ontario: Doubleday.

Lewin, K. (1975). *Field theory in social science: Selected theoretical papers*. Westport, CT: Greenwood Press.

Lincoln, Y. S., & Guba, E. G. (1985). *Naturalistic inquiry*. Thousand Oaks, CA: Sage.

McGrew, W. C. (1972). *An ethological study of children's behavior*. New York, NY: Academic Press.

Mergen, B. (Ed.). (1986). *Cultural dimensions of play, games, and sport*. Champaign, IL: Human Kinetics Publishers, Inc.

Mitchell, E. D., & Mason, B. S. (1937). *The theory of play*. New York, NY: A. S. Barnes and Company, Inc.

Morison, S. J., Ames, E. W., & Chisholm, K. (1995). The development of children adopted from Romanian orphanages. *Merrill-Palmer Quarterly, 41*(4), 411-430.

National Research Council. (1999). *The changing nature of work: Implications for occupational analysis*. Washington, DC: National Academy Press.

Neutens, J. J., & Rubinson, L. (1997). *Research techniques for the health sciences* (2nd ed.). Boston, MA: Allyn and Bacon.

Osipow, S. H. (1968). *Theories of career development*. New York, NY: Meredith Corporation.

Pedhazur, E. J., & Schmelkin, L. P. (1991). *Measurement, design, and analysis: An integrated approach*. Hillsdale, NJ: Lawrence Erlbaum Associates.

Piaget, J. (1952). *The origins of intelligence in children*. New York, NY: International Universities Press.

Piaget, J. (1971). *Structuralism*. Boston, MA: Routledge & Kegan Paul.

Polatajko, H. J. (1992). Muriel Driver Lecture 1992, Naming and framing occupational therapy: A lecture dedicated to the life of Nancy B. *Canadian Journal of Occupational Therapy, 59*(4), 189-200.

Polatajko, H. J. (2004). The study of occupation. In C. Christiansen, & E. Townsend (Eds.), *Introduction to occupation*. Upper Saddle River, NJ: Prentice-Hall.

Portney, L. G., & Watkins, M. P. (1993). *Foundations of clinical research: Applications to practice*. Norwalk, CT: Appleton and Lange.

Rapoport, R., & Rapoport, R. N. (1975). *Leisure and the family life cycle*. Boston, MA: Routledge & Kegan Paul Ltd.

Richards, I. A. (1926). *Principles of literary criticism* (2nd ed.). London: Routledge & Kegan Paul.

Roe, A. (1956). *The psychology of occupations*. New York, NY: Wiley.

Rudman, D. L., Cook, J. V., & Polatajko, H. (1997). Understanding the potential of occupation: A qualitative exploration of seniors' perspective on activity. *The American Journal of Occupational Therapy, 51*(8), 640-650.

Rymer, R. (1993). *Genie: A scientific tragedy*. New York, NY: HarperCollins Publishers, Inc.

Segal, N. L. (1999). *Entwined lives: Twins and what they tell us about human behavior*. Toronto, Ontario: Penguin Books.

Smyth, M. M., & Mason, U. C. (1998). Direction of response in aiming to visual and proprioceptive targets in children with and without Developmental Coordination Disorder. *Human Movement Science, 17*, 515-539.

Stant, M. A. (1972). *The young child: His activities and materials*. Englewood Cliffs, NJ: Prentice Hall, Inc.

Statistics Canada. (1999). General social survey: Overview of the time use of Canadians in 1998. Catalogue no. 12F0080XIE. Ottawa Minister of Industry.

Statistics Canada. (2002). 2001 Census. Retrieved April 4, 2002, from http://www.statcan.ca.

Sutton-Smith, B. (Ed.). (1976). *A children's games anthology: Studies in folklore and anthropology*. New York, NY: Arno Press.

Terkel, S. (1970). *Hard times: An oral history of the great depression*. New York, NY: Random House.

Terkel, S. (1975). *Working*. New York, NY: Avon Books.

Tieger, P. D., & Barron-Tieger, B. (1995). *Do what you are: Discover the perfect career for you through the secrets of personality type* (2nd ed.). Toronto, Ontario: Little, Brown and Company.

United States Department of Commerce, U.S. Census Bureau. (n.d.). United States Census 2000. Retrieved April 4, 2002, from http://www.census.gov.

University of California, San Diego, Social Sciences and Humanities Library. (n.d.). General Social Survey (GSS). Retrieved April 4, 2002, from http://ssdc.ucsd.edu/gss.

Van Alstyne, D. (1976). *Play behavior and choice of play materials of pre-school children*. Chicago, IL: The University of Chicago Press.

Vygotsky, L. S. (1978). *Mind in society: The development of higher psychological processes*. Cambridge, MA: Harvard University Press.

Waite, T. (1993). *Terry Waite: Taken on trust*. Toronto, Ontario: Doubleday Canada Limited.

Weber, M. (1930). *The protestant ethic and the spirit of capitalism* (T. Parsons, Trans.). New York: Scribner. (Original work published 1904).

Wheaton, B., & Gotlib, I. H. (1997). Trajectories and turning points over the life course: Concepts and themes. In I. H. Gotlib & B. Wheaton (Eds.), *Stress and adversity over the life course* (pp. 1-25). New York, NY: Cambridge University Press.

Wilcock, A. A. (1998). *An occupational perspective of health*. Thorofare, NJ: SLACK Incorporated.

Wood, D. J., Bruner, J. S., & Ross, G. (1976). The role of tutoring in problem solving. *Journal of Child Psychology and Psychiatry, 17*, 89-100.

Woodruff-Pak, D. S., & Papka, M. (1999). Theories of neuropsychology and aging. In V. L. Bengtson & K. W. Schaie (Eds.), *Handbook of theories of aging* (pp. 113-132). New York, NY: Springer Publishing Company.

Wright, L. (1997). *Twins and what they tell us about who we are*. Toronto, ON: John Wiley & Sons, Inc.

Yerxa, E. J., Clark, F., Frank, G., Jackson, J., Parham, D., Pierce, D., et al. (1990). An introduction to occupational science: A foundation for occupational therapy in the 21st century. In J. A. Johnson & E. J. Yerxa (Eds.), *Occupational science: The foundation for new models of practice* (pp. 1-17). New York, NY: The Haworth Press.

Recommended Reading

Banister, P., Burman, E., Parker, I., Taylor, M., & Tindall, C. (1994). *Qualitative methods in psychology: A research guide*. Philadelphia, PA: Open University Press.

Breakwell, G. M., Hammond, S., & Fife-Schaw, C. (Eds.). (1995). *Research methods in psychology*. Thousand Oaks, CA: Sage.

Clark-Carter, D. (1997). *Doing quantitative psychological research: From design to report*. Hove, England: Psychology Press.

Creswell, J. W. (1994). *Research design: Qualitative and quantitative approaches*. Thousand Oaks, CA: Sage.

DePoy, E., & Gitlin, L. N. (1994). *Introduction to research: Multiple strategies for health and human services*. St. Louis, MO: Mosby-Year Book .

Drew, C. J., Hardman, M. L., & Weaver Hart, A. (1996). *Designing and conducting research: Inquiry in education and social science* (2nd ed.). Toronto, Ontario: Allyn and Bacon.

Glaser, B. G., & Strauss, A. L. (1968). *The discovery of grounded theory: Strategies for qualitative research*. Chicago, IL: Aline.

Glesne, C., & Peshkin, A. (1992). *Becoming qualitative researchers: An introduction*. White Plains, NY: Longan.

Haworth, J. (Ed.). (1996). *Psychological research: Innovative methods and strategies*. New York, NY: Routledge.

Hayes, N. (Ed.). (1997). *Doing qualitative analysis in psychology*. Hove, England: Psychology Press.

Jackson, W. (1999). *Methods: Doing social research* (2nd ed.). Scarborough, ON: Prentice-Hall Allyn Bacon Canada.

Lincoln, Y. S., & Guba, E. G. (1985). *Naturalistic inquiry*. Thousand Oaks, CA: Sage.

Neutens, J. J., & Rubinson, L. (1997). *Research techniques for the health sciences*. (2nd ed.). Boston, MA: Allyn and Bacon.

Pedhazur, E. J., & Schmelkin, L. P. (1991). *Measurement, design, and analysis: An integrated approach*. Hillsdale, NJ: Lawrence Erlbaum Associates.

Portney, L. G., & Watkins, M. P. (1993). *Foundations of clinical research: Applications to practice*. Norwalk, CT: Appleton and Lange.

Chapter Nine: Methods of Inquiry Reflections and Learning Activities

Julie Bass-Haugen, PhD, OTR/L, FAOTA

Reflections

This chapter introduced a process you can use to ask and answer your own questions about occupation. As you read each chapter, you probably wondered about some of the things that were included in each chapter and some of the things that weren't. You were curious. Curiosity is a wonderful human trait. We were curious as children. "What can I make if I mix water and mud?" and "How does a wristwatch work?" Each question required us to use certain strategies to get an answer. We are also curious as adults. "What did our grandparents or great-grandparents do to survive the Depression?" and "Who were the key players in the civil rights movement?" Some things we were curious about as children serve as a springboard for our adult activities. Perhaps there was a child who asked, "How does a wristwatch work?" and then later developed a better wristwatch. Curiosity is the foundation for all advances in knowledge.

Curiosity is important in our learning about human occupation. The discipline of occupational science is still in its infancy, and thus, many basic questions need to be asked regarding human occupation. There is much we need to learn. Perhaps, if we answer these basic questions about occupation now, we can improve the human experience through occupation in the future.

Asking good questions or defining an area of inquiry is a challenge even for the seasoned researcher with years of experience! How do you begin? An important step is to learn as much as you can about a subject of interest through your own exploration. Reading, observation, reflection, and discussion are wonderful ways to turn on those light bulbs. Sometimes, our questions originate from our curiosity about things of personal interest. Sometimes, our questions emerge from studies and research conducted by other people. Sometimes, our questions are more practical and relate to problems that need solutions. Developing a topic of inquiry often starts with "hmmm... I wonder..." statements. I had quite a few questions as I read the chapters. I wondered about the evolution of work and leisure in non-Western cultures. I wondered if there was a greater appreciation of the meaning of occupation after a major medical diagnosis, like cancer. I wondered if perceptions of time were influenced by factors other than age (e.g., lifestyle, type of work, etc.). I wondered whether specific occupations were important for development. I could go on and on. What are your questions?

Once you have an interesting question to ask, the next step is to figure out how to answer it. The chapter outlined two primary strategies for engaging in inquiry: examine the existing knowledge on the topic and generate new knowledge on the topic. Let's look at each of these strategies in more detail for my topic of specific occupations important for development.

The OCF was introduced as a technique to help you refine your topic of inquiry. You might wonder, "Why do we have to refine the topic?" The initial topic proposed is usually too broad. For my topic of inquiry on occupations and development, I could put the words "occupation" or "development" in a library search engine, but I would likely get a gazillion hits. I need to be more specific and narrow my interests down. The OCF is one way to do this for topics related to occupation.

Each dimension of the OCF addresses a very important component of human occupation. In fact, it would be almost impossible to ask a good, focused question about human occupation without considering all three dimensions. The person dimension requires us to identify the specific aspect(s) of the person for further study. For my topic of inquiry, I could explore a specific aspect of personal development like "fine motor development," "self-esteem," or "abstract reasoning." The occupation dimension identifies different classifications of occupations to consider. For my topic of inquiry, I could investigate "independent dressing," "handwriting," or "imaginary play." The environment dimension describes several components of the environment that influence occupational performance. For my topic of inquiry, I could restrict my study to "the first grade classroom," "Montessori classrooms," or "Head Start programs." In a very short time, I can revise my unworkable topic of the relationship between occupation and development and propose a solid question like, "How does the childhood occupation of handwriting influence fine motor development for children in Montessori classrooms?" Now I have a starting point for reviewing existing knowledge on a topic or developing a plan to generate new knowledge.

The next step in the process is to identify disciplines that produce knowledge on this topic. We might find several sources of information for our questions by considering the dimensions of the OCF. For my question, I could explore child development, human movement, and education literature as well as the occupational science and occupational therapy literature. Finding the relevant literature requires you to put on your detective hat and start looking for clues. You also have to be honest about your past experience as a detective looking for literature. Are you a rookie detective who doesn't know where to begin to look for clues? Are you a seasoned detective who is already familiar with all the literature and search clues?

Some detective work can be done the old-fashioned way, especially if you feel you have a lot to learn. You can browse through real libraries, virtual libraries, databases, and the Internet to become more familiar with your topic and the search mechanisms. Your browsing might raise questions about your topic. Are the key words in the question found in the literature? Are there alternative key words that will lead to the relevant literature? What combinations of key words should be used to find the most relevant literature? Should the question be broader or narrower to find the best literature? Your browsing might also raise questions about different search methods. What is the primary focus of this search service? What type and quality of literature (e.g., professional journals, popular press, textbooks) is accessed with this search service? What are recommended search rules to obtain the best results from this search service? What exactly can I get from this search service (e.g., full text, abstract, reference)? I strongly encourage you to complete an on-line tutorial for each search service you use. You will generally find tutorials on the homepage for most search services.

Once you feel you have a better handle on your topic, then you can begin a more methodical approach to retrieving and reviewing the best literature on the topic. This methodical approach will require both a good process and good search methods. Many guidelines for literature review suggest that you keep a paper trail of where you have been and where you are going. This is the process. It requires that you use an organizer (e.g., three-ring binder, index cards, computer-based system) and create sections for important things you want to track (e.g., key words, search services, the steps taken, plans, and reference lists). This organizer is like a detective's notepad. You will also need to document the types of searches (e.g., internet, databases, government reports) and literature (e.g., original research, secondary sources, review articles) you have reviewed; these are the search methods. Good literature detectives also use simple clues that others might not consider (e.g., tracking an author's work over time, inspecting the reference list of an article, reviewing key words of relevant articles).

The last step in the review of existing knowledge is to examine the literature you have acquired in terms of your primary question. Again, you can use the OCF to determine where each piece of existing knowledge fits. For my question, perhaps I would find information on Montessori methods (i.e., the environment), handwriting (i.e., the occupation), and fine motor development in children (i.e., person). All of this literature can help you determine if there is existing knowledge or if new knowledge needs to be generated.

If the existing knowledge is insufficient, then you can generate new knowledge using a method of inquiry. There are many different methods to consider. In fact, a single question can sometimes be answered using a variety of methods. Usually, however, we select a single method as a place to begin, and if we remain really passionate about our question, we can pursue other methods later.

How do you get your question ready to conduct an inquiry? In this chapter, we learned that most questions related to human occupation can be framed in terms of the who, what, when, where, why, and how questions we used so often as children. Who, what, when, and where are words of inquiry that help us to describe something. How and why are words of inquiry that help us to explain something. My specific question about occupation and development is a "how" question. I could have proposed other questions about this topic. What childhood occupations are selected by Montessori teachers to address fine motor development goals? When do Montessori programs introduce handwriting as an occupation?

After I have a clear question, the next step is to develop the overall methods for the inquiry and select a specific design. This chapter distinguished between two primary types of designs: quantitative and qualitative. Quantitative designs may be further classified as descriptive or experimental. Descriptive quantitative designs are generally used to answer who, what, when, and where questions and describe or explore phenomenon and relationships. Experimental designs are used to answer why and how questions and explain cause and effect relationships. Qualitative designs may be further classified as ethnography, case study, phenomenology, and grounded theory. Each of these designs has specific areas of interest. Ethnography attempts to understand attitudes, beliefs, and values. Case study explores activity or phenomenon. Phenomenology examines experiences and meanings. Grounded theory identifies categories, relationships, and theoretical constructs.

In the previous paragraph, we have very briefly summarized methods of inquiry. Each of these inquiry methods has dozens of textbooks devoted to it. You can see that any serious inquiry with a goal to generate new knowledge would require that other resources be used. I also want to caution you that the language of research and inquiry is tricky business. The classifications presented above include terminology commonly used by some authors, but not others. That doesn't make one author right and the other wrong. It simply means that people have different backgrounds, perspectives, and viewpoints, and these differences are reflected in the way they present information. As you select a method of inquiry, it is important to document your source of information for this method.

You now have two strategies to use as you begin to act on your curiosity about human occupation: review existing knowledge and generate new knowledge. Each of these strategies will open many doors of knowledge for you. I also believe that the questions regarding human occupation you pose and start to answer today will improve the human experience tomorrow!

Journal Activities

1. Look up and write down dictionary definitions of curiosity, inquiry, and research. Highlight the components of the definitions that are most related to their descriptions in Chapter Nine.
2. Identify the most important new learning for you in this chapter.
3. Identify one question you have about Chapter Nine.
4. Reflect on the words of inquiry found in this chapter. Generate three basic questions related to human occupation that are related to the chapters you have read in this text. Start each question with one of the words below. Then, use the OCF to refine each question. Underline the key words in your questions and generate at least one alternative key word for each word underlined.
   - Who...
   - What...
   - When...
   - Where...
   - How...
   - Why...

Technology/Internet Learning Activities

1. Use a discussion database to share specific journal entries.
2. Use a good Internet search engine or your online library to find several databases for literature review.
   - Enter the phrase "PubMed" in your search line (PubMed at the National Library of Medicine).
   - Enter the phrase "ERIC" in your search line (Educational Resources Information Center).
   - Enter the phrase "PsycINFO," "Psychlit," or "Psychcrawler" in your search line (Psychology).
     - ✧ Document the location of the database and scan the database.
     - ✧ Complete the tutorial.
     - ✧ What is the purpose of this database?
     - ✧ What search strategies are recommended for conducting searches on this database?
     - ✧ What types of literature are searched on this database?
     - ✧ What are the retrieval capacities on this database? (e.g., reference? abstract? full text?)
     - ✧ Experiment with using the database.
     - ✧ Search for information on several topics of interest related to human occupation.
     - ✧ Keep a paper trail of your search.
     - ✧ Is the database user-friendly?
     - ✧ What features did you like about the database?
     - ✧ What aspects of the database were frustrating?
     - ✧ Were you able to find information on your topics?
     - ✧ Describe the strategies you used to keep a paper trail. Could you retrace your steps?
3. Use a good Internet search engine or your online library to find existing knowledge on a topic or question of interest. Select one of the questions generated in Journal Activity #4.
   - Open a database related to your topic or question.
     - ✧ Document the location of the database and scan the database.
     - ✧ Keep a paper trail of your search, key words, and document sources.
     - ✧ Search for information on your question using the key words and alternative key words.
     - ✧ What strategies led you to relevant literature on your question?
     - ✧ What strategies led you to roadblocks on your question?
     - ✧ Scan eight to 10 articles/documents that have relevance to your question.

    - ✧ Select three articles/documents for further review and obtain a full text version.
4. Visit your online academic library.
    - Record three to five databases available in your online library (other than the ones listed above).
    - For each database:
        - ✧ Describe the characteristics or focus.
        - ✧ Search for information on several topics of interest related to human occupation.
        - ✧ Is the database user-friendly?
        - ✧ What features did you like about the database?
        - ✧ What aspects of the database were frustrating?
        - ✧ Were you able to find information on your topics?

APPLIED LEARNING

Individual Learning Activity #1: Conducting an Inquiry of Existing Knowledge on a Topic

Instructions:

- Complete Journal Activity #4 and Technology/Internet Learning Activity #3.
- Complete a summary of the three articles/documents you found using the table.
    - ✧ Article/Document Reference: Include all information on the article/document needed for referencing and future retrieval (e.g., title, source, author, publisher and year of publication, Internet site, and date retrieved).
    - ✧ Type of Article: 1) Primary-original research (include brief summary of method and design); 2) Secondary-review of existing literature, theoretical papers, textbook chapters, reference books, government documents; 3) Tertiary-systematic or critical reviews; 4) Other—popular press.
    - ✧ Purpose of Article/Document: Identify the stated purpose of this article/document. Sometimes, you may need to infer the purpose if it is not directly stated.
    - ✧ Summary of Article/Document: Summarize the key points and conclusions of this article/document.
    - ✧ Comments: Record comments you have about the conclusions of the author, the quality of the article/document, and relevance of this article to your question.
- Identify three to five statements summarizing information you have so far related to your question and the literature you reviewed. Record the statements, supporting facts or ideas, and your supporting reference(s) for the statements in the table.
- Identify a statement that summarizes one piece of information related to your question. This statement may be similar to the topic sentence that begins a paragraph.
- Document any supporting ideas and details for each statement.
- Record the reference(s) that supports this statement.
- Identify two to three things you still do not know as it relates to your question and possible literature to explore.
    - ✧ Missing Information:

        Possible Sources:

    - ✧ Missing Information:

        Possible Sources:

✧ Missing Information:

Possible Sources:

✧ Missing Information (Example): Handwriting and fine motor development. Montessori methods and materials.

Possible Sources: Psychology database, Education database

Summary of Three Articles/Documents

A. Article/ Document Reference	*B. Type of Article/Document*	*C. Purpose of Article/Document*	*D. Summary of Article/Document*	*E. Comments*
# 1				
# 2				
# 3				

Summary of Three articles/Documents—Example

A. Article/ Document Reference	*B. Type of Article/Document*	*C. Purpose of Article/Document*	*D. Summary of Article/Document*	*E. Comments*
# 1. Handwriting Doesn't Have To Be a Lost Art. Montessori Life; v13 n4 p38-41 Fall 2001Woods, Carol A. ERIC database	Journal Article—(secondary article in refereed/peer reviewed journal) Project Description	Project description of one Montessori program	Writing is complex: involves cognitive, perceptual, motor. Montessori has methods and materials related to writing	Helped me understand a Montessori approach to handwriting. Not a research-based article.

Summary of Three to Five Statements You Can Make Based on the Literature

A. Information/Conclusions on Question	*B. Supporting Ideas*	*C. Reference(s)*
# 1		
# 2		
# 3		
# 4		
# 5		

Summary of Three to Five Statements You Can Make Based on the Literature—Example

A. Information/Conclusions on Question	*B. Supporting Ideas*	*C. Reference(s)*
# 1 Handwriting is a complex childhood occupation	It requires personal skills in the areas of motor, cognition, and perception	Woods (2001)

Individual Learning Activity #2: Proposing a Topic and Method of Inquiry to Generate New Knowledge

Instructions:

- Complete Individual Learning Activity #1.
- Review the missing information for your question in Individual Learning Activity #1.
- Identify two to three specific questions you have based on this missing information.
- Review the inquiry word you used for each question: who, what, when, where, why, how.
- Propose a method of inquiry for each specific question. Is the method of inquiry a good match for the type of question?
  - ✧ Quantitative Methods:
    - Designs: Descriptive, Experimental
  - ✧ Qualitative Methods:
    - Designs: Ethnography, case study, phenomenology, grounded theory

Summary of Two to Three Questions Appropriate for Further Inquiry to Generate New Knowledge

A. Question	*B. Method and Design*	*C. Summary of How You Would Use the Method and Design to Answer the Question*
#1		
#2		
#3		

Summary of Two to Three Questions Appropriate for Further Inquiry to Generate New Knowledge—Example

A. Question	*B. Method and Design*	*C. Summary of How You Would Use the Method and Design to Answer the Question*
#1 What are the specific handwriting activities in Montessori programs?	Quantitative method Descriptive design	I would survey 10 Montessori programs and obtain information on specific handwriting activities and samples of materials. I would evaluate the characteristics of these handwriting activities

ACTIVE LEARNING

Group Activity #1: Exploring a Collaborative Approach to Inquiry

Preparation:
- Read Chapter Nine.
- Complete Applied Learning Activities #1 and #2.

Time: 1 to 1.5 hours

Materials:
- Information from Applied Learning Activities #1 and #2
- Flip chart, chalkboard, white board, or virtual board

Instructions:
- Individually:
  - ✧ Review Applied Learning Activities #1 and #2.
  - ✧ Be prepared to share your results from Applied Learning Activities #1 and #2.
  - ✧ Complete the self-assessment of inquiry skills on p. 216.

Self-Assessment of Inquiry Skills

Rate your experience with this skill on a scale of 1 to 5.

1 = I don't think I have ever done this in my entire life.

5 = I have had so much experience with this, I have done it in my sleep.

Rate your proficiency with this skill on a scale of 1 to 5.

1 = I have so little of this skill I barely even know what it is.

5 = I have so much of this skill I could teach the course on it.

Inquiry Skills	*Experience*	*Proficiency*
Getting Started		
Generating ideas for a topic of inquiry	_____	_____
Asking a good question related to the topic of inquiry	_____	_____
Reviewing Existing Knowledge		
Finding the relevant literature using a variety of sources	_____	_____
Selecting the best literature that is relevant to your question	_____	_____
Analyzing the literature from a critical perspective	_____	_____
Summarizing the literature using written communication	_____	_____
Summarizing the literature using verbal communication	_____	_____
Generating New Knowledge		
Selecting a method and design that fits the question	_____	_____
Developing the method and design	_____	_____
Collecting information and/or data	_____	_____
Coding information or entering data	_____	_____
Analyzing information or data (e.g., computer or by hand)	_____	_____
Presenting data in tables or figures	_____	_____
Summarizing the results using written communication	_____	_____
Summarizing the results using verbal communication	_____	_____
Answering your question and developing your conclusions	_____	_____

- In small groups (3 to 4 people):
  - ✧ Share your individual results of the self-assessment.
  - ✧ Identify the strengths and challenges your group has related to inquiry skills.

Strengths	**Challenges**

  - ✧ Briefly share the results of Applied Learning Activities #1 and #2.
  - ✧ Select one question from Applied Learning Activity #2 for collaborative inquiry.
  - ✧ Record the individual summary from Applied Learning Activity #2 in the following table.
  - ✧ Collaborate to revise the question, method/design, and your ideas about how to conduct the inquiry.

Individual and Collaborative Summary on One Question of Inquiry to Generate New Knowledge

A. Question	*B. Method and Design*	*C. Ideas of How You Would Use the Method and Design to Answer the Question*
Individual		
Collaborative		

Discussion:

- Discuss the strengths and challenges of collaborative inquiry.
- Discuss how your question evolved from an individual to a collaborative question.
- Discuss how your group might assign tasks if you were to conduct this inquiry.
- Discuss additional support you would need in specific areas to conduct this inquiry.

An Occupation-Based Framework for Practice

Section II

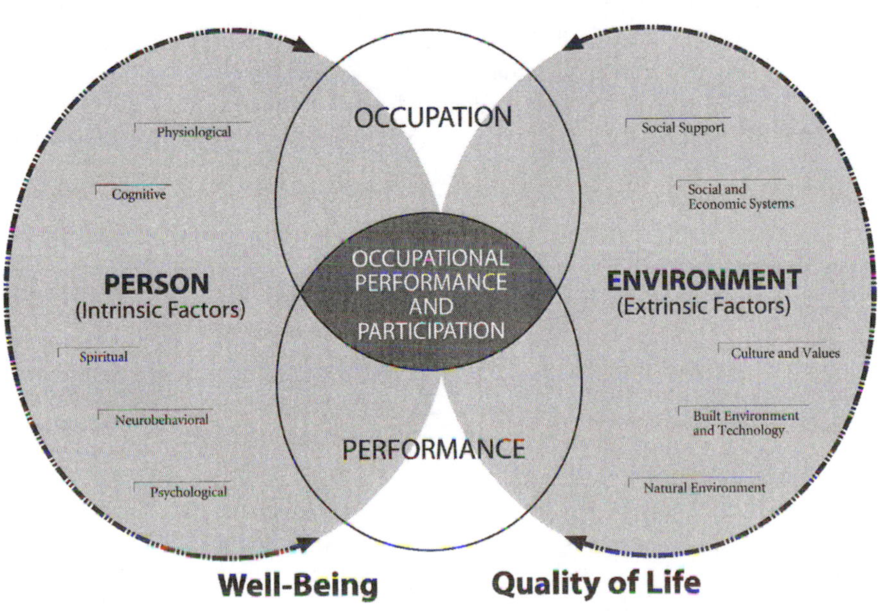

Chapter Ten Objectives

The information in this chapter is intended to help the reader:

1. Describe occupation-based practice and how it links practice to the ICF.
2. Describe the uniqueness of occupational therapy service.
3. Understand how the occupational therapist facilitates occupational performance by matching occupational goals to the person's capabilities and the available or enhanced environment.
4. Describe how the occupational therapist uses activity in a therapeutic context.
5. Describe how the environment can be enhanced to support occupational performance.
6. Describe the concepts central to the core of occupational therapy practice and how they relate to the scope of practice.
7. Describe the recent emphasis on evidence for practice and the implications for occupational therapy practice.

Key Words

ability: Lack of ability may constrain performance and limit engagement in activity and tasks, make it difficult to complete the tasks within time frame, or limit the ability to meet standards of performance.

action: Actions taken during a task may be a reflection of the individual's capabilities, skills, and experiences.

activity analysis: Activity analysis is a process in which the practitioner determines the performance demands of the activity by determining the performance demands of the activity and breaking the activity down to components parts. This involves analyzing each task in terms of its contextual, temporal, psychological, social, cultural, and meaning dimensions.

activity limitations: Activity limitations occur because the activity is not adapted to accommodate a change in capability, and likewise, participation restrictions occur because the environment does not accommodate the loss of capability and limitations in activity.

activity synthesis: The process of modifying activities or the environment to better match the goals and the capabilities of the client with the environment in which performance is to occur.

competency: Occupational therapist needs to demonstrate the ability to understand the interaction among the person, occupation, and environment. Being able to influence occupational performance requires a thorough understanding of a person's capabilities, how identity is influenced by occupations, the way in which actions and tasks may be modified with technology, and how all the environmental influences create barriers and enablers for performance.

evidence-based practice: Refers to intervention guided by a methodical review of the available research and expert opinion pertaining to an area of practice. Telling clients about the supporting evidence is necessary for giving adequate informed consent for treatment.

Knowledge is of no value unless you put it into practice.
Anton Chekhov

Chapter Ten

Introduction to Occupation-Based Practice

Penelope Moyers, EdD, OTR, FAOTA

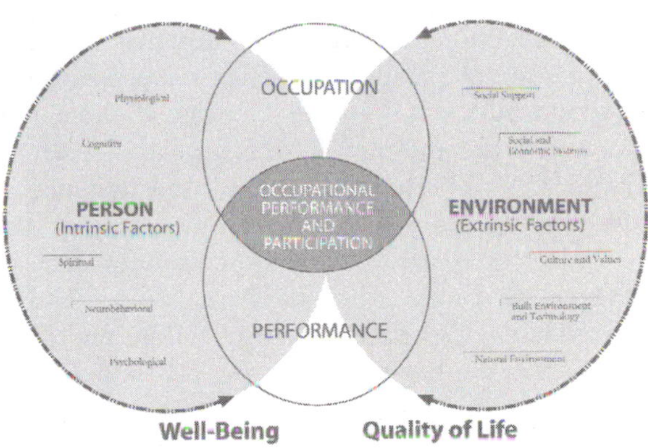

Setting the Stage

This chapter provides an overview of how occupational therapists and occupational therapy assistants implement occupation-based practice to address the occupational performance needs of their clients. Occupational therapists and occupational therapy assistants promote health and prevent disease through facilitating engagement in occupations that are personally meaningful and fulfilling and that provide opportunity to develop and allow expression of identity (Christiansen, 1999; Crabtree, 1998). Because of this focus on what the individual needs and wants to do, this chapter highlights how occupational therapists and occupational therapy assistants view health as the person's ability to actively participate in all aspects of daily living, as opposed to viewing health as an absence of disease or impairment.

Don't miss the companion Web site to *Occupational Therapy: Performance, Participation, and Well-Being, Third Edition.* Please visit us at http://www.cb3e.slackbooks.com.

Moyers, P. (2005). *Introduction to occupation-based practice.* In C. H. Christiansen, C. M. Baum, and J. Bass-Haugen (Eds.), Occupational therapy: Performance, participation, and well-being (3rd ed.). Thorofare, NJ: SLACK Incorporated.

Uniqueness of Occupational Therapy

Occupational therapists and occupational therapy assistants, through their emphasis on what the client can do, offer services to improve, maintain, or restore occupational performance that may have been challenged as the result of various problems or risks for these problems, such as injury, disease, congenital abnormalities, delayed development, behavioral health problems, poor task and environmental design, or lack of access to occupations and support from family or caregivers (Moyers, 1999). Occupational therapy practitioners understand a client's function in terms of the quality of performance exhibited during participation in meaningful occupations within relevant environments; the satisfaction engendered when engaging in these occupations; and the impact upon the client's overall state of physical, cognitive, and emotional health. Deterioration and dysfunction may partially occur as the result of situations in which the person is deprived of opportunities or is unable to engage in desired occupations because of barriers that prevent participation (Kielhofner, 1992). Deterioration and dysfunction may also result from engagement in occupations that are unhealthy and are socially or culturally unacceptable (Moyers & Stoffel, 2001). Clark, Wood, and Larson (1998) write, "Whereas some occupations and patterns of occupation are health promoting, others may be health compromising" (p. 18).

Occupational Performance

Understanding all aspects of occupational performance is the occupational therapy practitioner's unique contribution to health care or to social service provision. Because of this focus on helping people engage in desired and healthy occupations and helping people participate within their respective environments in the multiple activities and tasks that are a part of these valued occupations, the practice of occupational therapy is distinguished from the services of other health care practitioners and social service providers. Occupational therapy practitioners are concerned with both the observable aspects of performance as well as the more subjective aspects of performance (e.g., psychological and cognitive) (American Occupational Therapy Association [AOTA], 1999a).

While other disciplines may also focus on improving the function of their clients, it is recognized that the word *function* has multiple meanings, and achieving this objective of improved function may be accomplished using a variety of methods. According to the World Health Organization (WHO) (2001), "functioning is an umbrella term encompassing all body functions, activities, and participation" (p. 3). Occupational therapy services are unique because of the way in which occupational therapy practitioners collaborate with their clients, other health care practitioners, and other professionals (e.g., teachers, lawyers, engineers, social policy analysts, etc.) to carefully design therapeutic occupations to address the occupational performance problems or risks that could lead to dependence, declines in health, disability, or a reduced quality of life (Moyers, 1999). Occupational therapy practitioners offer a perspective that understands people as occupational beings (Jackson, Carlson, Mandel, Zemke, & Clark, 1998). People use occupations to develop an understanding of "who they are, what they might do, the contexts in which they might act, and who they might become" (Hocking, 2001, p. 464).

Maximizing Fit

Occupational therapy services can be understood as the process of maximizing fit amongst the person, the environment, and the occupation. In other words, the occupational therapy practitioner links the activities and tasks of the individual's valued and healthy occupations to the individual's capabilities and to the environmental context that would best facilitate and sustain successful performance. The occupational therapy practitioner understands what the individual needs and wants to do by determining the individual's roles, such as being a worker, parent, sibling, recreator, spouse or partner, student, etc. (Moyers, 1999). These roles contribute to the way in which the individual has formed his or her identity. We often know others by the roles that they fulfill, as well as describe ourselves to others by the roles we fulfill (Christiansen, 1999). It is not uncommon for introductions between people to consist of descriptions of what one does. From the perspective of understanding people as occupational beings, identity thus relies on the integration of values, interests, and roles so that the person may express that identity through occupational performance (Kielhofner, 1995). Occupations are the "vehicle for experiencing life meaning" (Hocking, 2001, p. 464).

Roles

Roles determine the occupations and their associated activities and tasks in which one engages (Kielhofner, 1995). The culture, society, and the organizations in which these roles are enacted determine to some degree the criteria for successful completion of these important occupations and the appropriate actions that make up these activities and tasks. However, the actions taken during a task may also be a reflection of the individual's capabilities, skills, habits, and experiences (Reed &

Sanderson, 1999). Most individuals have multiple roles and are faced with challenges to balance these various roles and their corresponding occupations (Kielhofner, 1995). Often, these roles come into conflict in terms of forcing the individual to make choices among various occupations in which to engage, to determine the extent to which the criteria for performance will be achieved, and to prioritize the occupations and their associated activities and tasks as the result of time limits. It may be that a person will choose to engage primarily in certain occupations and activities, thereby deliberately risking inability to complete the activities and tasks of other occupations on time or to the level of quality demanded by standards. Certain roles may take priority as reflected by the occupations and their activities in which the individual spends most of his or her time. These role priorities may change over time, such as when a child grows up and goes off to college, thereby substantially decreasing the parent's activities associated with caretaking. Individuals may give up roles or assume new roles as during periods of significant role transitions, such as retirement or having a first child. These transitions occur either voluntarily or involuntarily, as capabilities, interests, values, or environmental circumstances change.

Capabilities

Being able to perform these occupations and their associated activities and tasks depends upon the individual's capabilities. Lack of ability may constrain performance in terms of inability to engage in the activity and tasks altogether, inability to complete the tasks within time frames, or inability to meet standards of performance (Christiansen & Baum, 1997). For instance, a person's ability to use word processing to type a paper could be influenced by a problem with body structure or body function (a component of functioning and disability according to ICF terminology) (WHO, 2001). Hemiplegia resulting from a cerebrovascular accident that produces loss of voluntary motor control and a reduction in range of motion is an example of an impairment in body structure/body function that could lead to an activity limitation and to a participation restriction (a second component of functioning and disability according to ICF terminology) (WHO, 2001). Activity limitations occur because the activity is not adapted to accommodate a change in capability, and likewise, participation restrictions occur because the environment does not accommodate the loss of capability and limitations in activity.

In addition to the influence of body structure and function on a person's capabilities, the performance of an activity, such as word processing, could be influenced because the person never learned word processing skills. The person may also possess habits that do not include proper positioning of the fingers on the keyboard. Finally, the person may not have the experience over time in using word processing skills. The quality of the skill is never fully honed as a result of insufficient practice. Therefore, capabilities are heavily influenced by experience in the development of skills and habits.

Environment

The environment in which the occupation and its associated activities and tasks occur is important in terms of the way in which the environment enables or acts as a barrier to performance. Occupational performance results from the integral interaction among the person, activity, and environment. The environment consists of not only the physical and geographical environment, but also includes the cultural and social environments as well. Some physical environments are supportive of performance in that they include the tools, equipment, and space required to successfully complete the activity and tasks of a variety of occupations. Geography can be conducive to an occupation, such as the availability of lakes in the surrounding area for boating. People living in the Midwest have barriers created by geography when wanting to snow ski and, as a result, must travel to other states with mountain ranges. Living in a specific geographical area may contribute to illness and disease as the result of heavy air and water pollution or the high incidence of pollen and mold leading to asthmatic conditions.

The social environment may also be supportive in that help from others is available to augment aspects of the performance that the person is unable to complete independently. Many occupations and their associated activities and tasks are performed within a social group and thus are interdependent upon the performance of everyone involved. Occupational performance rarely occurs within a social vacuum as an individual's "occupations may range from providing support for others to creating unnecessary and excessive work. Between these extremes, occupations may be experienced as mutually enjoyed or beneficial or as providing a focus for others' actions and care" (Hocking, 2001, p. 465).

Societal policies and attitudes may positively support engagement by ensuring access to activities and financial support for participation. The culture also can support or inhibit performance in terms of creating value and meaning related to engagement in the occupation, determining when the performance should occur, and delineating how much time should be spent on the occupation's associated activities and tasks. The culture also impacts the social environment because of the customs and rituals that prescribe the manner in which actions are taken as well as the way in which the individual relates to others during the performance (Hasselkus & Rosa, 1997).

Activity Analysis and Synthesis

In addition to understanding the individual's capabilities and the environmental context in which performance occurs, the occupational therapy practitioner uses activity analysis and synthesis to specifically determine the fit between the person and the occupation and the way an occupation is enacted in a specific environment. Activity analysis is a process whereby the therapy practitioner determines the performance demands of the activity by first understanding the activity as a whole and then breaking the activity down into component parts (Buckley & Poole, 2000). For instance, occupations consist of multiple activities, which each can be broken down into discrete tasks. Occupational therapy practitioners analyze each task in terms of its performance, contextual, temporal, psychological, social, cultural, and meaning dimensions (Moyers, 1999).

In terms of the performance dimension, tasks require discrete actions that are dependent upon specific skills. These skills rely upon certain performance capabilities, such as cognitive, neurobehavioral, and physiological. For example, to study for a test, a student must be able to read, which requires maintenance of body posture, coordinated eye movements, visual acuity, visual perception, and information processing for cognitive understanding. Also, in this example, the contextual dimension of the task is related to circumstances that create the need for study, such as the individual being in school or in some kind of training program. There is a temporal dimension, as most students have a specific time frame in which to complete the studying task, some of which may be self-imposed. A psychological dimension may involve the student's emotions related to studying and to the test and possible concerns about how well the person predicts that he or she will ultimately perform. Taking tests depends upon the person's psychological capability for managing anxiety and other distracting emotions that interfere with studying.

In terms of the social dimension, studying can be an activity in which only the student participates or can occur within groups of varying sizes. For the most part, studying requires uninterrupted time in which the person is free from distractions to concentrate on the material. At the very least, studying is dependent upon the interaction between student and teacher. The cultural dimension could subtly influence the task in terms of the expectations of the teacher, family members, classmates, colleagues, employers, etc. Also, occupational therapy practitioners know that occupations and their activities possess many possible meaning dimensions related to the individual's standards regarding performance. The student may be defining success or failure in terms of very strict criteria (i.e., having to get an A grade) or by broader criteria where learning new information is valued more highly than actual performance on a test.

Based on a thorough understanding of the person's capabilities, environment, and occupation, the occupational therapy practitioner facilitates performance by matching the occupation to the person's capabilities and to the environment in which the person performs (Holm, Rogers, & James, 1998). Activity synthesis is the process of modifying activities or the environment to better match the goals and the capabilities of the client with the environment in which performance is to occur (Kramer & Hinojosa, 2000). When a client has difficulty with an activity or task and it is not expected that the client's capability will change, the activity and the environment are modified to enable performance. If the client's capabilities can be improved, the occupational therapy practitioner grades the activity, first by simplifying to match the capability and then by gradually grading the activity for increasing complexity to ultimately improve the capability (Kramer & Hinojosa, 2000).

In determining the best match among the client's capabilities, goals, occupation, and environment, the occupational therapist in conjunction with the client must decide if performance is ultimately safe and whether performance is adequate and efficient (Moyers, 1999). Acceptability of the performance is also assessed to determine if the person's performance meets personal and societal standards and cultural expectations. The performance should also be desirable in that the individual should experience a certain level of satisfaction and meaning.

Occupational Therapy Contribution

The occupational therapy perspective provides a unique contribution to the achievement of health care outcomes. Whether a person can engage in the activities of his or her own choosing, regardless of disease or impairment, is thus an ultimate measure of health. This occupational perspective includes an understanding of the client's need to engage in a healthy balance of meaningful and purposeful occupations involving self-care, work and productive activities, and play/leisure (and sleep) (Moyers, 1999). Occupational therapy practitioners additionally recognize how performance depends upon a healthy interaction with the environment, an influence that cannot be underestimated. Because of this understanding of the power of the environment, occupational therapy interventions not only help the person to balance engagement in multiple occupations for different purposes, but also to manipulate the environment and the occupation to support limited capabilities.

Balance of Occupations

The uniqueness of occupational therapy is based upon the occupational therapy practitioner's view of health as occurring within the client's context of daily living. Occupational therapy practitioners are concerned with the way in which clients are able to engage in valued occupations and to participate in the community regardless of disease or impairment. These valued occupations consist of a combination of purposeful and meaningful activities and tasks and reflect a balance among the occupational areas of rest, self-care, work, and play/leisure (Meyer, 1977; Moyers, 1999). This balance should not be construed to mean that time is equally spent among these four occupational areas, but that the individual's time spent in each of these areas is adequate for health, well-being, and life satisfaction (Yerxa, 1998a). This optimal time configuration is unique to each individual.

Dissatisfaction and poor health may partially arise from an imbalance among these occupational areas, as well as may contribute to further imbalances due to lack of energy and general malaise. People engage in occupations for a specific purpose, and according to Wilcock (1993), occupations "help individuals meet their bodily needs of sustenance, self-care and shelter and safety"; "...develop skills, social structures and technology aimed at superiority over predators and the environment"; and "...exercise and develop personal capabilities enabling the organism to be maintained and to flourish" (p. 20). Imbalance may occur as a result of difficulty engaging in a variety of occupations to meet these important purposes.

Inadequate health information or education, inappropriate habits, or an environment that fosters an imbalance, such as a work schedule that does not allow time off or a long enough lunch time, may also contribute to an imbalance of occupations. Imbalance can occur because the individual avoids engaging in occupational areas that are a mismatch with the person's capabilities, values, or interests. Poor planning or difficulty in coping with unexpected events may also contribute to occupational imbalances.

Often, an imbalance leads to a reduction in rest and relaxation. Without adequate rest, for instance, the individual is vulnerable to a number of illnesses (Porth, 1998). The amount of rest needed is dependent upon age, stress levels, amount of physical and mental activity, etc. Adequate time spent in self-care activities includes preventing tooth decay and skin problems resulting from poor hygiene, exercising regularly, eating a healthy diet, taking medications as prescribed, designing safe environments, etc. These self-care health habits are often referred to as lifestyle issues (Scaffa, 2001a) and are thus targeted for change to promote health and prevent disease. Because individuals need relief from the stress of work, play/leisure is important for promoting relaxation, increasing creativity, and ensuring physical and mental fitness (Schrier, 1994). However, without work, individuals have difficulty in not only meeting basic financial needs, but also in achieving satisfaction and a sense of life purpose and meaning (Yerxa, 1998a). Occupational therapy practitioners thus strive to help the client evaluate his or her balance of occupations to make decisions and implement strategies to obtain a more healthy balance of affective occupational experiences given the type of health problem, life dissatisfaction, or risks currently experienced (Primeau, 1996).

Healthy Interactions With the Environment

Occupational therapists design interventions to facilitate the interaction between the environment and the individual to create environments that maximize the fit between the person's capabilities and the demands of the occupation. Environmental modifications can augment or prevent declining or lost capabilities, thereby encouraging active participation in the community. As the baby boomers age, for instance, there is a growing need to design environments that accommodate changes in the person's capabilities over time. Occupational therapy practitioners will play an increasing role in this cultural shift that is occurring where attitudes toward aging and disability are becoming more positive. Universal design is thus a popular concept in the area of architecture and engineering and is an excellent opportunity for occupational therapists to collaborate to enhance occupational performance (AOTA, 1993). For instance, a shower stall that has built-in benches, grab bars, a skid resistant floor, and a hand-held spray option to enable showering while seated might be added to a home years prior to the predicted effects of aging or a progressive disease, thereby avoiding building structures that create barriers for people (Gitlin, Miller, & Boyce, 1999).

Occupational therapy practitioners, however, do not only modify the physical environment to enhance occupational performance, but also mobilize social support mechanisms, of which training caregivers is an example (Moyers, 1999). Advocating for clients in terms of developing social policy that supports inclusion in community activities is an example of a possible societal policy modification. All these environmental modifications, whether focused on social, physical, societal policy and attitudes, or cultural norms, are important for ensuring the client's interaction with the environment remains supportive of health and quality of life.

In addition to occupational therapy practitioners being interested in designing environments that support occupational performance, there is also an emphasis upon creating a "just right challenge" from the environment to enable an adaptive response (Yerxa, 1998b). Schkade and Schultz (1993) indicated that the environment creates stimuli that "impinge on an individual and set the stage for the occupational response" (p. 87). It is assumed in occupational therapy theory that individuals desire mastery (Bundy & Murrary, 2002). This desire for mastery in combination with an environment that presses for mastery motivates the person to change performance. The environment motivates change when offering challenges that are new to the person and that require patterns of action not yet experienced by that person (Schkade & Schultz, 1993, p. 87). The key to managing this press for change is to create environments that do not overwhelm the capabilities of the individual, but instead present the right amount of challenge. Yerxa (1998b) stated, "such coaching by occupational therapists could benefit all people who need to develop skills to survive, contribute, and achieve satisfaction in their daily life activities, whether or not they have impairments" (p. 863).

Practice of a Profession

Scope of Practice

Scope of occupational therapy practice evolves over time as the result of research, outcome studies, theoretical developments, and changes in societal need. Regardless of changes in the scope of practice, however, the core of occupational therapy remains constant. Hinojosa and colleagues (2000) defined this core as understanding occupation and purposeful activities and their influence on performance, possessing unique skills such as activity analysis and adaptation, engaging in critical and ethical reasoning, and having attitudes related to holistic intervention and beliefs in the right of self-determination (pp. CE-1-2).

Currently, the scope of practice is outlined in *The Guide to Occupational Therapy Practice* (Moyers, 1999). It indicates "occupational therapy practitioners are concerned with the engagement by persons in meaningful and purposeful occupations in the performance areas of ADL, work and productive activities, and play/leisure" (p. 258). To accomplish this objective of facilitating performance, the occupational therapy practitioner engages in a certain process generally involving referral, screening, evaluation, intervention planning, intervention implementation and reevaluation, and discharge and follow-up (Moyers, 1999, p. 263).

Occupational Therapy Process

To ensure the focus on what the client needs and wants to do, the occupational therapy process must include the following:

- Conducting an occupational history of the client's previous activities, determining the client's perception of what has happened, and assessing the client's roles (referral and screening)
- Determining the client's immediate and long-term goals regarding occupational performance (screening and evaluation)
- Evaluating strengths and limitations created by capabilities, environment, and activity (evaluation)
- Searching the evidence supporting intervention methods that reduce limitations and maximize strengths (intervention planning)
- Developing a client-centered intervention plan that specifies options and obtains client choice and informed consent (intervention and discharge planning)
- Implementing the client-centered intervention and discharge plans and reevaluating the subsequent change in occupational performance and community participation (intervention implementation and reevaluation)
- Modifying the client's goals and assessing the client's perception of what has changed (reevaluation, discharge/follow-up)

International Classification of Functioning, Disability, and Health

The occupational therapy process parallels the ICF health classification. For instance, when the occupational therapist facilitates the discussion of client goals, there is encouragement to initially focus on the activities the client wishes to perform and how the client would like to participate in the community (one of two ICF components of functioning and disability). The evaluation should assess all components of health, including body structure/body function (an ICF component of functioning and disability). However, this focus on body structure/body function is only appropriate as long as the assessment of capabilities remains fully focused on understanding how these capabilities interact with the environment and the occupation to create activity limitations and participation restrictions. Additionally, the occupational therapist must understand how the remaining ability can facilitate future occupational performance. The ultimate goal of understanding body structure/body function is to determine the way in which the person's capabilities may be enhanced, the activity modified, or the environment adapted for improved community participation. Focusing the evaluation on entirely one component of functioning, such as the capabilities of strength, range of motion, or coordination (all body structure/body function issues), leads to the danger of the occupational therapist misunderstanding the client's residual adaptive strategies for activity and community participation, as well as misunderstanding the way in which the client currently interacts within multiple environments (Mathiowetz, 1993; Trombly, 1995).

Interventions are planned collaboratively among the client, the occupational therapist, and others as appropriate that also target the two components of functioning and disability (body structure/body function and activity/participation) with an emphasis upon the activity and participation component (Moyers, 1999). Interventions that reduce impairments or restore body structure/body function are planned within the occupational therapy scope of practice as long as there is reasonable expectation that psychological, cognitive, neurobehavioral, and physiological capabilities will change and will result in improved occupational performance or a reduction in risk for declining performance. Typically, interventions that target both components of functioning and disability (body structure/body function and activity/participation) are combined with the emphasis changing throughout the therapy process (Moyers, 1999).

Practice Settings

Occupational therapists practice within a variety of settings throughout the continuum of health care and social service, including institutional, outpatient, and home and community settings (Moyers, 1999). The question is how can occupational therapists evaluate the actual performance of desired and meaningful occupations and design effective interventions to be implemented within the environment in which the performance normally occurs? There are really two issues here. The first is that a growing body of research illustrates that performance is heavily influenced by the context in which it is performed (Mathiowetz & Haugen, 1994). In other words, the environment significantly changes the way in which the occupation is performed. Without fully understanding the community in which the client lives, works, and plays, the occupational therapy practitioner will be unable to reduce or prevent participation restrictions. The client may be able to only perform an activity in restricted environments as the result of the occupational therapist's incomplete understanding of the influence of a variety of environments on performance.

Second, there is the decision of whether to use simulated or real activities and tasks during the evaluation and intervention processes (Hocking, 2001). Research again is suggesting that simulated activities may not elicit the same motivation to perform or similar motor patterns as the real occupation (Kielhofner, 1992). Simulated activities may in fact be perceived as novel tasks rather than familiar tasks as intended due to the differing demands in performance created by the interaction between this slightly different activity and this strange environment. It is not uncommon, for instance, to hear clients exclaim that cooking in the occupational therapy kitchen in a hospital outpatient clinic is not the same as cooking at home.

Baum and Law (1997, 1998) advocated for the reframing of occupational therapy from a biomedical to a sociomedical context as a way to facilitate occupational therapy practitioners taking an active role in building healthy communities through promoting engagement in meaningful and purposeful occupations for all citizens. Clark et al. (1998) write, "Just as particular occupations may promote health and well-being in individuals, so may the patterns of occupation that characterize particular cultures affect the health of towns, nations, cities, neighborhoods, and communities" (p. 18).

Working in the community requires the occupational therapy practitioner to collaborate with "persons in the client's environment (i.e., family members, teachers, independent living specialists, employers, neighbors, friends) to assist [him or her] in obtaining the skills and making the modification to remove barriers that create social disadvantage" (Baum & Law, 1998, p. 8). Working in the community typically requires the occupational therapy practitioner to have a broader understanding of who the client is. The client may be an individual, but also may be a group of individuals, an organization, or the community itself (Moyers, 1999). The setting in which practice is undertaken may require occupational therapy practitioners to engage in population-based practice in which the needs of many are addressed simultaneously. For instance, the occupational therapist may consult with city government in terms of determining accessibility issues and helping to formulate an improvement plan to accommodate the multiple needs of aging and disabled citizens.

Competence

Providers, payers, and health care service recipients are becoming more intolerant of the costs associated with poor intervention outcomes. Practitioners who have not consistently updated their knowledge and skills may become incompetent over time and, as a result, may be a factor in services that produce poor outcomes. Additionally, the move to community-based practice demands a different set of competencies than those expected of occupational therapy practitioners in traditional medical-model practice settings (Baum & Law, 1998). Baum and Law (1998) write, "A critical skill for occupational therapists is to learn to work in communities as members of teams that go beyond the traditional make-up of occupational therapist, physical therapist, speech-language pathologist, nurse, and physician" (p. 9).

Occupational therapists need to understand the interaction among the person, occupation, and environment. Being able to influence occupational performance requires a thorough understanding of a person's capabilities, how identity is influenced by occupations, the way in which actions and tasks may be modified with technology, and how all the environmental influences create barriers and enablers for performance. Competence in community-based practice means the occupational therapy practitioner has knowledge of social policy, social attitudes, and cultural norms and values, along with knowledge of community support mechanisms available for assisting occupational performance. Likewise, the situational analysis also requires new competencies involving client-centered practice, occupational history taking, occupation-based assessment, gathering evidence to support intervention recommendations, designing occupation-based interventions, and measuring the outcomes of these selected interventions.

The AOTA (1999b) has developed *Standards for Continuing Competence*, which address the need for the practitioner to demonstrate the appropriate knowledge, critical reasoning, interpersonal abilities, performance skills, and ethical reasoning needed for implementing the core of occupational therapy and for assuming other related roles (p. 599). The professional should judge his or her competence according to the current job responsibilities and needs of the community and the client and should determine one's educational needs in light of the *Standards for Continuing Competence*. Does the practitioner have the required knowledge, critical and ethical reasoning ability, and interpersonal and performance skills necessary to facilitate client achievement of specified outcomes in relevant community environments? There is need to maintain skills required for implementing the core of occupational therapy, to develop a specialized knowledge and skill base, and to obtain advanced abilities. For instance, although the core of occupational therapy does not change, the theoretical, research, and knowledge base continually expands; the technology related to compensation, to promoting a client's adaptation, or to analyzing an occupation and its associated activities change; and community issues evolve and become more complex.

Evidence

Evidence-based practice "refers to intervention guided by a methodical review of the available research and expert opinion pertaining to an area of practice" (Egan, Dubouloz, von Zweck, & Vallerand, 1998, p. 137). The ability of occupational therapists to select the best intervention approach and for occupational therapy practitioners to skillfully provide the appropriate services in the community according to the evidence indicating the intervention's effectiveness and efficacy is an aspect of competence (Moyers, 1999). Searching for and obtaining the evidence to support chosen interventions is important for client-centered practice. Telling clients about the supporting evidence is necessary for giving adequate informed consent (Tickle-Degnen, 2000). However, it is likely that evidence to support many interventions suggested as effective by theory or experience is not available and thus requires occupational therapists to not only consult with experts by examining practice guidelines and case studies, but to also measure and collect outcomes to support future use of the intervention in their particular practice area. The client is informed of this lack of research evidence and is told of the reliance on expert opinion and recommendation.

Because of the development of evidence-based practice in the medical profession, it is problematic to adopt the singular emphasis on randomized clinical trials as being the best evidence, when in fact much of occupational therapy practice is holistic in its implementation as a result of the complexity of occupational performance. Effective occupational therapy intervention requires manipulation of multiple interventions simultaneously, targeting both components of functioning and disability (body structure/body function and activity and participation) to facilitate occupational performance in relevant environments. Occupational therapists will need to develop ways to incorporate the results of many research methodologies, including qualitative research, into evidence-based practice decisions. Also, it is very clear that evidence-based practice depends on addressing the wishes of the client in making the ultimate determination of which methods are preferred in order to achieve the client's immediate and long-term occupational performance goals (Tickle-Degnen, 2000).

Intervention Strategies

In their emphasis on promoting occupational performance as an aspect of achieving health and life satisfaction, occupational therapy practitioners use specific intervention strategies categorized as remediation, prevention/promotion, compensation, adaptation, consultation, and education. Table 10-1 contains the definition of each of these general strategies and gives examples of specific interventions in each intervention category. The relationship to the ICF components of health classification is also included. These intervention strategies may be designed for the individual, groups of individuals, or populations. Occupational therapists and their clients collaboratively choose specific strategies based upon the evaluation results, the client's goals regarding occupational performance, and the evidence from research and expert opinion.

Regardless of the strategy chosen, the "hallmark of occupational therapy intervention is the use of occupations, activities, and tasks meaningful to the client in order to promote and maintain health and to improve occupational performance" (Moyers, 1999, p. 270). Occupations are chosen because of their potential to remediate impaired capabilities; to facilitate transfer of capabilities to multiple contexts; to enhance motivation to change and adapt; to promote self-exploration and development of identity; to match current capabilities; to provide opportunities to practice skills and develop habits; to provide feedback; to experience success, pleasure, and other emotions; and to interact with others (Moyers, 1999, pp. 270-272). Occupations are an important intervention tool due to growing realization through research that improving a person's capabilities does not necessarily guarantee improvements in occupational performance (Mathiowetz & Haugen, 1994). By deliberately ensuring the transfer of capabilities to actual performance in real environments, occupational therapy practitioners understand that linear relationships among impairments, activity limitations, and participation restrictions do not typically exist (Moyers, 1999, p. 276).

Summary

In conclusion, the occupational therapy process and outcomes are ultimately concerned with changing the client's occupational performance according to the client's goals. Intervention strategies generally include remediation, adaptation, compensation, prevention/promotion, consultation, and education. These strategies are selected based on the evidence supporting effectiveness; on the client's preference and goals; on the results of the evaluation exploring the interaction among the person's capabilities, the environment, and the activity; and on the competence of the occupational therapist. Occupational therapists target outcomes at both components of functioning and disability of the ICF (body structure/body function and activity/participation), particularly emphasizing reduction in or prevention of activity limitations and participation restrictions. A focus on activity and participation requires the therapist to re-examine effectiveness of using simulated tasks and environments and instead necessitates a thorough understanding of the community in which the client lives, works, and plays.

References

American Occupational Therapy Association. (1993). *Design for aging: Strategies for collaboration between architects and occupational therapists*. Bethesda, MD: Author.

American Occupational Therapy Association. (1999a). Definition of OT practice for the AOTA model practice act. *American Journal of Occupational Therapy, 53*(6), 608.

American Occupational Therapy Association. (1999b). Standards for continuing competence. *American Journal of Occupational Therapy, 53*(6), 599-600.

Baum, C. M., & Law, M. (1997). Occupational therapy practice: Focusing on occupational performance. *American Journal of Occupational Therapy, 51*(4), 277-288.

Baum, C., & Law, M. (1998). Nationally speaking: Community health: A responsibility, an opportunity, and fit for occupational therapy. *American Journal of Occupational Therapy, 52*(1), 7-10.

Buckley, K. A., & Poole, S. E. (2000). Activity analysis. In J. Hinojosa & M. L. Blount (Eds.), *The texture of life: Purposeful activities in occupational therapy* (pp. 51-90). Bethesda, MD: American Occupational Therapy Association.

Bundy, A. C., & Murray, E. A. (2002). Sensory integration: A. Jean Ayres' theory revisited. In A. C. Budy, S. J. Lane, & E. A. Murray (Eds.), *Sensory integration: Theory and practice* (2nd ed., pp. 3-33). Philadelphia, PA: F. A. Davis Company.

Christiansen, C. H. (1999). Defining lives: Occupation as identity: An essay on competence coherence, and the creation of meaning. *American Journal of Occupational Therapy, 53*(6), 547-558.

Christiansen, C., & Baum, C. (1997). Person-environment occupational performance: A conceptual model for practice. In C. Christiansen & C. Baum (Eds.), *Enabling function and well-being* (2nd ed., pp. 49-70). Thorofare, NJ: SLACK Incorporated.

Clark, F., Wood, W., & Larson, E. (1998). Occupational science: Occupational therapy's legacy for the 21st century. In M. E. Neistadt & E. B. Crepeau (Eds.), *Willard and Spackman's occupational therapy* (9th ed., pp. 13-21). Philadelphia, PA: Lippincott.

Crabtree, J. L. (1998). The end of occupational therapy. *American Journal of Occupational Therapy, 52*(3), 205-214.

Table 10-1

Occupational Therapy Intervention Strategies

Strategies	*Definition*	*Focus*	*Example Intervention Methods*	*ICF*
Remediation	Changing the person's capabilities: psychological, cognitive, physiological, and neurobehavioral	Restoring, maintaining, developing, or improving capabilities needed for occupational performance	Enabling activities, sensorimotor techniques, graded exercise and activities, physical agents, manual techniques	Body structure/body function
Adaptation	The internal process by which people respond to the demand for change. The person changes by incorporating new skills and habits into daily occupational performance	Skill and habit development or modification; creating the environmental "just-right" challenge	Practice, repetition, selection of challenging environments that motivate change while supporting skill and habit development	Activity participation
Compensation	Changing the activity and the environment to match the capabilities of the client	Modifying the task skill requirements, task procedures, or task objects. Making environmental modifications to support existing capabilities and to incorporate task modifications	Activity analysis and synthesis; applying ergonomic principles; using adaptive equipment, assistive technology, and other substitute task objects; training caregivers; changing the environment	Activity participation
Prevention Primary: targeted to those without any limitations or impairments Secondary: targeted to those at risk Tertiary: to limit the detrimental effects of illness or injury	Involves "anticipatory action taken to reduce the possibility of an event or condition from occurring or developing, or to minimize the damage that may result from the event or condition if it does occur" (Pickett & Hanlon, 1990, p. 81). Occupations that facilitate occupational performance while avoiding the creation of impairments, activity limitations, and participation restrictions	Safe task methods and task objects, efficient design of occupations, supportive and safe environments	Application of ergonomic, psychosocial, and cognitive intervention principles to the performance of occupations in multiple environments	Both components of functioning and disability and environmental factors

(continued)

Table 10-1

Strategies	*Definition*	*Focus*	*Example Intervention Methods*	*ICF*
Health promotion	Involves "the process of enabling people to increase control over and to improve their health" (WHO, 1986, p. iii)	Health promotion strategies center on the power of occupation as an important aspect of staying healthy	Purposeful and meaningful occupations; balance of rest, self-care, work, play/leisure; healthy interactions with the environment; lifestyle redesign; client education	Both components of functioning and disability and environmental factors
Education	Educating clients about ways to manage their occupational performance in a variety of environments	New skills, habits, task methods, and use of new task objects; health education	Teaching/training	Both components of functioning and disability and environmental factors
Consultation	Providing of information and expert advice	May be short-term or long-term Most often used when new programs are being developed or are undergoing significant change (Scaffa, 2001b, p. 14)	Program development and evaluation, supervisory models, organizational issues, and clinical concerns (Scaffa, 2001b, p. 14)	Both components of functioning and disability and environmental factors

Evidence Worksheet

Author	*Year*	*Concept*	*Importance for Practice*
Christiansen & Baum	1997	Ability	Lack of ability may constrain performance and limit engagement in activity and tasks, make it difficult to complete the tasks within time frame, or limit the ability to meet standards of performance
Reed & Sanderson	1999	Actions	Actions taken during a task may be a reflection of the individual's capabilities, skills, and experiences
Buckley & Poole Moyer	2000 1999	Activity analysis	Activity analysis is a process in which the practitioner determines the performance demands of the activity by determining the performance demands of the activity and breaking the activity down to components parts. This involves analyzing each task in terms of its contextual, temporal, psychological, social, cultural, and meaning dimensions
Moyers	2005	Activity limitations	Activity limitations occur because the activity is not adapted to accommodate a change in capability, and likewise, participation restrictions occur because the environment does not accommodate the loss of capability and limitations in activity
Kramer & Hinojosa	2000	Activity synthesis	The process of modifying activities or the environment to better match the goals and the capabilities of the client with the environment in which performance is to occur
Moyers	2005	Competency	Occupational therapist needs to demonstrate the ability to understand the interaction among the person, occupation, and environment. Being able to influence occupational performance requires a thorough understanding of a person's capabilities, how identity is influenced by occupations, the way in which actions and tasks may be modified with technology, and how all the environmental influences create barriers and enablers for performance
Egan et al.	1998	Evidenced-based practice	Refers to intervention guided by a methodical review of the available research and expert opinion pertaining to an area of practice. Telling clients about the supporting evidence is necessary for giving adequate informed consent for treatment
WHO	2001	Functioning	Functioning is an umbrella term encompassing all body functions, activities, and participation
Moyers	2004	Health	Being able to perform the activities of one's own choosing, regardless of disease or impairment
Porth	1998	Importance of rest	Without adequate rest, an individual is vulnerable to a number of illnesses
Moyers	1999	Occupational therapy service	Occupational therapy is unique because of the way its practitioners collaborate with their clients, other heath care practitioners, and other professions (teachers, lawyers, engineers, social policy analysts etc.) to design therapeutic occupations to address the occupational performance problems that can lead to dependence, declines in health, disability, or a reduced quality of life
Kielhofner	1995	People as occupational beings	Identity relies on the integration of values, interests, and roles so that the person may express that identity through occupational performance

(continued)

Author	*Year*	*Concept*	*Importance for Practice*
Moyers	2005	Performance dimensions	Skills rely upon performance capabilities (cognitive, psychological, physiological, and neurobehavioral)
Kielhofner	1992	Simulated activities	Simulated activities may not elicit the same motivation to perform or similar motor patterns as the real occupation
Wilcock	1993	What does occupation do?	Occupation helps individuals meet their bodily needs of sustenance, self-care, shelter, and safety. It develops skills, social structures, and technology aimed at superiority over predators and the environment. It also provides exercise, develops personal capabilities, and enables the organism to be maintained and to flourish
Holm, Rogers, & James Moyer Primeau Moyers Schkade & Schultz	1998 1999 1996 1999 1993	What the occupational therapist does	Based on a thorough understanding of the person's capabilities, environment, and occupation, the occupational therapy practitioner facilitates performance by matching the occupation to the person's capabilities and to the environment in which the person performs. Occupational therapy practitioners strive to help clients evaluate their balance of occupations to make decisions and implement strategies to obtain a more healthy balance of occupations. Occupational therapy practitioners mobilize social support mechanisms (i.e., train parents, personal assistants, caregivers). Provides a "just-right challenge" to enable an adaptive response or participation
Hocking	2001	Why people use occupations	Occupations help people understand who they are, what they might do, the context in which they might act, and who they might become

Egan, M., Dubouloz, C. J., von Zweck, C., & Vallerand, J. (1998). The client-centered evidence-based practice of occupational therapy. *Canadian Journal of Occupational Therapy*, 65(3), 136-143.

Gitlin, L. N., Miller, K. S., & Boyce, A. (1999). Bathroom modifications for frail elderly renters: Outcomes of a community-based program. *Technology and Disability, 10*, 141-149.

Hasselkus, B. R., & Rosa, S. A. (1997). Meaning and occupation. In C. Christiansen & C. Baum (Eds.), *Enabling function and well-being* (2nd ed., pp. 363-377). Thorofare, NJ: SLACK Incorporated.

Hinojosa, J., Bowen, R., Case-Smith, J., Epstein, C. F., Moyers, P., & Schwope, C. (2000). Standards for continuing competence for occupational therapy practitioners. *OT Practice*, 5(20), CE-1-CE-8.

Hocking, C. (2001). The issue is: Implementing occupation-based assessment. *American Journal of Occupational Therapy*, 55(4), 463-469.

Holm, M. B., Rogers, J. C., & James, A. B. (1998). Treatment of occupational performance areas. In M. C. Neistadt & E. B. Crepeau (Eds.), *Willard & Spackman's occupational therapy* (9th ed., pp. 323-390). Philadelphia, PA: Lippincott.

Jackson, J., Carlson, M., Mandel, D., Zemke, R., & Clark, F. (1998). Occupation in lifestyle redesign: The well elderly study occupational therapy program. *American Journal of Occupational Therapy*, 52(5), 326-336.

Kielhofner, G. (1992). *Conceptual foundation of occupational therapy*. Philadelphia, PA: F. A. Davis.

Kielhofner, G. (1995). Habituation subsystem. In G. Kielhofner (Ed.), *A model of human occupation theory and application* (2nd ed., pp. 63-81). Baltimore, MD: Williams & Wilkins.

Kramer, P., & Hinojosa, J. (2000). Activity synthesis. In J. Hinojosa & M. L. Blount (Eds.), *The texture of life: Purposeful activities in occupational therapy* (pp. 91-105). Bethesda, MD: American Occupational Therapy Association.

Mathiowetz, V. (1993). Role of physical performance component evaluation in occupational therapy functional assessment. *American Journal of Occupational Therapy, 47*(3), 225-230.

Mathiowetz, V., & Bass-Haugen, J. (1994). Motor behavior research: Implications for therapeutic approaches to central nervous system dysfunction. *American Journal of Occupational Therapy, 48*(8), 733-745.

Meyer, A. (1977). The philosophy of occupational therapy. *American Journal of Occupational Therapy, 31*, 639-642.

Moyers, P. (1999). The guide to occupational therapy practice. *American Journal of Occupational Therapy, 53*, 247-322.

Moyers, P. (2005). Introduction to occupation-based practice. In C. H. Christiansen, C. M. Baum, & J. Bass-Haugen (Eds.), *Occupational therapy: Performance, participation, and well-being* (3rd ed.). Thorofare, NJ: SLACK Incorporated.

Moyers, P. A., & Stoffel, V. C. (2001). Community-based approaches for substance use disorders. In M. Scaffa (Ed.), *Occupational therapy in community-based practice settings* (pp. 318-342). Philadelphia, PA: F. A. Davis.

Pickett, G., & Hanlon, J. J. (1990). *Public health: Administration and practice*. St. Louis, MO: Times Mirror/Mosby.

Porth, C. (1998). Stress and adaptation. In C. Porth (Ed.), *Pathophysiology: Concepts of altered health states* (pp. 1233-1242). Philadelphia, PA: Lippincott.

Primeau, L. A. (1996). Work and leisure: Transcending the dichotomy. *American Journal of Occupational Therapy, 50*(7), 569-577.

Reed, K., & Sanderson, S. (1999). *Concepts of occupational therapy* (4th ed.). Baltimore, MD: Lippincott, Williams & Wilkins.

Scaffa, M. E. (2001a). Paradigm shift: From the medical model to the community model. In M. E. Scaffa (Ed.), *Occupational therapy in community-based practice settings* (pp. 19-34). Philadelphia, PA: F. A. Davis Company.

Scaffa, M. E. (2001b). Community-based practice: Occupation in context. In M. E. Scaffa (Ed.), *Occupational therapy in community-based practice settings* (p. 318). Philadelphia, PA: F. A. Davis Company.

Schkade, J. K., & Schultz, S. (1993). Occupational adaptation: An integrative frame of reference. In H. Hopkins, & H. Smith (Eds.), *Willard and Spackman's occupational therapy* (8th ed., pp. 87-90). Philadelphia, PA: J. B. Lippincott.

Schrier, E. W. (1994). Work and play: A nation out of balance [Special issue]. *Health*, 8(6).

Tickle-Degnen, L. (2000). Evidence-based practice forum-Communicating with clients, family members, and colleagues about research evidence. *American Journal of Occupational Therapy*, 54(3), 341-343.

Trombly, C. A. (1995). Eleanor Clarke Slagle lectureship—1995. Occupation: Purposefulness and meaningfulness as therapeutic mechanisms. *American Journal of Occupational Therapy*, 49,(10), 960-972.

Wilcock, A. A. (1993). A theory of the human need for occupation. *Journal of Occupational Science: Australia, 1*(1), 17-24.

World Health Organization. (1986). The Ottawa charter for health promotion. *Health Promotion, 1*, iii-v.

World Health Organization. (2001). *International classification of functioning, disability and health* (ICF). Geneva, Switzerland: Author.

Yerxa, E. J. (1998a). Health and the human spirit for occupation. *American Journal of Occupational Therapy, 52*(6), 412-418.

Yerxa, E. J. (1998b). Dreams, decisions, and directions for occupational therapy. In M. E. Neistadt and E. B. Crepeau (Eds.), *Willard and Spackman's occupational therapy* (9th ed.) (pp. 861-865). Philadelphia, PA: Lippincott.

Chapter Ten: Introduction to Occupation-Based Practice Reflections and Learning Activities

Julie Bass-Haugen, PhD, OTR/L, FAOTA

Reflections

This chapter provided an introduction to an occupational therapy practice that is occupation-based. It used information from the previous chapters to strengthen your understanding of exactly what you will do in your occupational therapy practice and why you are doing it.

You are committed to a profession that has overlap with many related professions—nursing, psychology, physical therapy, speech pathology, special education, and social work. At times, it may appear that all of these professionals have the same body of knowledge and the same goals for their clients. We use similar terminology like function, health, activities of daily living, and independence. What is the unique role of occupational therapy? Well, the reason we spent nearly half this textbook on occupation is that occupational therapy's unique professional contribution is occupation. When we use a term like *function*, our primary concern is whether there is sufficient function to perform important and meaningful occupations, not whether there is function at the elbow joint. When we use a term like *health*, our primary concern is whether occupational engagement is supporting or compromising health, not whether blood pressure is in a healthy range.

As you go forward in your occupational therapy practice, your most important professional development activity is to develop a strong occupational base. If you don't do this, you may eventually become confused about your professional identity and lose your unique role on an interdisciplinary team. What are the unique contributions you will make as an occupational therapy practitioner? First, you will understand and communicate the clients' perspectives on their occupations. You will know how the ability and/or inability to do certain occupations are affecting their health and personal identity. You will know what they want to be able to do, what they view as important, and what they view as meaningful. Second, you will understand and communicate the "big picture" on performance. You will know what they are able to do, what specific personal characteristics (neurobehavioral, physiological, cognitive, psychological, and spiritual) are helping and hindering performance, and what specific environmental characteristics (natural environment, built environment and technology, culture and values, social supports, and social and economic systems) are helping and hindering performance. You will know how to analyze the multiple layers of occupational performance from the most basic actions to complex roles. Third, you will understand and communicate the evidence regarding occupation, performance, person, and environment. You will know how to evaluate clinical and research findings that relate to occupational performance. Fourth, you will understand and communicate the intervention options that are available to improve occupational performance. You will know how to select the right options at the right time for the right purpose. Fifth, you will base your assessment and interventions on the actual doing of occupations. You will not be satisfied to just talk about occupations; you will want to see real performance to understand the interaction of person, environment, and occupational performance. Finally, you began this process determining the client's perspective, and you will end this process the same way. You will determine how your clients are able to perform the things they want to do and how they feel about their performance.

Now, I challenge you to examine similar professions—nursing, physical therapy, speech pathology, special education, psychology, and social work. Think about their roles as you know them. Do you have any doubt now that occupational therapy has a unique role that is different from every other professional?

The occupational therapy practitioner has another unique skill as it relates to occupational performance. In the traditional occupational therapy literature, this skill is described as activity analysis and synthesis. When occupational therapy practitioners do an activity analysis, they analyze the activity and the person and environment characteristics used for performance. Think of a seemingly simple activity, such as brushing your teeth. Think about the way in which this activity is typically done. What are the different steps in teeth brushing, and what are some common variations in the steps? What personal factors are typically employed to brush your teeth? Do you need to have a certain amount of strength and range of motion and coordination? Do you usually do this activity in the standing position? Do you usually use your dominant hand? Do you use vision or sensation? Do you need to remember a certain sequence to the steps? What environmental factors are typically employed to brush teeth? What are the characteristics of the typical toothbrush and toothpaste? Where do you usually brush your teeth? How much lighting is necessary? Do you use a mirror? Is this an activity that is usually done independently or with the help of another person? Are their any cultural differences in performance of this activity?

By the time you get through this list of questions and others, you have done an activity analysis. You fully understand both the activity and typical performance of the activity. Now you can work with a specific person who has an occupational goal related to oral hygiene. You can take what you know about the activity through your activity analysis and compare it to the current performance of a specific person. Then, you are able to complete an activity synthesis. That is, you can modify the activity or the environment to meet the current capabilities of the person for performance. Let's continue the example of brushing teeth. What interventions would you try if a person had limited strength in the upper arms and hands? What interventions would you try if a person had limited vision? What interventions would you try if a person hadn't learned or couldn't perform all the steps necessary for good oral hygiene? How would you change or grade your interventions if any of these person factors improved or worsened?

In activity synthesis, the focus is on modification of the activity or environment to meet the current capabilities of the person. Occupational therapy practitioners use another strategy to help people reach occupational goals. They provide the "just-right challenge" for current personal capabilities. This "just-right challenge" encourages optimal use of person factors for performance. Let's go back once more to the example of brushing teeth. If a person had limited, but improving strength in the dominant upper arm, would you want to modify the activity to entirely eliminate the need for any upper arm strength? Probably not. You would want to figure out the "just-right challenge" to achieve the occupational goal of brushing teeth and, at the same time, maintain or improve strength in the upper arm. Perhaps you would encourage the person to use as much dominant arm strength as possible for brushing until tired. Then, you might encourage resting the arm on a counter in the seated position or switching to the nondominant arm to complete the activity. You might also recommend use of a battery-operated toothbrush to reduce performance demands. This is an example of using the best options from activity synthesis and "just-right challenge" for occupational performance.

This chapter also provided an introduction to intervention strategies that are commonly used in occupational therapy practice: remediation, adaptation, compensation, prevention, health promotion, education, and consultation. Usually, more than one strategy is used in a given situation. The selection of strategies depends on the occupational goals and performance issues, the type of situational analysis, and the setting. For each situation, you choose strategies that are the most effective, the most efficient, and the most likely to result in good overall outcomes.

Finally, this chapter introduced a number of resources that may guide your further learning. Evidence (or literature) on person, environment, and occupational performance assessments and interventions will help you make informed decisions for each step. The AOTA has published *The Guide to Occupational Therapy Practice* and *Standards for Continuing Competence* to provide specific standards and guidelines for occupational therapy practice and practitioners. There are many other sources of information, too. All of these resources are an important part of your occupational therapy tool kit, regardless of whether you are a student or experienced practitioner. Now, you are ready to adopt an occupation-based framework for your practice.

Journal Activities

1. Look up and write down dictionary definitions of function and functioning. Highlight the components of the definitions that are most related to their descriptions in Chapter Ten.
2. Identify the most important new learning for you in this chapter.
3. Identify one question you have about Chapter Ten.
4. Reflect on how you evaluate your current level of competence for each of the standards in the *Standards for Continuing Competence* (AOTA, 1999, pp. 599-600). For each standard, identify your strengths, identify areas needing improvement, and identify several short-term goals.
    - Knowledge—understanding and comprehension of the information required.
    - Critical reasoning—reasoning processes to make sound judgments and decisions
    - Interpersonal abilities—professional relationships with others
    - Performance skills—expertise, aptitudes, proficiencies, and abilities
    - Ethical reasoning—identify, analyze, and clarify ethical issues or dilemmas in order to make responsible decisions

Technology/Internet Learning Activities

1. Use a discussion database to share specific journal entries.
2. Use a good Internet search engine to find the Web site for the AOTA.
   - Enter the phrase "AOTA" or "American Occupational Therapy Association" in your search line.
   - Review the Web site.
   - What is the primary purpose of this site?
   - Identify the primary resource areas for occupational therapy practice at this site.
   - Review the *Core Values of the American Occupational Therapy Association.*
   - Identify the core values of the AOTA.
   - Discuss the importance of three core values in a strong occupation-based practice.
3. Use a good Internet search engine to find the Web site for the AOTA.
   - Enter the phrase "AOTA" or "American Occupational Therapy Association" in your search line.
   - Review the Web site.
   - Review the *Occupational Therapy Code of Ethics-2000.*
   - Identify the principles in the *Occupational Therapy Code of Ethics-2000.*
   - Discuss the importance of one principle in a strong occupation-based practice.
4. Use a good Internet search engine to find the Web net site for the AOTA.
   - Enter the phrase "AOTA" or "American Occupational Therapy Association" in your search line.
   - Review the Web site.
   - Review the *Standards of Practice for Occupational Therapy.*
   - Identify the standards in the *Standards of Practice for Occupational Therapy.*
   - Discuss the relationship between the *Standards* and the key concepts in this chapter on occupational therapy practice and process.
     - ✧ What are the similarites and differences?
5. Use a good Internet search engine to find the Internet sites for other professional organizations.
   - Enter the following phrases in your search line: "American Nursing Association," "American Physical Therapy Association," "American Speech Language Hearing Association," "National Association of Social Workers," "Council for Exceptional Children," "Society of Clinical Psychology."
   - Review each Web site.
   - Identify the roles and responsibilities for each profession. What does each professional do?
   - Discuss similarities and differences in these roles as compared to occupational therapy.

Applied Learning Activities

Individual Learning Activity #1: Defining the Client in Different Situations

Instructions:

- Read the section on Practice Settings in the chapter.
- Reflect on the cases presented in the table on p. 238.
- For each case, develop different definitions of the client using hypothetical examples (e.g., a population for Case #1 might be young adult bikers).
  - ✧ Reflect on how your occupational therapy services might change for each case.

Case	*Person*	*Population*	*Organization*
1	A 25 year old female college student who was in a recent biking accident		
2		A population of about 500 at-risk adolescents (12 to 18 years old) living in a small community	
3			A light manufacturing company that is concerned about the health and personal stress levels of its employees

Individual Learning Activity #2: Conducting an Activity/Task Analysis

Instructions:

- Select an occupation for a basic activity/task analysis (e.g., sewing a dress, mowing the lawn, making coffee or tea, studying for a test, playing a game of chess, making a bed).
- Analyze the occupation by the following characteristics and dimensions adapted from the *Guide to Occupational Therapy Practice* (AOTA, 1999).
- Explore the occupation in detail so that you fully understand all components and aspects of it.

Dimension	*Probes*	*Analysis*
Performance steps	What are the steps in performance?	
Performance person factors	What person factors are typically used for performance? Neurobehavioral? Physiological? Cognitive?	
Contextual	What are the physical (natural and built) characteristics of the task and broader environment?	
Temporal	When is this occupation done? What aspects of time are important in this occupation?	
Psychological	What aspects of personality, emotions, self-concept, self-esteem, identity are associated with this occupation?	
Social	What social roles are associated with this occupation? What is the role of social interaction in this occupation?	
Cultural	What values, beliefs, customs, and behaviors are associated with this occupation in one culture?	
Meaning	What is the meaning of this occupation for one person? Spirituality?	

Individual Learning Activity #3: Exploring Principles of Occupation Therapy Intervention

Instructions:

- Pretend you are a hospitalized 22-year-old student in an occupational therapy program who had a biking accident. You have a lot of pain, a broken shoulder and pelvis, a mild head injury, face abrasions, and unclear vision.
- Identify occupations that your occupational therapy practitioner could provide you to meet the following principles and meet your interests, needs, and values.
- Discuss the principles that were easiest and hardest to find an occupational match. Why do you think this was the case?

Principle	*Occupation*
• Remediate impaired capabilities	
• Transfer your capabilities in the hospital environment to a relevant context or environment	Example: Practice showering/bathing in variety of bathrooms to simulate showers/baths in apartment and parents' home
• Promote self-exploration and development of identity	
• Match current capabilities or obtain best person-environment fit	
• Practice skills and develop habits	
• Provide feedback on current level of performance	
• Experience success, pleasure, and other emotions	
• Interact with others	

Active Learning Activities

Group Activity: Exploring Strategies for Activity/Task Synthesis

Preparation

- Read Chapter Ten.
- Complete Applied Learning Activity #2.

Time: 45 minutes to 1 hour

Materials:

- Completed Applied Learning Activity #2
- Adaptive equipment catalogs
- Flip chart, black board, or white board

Instructions:

- Individually:
  - ✧ Review the results of your activity/task analysis from Applied Learning Activity #2.
  - ✧ Be prepared to summarize your activity/task analysis for your small group.
- In small groups:
  - ✧ Review the activity/task analyses for members of the group.
  - ✧ Select one occupation for further examination.
  - ✧ Select two specific impairments in person factors that would influence performance (e.g., vision, strength, endurance, memory, attention, etc.).

- ✧ Conduct an activity/task synthesis to explore how you might grade the activity/task, change the methods, and change the objects or environment.
- ✧ Summarize your ideas in a table similar to the one on p. 238.

Occupation	*Impairment in Person Factor*	*How Could You Grade the Activity/Task?*	*How Could You Change the Method?*	*How Could You Change the Objects or Environment?*
Making a sandwich	Cognitive—short-term memory loss	Change the number of cues Change the type of sandwich	Use familiar types of sandwiches Write out the steps	Put all needed items on counter Clear counter of other distractions
	Neurobehavioral—weakness in dominant arm	Change the level of use by the weak arm Change the number of steps completed	Use weak arm as assist for task completion Sit down to save energy	Provide stabilizer for bread Provide one-handed jar opener

Discussion:

- Discuss the ideas for activity synthesis that were the easiest to develop.
- Discuss the ideas for activity synthesis that were the hardest to develop.
- What resources and learning would strengthen your skills in activity synthesis?

Chapter Eleven Objectives

The information in this chapter is intended to help the reader:

1. Understand the importance of viewing the person, the organization, and the community from a top-down client-centered perspective.
2. Describe the intrinsic or personal performance capabilities or constraints that impact occupational performance.
3. Describe the environmental enablers or barriers that impact occupational performance.
4. Understand the hierarchy of abilities, actions, and tasks and how they support occupations.
5. Understand how roles support the performance of many occupations.
6. Understand how the PEOP model provides the structure for practitioners to identify and consider the factors that influence occupational performance.

Key Words

affordance: Humans perceive possibilities based upon both the places and objects in the environment, and these influence meaning and action (Gibson, 1979).

arousal: The process through which environment influences our actions. Three groups of variables are associated with arousal. These include psychophysical characteristics such as noise or light, ecological events such as a storm or rough terrain, or situations (Berlyne, 1960).

built environment: Physical environments can be built for accessibility, manageability, safety, aesthetics, comfort, and enjoyment. The suitability of the space to accommodate an individual's needs is central to physical or built environments. Built environments also include tools that support engagement in tasks and occupations. Tools that are usable within the person's capabilities are grouped under the category of assistive technology.

cognitive factors: Cognition involves the mechanism of language comprehension and production, pattern recognition, task organization, reasoning, attention, and memory (Duchek, 1991).

cultural environment: Culture refers to values, beliefs, customs, and behaviors that are transmitted from one generation to the next. Culture affects performance by prescribing norms for the use of time and space and influencing beliefs regarding the importance of activities, work, and play. It also influences choices in what people do, how they do it, and how important it is to them (Altman & Chelmers, 1984; Hall, 1973).

disability: The cause of disability has shifted from being viewed as a pathology that could be medically managed to one of an interaction between the characteristics of the individual and his or her impairments and the characteristics of the environment (Brandt & Pope, 1997).

environmental press: Places influence behavior by creating demand or expectations for behavior (Barris, Kielhofner, Levine, & Neville, 1985; Lawton, 1980; Murray, Barrett, & Hamburger, 1938).

human agency: People are naturally motivated to explore their world and demonstrate mastery within it. To do this, the person must effectively use the resources (personal, social, and material) available in his or her environment (Baum & Christiansen, 2005).

motivation: Successful experience supports motivation (Baum & Christiansen, 2005).

natural environment: The natural environment includes geographical features such as terrain, hours of sunlight, climate, and air quality. The natural environment can be a significant factor in determining whether or not an individual's physical limitations are disabling (Brandt & Pope, 1997).

neurobehavioral factors: The sensory (olfactory, gustatory, visual, auditory, somatosensory, proprioceptive, and vestibular) and motor systems (somatic, cerebellum, basal ganglia network, and thalamic integration) underlie all neuromotor performance (Baum & Christiansen, 2005).

occupational performance: Occupational performance is central to the development of occupational therapy models. It operates as a means of connecting the individual to roles and to the sociocultural environment (Reed and Sanderson, 1999).

occupations: Goal-directed pursuits that typically extend over time, have meaning to the performer, and involve multiple tasks (Christiansen & Baum, 1997).

performance: Performance is supported by a complex interaction of biological, psychological, and social phenomena that requires a satisfactory match between person, task, and situational characteristics (Engel, 1977; Meyer, 1922; Mosey, 1974; Reilly, 1962).

physiological factors: Endurance, flexibility, movement and strength are necessary requirements for occupations requiring moderate or sustained effort. People who are physically active are healthier and live longer than those who are sedentary (Minor, 1997).

psychological factors: Psychological factors describe the personality traits, motivational influences, and internal processes used by an individual to influence what they do, how events are interpreted, and how they contribute to a sense of self. Self-efficacy is an important psychological factor as it allows people to view themselves as competent. Persons who view themselves as competent view their overall well-being more favorably and continue working on tasks despite setbacks (Bandura, 1977, 1982; Baum & Christiansen, 2005; Gage & Polatajko, 1994).

roles: Positions in society having expected responsibilities and privileges (Christiansen & Baum, 1997).

social environment: Social support is an experienced rather than an observed phenomenon and is essential to maintain health. There are three types of social support that enable people to do what they need and want to do. These include practical support, informational support, and emotional support (Dunkel-Schetter & Bennett, 1990; McColl, 1997; Orth-Gomer, Rosengren, & Wilhelmsen, 1993; Pierce, Sarason, & Sarason, 1990; Thoits, 1997).

societal environment: The standing of an individual within the group shapes behavior and attitudes toward self. Social rejection and isolation can have devastating psychological consequences. Societal policies govern the availability of resources which controls access to services and work (Baum & Christiansen, 2005).

spirituality: Everyday places, occupations, and interactions are filled with meaning that is interpreted by the person based on his or her goals, values, and experiences. Spirituality is socially and culturally influenced but become internal to the individual through personal interpretation. As meanings contribute to personal understanding about self and one's place in the world, they are described as spiritual. People develop a self-identity and serve a sense of fulfillment as they master and accomplish goals that have personal meaning (Christiansen, 1997).

tasks: Combinations of actions sharing a common purpose recognized by the performer (Christiansen & Baum, 1997).

top-down client-centered strategy: An occupational performance approach requires the practitioner to determine what the client perceives to be issues that are causing difficulty in occupations that support productivity, work, personal care, home maintenance, sleep, and recreation of leisure (Trombly, 1995; Mathiowetz & Bass-Haugen, 1994; Fisher, 1998).

The purpose of science is not to analyze or describe but to make useful models of the world.
A model is useful if it allows us to get use out of it.
Edward De Bono

Chapter Eleven

Person-Environment-Occupation-Performance: An Occupation-Based Framework for Practice

Carolyn M. Baum, PhD, OTR/L, FAOTA and Charles H. Christiansen, EdD, OTR, OT(C), FAOTA

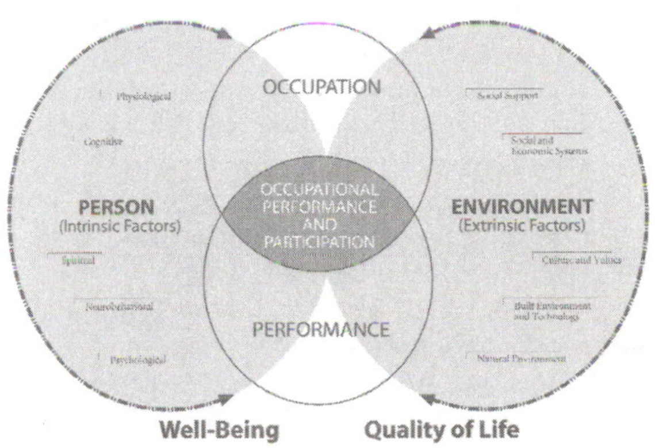

Setting the Stage

The first section of this book has introduced you to the principles, values, and knowledge that support our current understanding of occupation. Occupation is of interest to many disciplines because it is the science that helps us understand what people do in their everyday lives. This section will focus on how occupation forms the core of a specific profession, occupational therapy. Occupational therapists have a unique perspective—that of enabling people to engage in occupation when health conditions, societal conditions, or disabilities impair or threaten their ability to do that which is important and has meaning for them. Occupational therapists' work is focused on occupational performance and participation, or the point when and where the person, the environment, and what the person wants and needs to do intersect.

Baum, C. M, & Christiansen, C. H. (2005). Person-environment-occupation-performance: An occupation-based framework for practice. In C. H. Christiansen, C. M. Baum, and J. Bass-Haugen (Eds.), Occupational therapy: Performance, participation, and well-being *(3rd ed.). Thorofare, NJ: SLACK Incorporated.*

INTRODUCTION

The concept of occupational performance has become central to the development of models of occupational therapy. This process, which constitutes the doing of activities, tasks, and roles, operates as a means of connecting the individual to roles and to the sociocultural environment (Reed & Sanderson, 1999). This connection is sometimes depicted as a Venn diagram and sometimes with arrows showing the relationship of person, occupation, and environment.

The purpose of this chapter is to place the PEO model in a historical context and introduce its constructs. Practice models organize concepts, provide terms and definitions for labeling practice-related activities and situations, and help define problems, thus leading to strategies for problem-solving. There are six contemporary PEOP models emerging in the occupational therapy literature: The Person-Environment-Occupation-Performance model (Christiansen & Baum, 1991, 1997); the Ecology of Human Performance model (Dunn, Brown, & McGuigan, 1994); Model of Human Occupation (Kielhofner, 1995, 2002); Person-Environment-Occupation model (Law, et al., 1996); Canadian Model of Occupational Performance (Canadian Association of Occupational Therapists [CAOT], 1997); and Occupational Performance Model: Australia (Chapparo & Ranka, 1997).

Each of these models includes three central elements: person, occupation, and environment. Yet, all are different and are at different stages of development. Each is designed to be an ecological model, and they all recognize the importance of the stages of development as they influence motivation, skills, and roles. Moreover, they share views of human well-being that emphasize the complex interaction of biological, psychological, and social phenomena and the importance of a satisfactory match between personal, task, and situational characteristics in order for performance to be supported.

These concepts have been articulated by scholars in occupational therapy since early in the 20th century (Engel, 1977; Meyer, 1922; Mosey, 1974; Reilly, 1962) and form the basis for views of occupational therapy practice that can address multiple factors (people, occupations, and environments) in the occupation performance issues of individuals, organizations, communities, and society. All these models are supported by research and knowledge from the traditional behavioral and social sciences (such as anthropology, sociology, and psychology), as well as from work done in newer areas, such as rehabilitation science, disability studies, and occupation science. All provide a framework to guide intervention.

While all PEO models have elements in common, there are some distinct differences that make each one unique. This book is organized to present the Person-Environment-Occupation-Performance (PEOP) model, and this chapter provides the conceptual rationale underlying its unique approach to guiding occupational therapy intervention.

THE PERSON-ENVIRONMENT-OCCUPATION-PERFORMANCE MODEL

The PEOP model (Christiansen & Baum, 1991, 1997; Christiansen, Baum, & Bass-Haugen, 2005) is a client-centered model organized to improve the everyday performance of necessary and valued occupations of individuals, organizations, and populations and their meaningful participation in the world around them. This model began its development in 1985 and was first published in 1991. The inclusion of occupation, performance, and participation in the PEOP model reflects the complex interactions between the person and the environment in which people carry out the activities, tasks, and roles that are meaningful to them. To achieve a desired level of participation, people and groups require the support of enablers and must overcome barriers that limit their participation in activities, tasks, and roles that are important and meaningful to them. The model describes an interaction of person factors (intrinsic factors, including psychological/emotional factors, cognition, neurobehavioral, and physiological factors as well as spirituality) and environmental factors (extrinsic factors, including social support, societal policies and attitudes, natural and built environments, and cultural norms and values) that either support, enable, or restrict the performance of the activities, tasks, and roles of the individual, organization, or community.

In the PEOP model, occupational therapy intervention is viewed as a process of using a broad range of purposeful client-centered strategies that engage the individual or the group to develop or use resources that enable successful performance of the necessary and meaningful occupations. These strategies recognize that the satisfactory performance of occupations is a consequence of individual or group goals and characteristics and environmental characteristics that either limit or support participation. However, intervention strategies may or may not involve an individual's direct engagement in occupation, nor do they necessarily involve a physiological change, because in some cases, such as in modifying built environments to make them accessible and manageable, the client's active involvement may consist of working with the therapist to identify goals and strategies that will remove barriers and enable participation in tasks and roles that have meaning to the person.

Because the desired outcome of therapy is the individual's ability to live a satisfying or productive life, an appropriate strategy may include teaching a patient to supervise others in the performance of tasks. An individual, for example, might require (or request) a personal care attendant to assist with dressing and hygiene activities so that his or her time and energy can be saved for work, study, or other more personally satisfying occupations. This approach to practice emphasizes that occupational therapy almost never does things to people; it more frequently does things with people. Sometimes, effective therapy requires the client's active physical involvement, but it always requires the client's interest, attention, and cooperation. A term sometimes used to describe people who are interested, attentive, and cooperative is *engagement*.

The PEOP model is conceptually similar to other ecological models in occupational therapy (Dunn et al., 1994; Kielhofner, 1995; Law et al., 1996; Mathiowetz & Bass-Haugen, 1994). However, it differs in the degree to which the ideas in the model are defined, described, and emphasized. One defining characteristic of the PEOP model is that it emphasizes occupations (consisting of valued roles, tasks, and activities) and performance, thus requiring a top-down approach.

Why Does the Model Focus on Occupational Performance and Participation?

Occupational therapy's traditions and body of knowledge are well suited to identify intervention strategies that contribute to the occupational competence of a person. To be competent is to be able to perform. The word *occupational competence* brings to mind terms like self-reliance and the ability to participate within social groups in ways that are productive and satisfying. Competence implies goal attainment, whether the goal involves addressing the practical necessities of living or lifestyle choices in leisure, recreation, or play that are related to rest, renewal, or enjoyment. Occupational competence is similarly appropriate for describing engagement in activities that promote health and well-being. By focusing on the competent performance of occupations, the occupational therapy practitioner is relating intervention to the individual's everyday experiences of doing things in places and participating in activities for purposes that have meaning and value (Baum & Law, 1997).

What is a Top-Down Approach?

Emphasis on both occupational performance and participation requires the practitioner to employ a top-down client-centered strategy (Fisher, 1998; Mathiowetz & Bass-Haugen, 1994; Trombly, 1995). The practitioner must determine with the client what he or she perceives to be the important occupational performance issues that are limiting participation and causing difficulty in carrying out tasks and roles within the daily round of occupations, which include those related to productivity and work, personal care, home maintenance, sleep, and recreation or leisure. This approach requires the practitioner to collect assessment information about the physiological, psychological, cognitive, neurobehavioral, and spiritual factors that may be interfering with or supporting their performance and, as well, to identify environmental factors that may serve as enablers or barriers to performance.

Components of the Model

As its title suggests, the PEOP model has four major components. These four elements describe what people want or need to do in their daily lives (occupations); the actual act of doing the occupation (performance); and how psychological, physiological, neurobehavioral, cognitive, and spiritual factors (person) combine with the places in which occupations are undertaken (environment) to influence success. The interaction of capacity, environment, and chosen activity lead to occupational performance and participation.

A basic belief of the PEOP model is that people are naturally motivated to explore their world and demonstrate mastery within it. A widely used social science term for this process is *human agency*. An individual's ability and skill to do what he or she must do in order to meet personal needs is a measure of his or her competence. To do this, a person must effectively use the resources (personal, social, and material) available within the living environment. If an individual possesses the necessary emotional maturity and problem-solving skills, he or she will be capable of learning to identify and achieve goals that contribute to the attainment of life satisfaction.

A second important belief of this model is that situations in which people experience success help them feel good about themselves. This motivates them to face new challenges with greater confidence. The PEOP model proposes that through their daily occupations, people develop a self-identity and derive a sense of fulfillment. Fulfillment comes both from feelings of mastery as well as the accomplishment of goals that have personal meaning. Over time, these meaningful experiences permit people to develop an understanding of who they are and what their place is in the world. These concepts can be traced to some of earliest philosophical statements underlying the establishment of occupational therapy as a health-related discipline.

As its name implies, the major elements of the PEOP model include personal factors (i.e., the person), environ-

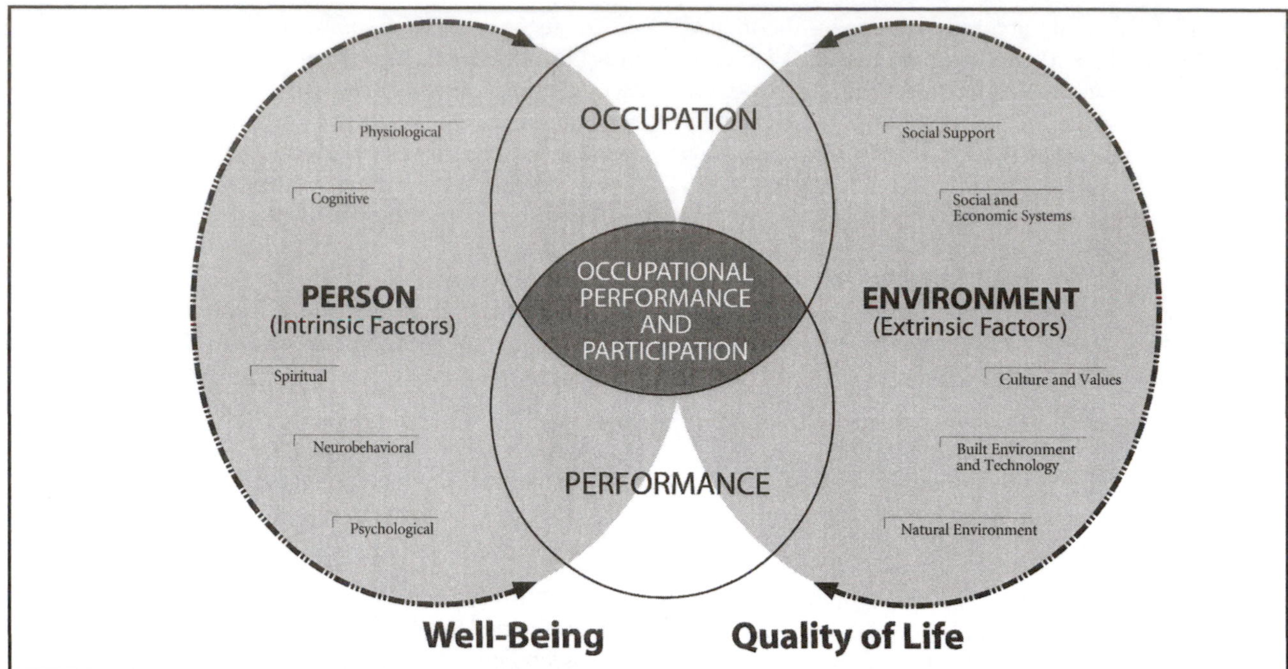

Figure 11-1. The Person-Environment-Occupation-Performance (PEOP) model.

mental factors, and characteristics of doing, which include both occupation and performance. In the following section, each of the principal elements of the PEOP model is introduced, and an overview of some of the major points that are pertinent to these individual parts of the framework are provided. Figure 11-1 provides a graphic overview of the model.

Occupational performance reflects the act of doing. It also serves as the central construct of participation and requires the understanding and linking of occupation and performance. Much of this book has centered on occupation and how the concept is central to the individual and involves what people need and want to do to support their roles in daily life. To be able to do requires that an action or a task be performed. Performance can come from either capacity intrinsic to the individual or by support provided by the environment or a combination of both. Doing (performance) itself is not enough. Why is it done, for whom is it done, what pleasures are derived from the act? Occupational therapy practitioners believe that this is done by the individual to express his or her uniqueness; it has purpose to the individual. When occupation and performance are joined in the term *occupational performance*, it describes the actions that are meaningful to the individual as he or she cares for him- or herself, cares for others, works, plays, and participates fully in home and community life.

Personal Factors: The Intrinsic Enablers of Performance

Underlying general abilities and skills are various supporting factors and mechanisms that are referred to as performance enablers. In this text, person-related factors contributing to performance are organized into the following categories: neurobehavioral, physiological, cognitive, psychological and emotional, and spiritual. These factors reside within the person and are therefore also known as intrinsic factors.

Neurobehavioral Factors

Various neurobehavioral factors must be considered for their potential to support or facilitate performance. The sensory (olfactory, gustatory, visual, auditory, somatosensory, proprioceptive, and vestibular) and motor systems (somatic, cerebellum, basal ganglia network, and thalamic integration) exhibit principles that underlie all neuromotor performance. The ability to control movement, to modulate sensory input, to coordinate and integrate sensory information, to compensate for sensorimotor deficits, and to modify neural structures through behavior are all important characteristics that influence and support occupational performance.

The sensory and motor systems facilitate adaptive and/or compensatory responses. The capacity of these systems to support occupational performance and participation must be determined. Interventions must be guided by basic neurobehavioral principles so that individuals can derive optimal benefit from therapy. The importance of the neurobehavioral factors were anticipated early in the development of occupational therapy when Meyer (1922) challenged proponents of the field to observe the restorative benefits of engagement in occupation on the behavior of those receiving services.

Physiological Factors

Physical health and fitness are necessary requirements for those occupations requiring even moderate exertion or sustained effort. People who are physically active are healthier and live longer than those who are sedentary (Minor, 1997). Abilities such as endurance, flexibility, movement, and strength are key to the performance of some tasks and are necessary for maintaining health. Physical inactivity (sedentary lifestyles) and the poor fitness that often results can lead to major health problems across the lifespan. The therapy for inactivity is to increase physical activity, and the method of this cure is determined by the needs, status, and preferences of the individual. Physical activity is defined as "any bodily movement produced by skeletal muscles that results in caloric expenditures" (Caspersen, Kriska, & Dearwater, 1994, p. 27). Occupations can be used to engage individuals to use their motor and memory skills, which will in turn enhance their performance of tasks, activities, and roles and at the same time maintain their physiological fitness.

Cognitive Factors

Cognition involves the mechanisms of language comprehension and production, pattern recognition, task organization, reasoning, attention, and memory (Duchek, 1991). When these mechanisms are intact, they support the person in learning, communicating, moving, and observing. When the mechanisms are deficient, they create functional limitations for the individual and the people with whom they live. Cognitive rehabilitation and cognitive strategies enable the individual to learn strategies to bypass the deficit and/or compensate for the loss.

The field of neuroscience is developing an understanding of how experiences generate changes in the nervous system that shape language, vision, coordinated movement, and cognition (Merzenich, Scheiner, Jenkins, & Wang, 1993). It should be the goal of occupational therapy practitioners to understand how the consequences of brain injury can be minimized so that the tasks of daily living, social interaction, family life, and vocational and educational pursuits can continue to be pursued.

Cognition is not just to be considered when one has a cognitive impairment. Therapists should also understand how engagement in specific occupations promotes and maintains cognitive skills throughout the lifespan. Recent research shows that as personal interactions and participation in social activities weaken, older adults are at greater risk for cognitive decline (Bassuk, Glass, & Berkman, 1999). Additionally, research demonstrates that intellectual engagement through participation in everyday activities buffers individuals against cognitive decline in later life (Hultsch, Hertzog, Small, & Dixon, 1999). Research conducted at the University of Southern California clearly shows the importance of physical, social, and intellectual activity in providing a protective response to maintain occupational performance (Jackson, Carlson, Mandel, Zemke, & Clark, 1998). The link between cognition and occupation is being strengthened and should be a central aspect of the interventions used to enhance and maintain health.

Psychological and Emotional Factors

Psychological factors are basic to doing (Bonder, 1993; Fidler & Fidler, 1973). Psychological factors describe the personality traits, motivational influences, and internal processes used by an individual to influence what they do, how these events are interpreted, and how they contribute to a sense of self.

Personality traits are determined by genetics and early formative experiences and influence preferences and dispositions that influence activity choices and reactions to experience. In the course of a typical day, people shift their attention from one goal to another, and, as a result, the nature of their occupations changes. Personality can be described as the interests, values, and attitudes of an individual that influence their attention, behavior, and interpretation of new events. Links between personality and activity preferences have been demonstrated conclusively by research in action psychology (Furnham, 1981; Little, Lecci, & Watkinson, 1992).

Interpretations of experience influence emotional state (or affect) and contribute to self-concept, self-esteem, and an individual's sense of identity. Self-efficacy is an important psychological factor because the experience of past success is what allows people to view themselves as competent (Bandura, 1977, 1982). Research has shown that people who perceive themselves as competent tend to view their overall well-being as more favorable. As a result, they are more likely to continue working on tasks despite early setbacks (Gage & Polatajko, 1994).

In addition to understanding how psychological factors influence motivation, shape identity, and contribute to effective performance, the occupational therapist is concerned with how a person's occupations contribute to his or her sense of well-being. A growing body of research shows links between patterns of occupation, occupational competence, and well-being (Christiansen, Backman, Little, & Nguyen, 1999; Palys & Little, 1983). Some of this research shows that engagement in occupation over time is a key factor in the creation of life meaning

(Christiansen & Matuska, 2004; Christiansen, 2000; McGregor & Little, 1998).

Spiritual Factors

The creation of meaning involves psychological factors but is sufficiently related to other intrinsic factors, such as cognition, to justify its identification as a unique personal factor that influences occupational performance through its interaction with environmental characteristics. Everyday places, occupations, and interactions are filled with meaning (Gustafson, 2001). This meaning comes from the nature of a situation and how a person interprets its significance based on his or her current goals, values, and past experiences. There are individual meanings and collective or shared meanings.

Shared meaning comes from shared experience. Our world is comprehensible to us only because others have validated our individual perceptions. Thus, meaning is socially and culturally influenced but becomes internal to the individual through personal interpretation. In a similar way, general agreement regarding the meaning of signs, symbols, and sounds underlies everyday language. Language, in turn, influences thought.

Signs are direct representations of conditions, objects, or events, while symbols convey more complex and personal meaning. A coffee pot is recognizable to most people as a device for making coffee, but it can also have a personal meaning related to the particular experiences of an individual. It might remind them, for example, of long talks over coffee in the kitchen of a deceased friend or relative.

The field of semiotics is based on the signs and symbols that influence everyday life through the meaning provided by objects and actions (Danesi, 1994). When these meanings contribute to a greater sense of personal understanding about self and one's place in the world, they can be described as spiritual (Christiansen, 1997). Symbols with spiritual meaning abound in our environment, enrich our engagement in occupations, and infuse them with special forms of meaning (Campbell, 1962, 1988).

Environment: The Context of Performance

Participation is always influenced by the characteristics of the environment in which it occurs. Research has shown that even the perception that an environment is supportive can influence well-being (Wallenius, 1999). Barris was one of the first writers in the field to attempt to organize dimensions of the environment within a conceptual framework (Barris, 1982; Barris et al., 1985), although the past decade has seen major advances in this area (Law, 1991; Letts et al., 1994).

Through a process identified by Berlyne (1960) as arousal, environments can influence our inclination to interact with or explore our environment. Arousal has both physiological as well as psychological characteristics related to one's level of alertness and has its most obvious effect on performance when people are bored and inattentive (under aroused) or anxious (over aroused). Three groups of environmental variables are associated with arousal. These include psychophysical characteristics such as loud noises and bright lights; ecological events that are related to one's well-being (such as a severe storm); and situations viewed as novel, surprising, or ambiguous (called collative characteristics). The degree of match between the characteristics of the environment and a person's interests and values may influence the inclination to explore or interact within that setting (Ryan & Deci, 2000). Barris notes that the characteristics of settings that influence arousal must be carefully considered, so that an optimal level (producing neither boredom nor anxiety) is attained (Barris, 1982, p. 638).

The personality theorist Murray (Murray et al., 1938) was one of the first to recognize that characteristics of places influence behavior by creating demands or expectations for behavior, either objectively or as subjectively perceived by the individual. His term for this phenomenon was *press*. The idea that places influence activities and meanings has been refined and extended by other investigators, including Lawton (1980), and has been given prominence in the occupational therapy literature by Barris and colleagues (1985; Hamilton, 2003; Rowles, 1991).

A similar ecological concept, called *affordance*, was proposed by Gibson (1979). Gibson believed that animals (including humans) perceive possibilities based on the characteristics of environments (places and objects) and these possibilities influence meaning and action. The concept of affordance has influenced architectural design and has powerful implications for the strategies occupational therapists can use to influence occupation-related performance and meaning.

During the past 10 years, the role of the environment has become central to all of the evolving disability models. This is because the "prevailing wisdom about the cause of disability has undergone profound change" (Brandt & Pope, 1997, p. 147). Prior to this time, disability was viewed as a pathology that could be medically managed and hopefully fixed. This approach excluded consideration of the environment. Recent approaches have viewed disability as the interaction between the characteristics of the individual (and his or her impairments) and the characteristics of the environment (Brandt & Pope, 1997). The environment becomes important because it is thought of as being an active part of the individual person, just as glasses enable a person to see, and a chair allows a person to sit, so be it with any person. A wheelchair enables a person to sit, to move, to socialize, to work, and to be where he or she wants to be to do what he or she wants to do.

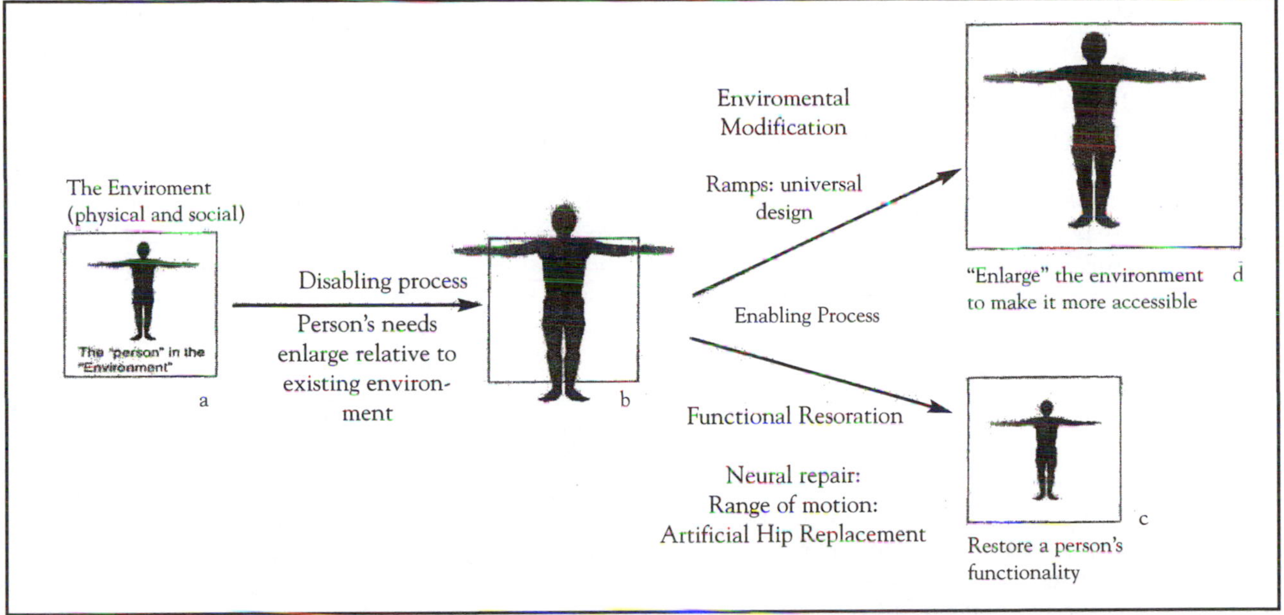

Figure 11-2. Conceptual overview of the enabling-disabling process. The environment, depicted as a square, represents both physical space and social structures (family, community, society). A person who does not manifest a disability (a) is fully integrated into society and "fits within the square." A person with potentially disabling conditions has increased needs (expressed by the size of the individual) and is dislocated from his or her prior integration into the environment (b) that is, it "doesn't fit in the square." The enabling (or rehabilitative) process attempts to rectify this displacement, either by restoring function in the individual (c) or by expanding access to the environment (d) (e.g., building ramps). (Reprinted with permission from [Enabling America: Assessing the Role of Rehabilitation Science and Engineering] © [1997] by the National Academy of Sciences, courtesy of the National Academies Press, Washington, D.C.)

This change in approach has coincided with the further development of PEO models in occupational therapy (Bass-Haugen & Mathiowetz, 1995; Christiansen & Baum, 1991, 1997; Christiansen, Baum, & Bass-Haugen, 2005; Dunn et al., 1994; Kielhofner, 1995; Law, et al., 1996). These view occupation, the person (and his or her impairments), and the environment as the contextual elements that dynamically influence the meaningful activities, tasks, and roles of daily life.

This change in focus does not mean that only environmental interventions are used. In fact, functional restoration remains central to all rehabilitation programs. Functional restoration, however, is not the only approach used. What is critical for all professionals in the rehabilitation field is to "understand the fundamental nature of the enabling-disabling processes. That is, how disabling conditions develop, progress, and reverse, and how biological, behavioral, and environmental factors can affect these transitions" (Brandt & Pope, 1997, p. 5). Figure 11-2 provides a conceptual overview of the enabling-disabling process developed as a part of the report *Enabling America: Assessing the Role of Rehabilitation Science and Engineering* prepared for the United States Congress by a committee of the Institute of Medicine (Brandt & Pope, 1997).

The Built Environment

The physical properties of environments are the most obvious and, thus, are the most likely to be given consideration when environmental influences on performance are discussed. Clearly, design is an important characteristic of the physical environment and is one that is deserving of even greater attention than it has received in the past. Physical environments must be considered for accessibility and manageability, as well as for safety and aesthetics. Design considerations can and should accommodate all these issues if they are to support an individual's performance of occupations and provide for comfort and enjoyment. Both the suitability of personal living space to accommodate unique individual needs as well as the negotiability of public places are relevant to the analysis of the physical or built environments.

All people use tools or appliances to support their engagement in activities. Computers in the work setting and racquets on the tennis court are common examples of tools used for work and recreational occupations. Able-bodied people who can easily move to the television or other appliances they use for relaxation or work commonly use remote control devices. Some people even use devices for rest and sleep (e.g., sleep masks, "white noise" masking machines, dark blinds, and night lights) to support or enhance these activities. Thus, the use of tools by people with disabilities is consistent with this practice except that the devices must be usable within the person's capabilities. Tools or appliances that fit this description are sometimes grouped under the category known as assistive technology devices (ATDs). Many of these devices can be directly purchased and easily used without training. Despite this, most people do not know of the vast number of such occupation-enabling resources that are available.

The Natural Environment

The natural environment, which includes geographical features such as terrain, hours of sunlight, climate, and air quality, can influence a person's occupational performance in many ways (Hamilton, 2003). Geographic factors can create occupational requirements (shoveling snow or keeping cool) that influence necessary tasks, required capabilities, and comfort or convenience. Allergies create discomfort and can be life threatening. Mountainous areas create mobility challenges that are not found in flatlands. Thus, the natural environment can be a significant factor in determining whether or not an individual's physical limitations are disabling (Brandt & Pope, 1997). For people with impairments, the natural environment may make a difference as to whether they can go to school, get to work during the heat of summer or the cold of winter, and/or engage in leisure activities that are important to them.

The Cultural Environment

Culture refers to the values, beliefs, customs, and behaviors that are passed from one generation to the next. This includes socially transmitted behavior patterns, arts, beliefs, institutions, and all other products of human work and thought (*Oxford English Dictionary*, 1989). Culture affects performance in many ways, including prescribing norms for the use of time and space, influencing beliefs regarding the importance of various tasks, and transmitting attitudes and values regarding work and play (Altman & Chelmers, 1984; Hall, 1973). Cultural factors also influence social role expectations, such as what men, women, children, and heads of families are expected to do.

People within cultures have orientations that influence their choices regarding what they do, how they do it, and how important it is to them. Cultural preferences must be respected and accommodated by therapy personnel as intervention is planned and delivered. Both knowledge and sensitivity to cultural influences on occupational performance are important to the effective delivery of care because they influence outcomes. These influences occur through the person's understanding of the purpose and importance of interventions, which affects cooperation and adherence.

Culture refers not only to individuals, but also to organizations. An organization has a culture that is reflected in the patterns of shared assumptions, values, and beliefs practiced among its members. An organization's culture helps the member's understand acceptable and unacceptable actions. Hospitals, academic institutions, schools, industry, and community organizations all have a culture, and these differ in the same manner that personalities differ among people.

The word *culture* is used in many ways. All meanings relate to everyday life. For example, we hear the term *popular culture*, and this refers to the everyday pastimes of a preponderance of people in a social group. Sometimes, the term *high culture* is used. Activities described in this manner are thought to be more serious, more profound, and more important than those of the popular or "pop" culture. High culture activities are often viewed as those that cultivate the mind and spirit. Another term sometimes used to describe cultural activities is *folk culture*. These include traditional or everyday activities or pastimes that communicate values and meanings through oral communication such as stories, jokes, and "wives tales." A more contemporary term for these communications is *urban myths* (McAdams, 1992).

Culture also reflects how people explain their health and medical conditions. An explanatory interview can be used to elicit illness-related perceptions, beliefs, and practices, all of which are central to understanding what the client understands about causes and treatments for different conditions. Such an interview explores the individual's cultural background, the nature of the presenting problem, need for help, and beliefs related to the physical or mental illness (Lloyd et al., 1998).

Societal Factors

Human beings are group-living, social animals. As a result, the standing of an individual within the group and the importance of interpersonal relationships provides a fundamental influence in shaping behavior and attitudes toward the self. Societal acceptance is universally sought, and social rejection and isolation can have devastating psychological consequences. Prejudicial attitudes, stereotypes, and the intolerance of differences are products of ignorance and remain a part of the social environment.

People with observable differences must contend with the attitudinal barriers that inhibit their acceptance by others. Because these attitudinal barriers exist even among informed, educated people (including health care professionals), the experience of disability must be studied and understood if such social barriers are to be eliminated. Understanding these barriers is also relevant for people with disability because they must learn to recognize and contend with the stigma (social prejudice) that accompanies them.

Societal attitudes and values also influence the policies that can support or limit the occupational performance of individuals. Every nation has policies that govern access to services, access to education, and laws that protect the rights of its citizens. These policies and laws have a major impact on how people with and without disabilities move about their environments, access jobs in the workplace, and have access to health and social services.

Social Interaction

Because people are social beings, what they do usually involves others or is done with social purposes in mind. Social support influences the outcomes of occupational pursuits and contributes to health and well-being on several levels. Some individuals choose to have more social networks than others. When a disability occurs, strategies for obtaining social support to enable participation become useful. Occupational therapy practitioners must understand social support mechanisms if they are to help others learn to use it effectively. The practitioner must know about networks, types and sources of support, and how to assess the patterns of social support used by his or her clients (McColl, 1997).

Social support is an experienced rather than an observed phenomenon (Dunkel-Schetter & Bennett, 1990) and is essential to maintain health (Orth-Gomer et al., 1993; Pierce et al., 1990). There are basically three types of social support (McColl, 1997; Thoits, 1997) that enable people to do what they need and want to do. These include practical support (defined as instrumental, aid, and tangible support), informational support (including advice, guidance, knowledge, or skill training), and emotional support (which communicates esteem and belonging and provides guidance). Each of these types of support is central to the idea of community and is necessary for a satisfactory person-environment fit. Social groups are built on the idea of cooperation, which requires a level of altruism or reciprocal assistance. Modern society requires and represents a level of interdependence among people that is often overlooked. For this reason, many observers have questioned and challenged the ideal of independence as the expressed aim of rehabilitation programs, noting that few individuals in the modern world can exist without the support of others.

Social and Economic Systems

Economic conditions and the availability of resources may be the factor that determines whether or not a person with a disability or chronic health condition can access a physician or other service provider, can have a means to move about his or her environment, or can even be in touch with people in his or her support network. Government and employment policies often dictate access to the resources that make doing possible. Central to the issues of those whose occupational performance is impaired or threatened is the need to have options for employment, income, and social contribution.

Democratic principles embrace the rights of all individuals to achieve economic self-sufficiency, live independently, and participate in all aspects of society. These should include access to personal assistance, health care that does not discriminate against those with disabling or chronic conditions, inclusion of students with disabilities into neighborhood schools, equal employment opportunities, the availability of acceptable housing, access to assistive technology, and the right to participate fully in processes of government. Unfortunately, in some countries, we have yet to see these principles fully implemented.

The World Institute on Disability (WID) has established the Center on Economic Development and Disability to build and strengthen an infrastructure that addresses these and other issues that seek to foster increased social and economic participation. It is the mission of this organization to advocate for the elimination of artificial and arbitrary barriers to employment, economic security, and independence. Similarly, the World Bank provides grants and loans to countries to address social and economic barriers within communities.

Occupational therapists interact with individuals who are at risk because of economic conditions. In addition to helping those individuals seek out resources to address their immediate needs, the occupational therapist can be an advocate for change in social and economic policies that create the societal limitations that impair the occupational performance of the total population. This level of change is at the societal level and might be as basic as working with city or regional councils to plan adequate housing for the growing population of older adults and as complex as seeking sponsors for legislation that will enable the participation and thus health of a large number of people in our communities, which in turn could make a contribution to the national economy.

The Doing of Everyday Life

The third component of the model bridges the person and environment through the process of personal agency or the transaction that occurs when people act with intention within environments in the performance of everyday occupations. Human occupation has many dimensions, which impose a structure based on time and intention, a hierarchy of complexity, and social and cultural influences that define expectations. These are described in the next sections.

Table 11-1

A hierarchy of occupation-related behaviors and supportive abilities

Term	*Example*
Roles: Positions in society having expected responsibilities and privileges	Parent Homemaker
Occupations: Goal-directed pursuits that typically extend over time, have meaning to the performer, and involve multiple tasks	Shopping
Tasks: Combinations of actions sharing a common purpose recognized by the performer	Making a grocery list Managing a grocery sack
Actions: Observable behaviors that are recognizable	Lifting Directing another to lift
Abilities: General traits or individuals characteristics that support occupational performance	Attention, motor control, language

The Structure of Occupations

Occupations have a purpose. They are performed with different outcomes in mind, ranging from those related to paid work and productive pursuits, such as education or home maintenance, to recreation, personal care, and rest. Occupations always entail a social dimension, either directly, as when they require cooperation or competition, or indirectly when they are performed for the purpose of establishing an identity as a competent person or to fulfill social role obligations. An important characteristic of occupations is their temporal dimension. This pertains to the frequency, duration, and time(s) when they are performed. For example, the morning routine is a recurring daily occupation with predictable tasks associated with hygiene and grooming. In contrast, ceremonies such as weddings, bar mitzvahs, and graduations are less frequent rituals infused with special meaning. It is important to recognize that while certain social rituals have shared meaning within cultural groups, individual occupations have personal meaning that changes dramatically with the context of an individual's life. Therefore, it is dangerous to make assumptions about the personal meaning that may be associated with a given occupational pursuit.

Adolph Meyer observed that occupations provide a necessary structure to our existence, noting that many people in mental institutions at the time had lost the temporal order in their daily lives (Meyer, 1922). Kielhofner (1977, 1978) provided a useful analysis of the temporal properties of occupation, noting that physical and mental illnesses frequently interfere with an individual's ability to manage time, either because his or her sense of time is distorted or because the time required to accomplish necessary tasks has changed. He further suggested that role changes require a corresponding adjustment in the manner in which a person organizes time. This phenomenon can be observed in retired people who have not prepared for the increased amount of leisure time available in their lives. The term *temporal adaptation* has been used to describe the process of adjusting to changing temporal requirements in daily life or throughout the lifespan (Kielhofner, 1977).

Occupational performance and participation is the doing of occupation. As indicated in Chapter One, the performance of occupation can be described in terms of the types of occupations that people do as well as according to their degree of complexity. We observe that recognizable actions form parts of tasks. The performance of selected tasks and engagement in occupations reflect both individual personality, the expectations of different social roles, and the challenges and roles of different stages or periods in the life course. Occupational choices are also influenced by lifestyle preferences, which are occupational expressions of preference based on available resources, interests, values, and personal philosophies.

Table 11-1 illustrates an occupational hierarchy, reflecting increasing levels of complexity (and time). Using this hierarchy, a basic unit of occupation can be described as an action, such as lifting, walking, or grimacing the face. These actions are supported by abilities or general traits that are a product of genetic makeup and learning (Fleishman, 1975; Peterson et al., 1997). When actions are part of specific goal-oriented activities like lifting a basket, walking across a room to close a door, or folding a towel, they become tasks. Tasks offer a second level of occupational complexity and are viewed as combinations of actions sharing some purpose recognized by the person performing the task. Tasks are supported by skills or proficiencies for performing the task (Christiansen & Baum, 1997).

A third level of occupational complexity is depicted through use of the term *occupation*. Occupations are segments of goal-directed behavior that are recognizable by others and typically include a number of related tasks performed over time. Examples of recognizable occupations are dressing and grooming, housekeeping, report writing, keeping accounts, horseback riding, and tennis. While occupations include specified tasks, it is difficult to describe the relationship between those terms more specifically because people differ in the manner in which they undertake or perform occupational pursuits. These differences can be described as occupational styles.

Descriptions of time use using specific terminology for units of action is complicated because of the ambiguity of terms used in the English language to describe daily endeavors. Recognizable and named actions reflect general public recognition of task sequence and goals rather than precise scientific demarcations of action. Moreover, it is a fact of existence that some tasks and occupations occur concurrently. Mothers frequently attend to household chores while attending to their infants; and the use of wireless phones has made staying in touch while doing other activities a ubiquitous (and frequently annoying) aspect of daily life.

Anthropologists theorize that language itself may have evolved as a result of social grooming, a personal care occupation that led early humans into close proximity and created the opportunity for symbolic communication and the evolution of formal thought (Pinters & Bloom, 1990; Tattersall, 1998). Nevertheless, the question can be raised: "When does task performance become engagement in occupation?" The answer may very well be that task performance becomes engagement in occupation when we recognize it as a part of an identifiable stream of goal-directed behavior.

Social and Occupational Roles

Roles typically involve the performance of many occupations. For example, in some cultures, a grandmother may be expected to bake cookies, care for grandchildren, tell stories, and give wise advice. Thus, roles can be defined as recognizable positions in society, each having a defined status and specific expectations for behavior. Roles can be occupational, familial, or sexual; thus, a person can have multiple roles at the same time (e.g., therapist, mother, and wife). The term *role model* confers a standard of behavior for any position that others are expected to emulate. It is important to consider that a complete view of occupational performance must consider the actions, tasks, occupations, and roles of individuals as they go about their daily lives.

The concept of role emanates from social psychology and the symbolic interactionist school of thought, advanced principally by George Herbert Mead (1934) and Harry Stack Sullivan (1953). Symbolic interaction proposes that roles, defined as positions in society that have expected responsibilities and privileges, form the very nucleus of social interaction. Successful social interaction requires role reciprocity, or the effective role performance of each member in a group. Roles affect development and personality through strong social approval when roles are enacted successfully and equally strong sanctions when role expectations are not met. Socialization can thus be described as the process of learning role behaviors.

Sarbin and Allen (1968) note that within the boundaries of each role, both society and the role occupant form expectations. Thus, one's satisfaction with the performance of valued roles is based on internal as well as external appraisals. This external influence is reflected in exemptions granted by society to people who are experiencing difficult life events. An example is the "sick role," described eloquently by Parsons (1975), which excuses people from fulfilling role responsibilities during illness, as long as certain conditions are met, including seeking and complying with medical advice. Unfortunately, when the sick role is adopted by or ascribed to individuals with disabling conditions, the passivity and compliance expected in the sick role may conflict with the goals of the rehabilitation process. This is especially likely in situations where occupational therapy is appropriately practiced because active participation, autonomy, and self-reliance are valued (Burke, Miyake, Kielhofner, & Barris, 1983).

Roles are dynamic, in that, throughout the lifespan, they are being acquired or replaced. For example, during adolescence, a major concern is vocational choice or determining the specific nature of one's worker role. Later, parental roles may be acquired, subsequently to be replaced when one's children reach adolescence and leave home. These developmental transitions are especially important because they involve the development of new skills or the integration of skills previously learned.

Roles are important for occupational therapists to understand because they outline the nature of occupations at various points in time. It can be asserted that occupational performance deficits have meaning principally in the context of an individual's role responsibilities. In describing occupational dysfunction, it is possible to refer to one's inadequate performance of social roles. When people cannot perform roles to a level of personal or social satisfaction because of deficits in abilities and skills due to disease or disability, the conflicting demands of multiple roles (role conflict), or unclear role expectations, dysfunction is present. Such disruption in the roles of daily living, termed *occupational performance dysfunction* by Rogers (1983), constitutes the appropriate type of problem for occupational therapy intervention.

Benefits of the Model

Organizing knowledge for occupational therapy practice using the PEOP model offers several advantages over more reductionistic approaches to practice. First, this perspective helps the practitioner to identify and consider the many factors that influence performance, as well as the many dimensions of occupation. It presents the viewpoint that the characteristics of individuals; the unique environments in which they function; and the nature and meaning of the actions, tasks, and roles of the person are necessary for understanding human occupation. Second, the model enables practitioners to incorporate existing ideas and traditions from occupational therapy within a framework. Finally, it provides a method for viewing and studying occupations and human behavior that combines knowledge about the impairments that impede performance; the environments that support performance; and an individual's needs, preferences, styles, and goals.

Models that focus on the individual's needs and goals rather than their impairment are called client-centered models (Law, Baptiste, & Mills, 1995). The PEOP model is a client-centered model. It focuses on the individual and that person's daily occupations that are limited as the result of a health condition, a disability, a poorly designed environment, or problems experienced due to a societal consequence.

The PEOP model requires that information from disciplines outside of occupational therapy be sought, used, recognized, and respected. The complexity of human occupation, the uniqueness of individuals, and the diversity of environments make this necessary because no single discipline is sufficiently broad to encompass the knowledge required for all these areas. Delivered effectively, health care is the product of teams, which include people who produce knowledge and understanding (basic and social scientists), people who teach the knowledge (professors and instructors), and people who apply that knowledge (health care providers, policy makers, and clients and their families). From occupational therapy's perspective, the purpose of the partnership is to facilitate the health and function of the person whose occupational performance and participation is threatened or impaired.

Summary

The role of occupational therapy practitioners is to help clients meet their goals for enhancing performance and reducing environmental barriers that limit their capacity to do what is important to them. The PEOP model provides a framework to systematically understand and assist clients, whether individuals, families, or organizations, to successfully meet their occupation-related goals.

Because people, occupations, and environments are complex, and the relationships among them are dynamic, many performance problems may be understood as having several explanatory factors or causes and will benefit from multiple points of intervention. The practitioner may work with the client to identify opportunities for building personal capabilities, modifying environments, or reconsidering occupational processes and goals. Each client, however, will have assets that may offset the problems that are interfering with occupational performance and participation.

Occupational therapy practitioners have a unique contribution to bring to health care, to health promotion, to disability prevention, to social problems, and to enhancing the quality of life. That contribution is a knowledge of and appreciation for humans as occupational beings. Through application of occupational performance models, practitioners can create problem-solving approaches that acknowledge and address the complexities of human beings within social systems. The PEOP model was created to assist the student and practitioner to do this. The model identifies factors relevant to occupational performance and participation and provides a means for identifying possible points of intervention for therapeutic problem solving. Perhaps most importantly, it helps to organize a unique and extensive body of knowledge in occupational science, health care, and occupational therapy.

References

Altman, I., & Chelmers, M. M. (1984). *Culture and environment.* New York: Cambridge University Press.

Bandura, A. (1977). Self-efficacy: Toward a unifying theory of behavioral change. *Psychological Review, 84*, 191-215.

Bandura, A. (1982). Self-efficacy mechanisms in human agency. *American Psychologist, 37*, 122-147.

Barris, R. (1982). Environmental interactions: An extension of the model of occupation. *American Journal of Occupational Therapy, 36*(10), 637-644.

Barris, R., Kielhofner, G., Levine, R. E., & Neville, A. M. (1985). Occupation as interaction with the environment. In G. Kielhofner (Ed.), *A model of human occupation: Theory and application* (pp. 42-62). Baltimore: Williams & Wilkins.

Bass-Haugen, J., & Mathiowetz, V. (1995). Contemporary task-oriented approach. In C.A. Trombly (Ed.), *Occupational therapy for physical dysfunction* (4th ed.). Baltimore, MD: Williams & Wilkins.

Bassuk, S. S., Glass, T. A., & Berkman, L. F. (1999). Social disengagement and incident cognitive decline in community-dwelling elderly persons. *Annals of Internal Medicine, 131*(3), 220-221.

Evidence Worksheet

Authors	*Year*	*Concept*	*Description*
Reed & Sanderson	1999	Occupational performance	Occupational performance is central to the development of occupational therapy models. It operates as a means of connecting the individual to roles and to the sociocultural environment
Meyer Engel Mosey Reilly	1922 1977 1974 1962	Performance	Performance is supported by a complex interaction of biological, psychological and social phenomena that requires a satisfactory match between person, task, and situational characteristics
Trombly Mathiowetz & Bass-Haugen Fisher	1995 1994 1998	Top-down client-centered strategy	An occupational performance approach requires the practitioner to determine what the client perceives to be issues that are causing difficulty in occupations that support productivity, work, personal care, home maintenance, sleep, and recreation of leisure
Baum & Christiansen	2005	Human agency	People are naturally motivated to explore their world and demonstrate mastery within it. To do this, the person must effectively use the resources (personal, social, and material) available in his or her environment
Baum & Christiansen	2005	Motivation	Successful experience supports motivation
Baum & Christiansen	2005	Neurobehavioral factors	The sensory (olfactory, gustatory, visual, auditory, somatosensory, proprioceptive, and vestibular) and motor systems (somatic, cerebellum, basal ganglia network, and thalamic integration) underlie all neuromotor performance
Minor	1997	Physiological factors	Endurance, flexibility, movement, and strength are necessary requirements for occupations requiring moderate or sustained effort. People who are physically active are healthier and live longer than those who are sedentary
Duchek	1991	Cognitive factors	Cognition involves the mechanism of language comprehension and production, pattern recognition, task organization, reasoning, attention, and memory
Baum & Christiansen Bandura 1982 Gage & Polatajko	2005 1977, 1994	Psychological factors	Psychological factors describe the personality traits, motivational influences, and internal processes used by an individual to influence what he or she does, how events are interpreted, and how they contribute to a sense of self. Self-efficacy is an important psychological factor as it allows people to view themselves as competent. Persons who view themselves as competent view their overall well-being more favorably and continue working on tasks despite setbacks

(continued)

Authors	*Year*	*Concept*	*Description*
Christiansen	1997	Spirituality	Everyday places, occupations, and interactions are filled with meaning that is interpreted by the person based on his or her goals, values, and experiences. Spirituality is socially and culturally influenced but become internal to the individual through personal interpretation. As meanings contribute to personal understanding about self and one's place in the world, they are described as spiritual. People develop a self-identity and serve a sense of fulfillment as they master and accomplish goals that have personal meaning
Berlyne	1960	Arousal	The process through which environment influences our actions. Three groups of variables are associated with arousal. These include psychophysical characteristics such as noise or light, ecological events such as a storm, or rough terrain or situations
Murray et al.	1938	Environmental press	Places influence behavior by creating demand or expectations for behavior
Lawton Barris et al.	1980 1985		
Gibson	1979	Affordance	Humans perceive possibilities based upon both the places and objects in the environment and these influence meaning and action
Brandt & Pope	1997	Disability	The cause of disability has shifted from being viewed as a pathology that could be medically managed to one of an interaction between the characteristics of the individual and his or her impairments and the characteristics of the environment
Christiansen et al.	2005	Built environment	Physical environments can be built for accessibility, manageability, safety, aesthetics, comfort, and enjoyment. The suitability of the space to accommodate an individual's needs are central to physical or built environments. Built environments also include tools that support engagement in tasks and occupations. Tools that are useable within the person's capabilities are grouped under the category of assistive technology
Brandt & Pope	1997	Natural environment	The natural environment includes geographical features such as terrain, hours of sunlight, climate, and air quality. The natural environment can be a significant factor in determining whether or not an individual's physical limitations are disabling
Altman & Chelmers Hall	1984 1973	Cultural environment	Culture refers to values, beliefs, customs, and behaviors that are transmitted from one generation to the next. Culture affects performance by prescribing norms for the use of time and space, influencing beliefs regarding the importance of activities, work, and play. It also influences choices in what people do, how they do it and how important it is to them

(continued)

Authors	*Year*	*Concept*	*Description*
Christiansen et al.	2005	Societal environment	The standing of an individual within the group shapes behavior and attitudes toward self. Social rejection and isolation can have devastating psychological consequences. Societal policies govern the availability of resources, which controls access to services and work
Dunkel-Schetter & Bennett	1990	Social environment	Social support is an experienced rather than an observed phenomenon and is essential to maintain health. There are three types of social support that enable people to do what they need and want to do. These include practical support, informational support, and emotional support
Orth-Gomer et al.	1993		
Pierce et al.	1990		
McColl	1997		
Thoits	1997		
Christiansen & Baum	1997	Roles	Positions in society having expected responsibilities and privileges
Christiansen & Baum	1997	Occupations	Goal-directed pursuits that typically extend over time, have meaning to the performer, and involve multiple tasks
Christiansen & Baum	1997	Tasks	Combinations of actions sharing a common purpose recognized by the performer
Christiansen & Baum	1997	Actions	Observable behaviors that are recognizable
Christiansen & Baum	1997	Abilities	General traits or individuals characteristics that support occupational performance

Baum, C. M., & Christiansen, C. H. (2004). Person-environment-occupation-performance: A model for planning interventions for individuals, organizations, and populations. In C. H. Christiansen, C. M. Baum, & J. Bass-Haugen (Eds.), *Occupational therapy: Performance, participation, and well-being* (3rd ed.). Thorofare, NJ: SLACK Incorporated.

Baum, C. M., & Law, M. (1997). Occupational therapy practice: Focusing on occupational performance. *American Journal of Occupational Therapy*, *51*(4), 277-288.

Berlyne, D. E. (1960). *Conflict, arousal and curiosity*. New York, NY: McGraw-Hill.

Bonder, B. R. (1993). Issues in assessment of psychosocial components of function. *American Journal of Occupational Therapy*, *47*(3), 211-216.

Brandt, E. N. Jr., & Pope, A. M. (1997). *Enabling America. Assessing the role of rehabilitation science and engineers*. Washington, DC: National Academy Press.

Burke, J., Miyake, S., Kielhofner, G., & Barris, R. (1983). The demystification of health care and demise of the sick role: Implications for occupational therapy. In G. Kielhofner (Ed.), *Health through occupation: Theory and practice in occupational therapy* (pp. 197-210). Philadelphia, PA: F. A. Davis.

Campbell, J. (1962). *The hero with a thousand faces*. New York, NY: Pantheon.

Campbell, J. (1988). *The power of myth*. New York, NY: Doubleday.

Canadian Association of Occupational Therapists. (1997). *Enabling occupation: An occupational therapy perspective*. Ottawa, ON: CAOT Publications.

Caspersen, C. J., Kriska, A. M., & Dearwater, S. R. (1994). Physical activity epidemiology as applied to elderly populations. *Bailleres Clinical Rheumatology*, *8*, 7-27.

Chapparo, C., & Ranka, J. (1997). *Occupational performance model (Australia)*, *Monograph 1* (pp. 189-198). Sydney: Total Print Control.

Christiansen, C. H. (1997). Acknowledging a spiritual dimension in occupational therapy practice. *American Journal of Occupational Therapy*, *51*, 169-172.

Christiansen, C. H. (2000). Identity, personal projects and happiness: Self-construction in everyday action. *Journal of Occupational Science*, *7*(3), 98-107.

Christiansen, C. H., Backman, C., Little, B. R., & Nguyen, A. (1999). Occupations and subjective well being: A study of personal projects. *American Journal of Occupational Therapy, 53*(1), 91-100.

Christiansen, C., & Baum, C. M. (Eds.). (1991). *Occupational therapy: Overcoming human performance deficits*. Thorofare, NJ: SLACK Incorporated.

Christiansen, C., & Baum, C. M. (Eds.) (1997). *Occupational therapy: Enabling function and well-being* (2nd ed.). Thorofare, NJ: SLACK Incorporated.

Christiansen, C. H., Baum, C. M., & Bass-Haugen, J. (Eds.). (2005). *Occupational therapy: Performance, participation, and well-being* (3rd ed.). Thorofare, NJ: SLACK Incorporated.

Christiansen, C. H., & Matuska, K. M. (2004). The importance of everyday activities. In C. H. Christiansen & K. M. Matuska (Eds.), *Ways of living: Adaptive strategies for special needs* (pp. 1-20). Bethesda, MD: AOTA Press.

Danesi, M. (1994). *Messages and meanings: An introduction to semiotics*. Toronto, ON: Canadian Scholars Press.

Duchek, J. (1991). Cognitive dimensions of performance. In C. Christiansen & C. M. Baum (Eds.), *Occupational therapy: Overcoming human performance deficits* (pp. 283-303). Thorofare, NJ: SLACK Incorporated.

Dunkel-Schetter, C., & Bennett, T. L. (1990). Differentiating the cognitive and behavioral aspects of social support. In B. R. Sarason, I. G. Sarason, & G. R. Pierce (Eds.), *Social support: An interactional view* (pp 267-296). New York, NY: John Wiley & Sons, Inc.

Dunn, W., Brown, C., & McGuigan, A. (1994). The ecology of human performance: A framework for considering the effect of context. *American Journal of Occupational Therapy, 48*(7), 595-607.

Engel, G. (1977). The need for a new medical model: A challenge for biomedicine. *Science, 196*, 129-136.

Fidler, G. S., & Fidler, J. W. (1973). Doing and becoming: Purposeful action and self-actualization. *American Journal of Occupational Therapy, 32*, 305-310.

Fisher, A. G. (1998). Uniting practice and theory in an occupational framework: 1998 Eleanor Clarke Slagle Lecture. *American Journal of Occupational Therapy, 52*, 509-521.

Fleishman, F. E. (1975). Toward a taxonomy of human performance. *American Psychologist, 27*, 1017-1032.

Furnham, A. (1981). Personality and activity preference. *British Journal of Social Psychology, 20*(1), 57-68.

Gage, M., & Polatajko, H. (1994). Enhancing occupational performance through an understanding of perceived self-efficacy. *American Journal of Occupational Therapy, 48*(5), 452-462.

Gibson, J. J. (1979). *The ecological approach to visual perception*. Boston, MA: Houghton Mifflin Company.

Gustafson, P. (2001). Meanings of place. Everyday experiences and theoretical conceptualizations. *Journal of Environmental Psychology, 21*(1), 5-16.

Hall, E. T. (1973). *The silent language*. Garden City, NJ: Anchor Books.

Hamilton, T. B. (2003). Occupations and places. In C. Christiansen & E. Townsend (Eds.), *Introduction to occupation: The art and science of living* (pp. 173-196). Upper Saddle River, NJ: Prentice-Hall.

Hultsch, D. F., Hertzog, C., Small, B. J., & Dixon, R. A. (1999). Use it or lose it: Engaged lifestyle as a buffer of cognitive decline in aging? *Psychology and Aging, 14*(2), 245-263.

Jackson, J., Carlson, M., Mandel, D., Zemke, R., & Clark, F. (1998). Occupation in lifestyle redesign: The Well Elderly Study Occupational Therapy Program. *American Journal of Occupational Therapy, 52*(5), 326-336.

Kielhofner, G. (1977). Temporal adaptation: A conceptual framework for occupational therapy. *American Journal of Occupational Therapy, 31*(4), 235-242.

Kielhofner, G. (1978). General system theory: Implications for the theory and action in occupational therapy. *American Journal of Occupational Therapy, 32*, 637-645.

Kielhofner, G. (1995). *A model of human occupation: Theory and application* (2nd ed.). Baltimore, MD: Williams & Wilkins.

Kielhofner, G. (2002). *A model of human occupation: Theory and application* (3rd ed.). Lippincott Williams & Wilkins

Law, M. (1991). The environment: A focus for occupational therapy. *Canadian Journal of Occupational Therapy, 58*, 171-179.

Law, M., Cooper, B. A., Strong, S., Stewart, D., Rigby, P., & Letts, L. (1996). The Person-Environment-Occupation Model: A transactive approach to occupational performance. *Canadian Journal of Occupational Therapy, 63*(1), 9-22.

Law, M., Baptiste, S., & Mills, J. (1995). Client-centred practice: What does it mean and does it make a difference? *Canadian Journal of Occupational Therapy, 62*, 250-257.

Lawton, M. P. (1980). *Environment and aging*. Monterey, CA: Brooks-Cole.

Letts, L., Law, M., Rigby, P., Cooper, B., Stewart, D., & Strong, S. (1994). Person environment assessments in occupational therapy. *American Journal of Occupational Therapy, 48*(7), 608-618.

Little, B. R., Lecci, L., & Watkinson, B. (1992). Personality and personal projects: Linking Big 5 and PAC units of analysis. *Journal of Personality, 60*(2), 501-525.

Lloyd, K. R., Jacob, J. S., Patel, V., St. Louis, L., Bhugra, D., & Mann, A. H. (1998). The development of the Short Explanatory Model Interview (SEMI) and its use among primary-care attenders with common mental disorders. *Psychological Medicine, 28*(5), 1231-1237.

Mathiowetz, V., & Bass-Haugen, J. (1994). Motor behavior research: Implications for therapeutic approaches to central nervous system dysfunction. *American Journal of Occupational Therapy, 48*(8), 733-745.

McAdams, D. (1992). Unity and purpose in human lives: The emergence of identity as a life story. In R. A. Zucker & A. T. Ratain (Eds.), *Personality structure in the life course* (pp. 323-376). New York, NY: Springer-Verlag.

McColl, M. A. (1997). Social support and occupational therapy. In C. Christiansen & C. Baum (Eds.), *Occupational therapy: Enabling function and well-being* (2nd ed.). Thorofare, NJ: SLACK Incorporated.

McGregor, I., & Little, B. R. (1998). Personal projects, happiness and meaning: On doing well and being yourself. *Journal of Personality and Social Psychology, 74*(2), 494-512.

Mead, G. H. (1934). *Mind, self and society*. Chicago, IL: University of Chicago Press.

Merzenich, M. M., Scheiner, C., Jenkins, W., & Wang, X. (1993). Neural mechanisms underlying temporal integration, segmentation, and input sequence representation: Some implications for the origin of learning disabilities. *Annals of the New York Academy of Sciences, 682*, 1-22.

Meyer, A. (1922). The philosophy of occupation therapy. *Archives of Occupational Therapy, 1*(1), 1-10.

Minor, M. A. (1997). Promoting health and physical fitness. In C. Christiansen & C. Baum (Eds.), *Occupational therapy: Enabling function and well being* (2nd ed.). Thorofare, NJ: SLACK Incorporated.

Mosey, A. C. (1974). An alternative: The biopsychosocial model. *American Journal of Occupational Therapy, 28*(3), 137-140.

Murray, H. A., Barrett, W. G., & Hamburger, E. (1938). *Explorations in personality*. New York, NY: Oxford University Press.

Orth-Gomer, K., Rosengren, A., & Wilhelmsen, L. (1993). Lack of social support and incidence of coronary heart disease in middle-aged Swedish men. *Psychosomatic Medicine, 55*(1), 37-43.

Oxford English Dictionary. (1989). (2nd ed.). Oxford: Oxford University Press.

Parsons, T. (1975). The sick role and the role of the physician reconsidered. *Health & Society*, 257-278.

Palys, T. S., & Little, B. R. (1983). Perceived life satisfaction and the organization of personal project systems. *Journal of Personality and Social Psychology, 44*, 1221-1230.

Peterson, N., Mumford, M., Borman, W., Jeanneret, P., Fleishman, E., & Levin, K. (1997). *O*Net final technical report* (vol. 1-3). Salt Lake City, UT: National Center for O*Net Development, US Department of Labor.

Pierce, G. R., Sarason, I. G., & Sarason, B. R. (1990). General and relationship-based perceptions of social support: Are two constructs better than one? *Journal of Personality and Social Psychology, 612*(6), 1028-1039.

Pinters, S., & Bloom, P. (1990). Natural language and natural selection. *Behavioral and Brain Science, 13*, 707-784.

Reed, K. L., & Sanderson, S. (1999). *Concepts of occupational therapy* (4th ed.). Philadelphia: Williams and Wilkins.

Reilly, M. (1962). Occupational therapy can be one of the great ideas of 20th century medicine. *American Journal of Occupational Therapy, 16*, 300-308.

Rogers, J. C. (1983). Clinical reasoning: The ethics, science and art. *American Journal of Occupational Therapy, 37*, 601-616.

Rowles, G. D. (1991). Beyond performance: Being in place as a component of occupational therapy. *American Journal of Occupational Therapy.45*(3), 265-271

Ryan, R. M., & Deci, E. L. (2000). Self-determination theory and the facilitation of intrinsic motivation, social development, and well-being. *American Psychologist, 55*, 68-78.

Sarbin, T. R., & Allen, V. L. (1968). Role theory. In G. Lindsey & E. Aronson (Eds.), *Handbook of social psychology* (2nd ed.). Reading, MA: Addison-Wesley.

Sullivan, H. S. (1953). *Conceptions of modern psychiatry*. New York, NY: W. W. Norton.

Tattersall, J. (1998). *Becoming human: Evolution and human uniqueness*. New York, NY: Harcourt Brace.

Thoits, P. A. (1997). Stress, coping, and social support process: Where are we? What next? *Journal of Health and Social Behavior*, Spec No., 53-79.

Trombly, C. A. (1995). Occupation: Purposefulness and meaningfulness and therapeutic mechanisms. *American Journal of Occupational Therapy, 49*, 960-972.

Wallenius, M. (1999). Personal projects in everyday places: Perceived supportiveness of the environment and psychological well being. *Journal of Environmental Psychology, 19*(2), 131-143.

Chapter Eleven: Person-Environment-Occupation-Performance Reflections and Learning Activities

Julie Bass-Haugen, PhD, OTR/L, FAOTA

REFLECTIONS

If you have been working through the chapters in sequential order, you've been immersed in occupation lately. You've learned that occupations are integral to the human experience. They are more than just the "doing" of activities. Occupations are a means to achieve many things that are important in life: meaning, health, well-being, and personal growth. I know as I read these chapters I frequently paused to consider the importance of occupations in my own life. I hope you had a chance to do the same. I am guessing if you made it to this chapter, however, you have some beliefs and passion about the importance of occupation in other people's lives as well. In fact, I would guess by now you believe all individuals need occupations that bring meaning to their lives, promote well-being and quality of life, and enable participation in society. You care about people you know and people you don't know who have occupational issues of concern. You feel a vocational calling to work with people who have not reached their occupational goals. Occupational therapy is the core profession for doing this kind of work, and you are developing a passion for occupational therapy.

In Section II, you began your serious study of occupational therapy practice. You already know there is much depth and breadth to the profession of occupational therapy. You know occupational therapy practitioners work with people of all ages, with all levels of abilities, and in numerous settings. But what exactly do they do, how do they do it, and why do they do it? It is important at this stage to find a framework you can use for all your learning related to occupational therapy.

The PEOP model and other PEO models can serve as frameworks or "cookbooks" for your occupational therapy practice. They identify the basic "ingredients" for every occupational therapy "recipe"—person, environment, occupation, performance. If you don't include these ingredients in your occupational therapy recipe, something will go wrong! This edition of the cookbook, however, is written for master chefs. The specific amounts of these ingredients are not identified, and instructions don't seem written for the novice. If you learn to cook using this kind of cookbook, you are taking a leap of faith. You accept the fact it will be hard at first because you want to be more than a short order cook—you want to become a master chef. You can live with a little ambiguity now. You know that soon you will have the knowledge and experience to make wonderful, unique creations using only these ingredients. You will understand the characteristics of each ingredient and how these ingredients interact together in every recipe... enough of this culinary analogy!

The PEOP model is also based on two important beliefs about humans. The first belief is that each and every person has motivation, drive, and desire to do things and to do them well. This is quite a statement, especially if you consider the range of abilities, personalities, and behaviors of people we know. This is an essential statement, though, for occupational therapy practitioners who make a commitment to work with all people having occupational needs. The second belief is that each and every person needs to experience success to feel right with the world. This statement has huge implications for how we design our occupational therapy interventions. Participation, well-being, and quality of life are the outcomes of optimal interactions of the person, environment, occupation, and performance. Now, let's take a closer look at each of the components of the model.

Five personal factors were identified as intrinsic enablers of performance: neurobehavioral, physiological, cognitive, psychological and emotional, and spiritual. It is easy to take a list of factors like this for granted and to fail to appreciate its importance. We have a tendency to say, "Yeah, yeah, yeah, I know all of these factors." However, there are times (e.g., after a long, busy day) I realize our personal factors are truly amazing. How is it that all these personal factors can work together so I can do my occupations? Think about a few of your occupations. Think of your drive to work or school. How is it that we can coordinate all the personal factors that we need to drive and still have personal factor reserves to internally make all our plans for the day? Think of the multitasking you do at home. How is it that we can coordinate all the personal factors that we need to review terminology for a course, fold laundry, and keep stress under control as we prepare for a test? The human body is a marvelous thing.

We are fortunate when our personal factors are working well. However, we also have experienced times when one or more personal factors are not working at their peak. Have you ever had a broken bone or sprain? Have you ever felt foggy in your thinking because of a head cold? Have you ever felt a little "blue" because of some stressful times? In these kinds of situations, we see a clear effect on our occupations and performance. Our performance is less than optimal, or sometimes we can barely do even one occupation at a time. These simple examples make it easier to appreciate the effects of significant personal impairments, like rheumatoid arthritis, stroke, and depression, on occupational performance. Many people receiving occupational therapy services have personal factors that limit their occupational performance.

Four environmental factors were identified as extrinsic enablers of performance: the natural environment, built environment and technology, culture and values; social supports and social and economic systems. You will find a variety of terms used in the literature to represent these environmental factors. The basic idea, however, is that there are lots of things outside of ourselves (and sometimes outside our control) that positively or negatively influence our occupational performance. These environmental factors may be subtle or significant. Have you ever been late to school because of a storm or road construction? Have you ever experienced peer pressure to do something (or not do something)? Have you ever had someone support you at a critical time in your life? Have you ever been restricted in what you could do by a policy or your finances? If you have experienced any of these situations, you've experienced an environmental influence. These examples might seem minor in the big scheme of things. However, we know of individuals who encounter significant environmental obstacles to occupational performance.

Environmental factors may cause huge barriers to occupational performance for disadvantaged populations. We have made considerable progress in addressing some environmental factors in recent decades. It wasn't long ago that children with certain characteristics (e.g., race, disability status) were not allowed in some schools. People who used wheelchairs couldn't navigate in their community because of curbing, parking, and stairs at the entrance of every building. Young women did not have the opportunity to participate in collegiate competitive sports because of educational policies. We are grateful that some of these environmental issues have been addressed. However, there are still many environmental obstacles for occupational performance. People with mental illness are subjected to policies and practices that limit employment and access to health care. Elders experience isolation and occupational deprivation because of transportation, housing, or support system issues. These are just a few of the many environmental influences.

The last major components of the PEOP model are occupations and performance. You have already learned much about occupation. You know there are a variety of classification systems and terms to represent occupations (e.g., activities and participation in the ICF). Performance was described as the doing of occupation. It can be analyzed at different levels and from observable behaviors. Imagine that you are observing me as I prepare breakfast for my family on a Saturday morning. Meal preparation is the occupation. How would you describe my performance? Can you break up your description of my performance according to different layers? Actions, activities, tasks, occupation, daily life, and roles are part of an occupational hierarchy that may be useful in describing performance. For meal preparation, you might observe me reaching (i.e., action) as I fill the coffee pot with water (i.e., activity) to make coffee (i.e., task) as part of breakfast preparation (i.e., occupation) for some parent/child quality time (i.e., role). I must forewarn you though that these terms overlap and are even used in different ways by other people. However, applying these terms to a specific example is a useful exercise in itself. It helps us understand the multidimensional aspects of occupational performance.

What does the PEOP model mean in terms of how you approach occupational therapy practice? I think a good occupational therapy practitioner has a P-E-O-P mantra going inside the head at all times—"P-E-O-P, P-E-O-P." When I am trying to learn as much about a particular situation, I am thinking, "What do I need to know about this person? What do I need to know about this person's occupations and performance? What do I need to know about this person's environment? How do these components interact?" This model requires that we keep our focus on the person's perspective (i.e., a client-centered approach). It also requires that we use numerous resources inside and outside the discipline of occupational therapy to plan our interventions. Now that you have the primary "cookbook" for your occupational therapy practice, it is time to learn more about each of these ingredients and get some experience.

Journal Activities

1. Look up and write down a dictionary definition of model. Highlight the component of the definition that is most related to its descriptions in Chapter Eleven.
2. Identify the most important new learning for you in this chapter.
3. Identify one question you have about Chapter Eleven.
4. Reflect on a biography of a person you have read/viewed in recent years. Write a brief summary of this person using the PEOP model. Note his or her strengths and challenges for each component of the PEOP model. How did these components interact for this person? How did these components influence participation, well-being, and quality of life?

Technology/Internet Learning Activities

1. Use a discussion database to share specific journal entries.
2. Use a good Internet search engine to find the document, "Enabling America: Assessing the Role of Rehabilitation Science and Engineering" (1997).
   - Enter the phrase "Enabling America" in your search line.
   - Read the executive summary of the document.
   - Identify the organization that prepared this document.
   - What are the priorities for rehabilitation science and engineering according to this report?
   - How many Americans have a disabling condition?
   - What are the national economic costs associated with disability?
   - Describe the enabling-disabling process and its components (hint: See Figure 11-1 and Table 11-1.)
   - Propose a role for occupational therapy in this process.
3. Use a good Internet search engine to find the *International Classification of Functioning, Disability, and Health* (ICF) by the WHO.
   - Enter the phrase "International Classification of Function WHO" in your search line.
   - Review the home page for the ICF.
   - What is the purpose of the ICF?
   - What resources are available on the ICF Web site?
   - Review the online version of the ICF.
   - Identify the main categories of the ICF.

Main Categories

- Identify the main classifications (chapters) of activities and participation in ICF.
  - ✧ Rank ICF activities and participation classifications (chapters) that have the most and least relevance for occupational therapy (1 = primary relevance; 2 = secondary relevance).

Activities and Participation	*Rank*	*Activities and Participation*	*Rank*

- Examine the ICF checklist provided on the Web site.
  - ✧ Propose how you might use the ICF checklist in your occupational therapy practice.

4. Use a good Internet search engine to find the Web site for the World Institute on Disability.
   - Enter the phrase "World Institute on Disability" in your search line.
   - Scan the Web site.
   - What is the purpose or mission of the World Institute on Disability?
   - Describe the programs of the World Institute on Disability.
   - Identify the environmental influences addressed by this organization.
   - Propose a role for occupational therapy in this organization.

Applied Learning

Individual Learning Activity #1: Conducting a Self-Assessment of Person, Environment, and Occupational Performance

Instructions:

- Reflect on your personal factors at this point in time. Identify your strengths and challenges for each personal factor.
- Reflect on your environmental factors at this point in time. Identify your strengths and challenges for each environmental factor.
- Reflect on your occupational performance for studying and exercising. Think of times when your occupational performance is optimal and not optimal. Describe the "best case scenario" for your personal and environmental factors when your occupational performance is optimal. Describe the "worst case scenario" for your personal and environmental factors when your occupational performance is not optimal.

Factors	*Strengths*	*Challenges*
Person Factors—neurobehavioral, physiological, cognitive, psychological and emotional, and spiritual		
Environment Factors—natural and built environment, cultural norms and values, social supports, and societal policies and attitudes		

Occupational Performance Area	*Best Interaction of P and E*	*Worst Interaction of P and E*
Studying		
Exercise		

Individual Learning Activity #2: Examining the Layers of Occupational Performance.

Instructions:

- Identify an occupation you want to examine in more detail.
- Reflect on all aspects of your performance for this occupation.
- Describe two examples of the layers of occupational performance for this occupation.

Action	*Activity*	*Task*	*Occupation*	*Role*

Active Learning

Group Activity #1: Exploring Support Systems as an Environmental Factor

Preparation: Read Chapter Eleven.
Time: 30 to 45 minutes
Materials: Flip chart, chalkboard, white board, or virtual board
Instructions:

- Individually:
  - Complete a self-assessment of one environmental factor: your support systems.
  - Be prepared to share your results from the self-assessment.

A Self-Assessment of Support Systems

	Informational	*Practical*	*Emotional*
Who were your past support systems in this area?			
Who are your current support systems in this area?			
How could you strengthen your support system in this area?			

- In small groups:
  - Share the results of your self-assessment.
  - Summarize the support systems for your group.
  - Summarize the strategies to strengthen support systems for your group.
  - Generate ideas for support systems to use in your occupational therapy practice. Include ideas related to your needs as a practitioner and the needs of your clients.

Support Systems

	Informational	*Practical*	*Emotional*
A summary of the support systems used by individuals in the group			
A summary of strategies to strengthen support systems			
Ideas on support systems to consider in my occupational therapy practice			

Discussion:

- Discuss how support systems make a difference in your own life and the lives of people you know.
- Discuss some strategies you might use when working with people who do not have good support systems.

Group Activity #2: Interviewing Someone About PEOP Characteristics

Preparation: Read Chapter Eleven.
Time: 45 to 60 minutes
Instructions:

- Individually:
  - ✧ Review the PEOP components.
  - ✧ Develop some interview questions to learn about PEOP components of a person. You will want to explore strengths and challenges for the personal and environmental factors; occupations having importance and meaning; current performance of occupations; and the interactions of person, environment, occupations, and performance. Note: Develop questions that use layperson language.
- In small groups (2 to 3 people):
  - ✧ Interview a person to understand the PEOP components that are important.
  - ✧ Take notes during the interview.
  - ✧ Write a brief summary of this person using a PEOP framework.

Discussion

- How would you describe this person to an occupational therapy practitioner?
- What were the greatest challenges in conducting this interview?
- How did it feel to be in the role of interviewer?
- How did it feel to be in the role of interviewee?

Chapter Twelve Objectives

The information in this chapter in intended to help the reader:

1. Develop a global understanding of physiological function and dysfunction within the body.
2. Appreciate the influence of physical fitness on body function, wellness, and occupational performance.
3. Define psychology constructs and appreciate their impact on occupational performance.
4. Describe cognitive factors such as attention and memory and explain how they form a basis for engagement in meaningful activity.
5. Identify the importance of the impact of neurobehavioral factors on human performance.
6. Describe different types of genetic conditions in occupational therapy practice.
7. Appreciate the interaction between human genetic factors and environment and their influence on health status and well-being.
8. Define spirituality and appreciate its influence on well-being through occupations.

Key Words

affect: Emotions or feelings that are associated with evaluation of self.
attention: Ability to concentrate our perceptual experience on a selected portion of the available sensory information.
chromosomes: Microscopic structures inside the nucleus of the cells.
cognition: Acquisition and use of knowledge or the process of thinking.
cognitive rehabilitation: Systematic intervention, based on assessment, that may use the range of approaches from remedial to compensatory to address the variety of cognitive limitations experienced by a client.
genes: Individual units of hereditary material.
genetics: Subject concerned with variation and heredity in all living organisms.
medical genetics: The science of human biological variation as it relates to health and disease.
motivation: Drive toward action.
neuroscience: Study of the nervous system structure, function, and development.
physiology: Study of biological function.
process memory: Reproducing or recalling what has been learned.
psychology: Study of the behavior of individuals and their mental processes.
self-concept: The way in which individuals perceive themselves.
self-efficacy: Individuals' belief in their capacities of performance toward a specific task.
self-esteem: The relative value in which the individual holds the attributes that contribute to self-concept.
spiritual dimension: An individual's beliefs and practices that reflect significant connections with self, with others, with nature, and with a higher power or source of ultimate meaning.
structural memory: Memory store; short, long, sensory.

Everything you need you already have. You are complete right now, you are a whole, total person, not an apprentice person on the way to someplace else. Your completeness must be understood by you and experienced in your thoughts as your own personal reality.
Beverly Sills

Chapter Twelve

Personal Performance Capabilities and Their Impact on Occupational Performance

Jennie Q. Lou, MD, MSc, OTR and Shelly J. Lane, PhD, OTR/L, FAOTA

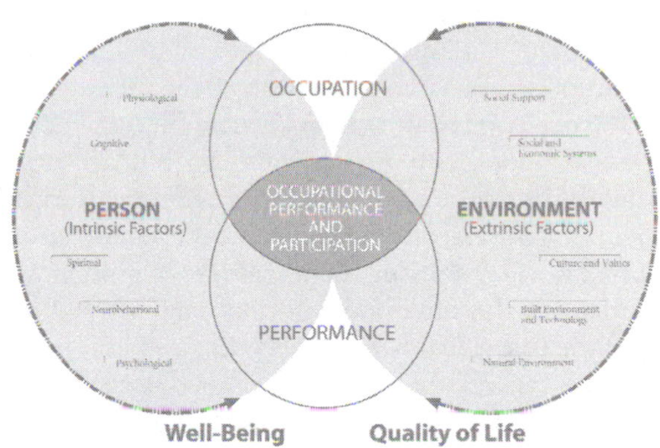

Setting the Stage

This chapter focuses on the intrinsic factors, or factors within the individual, that underpin the capacity of the individual to perform activities central to daily life. It is often these factors that practitioners speak about when they are using an intervention to support recovery. As described in the previous chapters, the Person-Environment-Occupation-Performance (PEOP) model has three major components. These three elements describe what people do, or want or need to do, in their daily lives (occupations) and how psychological, physiological, neurobehavioral, cognitive, and spiritual factors (person) combine with the situations in which occupations are undertaken (environment) to influence successful occupational performance (the interaction of capacity, environment, and choice in activities).

Don't miss the companion Web site to *Occupational Therapy: Performance, Participation, and Well-Being, Third Edition.* Please visit us at http://www.cb3e.slackbooks.com.

Lou, J. Q. & Lane, S. J. (2005). Personal performance capabilities and their impact on occupational performance. In C. H. Christiansen, C. M. Baum, and J. Bass-Haugen (Eds.), Occupational therapy: Performance, participation, and well-being *(3rd ed.). Thorofare, NJ: SLACK Incorporated.*

Introduction

An occupational performance intervention approach requires occupational therapy practitioners to employ a top-down client-centered strategy (Trombly, 1995). We must determine with our clients what they perceive to be the important occupational performance issues that are causing them difficulties in carrying out their daily activities and roles in the areas of work, self-care, and leisure. This approach requires occupational therapy practitioners to collect assessment information about the physiological, psychological, cognitive, neurobehavioral, and spiritual factors that may be supporting or interfering with their performance and to identify environmental factors that may serve as enablers or barriers to performance.

To understand performance, occupational therapy practitioners must consider the personal characteristics of individuals; the unique environment in which they perform their tasks and activities; and the nature and meaning of the actions, tasks, and roles to the individual. Identification and consideration of the many factors that influence performance help occupational therapy practitioners understand the client's capabilities within the multiple dimensions of occupation. In other words, studying occupational and human behavior requires us to combine knowledge about the impairments that impede performance; the environments that support performance; and the individual needs, preferences, styles, and goals.

The *International Classification of Function, Disability, and Health* (ICF) is a classification system designed to provide a common framework for all disciplines in the understanding of function and disablement. It does so using three domains: the body, the person, and the society (World Health Organization [WHO], 2001). Thus, aspects of it parallel the PEOP model presented in this text. According to ICF, disablement can occur at any of these three domains, with loss of body function or structure classified as impairment. As can be seen in the ICF model (Figure 12-1), impairments potentially lead to limitations in activities and restriction of participation (WHO, 2001). In embracing an understanding of occupational performance, it is critical for occupational therapy practitioners to understand what ICF terms the body domain and what the PEOP model classifies the person factors because it is here where we find the link between impairment, activities, and participation.

In this chapter, we will introduce some of the principle personal factors that are pertinent to the individual within the PEOP model: physiological, psychological, cognitive, neurobehavioral, genetic, and spiritual factors. These comprise the "body structure and function" portion of ICF, and they shape individuals' performance of tasks or actions (activities) in a particular environment. Through the discussion and case studies, we will illustrate how different personal factors may influence successful occupational performance.

Physiological Factors

Physiology is the study of biological function, how the body works, from cell to tissue, tissue to organ, organ to system. Physiology is the study of mechanisms, how things work, the study of function (Fox, 1996). Truly encompassing the function component of "body structure and function" in ICF, physiology is a major player in the personal performance capabilities as depicted in the PEOP model. A study of physiology includes a study of all tissues, organs, and systems within the body and the functions associated with them. There are 11 major organ systems within the human body, each with its own function. They are defined in Table 12-1.

As occupational therapy practitioners, we typically learn the basics of physiology, appreciate the ramifications of function within these systems, and deal with the impact of illness on those physiologic functions we can observe. We are, perhaps, most accustomed to dealing with the impact of disease on nervous, muscular, and skeletal systems. However, clinically, we are also faced with the impact of such things as spinal cord injury or typical aging on the integumentary system, as well as stress and illness on the endocrine and lymphatic systems. Many of us may consider the impact of health and disease on such things as attention and other cognitive functions as well, but often without depth of understanding.

Physiology and Physical Fitness

The concept of physical fitness works well into our discussion of physiology because it represents wellness. As noted by Minor (1997, p. 256), "Health-related physical fitness is a multifactorial phenomenon consisting of 1) cardiorespiratory function, 2) muscle strength, 3) muscle endurance, 4) flexibility, and 5) body composition." As such, it encompasses all systems described above in their healthy, functional state. Further, the President's Council on Physical Fitness and Sport (1992) defined physical fitness in a way we, as occupational therapy practitioners, might also define it: "the ability to carry out daily tasks with vigor and alertness, without undue fatigue, and with ample energy to engage in leisure time pursuits and to meet the above average physical stresses encountered in emergency situations." The concept of physical fitness then provides us a focus on wellness within the physiological systems and a means by which we can use physical activity to promote health and support performance. It is also an important consideration for clients faced with disability and disease. Physical deconditioning can complicate the rehabilitation process. For example, a client

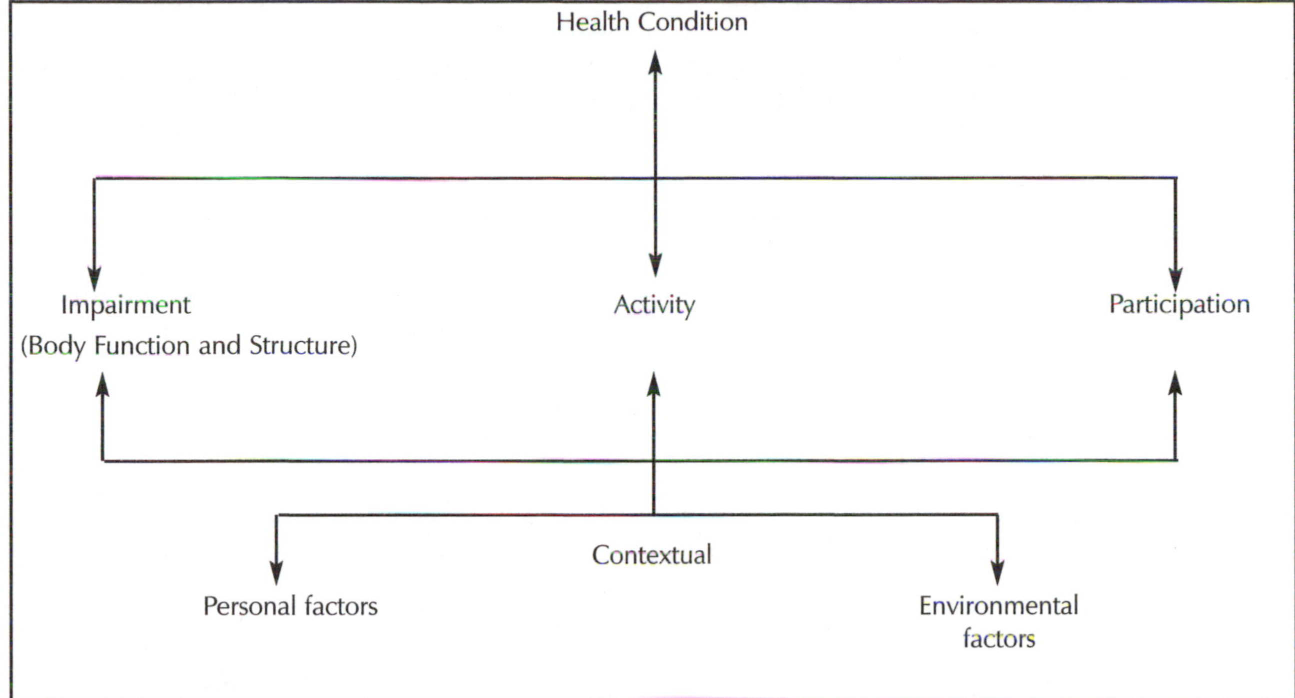

Figure 12-1. ICF model. (Reprinted with Permission of the World Health Organization, all rights reserved by the Organization. The International Classification of Function, Disability and Health, page 18 WHO, 2001 http://www.who.int/classification/ref.)

Table 12-1

Physiologic Systems and Functions

System	*Components*	*Function*
Integumentary	Skin, hair, nails	Forms a covering for the body, plays a role in protection and temperature regulation, and holds receptors needed for sensory intake
Skeletal	Bones, joints, cartilage	Protects and supports the body organs, movement and anchorage of muscles, mineral storage, production of red bone marrow
Muscular	Three types of muscle: skeletal, cardiac, smooth	Movement of the body, maintenance of body form and shape (posture), production of body heat
Nervous	Brain, spinal cord, peripheral nerves, sensory end organs	Reception of stimuli, transmission to the central nervous system, processing and integration of input; preparation for output; development of command for execution
Endocrine	Glands, hormones	Secrete hormones and chemical messengers that coordinate and direct such activities as growth, metabolism of minerals and nutrients, homeostatic functions, and sexual development
Circulatory	Heart, vessels	Pumps blood throughout the body, which transports nutrients and oxygen to all cells; carries waste away
Lymphatic	Lymph vessels, nodes, spleen, tonsils, and thymus; lymph fluid	Defense of body against pathogens

(continued)

Table 12-1

System	*Components*	*Function*
Respiratory	Lungs, pharynx, larynx, trachea, bronchial tree	Exchange of oxygen into the body and carbon dioxide from the blood; sound production
Digestive	Stomach, intestines, liver, gallbladder	Ingestion and breakdown of food for absorption, elimination of waste products from digestion
Urinary	Kidneys, ureters, bladder	Excretion of salts and excess water from blood, maintain acid-base balance, secrete waste in the form of urine
Reproductive	Testes, ovaries, genital tracts and ducts, external genitals	Enable reproduction, manufacture hormones needed for development of reproductive organs and secondary sex characteristics

Modified from Herlihy, B., & Maebius, N. K. (2000). *The human body in health and illness*. Philadelphia: W. B. Saunders Co; and Scott, A. S., and Fong, E. (2004). *Body structures & functions*. Clifton Park, NY: Thomson/Delmar Learning.

faced with a spinal cord injury following an automobile accident may spend a considerable amount of time in bed while vital physiologic functions become stabilized. During this period of time, his or her physical fitness from a muscular and cardiorespiratory perspective will have become compromised. As a result, when the client comes to you several weeks later for rehabilitation, you will now not only be dealing with issues related to the spinal cord injury, you will now also be dealing with diminished heart and lung function along with muscle weakness in the muscles that continue to receive signals.

According to Minor (1997), there are five basic components of physical fitness: cardiorespiratory function, muscle strength, muscle endurance, flexibility, and body composition. These form the basis for human performance and, as such, are what you need to consider in both wellness and disease or disability because they are what will either prevent or allow participation in activities.

Cardiorespiratory Function

This will include the circulatory and respiratory systems in Table 12-1. Cardiorespiratory fitness is defined as the ability to take in, transport, and use oxygen. As practitioners, it is important for us to be aware of the fact that this system is very sensitive to our needs and that the system works harder when the body is in different positions. The least stressful position for cardiorespiratory functions is supine, next is sitting, then standing. We ask more from our cardiorespiratory functions as we walk, run, etc. This seems quite logical, but needs to be kept forefront in our minds when we are dealing with a client who is not in good cardiorespiratory condition, especially when we begin to get him or her into a sitting position from the supine position, which has been maintained for several weeks. It may take the cardiorespiratory functions a bit of catch up time to function optimally, and we need to be cautious as practitioners to look for signs of overload to this system.

Muscle Strength

Muscle strength is the amount of force that can be exerted by one or a group of muscles in one voluntary contraction. It is measured and developed using static (isometric) and dynamic (isotonic) means, but simply working on strength training is not generally the purview of an occupational therapy practitioner. However, it is important to know that static muscle strength is important in the development of posture and balance, while both forms of muscle strength play a role in all activities in which we engage, so the development of adequate muscle strength is a critical component of overall fitness.

Muscle Endurance

Muscle endurance is defined as the ability to repeat muscle contractions or maintain a single contraction as needed for a prolonged period of time. We need endurance in different ways in different muscles. Our postural control muscles must maintain posture against gravity for prolonged periods of time, and our fine motor muscles, depending on what tasks we undertake, may need to repeatedly contract in the same way for prolonged periods of time. Our ability to perform such activities will depend on our muscular endurance. Muscle endurance is also tied to cardiorespiratory functions, as you might imagine.

Flexibility

Defined as the range of motion at a joint, or at a sequence of joints, flexibility will be influenced by the soft tissue around the joint(s), condition of the joint(s) themselves, and fat or excess muscle around the joint(s). Limited range of motion can clearly interfere with our ability to engage in many activities, including the very simple things, such as combing the back of our hair or tying our shoes.

Body Composition

This component of fitness refers to the fat and nonfat elements of the body. Both too little and too much body fat are thought to interfere with optimal body function and, as such, may interfere with our ability to engage in meaningful occupation.

What will you, the occupational therapy practitioner, do with this information on fitness? You will want to always consider the issues as they relate to wellness because you should always be considering ways to incorporate concepts of wellness and the promotion of wellness into your intervention. From this perspective, you can work with your clients to establish fitness goals once you understand fitness yourself, and then work with them on ways to increase the fitness complexity of activities they enjoy to meet their own fitness goals.

You will also want to be aware of what to look for in your clients that would indicate compromised function in these fitness components. There are times when your assessments and interventions will likely address aspects of fitness from an occupation/activity perspective, or occasionally from a component perspective as they have been described here. Thus, you may be working with a client on muscle strengthening and endurance, but this could be incorporated into your client's functional activity of bread baking as your client works to knead and roll the dough. You will, of course, keep in mind that this task will challenge the cardiorespiratory functions for some of your clients, and you will need to keep an eye on them for signs of cardiorespiratory changes.

Physiologic Systems and Disruption of Occupational Performance

Disturbance to any of these physiologic systems can cause changes in body structure and/or function, therefore affecting an individual's activities and participation. Disruption of physiologic systems can take place on either a primary or secondary level. When the problem is of a primary nature, occupational therapy practitioners are aware of it; therefore, it can be of primary importance in intervention. When the disruption is of a secondary nature, the practitioner must be astute in identifying both the nature of the disruption and its impact.

Primary disruptions are easy to identify in many cases. They are often, although not always, the reason for referral to a practitioner. For instance, a client may be referred to an occupational therapy practitioner following a burn, a spinal cord injury, or a stroke. The practitioner will be immediately able to determine the physiological impairment and, in conjunction with the client, the impact this impairment has or will have on the client's ability to engage in meaningful occupations as he or she looks to return to routine environments and activities.

The impact on participation in meaningful occupations of some direct physiological disruptions may be less obvious, and the practitioner may need to lobby to obtain referrals on clients in some cases. For instance, several disorders of the endocrine system have clinical findings that include an impact on such characteristics as appetite, weight, energy level, and fatigue resilience. These characteristics undergird a client's ability to engage in daily occupations, including self-care, leisure, and work. If an endocrine disorder is disrupting the ability of a client to meaningfully engage in daily activities, it becomes the purview of the occupational therapy practitioner invested in the overall health and well-being of the client to investigate the possibility of intervention with the client.

Physiologic systems may also be disrupted secondarily by disease or injury. An excellent example of this stair step disruption exists in the case of an individual with a traumatic brain injury who later develops heterotrophic ossification. In this case, the practitioner may already be working with the client on the cognitive impairments that have developed due to the brain injury, but must now consider the additional impact that the skeletal impairments will impart on occupational performance. Failure to recognize and consider these additional physiologic disruptions will mean that occupational performance cannot be restored.

Psychological Factors

Psychology is defined as the scientific study of the behavior of individuals and their mental processes. Psychology has both an applied side and a basic science side. The goals for basic research in psychology are to describe, explain, predict, and control behavior. The applied psychological research has a fifth goal—to improve the quality of human life. Occupational therapy practitioners are mainly interested in the application of psychology because it addresses the quality of human life: Why do people feel, think, and act the way they do? Why do people become stressed? What causes psychological disturbances, such as depression or schizophrenia? How can we improve the quality of life of our clients?

The science of psychology covers many areas of interest. Psychological studies examine the mechanisms underlying age-related (developmental) changes in memory, learning, reasoning, problem solving, and information processing and the roles of psychological and physiological characteristics in age differences and age changes in cognitive performance. Because occupational therapy practitioners believe psychological factors are basic to doing (Bonder, 2004; Fidler & Fidler, 1963), they are concerned with how psychological factors, including the internal experiences and personal reactions, shape individuals' performance. Occupational therapy practitioners are also interested in the psychological mechanisms through which the individual manages relationships between the environment and self. Occupational therapy practitioners believe psychological factors such as self-concept, self-esteem, and affect influence the individual's perception of self (Fidler & Fidler, 1963). In addition to looking at how these factors contribute to successful performance, occupational therapy practitioners are also fascinated with how a person's occupation contributes to their sense of well-being (Christiansen & Baum, 1997).

Occupational therapy practitioners consider that individuals' decisions about what they want to do, how they assess their satisfaction with their activities, and even what they experience as essential undertakings are based on psychological factors that include individual needs, perceptions, and evaluations of the world in the context of personal experience (Fidler & Fidler, 1978). When an individual is experiencing an activity limitation of participation restriction, regardless of the reason, psychological factors are central to his or her reaction to the situation. Thus, all occupational performance is shaped by psychological influences. For example, spinal cord injury causes not only physical limitations, but also psychological consequences. Occupational therapy will be ineffective if it fails to address both aspects; conversely, integration of all aspects of performance can result in more productive outcomes.

There are many ways to define psychological constructs (Bonder, 2004). Psychological constructs are terms used to describe internal experience, personal reaction to the external environment, and psychological mechanisms by which the individual addresses relationships between the environment and the self. As reflected in the PEOP model, psychological constructs can be categorized into three classes: intrinsic, extrinsic, and the outcomes of the relationship between self and the environment.

Intrinsic Factors

Intrinsic psychological factors include self-concept, self-esteem, and affect. Self-concept is the way in which individuals perceive themselves. Self-concept is descriptive rather than evaluative. It is reflected in individuals' statements about who they are both in terms of roles (daughter, student, etc.) and attributions (considerate, intelligent, etc.). When a person has a self-concept that is inconsistent with the way others see the individual, it may lead to psychological difficulties, as the individual may be disappointed in interactions with others. This can easily be seen as the self-concept unfolds during adolescence. A young girl perceiving herself as "looking cool" in the clothes she has chosen to wear to the dance can be crushed by overhearing her peers referring to her outfit as "so last year" or out of date.

Self-esteem refers to the relative value (positive or negative) in which the individual holds the attributes that contribute to self-concept. For example, an individual who describes him- or herself as "smart" might evaluate that as either positive or negative. An adolescent whose self-concept includes a perception of self as intelligent might believe that this is not valued by peers and might therefore evaluate the attribute negatively, lowering self-esteem. On the other hand, an adult might feel that intelligence is an admirable characteristic and, therefore, experience increased self-esteem because of a positive perception that he or she possesses the attribute. As with self-concept, self-esteem is mainly internal to the individual; however, inconsistency between the way others value the individual and ways the individual values him- or herself can become problematic.

Affect is the emotion or feelings that are associated with evaluation of self. The adolescent in the example above might feel unhappy about his or her perceived disadvantage, while the adult might find his or her intelligence a source of happiness. Affect or emotion can also contribute to psychological problems, as when it is inconsistent with the event or idea that caused it or it is excessive or inadequate to the situation. For example, an individual who is frequently sad may be unpleasant to others and, as a result, have a deprived social life.

Extrinsic Factors

The environment provides many external cues to internal processes. The relationship of self to the environment is an equally important consideration in occupational therapy. For example, among adolescents, social cues from peers and their interpretation by the individual can have a significant impact on self-esteem. Societal values, such as the importance of work, may affect the self-identity of an individual who finds him- or herself unemployed. Cultural values and norms provide direction to individuals about how to feel or how to perceive events. For example, a woman may feel bad about being smart to the extent that her culture indicates this to be an undesirable trait for women.

An important aspect of interaction of the individual with the environment relates to perception about where control over events rests, or locus of control. Some individuals believe they can control, to a large extent, what happens to them. That is, they have an internal locus of control. Others believe the environment largely controls them (i.e., an external locus of control). Both behavior and assessment of events will be influenced by locus of control. For example, an individual with an internal locus of control may attribute success on the job to talent, while an individual with an external locus of control may attribute similar success to luck.

Outcomes of the Relationship Between Self and the Environment

The desired outcomes of self-evaluation and of perceptions about personal relationship to the environment are optimal occupational performance, health, and well-being. Well-being often results when an individual enjoys positive self-esteem because of optimal match between personal perception and feedback from the environment. When an individual does not experience well-being, an expression of dissatisfaction will be evident. This might be an expression of negative affect or of defense mechanisms such as denial or projection. To resolve such a situation, the individual may undertake to change behavior, change the environment, or revise his or her perceptions. An inability to resolve these discrepancies may lead to psychological dysfunction.

Motivation is described as the drive toward action, and it is related to the individual's wish for well-being. Motivation leads the person to interact with the environment in ways that can produce well-being (Mowen, 2000). Lack of motivation, or motivation to unproductive or ineffective action, can lead to dissatisfaction.

Self-efficacy is another outcome of effective interaction between the self and the environment. Self-efficacy is an individual's belief in his or her capabilities of performance toward a specific task (Gage & Polatajko, 1994). When individuals are able to interact with the environment in ways that produce desired results (i.e., a sense of well-being and heightened self-esteem), they will perceive themselves as capable and effective people.

Occupational therapy practitioners must take all psychological factors into consideration in practice. Individuals experiencing a physical impairment may experience associated psychological reactions, and occupational therapy intervention must be sensitive to these issues. Many disorders considered primarily physical in nature often have psychological features that must not go unnoticed. Traumatic brain injury (TBI) is a very appropriate example. Although it is often difficult to directly assess the emotional consequences of TBI because of the accompanying cognitive or physical limitations that make standard instruments unreliable, clinical depression, with all associated signs and symptoms such as sadness, tearfulness, lethargy, and guilt, are frequently observed in people with TBI. Failing to consider the psychological issues in individuals with TBI will obviously lead to ineffective intervention.

In conclusion, impairment at the body structure and body function level can lead to altered self-concept, lowered self-esteem, depression, and anxiety and, therefore, can cause limitations in activities and restriction in participation. These secondary consequences of an acquired disability must be addressed to enhance motivation of the client to participate in all aspects of rehabilitation. Psychological factors or constructs are not independent of each other; they interact in complicated ways that influence human occupations. Impaired psychological factors may cause more significant activity limitations in individuals who suffer from persistent mental illnesses such as major depression or schizophrenia; however, psychological factors influence performance in all humans at all stages across the lifespan and must always be considered in occupational therapy assessment and intervention.

COGNITIVE FACTORS

As noted by Duchek (1991), in its broadest form, cognition is "the acquisition and use of knowledge or the process of thinking" (p. 286) or the process of knowing (Cicerone et al., 2000). The functions subsumed under cognition are broad reaching, with the potential to impact the performance capabilities of clients across all other personal factors. Higher functions such as those involved in visual processing, language, sensory and motor processing, reasoning, problem solving, attention, and memory form the components of cognition. They rely on relatively large numbers of neural actions and interaction and may themselves have complex internal structures. Importantly, the neural operations that take place to produce these various cognitive functions can vary within different contexts. Cognitive functions are organized hierarchically, with the more complex drawing on collections of more fundamental functions. The more complex may have emergent properties that cannot be predicted based on simple interactions among simpler functions (Gazzaniga, Ivry, & Mangun, 2002).

Cognitive rehabilitation is a broad a term as is cognition, encompassing approaches focused on remediation through the development of compensatory skills. Such rehabilitation may focus on any and all areas of cognitive function, including attention, memory, perception, and comprehension, to list just a few. It has been suggested that cognitive rehabilitation be directed at achieving improvement in the performance of meaningful daily activity or meaningful occupations (Cicerone et al., 2000). The breadth of both cognition and cognitive rehabilitation makes study in these areas nearly overwhelming. Here, we will discuss just two of the above-mentioned cognitive processes to provide a perspective for the pervasive nature of cognitive factors on occupational performance: attention and memory. This is not to downplay the importance nor the pervasive nature of the other cognitive processes noted above. We will begin with attention.

Attention

Attention refers to our ability to concentrate our perceptual experience on a selected portion of the available sensory information and, in doing so, to achieve a clear and vivid impression of the environment. Attention reflects a narrowing of focus or the ability to focus mental effort and sustain and shift focus as needed. Attention is the initial step in the process of receiving information from the environment and is also the primary step in the memory process. Attention has several aspects, including alertness (physical and mental level of arousal needed to respond), selection (ability to decide upon what to focus our attention and what to ignore; includes ability to shift attention), and allocation (based on the idea that there is a limited capacity for attention and we make decisions as to how much of our capacity to allocate to specific activities, leaving more or less "left over" for split attention to something else) (Duchek, 1991).

Attentional deficits include such characteristics as insufficient alertness, inability to selectively attend or sustain attention over long periods of time, and inability to shift attention (Ben-Yishay & Diller, 1981). Any and all of these characteristics may impair memory and learning and, therefore, daily function. Attention deficits may be the result of an injury, as with TBI; a disorder, as with attention deficit disorder; or something as natural as the process of aging (Bruhn & Parsons, 1971; Turhim, 1993; Van Zomeren & Van DenBurg, 1985). In addition, medications often have, as side effects, detrimental influences on attention and attentional mechanisms. Because attention is the initial stage of information processing, attentional deficits can have profound negative effects on the performance of activities and occupations.

Through a systematic review of intervention for stroke-induced attentional problems, Lincoln and colleagues (2002) concluded that there was some support for the use of training to improve both alertness and sustained attention. However, they were able to identify only two studies that met their strict criteria. Cicerone and colleagues (2000) examined a broader array of literature on this topic and reached a similar conclusion. These authors further indicated that attention training should focus on the performance of functional tasks and may not be useful during the acute recovery phase. It is during this phase that spontaneous recovery of skills occurs and intervention effects cannot be determined.

Memory

Memory has both structure and process components. The structure component is our memory store and includes what we refer to as short, long, and sensory memory. The process of memory involves reproducing or recalling what has been learned, particularly through the use of associative mechanisms.

Memory processes involve our abilities to organize the information for later retrieval, and we use various strategies in accomplishing this task. For instance, as occupational therapy students in anatomy, you may have learned your cranial nerves by using a verbal mnemonic such as On Old Olympus' Towering Top A Finn And German Viewed Some Houses (Olfactory, Optic, Oculomotor, Trochlear, Trigeminal, Abducens, Facial, Acoustic [also known as Vestibulocochlear], Glossopharyngeal, Vagus, Spinal Accessory, Hypoglossal). Visual imagery is another tool that can be used in processing pieces of information, such as in linking a visual image to a name to enable your ability to remember it. As might be apparent at this point, memory storage processes are linked to retrieval.

Sensory memory is very short-term storage of basic information as it enters the nervous system. It remains modality specific (e.g., visual or auditory specific). From the very short-term storage depot, sensory memory is transferred for analysis, or it decays (Duchek, 1991).

Short-term memory is often referred to as working memory and has limited capacity. Generally, the capacity in short-term memory is for seven items or seven chunks of material, and, therefore, working memory can be increased by chunking information into groups. Our ability to hold information in short-term memory lasts for about 30 seconds, but if rehearsal takes place, the length of storage can be increased. The rehearsal serves to refresh the memory store repeatedly. In practice, rehearsal is one of the most commonly used strategies that occupational therapy practitioners recommend to clients with memory deficits. It is important to remember that the improved short-term memory contributed to rehearsal is subject to interruption and loss of the memory trace.

Long-term memory is a form of memory storage assumed to be permanent, although it has been suggested that we may lose the ability to access some of our long-term memories. The organization of this structural memory has been suggested to be complex, such that it houses different information in different ways, and allows us to search only parts of this vast store of knowledge, depending on what we are looking to find. For instance, some time ago, Tulving (1972) suggested that we stored both episodic and semantic memories, where episodic memory consisted of personal events with some temporal reference and retrieval was generally guided by time tags, while semantic memory was that of general knowledge, with retrieval guided by dimensions such as meaning, associations, or rules.

A second useful means of dividing memory stores is procedural versus declarative memory. Using this categorization, procedural knowledge is the knowledge of "how"—a representation of a set of procedures that are easily shown, but not easily described. For example, you would remember how to ride a bicycle very well even though you first learned it more than 10 years ago and had not been riding it for 5 years. In contrast, declarative memories are knowledge of facts. They are relatively easy to describe verbally and tend to be well-organized memories. You likely remember important dates in your life, such as birthdates for yourself, your significant other, your children and/or parents, and other close friends and relatives. Such declarative memories may be stored by month, or perhaps by your relationship to the person.

Although neither of these categorical divisions of long-term memory holds up under the strictest scrutiny, they are both useful when looking at disorders of memory. Memory deficits arise from several disorders such as head injury, chronic alcohol abuse, or Alzheimer's disease. It is the most common consequence of brain injury (Erikson & Scott, 1977). Memory loss is also a function of normal aging. Typical aging seems not to affect sensory memory, nor the passive retention of information in short-term memory (Bee & Bjorklund, 2000). In contrast, manipulating the information placed in short-term memory is subject to the effects of natural aging (Salthouse, 1994; Smith, 1996). Aging effects on long-term memory are seen in slower retrieval, particularly with recall type of memory (Gutman, 2001; Labouvie-Vief & Schell, 1982). Aging also appears to have a greater impact on episodic long-term memory, while semantic remains largely intact. In contrast, Alzheimer's disease leads to deficits of both short- and long-term memory and deficits with episodic tasks involving new information processing. Memory involving automatic processes remains, and procedural memory can also be retained.

Engagement in meaningful activity can be profoundly impacted by memory deficits. Memory processing, storage, and retrieval deficits will impact clients at the very heart of their insight, awareness, and motivation in any intervention program. Occupational therapy practitioners must understand the structure and the process of memory and that the breakdown of memory process can happen at any level. For example, if an individual is unable to attend, the information may never enter the system. Some patients are able to process information in short-term or working memory, but never encode the material into long-term storage. Others can store the information but have a deficit in the retrieval process.

Intervention using simple techniques such as teaching mental imagery, encoding, attention, and relaxation, as well as the use of memory aids such as lists, have been shown to be beneficial (Berg, Konig-Haanstra, & Deelman, 1991; Burack & Lachman, 1996; Gutman, 2001; Stiggsdotter & Backman, 1989; Wilson, 1982; Yesavage, Lapp, & Sheikh, 1989). It is worth mentioning here that individuals with memory deficits may also have difficulty forgetting information that is no longer needed, resulting in unnecessary information overload. We need to keep this in mind when we teach and recommend memory strategies in intervention. We must avoid information overload and, in turn, cause more impairment of memory. Occupational therapy practitioners must understand all cognitive components influencing personal performance capabilities in order to successfully intervene.

Memory interventions were the subject of a recent critical analysis and review (Majid, Lincoln, & Weyman, 2002), a literature review (Cicerone et al., 2000), and a meta-analysis (Loya, 2001). While Majid and colleagues found mixed results in randomized controlled trials, both Loya and Cicerone et al. felt there was sufficient evidence to support the use of compensatory memory training. Cicerone and coworkers suggested that these techniques were effective if mild deficits were present, if clients had some independence in daily living skills, and if clients were participatory in choosing the memory deficits upon which they wished to focus. Motivation was noted to be an important contributor to successful outcome. Cicerone and colleagues caution that there is no evidence suggesting that such remediation is successful with clients experiencing more significant memory deficits.

In summary, the cognitive factor is made of higher functions of the nervous system, including those involved in visual processing, language, sensory and motor processing, reasoning, problem solving, attention, and memory. We have specifically addressed only two, attention and memory, here. This means we have barely scratched the surface of what we need to really understand about cognition in the practice of occupational therapy. However, this is a good place to begin because these aspects of cognition are not independent of each other, nor are they separate from the other functions listed here. A recent view of attentional processes suggests that cognition and attention arise from the same neural framework, both dependent on the coupling of person and environment (Lacoboni, 2000). This conceptualization fits well with the PEOP model and reinforces our need to examine the person factors (in this case, cognitive) along with the environmental factors when we are working on occupational performance.

NEUROBEHAVIORAL FACTORS

Neuroscience is the study of the nervous system structure, function, and development and includes the brain, the spinal cord, and networks of nerve cells (neurons) throughout the body. Neuroscientists use tools ranging from computers to special dyes to examine molecules, nerve cells, networks, brain systems, and behavior to advance the understanding of human thought, emotion, and behavior. From these studies, we learn how the nervous system develops and functions normally and what goes wrong in neurological disorders.

Neuroscience is now an interdisciplinary field that integrates biology, chemistry, and physics with studies of structure, physiology, and behavior, including human emotional and cognitive function that is necessary for everyday life. Through their research, neuroscientists work to describe the human brain and how it functions normally; to determine how the nervous system develops, matures, and maintains itself throughout the lifespan; and to find ways to prevent or cure many devastating neurological and psychiatric disorders.

Neuroscience research includes genes and other molecules that are the basis for the nervous system, individual neurons, and ensembles of neurons that make up systems and behavior. At the molecular level, neuroscientists use tools such as antibodies and gene probes to isolate and identify proteins and other molecules responsible for brain function. Molecular biologists isolate and describe the genes that produce the proteins important to neuron function. Neuroanatomists study the structure and organization of the nervous system. With special dyes, they detect specific neurotransmitters and mark neurons and synapses with specific characteristics and functions. Developmental neuroscientists study how the brain grows and changes. They define chemicals and processes neurons use to seek out and connect with other neurons and maintain connections. Behavioral neuroscientists study the processes underlying behavior in humans and in animals. Their tools include microelectrodes, which measure electrical activity of neurons, and brain scans, which show parts of the brain that are active during activities such as seeing, speaking, or remembering.

Cognitive neuroscience is a relatively new interdisciplinary field of study that uses the expertise of cognitive psychologists and researchers in the brain sciences and computer science to study the way the brain and mind use knowledge to guide thought and action. Cognitive neuroscience is about how information is acquired (sensation), interpreted to confer meaning (perception/recognition), stored or modified (learning/memory), used to ruminate (thinking/consciousness), used to predict the future state of the environment and the consequences of action (decision making), used to guide behavior (motor control), and used to communicate (language). In other words, cognitive neuroscience seeks to integrate what is known at the microscopic and molecular levels of single neurons and neuronal networks with the systems level represented by behavior (Churchland & Sejnowski, 1988). Cognitive neuroscientists study functions such as perception and memory in animals by using behavioral methods and other neuroscience techniques. In humans, they use noninvasive brain scans, such as positron emission tomography and magnetic resonance imaging, to uncover routes of neural processing that occur during language, problem solving, and other tasks.

Advanced computer systems are enabling neuroscientists to devise models of neurons and their connections in the brain—how humans perform complex tasks. This work may lead to computer programs that understand speech and respond to spoken questions.

Clinical neuroscientists such as psychiatrists, neurologists, and other medical specialists use basic research findings to develop diagnostic methods and ways to prevent and treat neurological disorders that affect millions of people.

A detailed introduction to the nervous system is beyond the scope of this chapter. Interested readers may find the following useful, although there are many other books with equally as much information that may be of use as well:

Cohen, H. (1999). *Neuroscience for rehabilitation* (2nd ed.). Baltimore, MD: Lippincott, Williams & Wilkins.

Gutman, S. A. (2001). *Quick reference neuroscience for rehabilitation professionals*. Thorofare, NJ: SLACK Incorporated.

Lundy-Ekman, L. (1998). *Neuroscience fundamentals for rehabilitation*. Philadelphia, PA: W. B. Saunders Co.

The above texts combine a good deal of functional information with their neuroanatomy, and all are written for the world of occupational and physical therapists. The reader will find Lundy-Ekman to have less text but very useful and plentiful color diagrams and figures. Cohen is more densely packed with information with black-and-white line drawings.

The following texts have tombs of knowledge and are excellent resources, but neither would be considered an entry-level book:

Kandel, E. R., Schwartz, J. H., & Jessell, T. M. (2000). *Principles of neural science* (4th ed.). New York, NY: McGraw-Hill.

Zigmond, M. J., Bloom, F. E., Landic, S. C., Roberts, J. L., & Squire, L. R. (1999). *Fundamental neuroscience*. Boston, MA: Academic Press.

These following texts contain general knowledge of neuroscience, and they are somewhat easier to read:

Gilman, S., & Newman, S. W. (1992). *Essentials of clinical neuroanatomy and neurophysiology* (9th ed.). Philadelphia, PA: F. A. Davis.

Haines, D. E. (1997). *Fundamental neuroscience*. New York, NY: Churchill Livingstone.

Kandel, E. R., Schwartz, J. H., & Jessell, T. M. (1995). *Essentials of neural science and behavior*. Norwalk, CT: Appleton & Lange.

Kingsley, R. E. (2000). *Concise text of neuroscience*. Philadelphia, PA: Lippincott, Williams & Wilkins.

In this chapter, we will talk about the importance of the impact of neurobehavioral factors on human performance. Humans contain roughly 100 billion neurons, the functional units of the nervous system. Neurons communicate with each other by sending electrical signals long distances and then releasing chemicals called neurotransmitters, which cross synapses, the small gaps between neurons. Critical components of the nervous system are molecules, neurons, and the processes within and between cells. These are organized into large neural networks and systems controlling functions such as vision, hearing, breathing, and, ultimately, all of human behavior. The importance of the neurobehavioral factors was introduced early in the development of occupational therapy when Meyer (1922) observed the restorative benefits of engagement in occupation on the behavior of those receiving services. As suggested by the PEOP model, various neurobehavioral factors must be considered for their potential to shape functional performance. For example, the sensory (olfactory, gustatory, visual, auditory, somatosensory, proprioceptive, and vestibular) and motor systems (somatic, cerebellum, basal ganglia network, thalamic integration) provide basis for all neuromotor performance. Occupational therapy practitioners must understand their clients' ability to control movement, to modulate sensory input, to coordinate and integrate sensory information, to compensate for sensorimotor deficits, and to modify neural structures through behavior. These are all important characteristics that influence and support occupational performance. During occupational therapy assessment, the capacity of the sensory and motor system must be determined to facilitate adaptive and/or compensatory responses. Occupational therapy interventions must be guided by basic neurobehavioral principles to generate optimal benefit from therapy.

Neuroscience research holds great promise for understanding and treating spinal cord injury, stroke, schizophrenia, Alzheimer's disease, and other conditions. The field of neuroscience is helping occupational therapy practitioners understand how experiences generate changes in the nervous system that shape language, vision, coordinated movement, and cognition (Merzenich, Schreiner, Jenkins, & Wang, 1993). The goal of occupational therapy is to minimize the consequences of neurological insult in those whose injuries adversely limit their activities and restrict their participation.

Genetic Factors

Genetics is a diverse subject that is concerned with variation and heredity in all living organisms. Within this broad field, human genetics is the science of variation and heredity in human beings. Medical genetics is the science of human biological variation as it relates to health and disease (Lou, 2002a).

Medical genetics is a branch of medicine dealing with the inheritance, diagnosis, and treatment of diseases due to different types of genetic effects (i.e., single gene mutations, chromosome abnormalities, and multifactorial predisposition). In other words, medical genetics include the studies of the pattern of inheritance of diseases in families, the mapping of disease genes to specific locations on chromosomes, analyses of the molecular mechanisms through which genes cause disease, and the diagnosis and treatment of genetic disease. Medical genetics also includes genetic counseling, which involves the communication of information regarding risks, prognoses, and treatment to clients and their families.

The genetic information, in the form of genes, is passed down through the family from ancestors such as great-grandparents, to grandparents, to parents, and to their children. If this inherited information is changed, it may cause a genetic disorder resulting in impairment of body structure/function, limitation in activities, and restriction of participation. Many of the health or developmental problems seen at birth are due to either a direct change in the genetic information or a combination of the inherited genetic information and environmental causes such as diet, chemical exposure, or lifestyle. Genetic disorders may also first be noticed in childhood, adolescence, or in adulthood.

The successes of the Human Genome Project have enabled researchers to pinpoint errors in genes, the smallest units of heredity that cause or contribute to disease (Collins, 1999; Collins & McKusick, 2001). We now know that heritable variations in genes contribute to not only rare conditions, but to a host of common conditions such as heart diseases, diabetes, Alzheimer's disease, and many types of cancer and mental illnesses. In other words, scientists now believe that all diseases have a genetic component, whether inherited or resulting from the body's response to environmental stresses like viruses or toxins, or a combination of both (Nathan, Fontanarosa, & Wilson, 2001).

Table 12-2 lists the top 10 causes of death in 1998. With the exception of injury, nine of the top leading causes of mortality all have genetic components.

The following provides a very brief introduction to some basic concepts in medical genetics, and the different types of genetic conditions that occupational therapy practitioners often encounter in their practice.

Table 12-2 Top 10 Leading Causes of Mortality in 1998

1. Heart disease (31.0%)
2. Cancer (23.2%)
3. Stroke (6.8%)
4. Chronic obstructive pulmonary disease (4.8%)
5. Injury (4.2%)
6. Pneumonia/influenza (3.9%)
7. Diabetes (2.8%)
8. Suicide (1.3%)
9. Kidney disease (1.1%)
10. Chronic liver disease (1.1%)

Adapted from Jorde, L. B., Carey, J. C., White, R. L., & Bamshad, M. J. (2000). *Medical genetics* (2nd ed.). St. Louis, MO: Mosby.

Chromosomes and Genes

Chromosomes are microscopic structures that are present inside the nucleus of the cells. There are 46 chromosomes in each somatic cell (all human cells except the reproductive cells) of our bodies. Mature reproductive cells, eggs and sperms, contain only 23 chromosomes. Chromosomes contain the genes or packages of hereditary information, which are passed down from one generation to the next. It is estimated that humans have about 30,000 genes. The chromosomes come in 23 pairs with one member of each pair having been donated by the individual's mother and the other being donated by the individual's father. Only one of the 23 pairs of chromosomes differs in males and females. These are the sex chromosomes. While females have two "X" chromosomes, males have an "X" and "Y" chromosome. The other 22 chromosomes are called autosomes. The chromosomes, in turn, are made of genes, which are the individual units of hereditary material. Similar to chromosomes, genes come in pairs, with one member of each pair also coming from either parent. When individuals make sperm or egg cells, they pass down half of their chromosomes and, thus, half of their genes to their children. The genes provide the cells with a set of instructions for growth and development through their products, which are called proteins. The proteins are the building blocks of our structure and are primarily made of amino acids. The genes, which are made of long chains of DNA, are made of molecules called nucleotides. The nucleotides are made of sugar, phosphate, and a nitrogen-containing molecule called base. There are four types of bases: Adenine (A), Thymine (T), Guanine (G), and Cytosine (C). (They may be remembered as A, T, G, and C). Genes work or function by using three bases, called a triplet or trinucleotide, as a mold or pattern to determine the sequence of amino acids. A mutation in the gene results in a change in the sequence of bases (loss, addition, or misspell of the bases) causing disruption of the function of the gene.

Types of Genetic Conditions

Clinically, there are four types of genetic conditions we often see in our practices: single gene disorders, chromosomal abnormalities, multifactorial traits and disorders, and mitochondrial disorders.

1. Single gene (Mendelian or monogenic) disorders: Produced by the effects of one gene or gene pair. Such traits are transmitted in simple patterns as originally described by Mendel.
   a. Autosomal dominant disorders: Dominant inheritance means one copy of the abnormal gene is sufficient to cause disease. Autosomal dominant disorders are transmitted on the nonsex chromosomes (i.e., chromosomes other than the X or Y) and are expressed when only a single copy of the mutant gene is present. Huntington's disease is an example of an autosomal dominant disorder.
   b. Autosomal recessive disorders: Recessive inheritance means two abnormal copies of the relevant gene must be present in the affected individual. Autosomal recessive disorders are transmitted on the nonsex chromosomes and are only expressed when both copies of a gene are mutant. Cystic fibrosis is an example of autosomal recessive disorder.
   c. X-linked disorders are transmitted on the X chromosome. An example of an X-linked disorder is Duchenne muscular dystrophy.

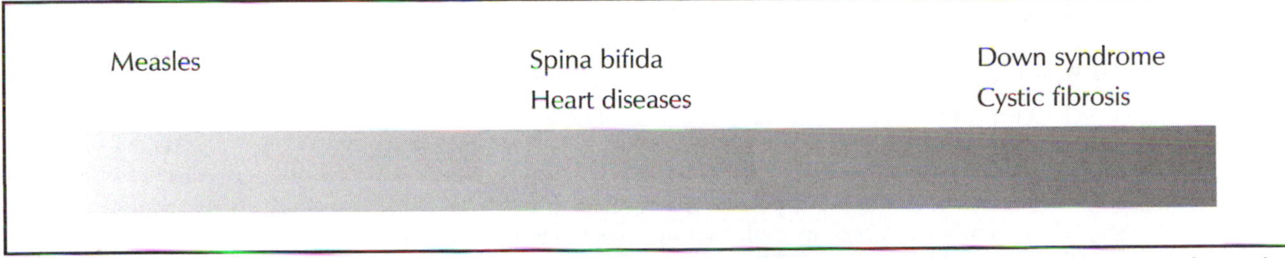

Figure 12-2. The continuum of genetic influence. (Reprinted with permission from Lou, J. Q. (2002b). (Ed.). *Medical genetics: Challenges and opportunities for health professionals.* Dubuque, IA: Kendall/Hunt Publishing Company.)

Table 12-3

Examples of Inheritable Traits and Disorders

	Examples
Completely heritable (or nearly completely)	Gender, eye color, skin color, cystic fibrosis, muscular dystrophy, and many forms of deafness
Partially heritable	Height, cognition, body mass, personality traits (at least many traits), diabetes, asthma, schizophrenia
Not heritable (or only very weakly)	Distance a person lives from work

Reprinted with permission from Lou, J. Q. (2002b). Genetic, Human Genome Project and occupational therapy practice. *Occupational Therapy in Health Care, 14*(2), 67-78.

2. Chromosome abnormalities are deviations from the normal chromosome number or structure. Examples include Down syndrome and Turner syndrome.
3. Multifactorial traits and disorders result from the combined effects of multiple genetic and nongenetic influences. Examples include spina bifida, common types of cancer, and atherosclerotic heart disease.
4. Mitochondrial disorders are a relatively small number of diseases caused by alterations in the small cytoplasmic mitochondrial chromosome. Examples include certain types of blindness, hearing loss, and certain neurological conditions.

Of these major classes of diseases, the single-gene disorders have probably received the greatest amount of attention. While some genetic disorders, particularly the single gene conditions, are strongly determined by genes, many others are the result of multiple genetic and nongenetic factors. We can therefore think of genetic diseases as lying along a continuum (Figure 12-2), with disorders such as cystic fibrosis and Duchenne muscular dystrophy situated at one end (strongly determined by genes) and conditions such as measles situated at the other (strongly determined by environment). Many of the most prevalent disorders, such as many birth defects and common diseases such as diabetes, hypertension, heart disease, and cancer, lie somewhere in the middle of the continuum. These diseases are the products of varying degrees of both genetic and environmental influences. Table 12-3 provides examples of inheritable traits and disorders on the continuum.

Strategies to Deal With Genetic Disorders

Occupational therapy practitioners encounter individuals with genetic conditions daily, regardless of the settings within which we practice. We must become familiar with the approaches in intervening genetic disorders and understand our roles in dealing with them.

Prevention

Some people are more at risk than others for developing a condition that is due to the combination of environmental factors with the genetic information they have inherited. They are "genetically predisposed" to develop these disorders. However, the presence of an environmental "trigger" is necessary for the person to be affected with the condition. In some cases, prevention of the disorder can be achieved by preventing the person from being exposed to the particular environmental factor that will trigger the disorder. For example, it is possible to prevent about 70% of the cases of spina bifida in babies by taking folic acid before and during early pregnancy (Jorde, Carey, White, & Bamshad, 2000).

Early Diagnosis and Treatment

In some genetic disorders, early diagnosis, sometimes even before the symptoms appear, can lead to specific treatment. For example, all newborn babies in America are screened for phenylketonuria (PKU) by a simple blood test. Diagnosis and treatment within the first month of life are crucial to avoid intellectual disability. Also, some forms of cancer that have a genetic component (e.g., breast cancer and bowel cancer) can be detected early enough for treatment to take place (Lou & Culver, 2002).

Genetic Counseling

Genetic counseling is available to families and individuals who have concerns about a disorder in their family that may have a genetic basis. A team of health professionals, which may include clinical geneticists, genetic counselors, and other health care professions, work together to provide information and supportive counseling. Families may then be better able to understand and adjust to the diagnosis of a genetic disorder (Lazzarini & Lou, 2002).

Support Groups

Support groups provide affected individuals and families with information about the disorder, community resources, and understanding and empathy. There are also a number of "umbrella" organizations for genetic support groups (e.g., Genetic Alliance [www.geneticalliance.org] and National Organization for Rare Disorders [NORD] [www.rarediseases.org]) that provide support and information for those families and individuals affected by a disorder so rare that there is no specific support group.

With genetics as the common link to disease, aging, and personality, occupational therapy practitioners in traditional, community-based, and emerging practice areas will all find themselves and their clients affected by the ethical, legal, social, and financial implications (ELSI) of the advances in genetics. Occupational therapy professionals must appreciate clinical expression (body function and body structure) of most conditions and how the genetic influence affects individuals' performance (activities and participation).

Modern medicine is placing an increasing emphasis on the importance of prevention. Because genetics provides a basis for understanding the fundamental biological makeup of the organism, it naturally leads to a better understanding of the disease process. In many cases, this knowledge can lead to the actual prevention of the disorder. It also leads to more effective disease treatment. Prevention and effective treatment are among the highest goals of medicine.

In occupational therapy, understanding a client's genetic makeup and predisposition for conditions can also prove valuable for treatment planning and developing intervention strategies for clients. With updated information in hand, occupational therapy practitioners can tailor goals toward the individual more effectively. Expanding knowledge of genetics will promote an individualized approach to health care focused on maintaining health, rather than treating diseases. This important challenge provides an exciting opportunity for occupational therapy professionals to appropriately use genetic information in health promotion and disease prevention activities (Kyler & Thomas, 2002; Lou, 2002b; Schroeder-Smith, Tischenkel, DeLange, & Lou, 2002).

Every domain of occupational therapy can in some way address the host of physical, cognitive, and psychosocial issues that individuals and families may face as genetic conditions affect their lives. As society addresses the ELSI of the Human Genome Project, occupational therapy professionals must develop and maintain competencies in genetics so they may fulfill occupational therapy's evolving role in meeting the challenges of the changing health care system (Kyler, 2000; Lou, 2002b). This position is clearly illustrated by AOTA's position statement:

> The American Occupational Therapy Association (AOTA) promotes the concept of genetics literacy among occupational therapy practitioners to help ensure competent occupational therapy services as part of individual, group, and population-based interventions. AOTA is committed to assisting practitioners learn and apply genetic information to practice, and in so doing, proactively assures that recipients of occupational therapy services are not denied full access to the benefits of society by the revelation of genetic information. (Commission on Practice for the American Occupational Therapy Association, 2001)

Spiritual Factors

Humans are not simply physical beings living in a physical world; they are also spiritual beings in a world full of symbolic meaning. Health care and medicine have been slow to recognize and acknowledge that the beliefs and meanings permeating daily life can influence a person's health status. Many have argued that prayer and other forms of metaphysical expression cannot be studied scientifically because direct observation of such phenomena cannot occur. Yet, more than half of the American public believes that faith and prayer can influence healing and recovery (King & Bushwick, 1994). Although rigorous studies of spirituality and its influence on health have been limited, several long-term studies are underway.

While no consensus definition of spirituality has emerged among health care researchers, there seems to be agreement in occupational therapy and other disciplines that the concept is broad and includes but goes beyond those beliefs and behaviors associated with traditional religious practices and a belief in God. In this broader definition, spirituality includes connections with one's self, with others, with nature, and with a higher power or source of ultimate meaning (Plotnifkoff, 2003). Egan and DeLaat (1994) were among the first occupational therapists to suggest the need for including spirituality as a dimension of the person that influences health and well-being. They asserted that spirituality is expressed through engagement in everyday occupations and concluded that spirituality is the essence or core being of the self. Christiansen (1997) agreed that spirituality has a central role in everyday existence and that it includes religious beliefs and practices but goes beyond these to embrace any activity that offers opportunity to connect one's existence to something that has greater meaning and more enduring significance than the self. Similarly, an individual's spirit becomes a life-giving force that provides motivation and direction and impels one to act with certain purposes in mind within an overall context of meaning.

In the PEOP model, and in occupational therapy generally, meaning is thought to influence health through its connection to occupation. Recent research by Persson (2001) suggests that this occurs through patterns of activity and values. Spiritual expression is one dimension of meaning-making through occupation. However, as noted by Urbanowski & Vargo (1994), because of its pervasive and individual nature, spirituality is difficult to define in a manner that allows it to be used in the selection of occupations that will enhance well-being for any given individual.

Abraham Maslow, known best for his need driven theory of motivation, identified higher order or "being" needs as essential for people who become self-actualized (Maslow, 1968). His studies suggested that people who were self-actualizers were able to transcend self-interest, identify a connection with others and the larger universe, were motivated less by self-interest and more by ultimate goodness, and view life as sacred, looking for the sacred in all aspects of their lives. Maslow found that these types of individuals were more inclined to have had peak experiences and to find awe, joy, mystery, humility, sacrifice, and inspiration among their happiest and most significant moments in life (Fuller, 1994; Maslow, 1970a). Maslow was clear that these spiritual dimensions were distinct from organized religion and believed that spirituality enhanced life experience, served as a driving source of motivation, and provided the means through which meaning derived through self-development could be connected to the larger universe; thus, promoting health and wellness (Maslow, 1970b).

The implied connection between meaning and an integrated, robust sense of self with health has been suggested in several psychological models, particularly those pertaining to the area of life stress and coping. The common thesis underlying these models has been that just as healthy bodies provide organized systems of defense to injuries and disease using available resources in an integrated manner, so too do healthy people have lifestyles with behavioral patterns that permit the optimal use of resources in a coordinated, integrated, and effective manner. A large body of literature has accumulated in the past two decades that links certain behavioral tendencies or personality types with measures of health. For example, Kobasa (1979) identified the characteristics of the hardy personality, which she identified as having a life commitment, a sense of being in control, and a tendency to view stressful circumstances as opportunities for growth and challenge, rather than as threats. This research is similar to the idea of a sense of coherence advanced by Aaron Antonovsky, an Israeli psychologist. Antonovsky's Salutogenic model (Antonovsky, 1975) suggests that people who have a central meaning associated with their lives, who perceive their lives as understandable, and who believe they have the resources to manage daily needs and threats will be better able to ward off illness and disease than those who do not demonstrate these characteristics. Research on the sense of coherence has also demonstrated evidence showing that these characteristics are associated with measures of better health (Ivimäki et al., 2002).

Evidence that supports the hypothesized relationship between spiritual practices and behaviors and health status has accumulated. A systematic review of more than 1,100 studies on the religion/health relationship showed a relationship between greater religious involvement and better mental health, better physical health, or lower use of health services (Koenig, McCullough, & Larson, 2000). Some of these studies have been criticized for methodological weaknesses (Sloan, Baglella, & Powell, 1999) such as those showing a correlation of health status with church attendance that fail to control for the likelihood that those attending church services may be self-selected because their functional status enables them to participate more than people with illness or chronic disease and disability.

Ryff and Singer (1998; Singer & Ryff, 1999) have shown that people who have a sense of meaning and purpose in life and who possess a personal awareness of self-realization and growth also enjoy better physical health. Studies of self-worth or self-esteem or those that measure the extent that an individual is able to perceive meaning and integrate life experiences have also shown to be related to better physical health (Akkasilpa, Minor, Goldman,

Magder, & Petri, 2000). Similarly, studies of intimacy and closeness to others have shown relationships to health and well-being (Fratiglioni, Wang, Ericsson, Maytan, & Winblad, 2000; Hafen, Karren, Frandsen, & Smith, 1996). A few studies have shown a positive relationship between perceived meaning in life activities and well-being (Christiansen, Backman, Little, & Nguyen, 1999; Little, 1998). In sum, the research cited above tends to validate the concept that spirituality and meaning are important personal dimensions in models of health and well-being that are expressed in everyday activities and lifestyles.

How might a sense of meaning and purpose lead to lifestyles that are health promoting? It is likely that people who possess higher levels of meaning and purpose are likely to choose daily occupations and engage in behaviors that create physiological advantages (such as lower serum cholesterol or blood pressure) and allow them to avoid behaviors and practices that can be harmful to health over time (such as over-eating, smoking, and excessive alcohol consumption). Conversely, it is possible that harmful daily practices are motivated by the desire to escape lives that are lacking in meaning, purpose, or opportunities for self-realization.

From the standpoint of occupational therapy practice, it is important for therapists to be aware of the growing literature that supports the importance of spiritual meaning and to help their patients clearly identify opportunities for creating meaning through participation and engagement in activities that align with their stories, beliefs, and life purposes. In recognizing this potential, Howard and Howard (1997) noted that occupational therapists can bring spirituality into practice when they create opportunities to enable patients to be engaged in meaningful activity and to connect with others.

Conclusion

This chapter has emphasized personal factors influencing occupational performance. Occupational therapy practitioners strive to identify all the factors that contribute to optimal performance if they are to provide their clients with the best possible intervention and if they are to achieve the best possible outcomes. They must consider these personal factors simultaneously; to break them up as has been done in the past, into physical factors, psychosocial factors, medical factors, etc., is to do our clients a disservice. We have attempted to point out how the various personal factors have both their own great depth in science, but also how they each overlap the other when we look at them from the occupational performance perspective. The following case briefly illustrates the depth of personal factors as well as their interlinkages.

Case Study: Child With Autism

Austin is a 3½-year-old child currently carrying a diagnosis of pervasive developmental disorder. He has been enrolled in an ABA intervention program to focus on the development of specific skills and has been receiving occupational and speech therapy services in his home for about 1 year. There is currently some friction between service providers about the best way to continue the provision of services.

According to his parents, Austin has poor receptive and expressive language skills, although he can sing some songs (Old MacDonald) and identify familiar people in pictures. He can feed himself, but would prefer to play with his food. He does not play with toys, but rather carries them from place to place, lays them down and stares at them, and then moves to another place. His parents currently see Austin as a child with very inconsistent behaviors; one minute he can be very loving and the next very aggressive. He seems sometimes to enjoy activities and sometimes to dislike the same activities. His behavioral outbursts are severe, and this prevents him from having playmates and prevents his parents from taking him to places where other children are playing. It also prevents his parents from enrolling him in a regular preschool or play group. They are equally uncomfortable leaving him with a baby-sitter.

His parents are beginning to look to transitioning Austin to placement within a school setting, and as such it is an ideal time to look at Austin using the PEOP model.

Occupational History

Austin, age 3½; gross motor milestones on time; fine motor milestones slightly delayed; began finger feeding at 12 months but has since stopped; at present is an agile climber, seeks movement activities; enjoys wet or messy activities; mouths most toys and objects, somewhat indiscriminately; enjoys books, especially those that make sounds;

(continued)

plays some social games with adults, enjoying those in which he can anticipate the outcome; makes limited eye contact and typically does not respond to name.

Factors	Examples of Intrinsic Performance Enablers	Examples of Intrinsic Constraints on Actions, Tasks, Roles, and Occupations
Physiological	Intact physiologic systems Good general health	No constraints
Psychological	Engaging and affectionate with familiar adults Responds well behaviorally to structured tasks in which he can anticipate subsequent steps	Limited cooperation for tasks in which he is not interested Can have aggressive outbursts when frustrated
Cognitive	Visual learning strength Enjoys books, especially those that make sounds Will sing songs Can name familiar people in pictures	Expressive language delays (10 to 15 word vocabulary) Receptive language delay Short attention span Excessive mouthing Limited eye contact Cognitive potential unclear at this point
Neurobehavioral	Enjoys movement activities with intense vestibular inputs	Ataxia Underresponsive to touch and movement Overresponsive to some visual input
Genetic	No familial history of autism or related disorders	
Environmental	Caregivers willing to work with him in an ABA program Receiving other services (Education, OT, ST)	Disagreement between ABA trainers and educators and related service personnel on best means of working with him (ABA vs. traditional preschool environment for children with special needs) No opportunity for socialization in current environment due to intervention within home using ABA format

Impairment of body structure and function: Austin has no impairments here.

Activity limitation: Austin has many activity limitations resulting from the constraints noted above. At present, his parents' main concern is communication, as this leads to frustration for them. The failure to communicate effectively also precipitates concerns for the future in terms of school placement, child care, and socialization. Activity limitations cross both play/leisure and self-care.

Participation restriction: Austin has many participation restrictions as well, due to the noted constraints. His behavior is a major barrier to participation in social events, integration into a regular preschool classroom, and participation in play activities on the local playground, and thus improved behavior has become a parental goal.

We find that Austin's cognitive, psychological, and neurobehavioral factors place primary constraints on his ability to engage in activities, tasks, and roles of childhood. In addition, they appear to be limiting his ability to participate in typical childhood environments. Austin's parents are concerned about these limitations. This would be a logical place to begin assessment and intervention, expanding on our knowledge of his strengths and needs in these areas and meshing them with parental desires.

There are also barriers presented by the environmental issues at play here. Austin's parents have enrolled him in an intervention program, ABA, which is not universally accepted and supported. This has created its own friction among the service providers working with this family and has led to additional complications for Austin and his family. Thus, for Austin, we see not only the complex interaction of the personal factors that have been addressed in this chapter, but also the interaction of personal factors with environmental factors. In this case, both work to limit his ability to participate fully in the occupations of childhood. To address these issues of participation, the occupational therapy practitioner will need to work from both sides of this model, addressing Austin's personal performance constraints and the environmental barriers he and his family are facing. The best approach will likely involve a team effort.

Evidence Worksheet

Authors	*Year*	*Topic*	*Method*	*Conclusion*
Adler, Holland, Enseleit, & Strakowski	2001	Age-related changes in regional activation during working memory in young adults	Case control cohort study	Increasing age is associated with increased activation of hippocampus even in young patients without evidence of working memory deficits and performing functional tasks may elicit changes that precede overt evidence of working memory deficits
Anderson et al.	2000	The effects of divided attention on encoding- and retrieval-related brain activity	Case control cohort study	These results indicate that prefrontal functional specificity of episodic memory is reduced by aging
Baker, Cesa, Gatz, & Mellins	1992	Genetic and environmental influences on positive and negative affect: support for a two-factor theory	Twin study	The results document differential genetic and environmental influences on positive and negative affect, providing further support for their being separate components of well-being
Bell, Bryson, Greig, Corcoran, & Wexler	2001	Neurocognitive enhancement therapy with work therapy: effects on neuropsychological test performance	Randomized controlled trial	Computer training for cognitive dysfunction in patients with schizophrenia can have benefits that generalize to independent outcome measures. Efficacy may result from a synergy between NET, which encourages mental activity, and WT, which allows a natural context for mental activity to be exercised, generalized, and reinforced
Bergeman, Plomin, Pedersen, & McClearn	1991	Genetic mediation of the relationship between social support and psychological well-being	Adoption/twin study	The results indicated that the relationship between the perceived adequacy of social support and psychological well-being (depression and life satisfaction) was mediated in part by genetic factors
Brown, Harwood, Hays, Heckman, & Short	1993	Cognitive rehabilitation and improving attention in patients with schizophrenia	Cohort; randomized to one of two treatment groups	No treatment effect; improvements in both groups for measures of attention. Suggest that the individualized intervention in a structured environment as the critical aspect leading to improvement. No improvements in problem solving *(continued)*

Authors	*Year*	*Topic*	*Method*	*Conclusion*
Burack & Lachman	1996	List making and recall in young and elderly adults	Cohort study	List making was an effective strategy for elderly adults, improving ability to recall information even without reference to list. List making did not make a difference for younger adults
Finkel, Pedersen, Berg, & Johansson	2000	Quantitative genetic analysis of bio-behavioral markers of aging in Swedish studies of adult twins	Twin study	Results indicate one aging theory cannot account for changes in all markers of aging. Aging of various systems occurs as a result of different combinations of genetic and environmental influences
Giles & Clark-Wilson	1988	The use of behavioral techniques in functional skills training after severe brain injury	Single case studies	Functional skills training following acquired brain injury depends on motivation; reinforcement that increases motivation is most useful. It is important that patients make independent choices (intrinsic motivation)
Loya	2001	A meta-analysis of memory rehabilitation among adolescent and adult traumatic brain injury survivors	Meta-analysis	Medium or better effect size from intervention

References

Adler, C. M., Holland, S. K., Enseleit, S., & Strakowski, S. M. (2001). Age-related changes in regional activation during working memory in young adults: An MRI study. *Synapse, 42*, 252-257.

Akkasilpa, S., Minor, M., Goldman, D., Magder, L. S., & Petri, M. (2000). Association of coping responses with fibromyalgia tender points in patients with systemic lupus erythematosus. *The Journal of Rheumatology, 27*(3), 671-674.

Anderson, N. D., Iidaka, T., Cabeza, R., Kapur, S., McIntosh, A. R., & Craik, F. I. (2000). The effects of divided attention on encoding- and retrieval-related brain activity: A PET study of younger and older adults. *Journal of Cognitive Neuroscience, 12*, 775-792.

Antonovsky, A. (1975). *Health, stress and coping*. San Francisco, CA: Jossey-Bass.

Baker, L. A., Cesa, I. L., Gatz, M., & Mellins, C. (1992). Genetic and environmental influences on positive and negative affect: Support for a two-factor theory. *Psychology and Aging, 7*, 158-163.

Bee, H. L., & Bjorklund, B. R. (2000). *The journey of adulthood* (4th ed.). Upper Saddle River, NJ: Prentice Hall.

Bell, M., Bryson, G., Greig, T., Corcoran, C., & Wexler, B. E. (2001). Neurocognitive enhancement therapy with work therapy: Effects on neuropsychological test performance. *Archive General Psychiatry, 58*, 763-768.

Ben-Yishay Y., and Diller, L. (1981) Rehabilitation of cognitive and perceptual defects in people with traumatic brain damage. *International Journal of Rehabilitation Research, 4*(2), 208-10.

Berg, I., Koning-Haanstra, M., & Deelman, B. G. (1991). Long-term effects of memory rehabilitation: A controlled study. *Neuropsychological Rehabilitation, 1*, 97-112.

Bergeman, C. S., Plomin, R., Pedersen, N. L., & McClearn, G. E. (1991). Genetic mediation of the relationship between social support and psychological well-being. *Psychology and Aging, 6*, 640-646.

Bonder, B. R. (2004). *Psychopathology and function*. Thorofare, NJ: SLACK Incorporated.

Brown, C., Harwood, K., Hays, C., Heckman, J., & Short, J. E. (1993). Effectiveness of cognitive rehabilitation for improving attention in patients with schizophrenia. *Occupational Therapy Journal of Research, 13*(2), 71-86.

Bruhn, P., & Parsons, O. (1971). Continuous reaction time in brain damage. *Cortex, 7*, 278-291.

Burack, O. R., & Lachman, M. E. (1996). The effects of list-making on recall in young and elderly adults. *Journal of Gerontology: Psychological Sciences, 51B*(4), P226-P233.

Christiansen, C. H. (1997). Acknowledging a spiritual dimension in occupational therapy practice. *American Journal of Occupational Therapy, 51*(3), 169-172.

Christiansen, C. H., Backman, C., Little, B. R., & Nguyen, A. (1999). Occupations and subjective well-being: A study of personal projects. *American Journal of Occupational Therapy, 53*(1), 91-100.

Christiansen, C., & Baum, C. (1997). *Occupational therapy: Enabling function and well-being*. Thorofare, NJ: SLACK Incorporated.

Churchland, P. S., and Sejnowski, T. J. (1988). Perspectives on cognitive neuroscience. *Science, 242*(4879), 741-745.

Cicerone, K. D., Dahlberg, C., Kalmar, K., Langenbahn, D. M., Malec, J. F., Bergquist, T. F., et al. (2000). Evidence-based cognitive rehabilitation: Recommendations for clinical practice. *Archives of Physical Medicine and Rehabilitation, 81*, 1596-1615.

Collins, F. (1999). Medical and societal consequences of the Human Genome Project. *New England Journal of Medicine, 241*, 28-37.

Collins, F., & McKusick, V. A. (2001). Implications of the Human Genome Project for medical science. *Journal of American Medical Association, 255*, 540-544.

Commission on Practice for American Occupational Therapy Association (2001). *Position paper: Genetics and occupational therapy practice*. Bethesda, MD: American Occupational Therapy Association.

Duchek, J. (1991). Cognitive dimensions of performance. In C. Christiansen & C. Baum (Eds.), *Occupational therapy: Overcoming performance deficits* (pp. 284-303). Thorofare, NJ: SLACK Incorporated.

Egan, M., & DeLaat, M. D. (1994). Considering spirituality in occupational therapy. *Canadian Journal of Occupational Therapy, 61*(2), 95-101.

Erikson, R., & Scott, M. (1977). Clinical memory testing: A review. *Psychological Bulletin, 84*, 1130-1149.

Fidler, G. S., & Fidler, J. W. (1963). *Occupational therapy: A communication process in psychiatry*. New York, NY: Macmillan.

Fidler, G. S., & Fidler, J. W. (1978). Doing and becoming: Purposeful action and self-actualization. *American Journal of Occupational Therapy, 32*, 305-310.

Finkel, D., Pedersen, N. L., Berg, S., & Johansson, B. (2000). Quantitative genetic analysis of biobehavioral markers of aging in Swedish studies of adult twins. *Journal of Aging Health, 12*, 47-68.

Fox, S. I. (1996). *Human physiology*. Dubuque, IA: Wm. C. Brown Publishers.

Fratiglioni, L., Wang, H.-X., Ericsson, K., Maytan, M., & Winblad, B. (2000). Influence of social network on occurrence of dementia: A community-based longitudinal study. *The Lancet, 355*, 1316-1319.

Fuller, A. R. (1994). *Psychology and religion: Eight points of view*. Lanham, MD: Rowman & Littlefield.

Gage, M., & Polatajko, H. J. (1994). Enhancing occupational performance through an understanding of perceived self-efficacy. *American Journal of Occupational Therapy, 48*, 783-790.

Gazzaniga, M. S., Ivry, R. B., and Mangun, G. R. (2002). *Cognitive neuroscience: The biology of the mind*. New York: Norton.

Giles, G. M., & Clark-Wilson, J. (1988). The use of behavioral techniques in functional skills training after severe brain injury. *American Journal of Occupational Therapy, 42*(10), 658-665.

Gutman, S. A. (2001). *Quick reference neuroscience for rehabilitation professionals*. Thorofare, NJ: SLACK Incorporated.

Hafen, B. Q., Karren, K. J., Frandsen, K. J., & Smith, N. L. (1996). *Mind/body health: The effects of attitudes, emotions and relationships*. Needham Heights, MA: Allyn & Bacon.

Howard, B. S., & Howard, J. R. (1997). Occupation as spiritual activity. *American Journal of Occupational Therapy, 51*(3), 181-185.

Ivimäki, M., Elovainio, M., Vahtera, J., Nurmi, J.-E., Feldt, T., Keltikangas-Järvinen, L., et al. (2002). Sense of coherence as a mediator between hostility and health: 7-year prospective study on female employees. *Journal of Psychosomatic Research, 52*, 239-247.

Jorde, L. B., Carey, J. C., White, R. L., & Bamshad, M. J. (2000). *Medical genetics* (2nd ed.). St. Louis, MO: Mosby.

King, D. E., & Bushwick, B. (1994). Beliefs and attitudes of hospital inpatients about faith healing and prayer. *Journal of Family Practice, 39*, 349-352.

Kobasa, S. C. (1979). Stressful life events, personality, and health: An inquiry into hardiness. *Journal of Personality and Social Psychology, 37*, 1-11.

Koenig, H. G., McCullough, M., & Larson, D. B. (2000). *Religion and health: A century of research reviewed*. New York, NY: Oxford University Press.

Kyler, P. (2000). Why are the ethics of genetics important to occupational therapists? *OT Practice, 5*, 23-24.

Kyler, P., & Thomas, M. J. (2002). Implications of the Human Genome Project for occupational therapy. *OT Practice*, Feb. 14, CE1-CE8.

Labouvie-Vief, G., & Schell, D. A. (1982). Learning and memory in later life. In B. B. Wolman (Ed.), *Handbook of developmental psychology* (pp. 828-846). Englewood Cliffs, NJ: Prentice Hall.

Lacoboni, M. (2000). Attention and sensorimotor integration. Mapping the embodied mind. In A. W. Toga & J. C. Mazziotta (Eds.), *Brain mapping: The systems* (pp. 463-490). San Diego, CA: Academic Press.

Lazzarini, A., & Lou, J. Q. (2002). Genetic counseling. In J. Q. Lou (Ed.), *Medical genetics: Challenges and opportunities for health professionals*. Dubuque, IA: Kendall/Hunt Publishing Company.

Little, B. R. (1998). Personal project pursuit: Dimensions of personal meaning. In P. T. P. Wong and P. S. Fry (Eds.), *The human quest for meaning: A handbook of theory, research and application*. Hillsdale, NJ: Lawrence Erlbaum.

Lincoln, N. B., Majid, M. J., & Weyman, N. (2002). Cognitive rehabilitation for attention deficits following stroke (Cochrane Review). In: Cochrane Library, Issue 1, 2002. Oxford: Update Software.

Lou, J. Q. (2002a). Genetic, Human Genome Project and occupational therapy practice. *Occupational Therapy in Health Care, 14*, 3.

Lou, J. Q. (2002b) (Ed.). *Medical genetics: Challenges and opportunities for health professionals*. Dubuque, IA: Kendall/Hunt Publishing Company.

Lou, J. Q., & Culver, K. W. (2002). Screening, diagnosis, and treatment of genetic diseases. In J. Q. Lou (Ed.), *Medical genetics: Challenges and opportunities for health professionals*. Dubuque, IA: Kendall/Hunt Publishing Company.

Loya, G. J. (2001). Efficacy of memory rehabilitation among adolescent and adult traumatic brain injury survivors: A meta-analysis. *Dissertation Abstracts International: Section B: the Sciences and Engineering, 61*(7B), 3850.

Maslow, A. H. (1968). *Toward a psychology of being*. New York, NY: John Wiley.

Maslow, A. H. (1970a). *Religions, values, and peak experiences*. New York, NY: Viking.

Maslow, A. H. (Ed.). (1970b). *New knowledge in human values*. Chicago, IL: Regnery.

Majid, M. J., Lincoln, N. B., & Weyman, N. (2002). Cognitive rehabilitation for memory deficits following stroke (Cochrane Review). In Cochrane Library, Issue 1, 2002. Oxford: Update Software.

Merzenich, M. M., Schreiner, C., Jenkins, W., & Wang, X. (1993). Neural mechanisms underlying temporal integration, segmentation, and input sequence representation: Some implications for the origin of learning disabilities. *Annals of the New York Academy of Sciences*, 682, 1-22.

Meyer, A. (1922). The philosophy of occupational therapy. *Archives of Occupational Therapy, 1*(1), 1-10.

Minor, M. A. (1997). Promoting health and physical fitness. In C. Christiansen & C. Baum (Eds.), *Occupational therapy: Enabling function and well-being* (2nd ed., pp. 256-287). Thorofare, NJ: SLACK Incorporated.

Mowen, J. C. (2000). *The 3M model of motivation and personality: Theory and empirical applications to consumer behavior*. Boston, MA: Kluwer Academic Publishers.

Nathan, D. G., Fontanarosa, P. B., & Wilson, J. E. (2001). Opportunities for medical research in the 21st century. *Journal of American Medical Association, 285*, 533-534.

Persson, D. (2001). *Aspects of meaning in everyday occupations and its relationships to health-related factors*. Unpublished doctoral dissertation, Lund University, Sweden.

Plotnifkoff, G. A. (2003). Spiritual assessment and care. In D. Rakel (Ed.), *Integrative medicine* (pp. 775-780). Philadelphia, PA: Saunders.

President's Council on Physical Fitness and Sport (1992). Healthier US: The President's Health and Fitness Initiative. Retrieved July 26, 2006, from http://www.fitness.gov/index.html.

Ryff, C. D., & Singer, B. H. (1998). The contours of positive human health. *Psychological Inquiry, 9*, 1-28.

Salthouse, T. A. (1994). The nature of the influence of speed on adult age differences in cognition. *Developmental Psychology, 30*, 240-259.

Schroeder-Smith, K., Tischenkel, C., DeLange, L., & Lou, J. Q. (2002). Duchenne muscular dystrophy in females: A rare genetic disorder and occupational therapy perspectives. *Occupational Therapy in Health Care, 14*(3).

Singer, B., and Ryff, C.D. (1999). Hierarchies of life histories and associated health risks. *Annals of the New York Academy of Sciences*, 896, 96-115

Sloan, R. P., Baglella, E., & Powell, T. (1999). Religion, spirituality, and medicine. *The Lancet, 353*, 664-667.

Smith, A. D. (1996). Memory. In J. E. Birren & W. K. Schair (Eds.), *Handbook of psychology of aging* (4th ed., pp. 236-250). San Diego, CA: Academic Press.

Stiggsdotter, A., & Backman, L. (1989). Comparison of different forms of memory training in old age. In M. A. Luszca & T. Nettelbeck (Eds.), *Psychological development: Perspectives across the life span*. Amsterdam, The Netherlands: Elsevier.

Trombly, C. (1995). *Occupational therapy for physical dysfunction*. Baltimore: Williams & Wilkins.

Tulving, E. (1972). Episodic and semantic memory. In E. Tulving & W. Donaldson (Eds.), *Organization of memory*. New York, NY: Academic Press.

Turhim, S. (1993). Medical therapy of ischemic stroke. In W. A. Gordon (Ed.), *Advances in stoke rehabilitation* (pp. 3-15). London: Andover Medical Publishers.

Urbanowski, R., & Vargo, J. (1994). Spirituality, daily practice and the occupational performance model. *Canadian Journal of Occupational Therapy, 43*, 51-52.

Van Zomeren, A. H., & Van DenBurg, W. (1985). Residual complaints of patients two years after severe head injury. *Journal of Neurology, Neurosurgery, and Psychiatry, 48*, 21-28.

Wilson, B. (1982). Success and failure in memory training following a cerebral vascular accident. *Cortex, 18*, 581-594.

World Health Organization. (2001). International Classification of Functioning, Disability and Health (ICF). Retrieved January 29, 2002, from http://www3.who.int/icf/icftemplate.cfm.

Yesavage, J., Lapp, D., & Sheikh, J. A. (1989). Mnemonics as modified for use by the elderly. In L. W. Poon, D. Rubin, & B. Wilson (Eds.), *Everyday cognition in adulthood and late life*. Cambridge, England: Cambridge University Press.

Chapter Twelve: Personal Performance Capabilities Reflections and Learning Activities

Julie Bass-Haugen, PhD, OTR/L, FAOTA

REFLECTIONS

The PEOP model has P for person as its first letter. Even though occupational performance is a focus of this model, I don't think it is any accident that the P for person comes first. After all, practice models are designed to help us in our work with people. If our practice is targeted at people, then we must understand the person.

In this chapter, a generalist's brush paints a broad stroke of the person factors of importance. Many of you are using a variety of textbooks and resources as you study occupational science and occupational therapy. You may find person factors are represented other ways in your resources. Does this make one right and one wrong? Not at all. As you learned from your study of occupations, developing a classification system is not easy. This is true of person factors as well. The important thing is that you, as an occupational therapy practitioner, understand how different factors influence and are influenced.

Here's an example to consider. Let's say you are working with a person who states there is nothing she loves more on a daily basis than a good hot shower but this same person reports she has not been able to take a shower recently. This is an issue not only for her, but also her family and the interdisciplinary health care team who is concerned about hygiene. What do you want to know about this situation? Specifically, what do you want to know about this person? How can you set reasonable goals and select intervention strategies until you understand the person factors that contributed to this recent history? What if I told you that she had a skin condition that improved (or worsened) when exposed to water? What if she had a respiratory condition that improved (or worsened) with humidity? What if she had a weak right leg? What if her self-esteem was influenced by her hygiene routine? What if this occupation was the single-most important thing on her mind right now and that squeaky-clean hygiene was an important cultural norm for her? What if she remembered (or couldn't remember) all the steps in her showering routine? What if she had lost sensation in her right arm? What if she had a wound on her leg?

Now, I would guess you appreciate the importance of each of these person factors. I am also guessing that you would want to know more. What is this skin condition? How is it being treated? How bad is it? What happens if it is not taken care of? What does it mean that showering is the single-most important thing on her mind? Is she going to take showers anyway regardless of what the health care team recommends? How will her self-esteem be affected positively or negatively by the outcome of our work together? Each piece of information you gather about the person helps as you develop an intervention plan. This information is considered again and again as you implement the intervention plan, evaluate its effectiveness, and determine when to discontinue occupational therapy services.

The PEOP model includes five primary person factors: physiological, psychological, cognitive, neurobehavioral, and spiritual. Each factor has many subfactors that provide more detail about personal characteristics. The PEOP model is a starting point for your learning about the person. You will continue to build knowledge about personal factors over your entire professional life. At this point, it is sufficient to get the big picture and some specific examples of the level of detail you will learn along the way.

The *International Classification of Function, Disability, and Health* (ICF) by the World Health Organization is a good organizing framework for a discussion about person factors. There are two primary domains in ICF that address person factors: body structure and body function. When there is a loss of body structure or function, an impairment results. The term *impairment* refers to any limitation in person factors and is important to distinguish from other terms like disability and handicap. Five person factors from ICF were considered in this chapter: physiological, psychological, cognitive, neurobehavioral, and genetic.

Physiological factors include the functions of all systems in the human body. There are 11 major organ systems in the body, and each one has an essential role. Can you name them? When one or more organ systems are not working properly, a primary disease process may be identified (or a secondary cause), and occupational performance may be compromised.

Fitness is the ideal status of our physiological factors. Take a moment and think of people who you consider physically fit. What are the images you have? I was thinking of those well-proportioned fitness gurus, and I envisioned people with lots of stamina who are strong, flexible, energetic, and have a healthy heart and lungs. I think it is interesting that the President's Council on Fitness and Sport (1990) describes fitness a slightly different way: "the ability to carry out daily tasks with vigor and alertness..." Thus, this Council emphasizes the occupational performance aspects of fitness. Occupational therapy practitioners consider five primary components of fitness: cardiorespiratory, muscle strength, muscle endurance, flexibility, and body composition. Each of these areas has specific definitions and measures of fitness.

Psychological factors are the mental processes that are shaped by both intrinsic and extrinsic factors and influence our behavior. Take another moment and think of people who you consider psychologically fit. What are the images you have? This is harder. I envision people who know and like themselves, generally feel positive about themselves and life, believe in themselves and their capabilities, have a balanced perspective on social and cultural influences, and strive to maintain their psychological fitness. Occupational therapy practitioners consider specific psychological factors in practice, including self-concept, self-esteem, affect, response to external social and cultural influences, locus of control, motivation, and self-efficacy.

Cognitive factors include all the simple and complex aspects of thinking. Take yet another moment and think of people who you consider cognitively fit. What are the images you have? This is still harder! I envision people who effectively process a lot of information and wisely act on that information. Beyond that, it is hard for me to envision the absolute essentials for cognitive fitness! Occupational therapy practitioners consider numerous cognitive factors in practice, including visual processing, language, sensory and motor processing, reasoning, problem solving, attention, perception, comprehension, and memory. As you can see, this list is long, and each concept is a chapter or text in itself. Attention and memory were discussed in more detail as examples of cognitive factors.

Do you ever remember a parent or teacher asking for your attention. "Pay attention!" "I need your attention!" What did they mean? Several different meanings are possible. Sometimes, this expression means "wake up your senses" (i.e., alertness). At other times, it means "focus on what I am asking you to do and not what you are currently doing" (i.e., selection). Finally, it may mean "give me the just-right amount of energy for this task" (i.e., allocation). Attentional deficits are seen in many clinical conditions and may have significant effects on occupational performance.

Memory is a complex cognitive factor with two primary components: structure and process. Structure is simply the type of memory storage, and process is how the memory is stored. Think of all the things that happen as part of memory. You remember where you put your keys this morning. You remember a phone number that is given to you by someone. You remember how to make chili without referring to a recipe. You remember a favorite birthday party or outing from childhood. These are only a handful of examples from the millions of memories we must have in our brains. The structure of memories varies depending on its use. Let's take a simple memory activity like remembering a phone number. If you are given a new phone number, sensory memory does an initial registration of this information (i.e., sensory store). To remember this number, we begin to rehearse the number over and over to prevent its loss (i.e., short-term memory). If this new phone number is for a family member or old friend who has just moved, you will begin to commit this phone number to permanent storage (i.e., long-term memory). This example of memory is knowledge-based (i.e., semantic or declarative). My memory of a birthday party is event-based (i.e., episodic) while how to make spaghetti is how-to-based (i.e., procedural).

Memory deficits occur for any number of reasons. They are associated with the normal aging process and are evident in clinical conditions like traumatic brain injuries and Alzheimer's disease. Memory deficits may have significant effects on occupational performance. I can't think of a single activity during my typical day that does not require some memory ability. Can you? Occupational therapy practitioners use compensatory memory training to improve occupational performance of individuals with memory deficits. The strongest candidates for this type of training are motivated individuals with mild deficits who can independently perform some skills and can identify specific areas of need.

The next two person factors discussed in the chapter (neurobehavioral and genetic factors) are not regarded as important for occupational therapy practice by some people. Imagine that! Why would this assumption be made? I guess it is natural to believe that things that cannot be seen (e.g., genes, nerves) have no relevance for things that are seen (e.g., people, occupations, environments). Let's look at a couple of simple examples to see why this assumption does not hold. Say I am working with a person who has no sensation in a limb and who wants to resume showering. Will my intervention plan for showering be shaped at all by the nature of the sensation loss? Will it make a difference if the sensation loss is temporary due to a peripheral nerve injury or permanent due to a central nervous system disorder? If you said yes, you are recognizing that you need to know something about the central nervous system and the peripheral nervous system, two neurobehavioral factors that you cannot see.

Genetic factors are also important to understand. Say I have just received a referral to work with a child who has lower extremity weakness. I learn that this child is the oldest in a family of five children. As I work with the child and family to address occupational needs and environmental barriers, is it important that I know anything else about the nature of the lower extremity weakness? Will it make a difference if the weakness is due to a genetic condition, like Duchenne's muscular dystrophy? If you said yes, you are recognizing that you need to know something about a specific genetic disorder and its pattern of inheritance in a large family.

We have covered a lot in this chapter. You are beginning to appreciate the many complex person factors that influence occupational performance. These factors are important to consider as information is gathered in a particular situation and is used to develop an intervention plan. As an occupational therapy practitioner, you will continue to learn about person factors throughout your career. This knowledge will be important not only in your practice but in your personal life as well.

Journal Activities

1. Look up and write down a dictionary definition of physiology, psychology, cognition, neurobehavioral, and spiritual. Highlight the components of the definitions that are most related to their descriptions in Chapter Twelve.
2. Identify the most important new learning for you in this chapter. (5 min)
3. Identify one question you have about Chapter Twelve. (5 min)
4. Observe a person doing an occupation for 30 minutes to 1 hour. Take notes and reflect on observable characteristics and behaviors that give you information on person factors. Use the PEOP person factors and/or ICF body structure/body function classifications to record your observations. Write a summary of your conclusions about the person factors for this individual.

Technology/Internet Learning Activities

1. Use a discussion database to share specific journal entries.
2. Use a good Internet search engine to find the *International Classification of Functioning, Disability and Health* (ICF) by the WHO.
   - Enter the phrase "International Classification of Function WHO" in your search line.
   - Review the home page for the ICF.
   - Review the online version of the ICF.
   - Identify the main classifications (chapters) of body functions in ICF.
     - ✧ Rank ICF body function classifications (chapters) that have the most and least relevance for occupational therapy (1 = most relevant; 2 = moderately relevant; 3 = least relevant).

Body Function	*Rank*	*Body Function*	*Rank*

- ✧ Examine subclassifications for one body function classification (chapter) of interest and relevance in occupational therapy. Identify one strategy for measuring or obtaining information on this subclassification for one person.

Body Function	*Subclassification*	*Measurement/Information Strategy*
2-Sensory Functions and Pain	b270 Sensory functions related to temperature and other stimuli	Sensory testing (e.g., Semmes-Weinstein monofilaments)

- Identify the main classifications (chapters) of body structures in ICF.
    - ✧ Rank ICF body structure classifications (chapters) that have the most and least relevance for occupational therapy (1 = most relevant; 2 = moderately relevant; 3 = least relevant).

Body Function	*Rank*	*Body Function*	*Rank*

- ✧ Examine subclassifications for one body structure classification (chapter) of interest and relevance in occupational therapy. Identify one strategy for measuring or obtaining information on this subclassification for a person.

Body Function	*Subclassification*	*Measurement/Information Strategy*
7-Structures Related to Movement	S730-Structure of upper extremity	Radiology reports on x-rays in medical chart

3. Use a good Internet search engine to find the President's Council on Physical Fitness and Sport.
    - Enter the phrase "President's Council on Physical Fitness and Sport" in your search line.
    - Review the home page for the Web site.
    - Examine the information on physical activity and health.
        - ✧ Why is physical activity identified as an important factor in determining health status?
    - Propose a role for occupational therapy on this council.

Applied Learning

Individual Learning Activity #1: Exploring the Contribution of Specific Physiological, Psychological, and Cognitive Factors to Occupational Performance

Instructions:

- Identify one of your favorite occupations.
- Conduct a brief activity analysis of this occupation as you typically perform it.
- Summarize the role of five specific personal factors in specific aspects of your performance for this occupation.

Example: Favorite Occupation—Acting. Flexibility is necessary for stunts and dance scenes.

Favorite Occupation:

Person Factor	*Example of Person Factor in Occupational Performance*
Cardiorespiratory	
Muscle strength	
Muscle endurance	
Flexibility	
Self-concept	
Self-esteem	
Affect	
Locus of control	
Motivation	
Self-efficacy	
Attention	
Memory	
Visual processing	
Language	
Sensory motor processing	
Reasoning	
Problem solving	

Individual Learning Activity #2: Exploring Major Organ Systems

Instructions:

- Review Table 12-1, which summarizes the 11 major organ systems.
- Reflect on the function of each system as it relates to occupational performance.
- For each system:
  - ✧ Give one example of how optimal functioning of the system supports occupational performance.
  - ✧ Identify one example of a medical condition that affects the system and give an example of how occupational performance may be limited when there is dysfunction in the system due to this condition.
  - ✧ Summarize your examples in the table provided on p. 295.

System	*Example of OP—Optimal Function*	*Example of OP—Dysfunction*
Integumentary	Testing the water temperature in preparation for bathing is done safely	Scleroderma may limit elasticity of skin and limit free movement during writing activity
Skeletal		
Muscular		
Nervous		
Endocrine		
Circulatory		
Lymphatic		
Respiratory		
Digestive		
Urinary		
Reproductive		

Individual Learning Activity #3: Exploring Spirituality as a Personal Factor

Instructions:

- Reflect on characteristics of spirituality in your life at this time.
- Draw a figure/model to portray your spiritual self. Include the following:
  - Connections (or relationships) between yourself, others, higher beings, and nature
  - Qualitative nature or characteristics of these connections or relationship
  - Five to ten words (or phrases or images) that represent your answer to the question, "what is the purpose or meaning of your life?"
  - Five to ten words (or phrases or images) that represent the most important beliefs and values you hold
- Write a brief summary of your spiritual self as portrayed in the figure/model.

Active Learning

Group Activity #1: Jigsaw Learning About the Personal Factors Associated With a Medical Condition

Preparation:

- Read Chapter Twelve.
- Assign each group member to study a specific medical condition (e.g., Down syndrome, spina bifida, cerebral palsy, schizophrenia, multiple sclerosis, stroke [cerebral vascular accident], Parkinson's disease, rheumatoid arthritis, heart disease, anorexia, asthma, depression, Alzheimer's disease).

Time: 45 minutes to 1 hour

Materials: Summary handout on the condition for each member of the small (or large) group

Instructions:

- Individually:
  - Complete an independent study of the medical condition.
  - Use a variety of medical and health resources to learn about the condition.

   ✧ Use the ICF by the WHO to examine the condition's effect on personal factors.
   ✧ Identify the primary body structures and body functions affected by this condition.
   ✧ Propose three occupations (activities and participation) that may be limited by this condition.

Condition
Brief Summary and Characteristics
Body Structures (primary structures only)
Body Functions (primary functions only)
Occupations (activities and participation)
References

- In small or large groups:
   ✧ Share the results of your learning about the condition.
   ✧ Provide a handout to your peers summarizing your findings on this medical condition.

Discussion:

- Was it difficult to identify the primary body structures and functions involved from the description of the medical condition?
- Do you know anyone with one of these medical conditions? If yes, how does the description of person factors and occupations fit and not fit with the experiences of the person you know?
- What is the most important information for you as you plan occupational performance interventions: the medical condition itself or the person factors that are impaired? Why?

Group Activity #2: Sharing Personal Spiritual Characteristics

Preparation:

- Read Chapter Twelve.
- Complete Individual Learning Activity #3.

Time: 30 to 45 minutes

Materials: Bring figure/model completed in Individual Learning Activity #3

Instructions:

- Individually:
   ✧ Complete Individual Learning Activity #3. Bring a copy of your figure/model.
   ✧ Prepare a summary of the components of your figure/model that you are willing to share.
- In small groups:
   ✧ Share your figure/model and a summary of your spiritual self.

Discussion:

- Describe the experience you had in trying to create a figure/model that represented your spiritual self.
- Discuss the similarities and differences in the figures/models.
- Discuss some strategies you might use to understand the spiritual factors of your clients.

Chapter Thirteen Objectives

The information in this chapter is intended to help the reader:

1. Gain an understanding of the role of the environment in successful occupational performance.
2. Understand the theoretical environmental models that support the PEOP model.
3. Understand the strategies used to modify the physical environment.
4. Understand the major environmental determinants that impact occupational performance.
5. Describe environmental modifications that can be used in the social environment.
6. Describe intervention strategies that address both the social and the physical environment.
7. Describe how environmental changes can assist caregivers of people who have disabilities.

Key Words

disabling process: A misfit between a person's abilities and the environment in which they perform their daily activities.

enabler: An environmental feature or attribute that supports a person's ability to perform his or her daily activities.

environmental attributes: Aspects of the environment that can influence an individual's occupational performance in either a negative or positive way.

environmental press: Demands placed on an individual by the environment.

Always design a thing by considering it in its next larger context—a chair in a room, a room in a house, a house in an environment, an environment in a city plan.
Eliel Saarinen

Chapter Thirteen

Environmental Enablers and Their Impact on Occupational Performance

Susan L. Stark, PhD, OTR/L and Jon A. Sanford, MArch

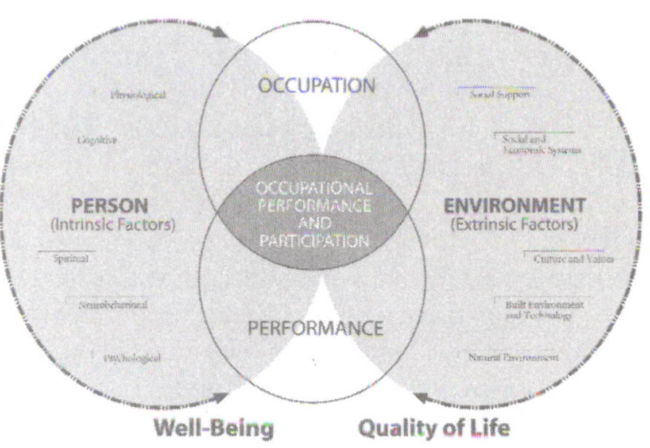

Setting the Stage

This chapter introduces the important concepts and theories about environment and how the environment influences occupational performance. The discussion will include a historical review of environment in both occupational therapy and rehabilitation. Specific models of intervention will be described and applied to a case study to assist the reader in understanding how the environment can influence occupational performance.

Stark, S. L., & Sanford, J. A. (2005). Environmental enablers and their impact on occupational performance. In C. H. Christiansen, C. M. Baum, and J. Bass-Haugen (Eds.), Occupational therapy: Performance, participation, and well-being *(3rd ed.). Thorofare, NJ: SLACK Incorporated.*

INTRODUCTION

This chapter emphasizes the important role of the environment in occupational performance. Occupational performance is the result of complex interactions between intrinsic person factors and extrinsic factors of the environment and what people need and want to do. Environmental attributes interact with human capabilities to enable performance, while others present barriers to an individual's attempts at meaningful interactions with his or her surroundings. In this chapter, we will explore this balance and the relationship between humans and the context within which they perform their occupations.

As described throughout this text, occupational performance is the result of complex interactions among person, environment, and occupation. This chapter will describe the important role of the environment in those interactions.

Environment is the context that is external to the person (Carver & Rhodda, 1978) and in which activity occurs. Environments consist of physical elements, both built and natural (doors, ramps, pathways), and social influences (policy, culture, support, and attitudes). As such, the environment is the context for people's performance and includes everything that a person encounters during participation as a human being in society.

Environmental influences, depending on how they affect a person, can facilitate or hinder occupational performance. As a result, there is increasing recognition of the importance of environmental factors in contributing to occupational performance, particularly among more vulnerable populations such as people with disabilities (Barris, 1982; Christiansen & Baum, 1991, 1997; Dunn & McGuigan, 1994; Dunn, Brown, McClain, & Westman, 1994; Law, 1991). This view of the environment has not only greatly impacted the concept of disability, but also rehabilitation professionals' views of the disablement processes.

Typical medical models of health attribute the inability of individuals to perform their daily activities to the functional limitations caused by impairments. Environmentally influenced models suggest that disability is a construct imposed by circumstances. Impairments do not become disabilities until they converge with the environment and the person cannot do what he or she needs or wants to do.

Conceptually, disability can be viewed as an expression of the misfit between person and environment. The outcomes of a person-environment match can be far reaching, beyond simply improving the performance of individuals with disabilities. As a result, modifying the environment has become an important intervention strategy to help manage chronic health care conditions; maintain or improve functioning; increase independence; ensure safety, ease of use, security, self-esteem, and self-confidence; reduce the need to relocate to institutional facilities; and even reduce the costs of personal care services. A growing body of evidence has demonstrated these positive impacts. For example, Connell and Sanford (2001) found that people with disabilities who modified their homes had little to moderate difficulty and dependence in the conduct of daily activities. Gitlin and colleagues (2001) concluded that home modifications slowed the rate of functional dependency and enhanced caregiver self-efficacy. Mann and colleagues (1999) reported that the rate of decline in independence of older adults and costs for personal assistance and health care were reduced through increased use of assistive technology and environmental interventions.

We all live our lives interacting with the physical and social environment. Therefore, it is not surprising that the environment is conceptualized, studied, and written about by numerous disciplines, including architecture, environmental science, geography, psychology, social policy, and landscape and interior design as well as occupational science. The body of knowledge that comprises many of these disciplines will be reviewed in this chapter to develop a better understanding of environmental contributions to occupational performance and to provide the foundation to begin building interventions that support occupation.

Specifically, the first part of this chapter will focus on the historical view of the environment in both occupational therapy practice and in traditional rehabilitation models. This discussion will be followed by an in-depth discussion of four models of person-environment interaction that can form the basis of a comprehensive understanding of the person-environment interaction. Each model represents a different perspective on this interaction, yet all four are important in understanding environmental contributions to successful occupational performance and each provides the foundation for environmental intervention. Having provided the foundation for environmental intervention, the third part of the chapter will present aspects of the physical and social environment that affect occupational performance. The last part of this chapter will explore a case study using the Person-Environment-Occupation-Performance (PEOP) situational analysis that explores the extrinsic factors that influence performance.

The Evolution of Environment in Occupational Therapy and Rehabilitative Models

Occupational Therapy Models

Historically, occupational therapy literature has recognized the importance of creating opportunities for meaningful interactions with the environment as the basis for promoting health through occupation (Meyer, 1922; Reilly, 1962). Although these visionaries challenged the profession to address the environment, it was not until the 1970s and 1980s that occupational therapists began to talk about the environment as central to the experience of occupation. The first to do so was Dunning (1972) who talked about space as important to consider in analyzing how an activity can be performed. Kiernat (1972) conceptualized the environment as an occupational therapy modality that is purposely manipulated to either challenge or support the client's competencies. In turn, the client's abilities expand in order to maintain a comfortable level of fit with the environment. Later, Reed and Sanderson (1980, 1983, 1992) divided the environment into three constructs: physical, psychobiological, and societal. They viewed the environment as interacting forces that shape the performance of individuals as they engage in occupation. The first occupational therapy model that focused on the environment was published in 1982. It was at that time that Howe and Briggs (1982) proposed the Ecological Systems model. They viewed the environment as composed of nested layers. The immediate settings were embedded in the social networks, and then both were in an ideological system. Beginning in 1985, more explicit models began to emerge, and all have included the environment as critical elements in their models. In Table 13-1, you can see that there is beginning to be agreement that the environment influences the development and maintenance of the person; however, how the environment is conceptualized is somewhat model dependent.

The Evolution of Rehabilitation Models That Include the Environment

At the same time that concepts of the environment were emerging in occupational therapy, work was going on in the area of disability policy. Some of the changes to rehabilitation models are directly related to occupational therapists serving in the policy arena and working with other colleagues and consumers of rehabilitation services to shape new models. Prior to 1993, models of disability viewed pathology and disability interchangeably and excluded the consideration of the environment as a determinate of function. The models that view disability resulting from the interaction between the characteristics of the individual and the barriers in the environment are just beginning to emerge (Brandt & Pope, 1997).

The National Medical Rehabilitation Research Center (NMRRC) report to Congress in 1993 introduced the idea of social participation and clearly articulated the role of the environment in both the definition of disability and societal limitations (Table 13-2).

In 1997, the Institute of Medicine (IOM) formed a panel in response to a request from the U.S. Congress to prepare a report that would assess the current knowledge base in rehabilitation science and engineering. Their task was to evaluate the utility of current rehabilitation models, to describe and recommend mechanisms for the effective transfer and clinical translation of scientific findings to promote health and heath care for people with disabling conditions, and to critically evaluate the current federal programmatic efforts in rehabilitation science and engineering. A panel was constructed that included scientists from public health, sociology, rehabilitation, engineering, public policy, medicine, and both occupational and physical therapy (Brandt & Pope, 1997). This report proposed a new model, the Enabling-Disabling Process model, in which the environment represents both physical space and social structures. It suggests that people with disabling conditions are dislocated from their prior integration in an environment. The model depicts the rehabilitation process as an attempt to rectify this displacement by either restoring the individual's function or expanding access to the environment that removes barriers that limit performance (Figure 13-1).

Concurrent with the NCMRR and IOM reports to the U.S. Congress, the World Health Organization (WHO) was initiating the revision of the *International Classification of Impairments, Disability and Handicaps* (ICIDH). The ICIDH classification was developed in 1980 as a means of classifying the consequences of disease. With the revision of the International Classification of Disease (ICD-10), which addresses functional states of health conditions, it was important to go beyond the functional status of the individual to guide and plan for the needs of people as they strive to return to active participation in meaningful lives. The ICIDH was revised during a 7-year process involving 65 countries and rigorous scientific examination of the document. The result of the revision process was approved by the WHO in 2001. The new publication, the *International Classification of Functioning, Disability and Health* (ICF), has been accepted as the international standard to describe and measure health and disability (WHO, 2001).

While traditional health indicators are based on the mortality (i.e., death) rates of populations, the ICF shifts focus to "life" (i.e., how people live with their health con-

Table 13-1 Occupational Therapy Models That Address Environmental Factors

Year	*Authors*	*Model*	*Role of Environment in the Model*
1985, 1995, 2002	Kielhofner	Model of Human Occupation	Environment includes objects, person, and events with which the person interacts. The environment affords or presses occupational behavior
1991, 1997	Christiansen & Baum	Person-Environment Occupation-Performance Model	The environment enables or acts as a barrier to occupational performance. The environment was described to include social support, social policies and attitudes, culture, and physical and natural attributes
1992	Polatajko	Occupational Competence Model	Occupational competence is the product of the dynamic interaction between the environmental demand and the individual's ability. The environmental dimensions include physical, social, and cultural
1992	Stewart	Model for the Practice of Occupational Therapy	The occupational therapy process involves interaction between client, therapist, environment, and activities
1992	Schkade & Schultz	Occupational Adaptation Model	Performance calls for an occupational environment to support the occupational response and includes the contest in which occupations occur (self-maintenance, play, and leisure)
1994	Dunn, Brown, et al.	Ecology of Human Performance Model	Environmental cues are used by a person to support the performance of tasks
1995, 2000	Hagedorn	Competent Occupational Performance in the Environment Model	Environmental demand is defined as the challenge presented by the environment, which provides the press that supports occupational performance
1995	Bass-Haugen & Mathiowetz	Contemporary Task Oriented Approach Model	The environmental and performance context (physical, socioeconomic, and cultural) as well as personal characteristics are important in determining occupational and role performance
1996	Law et al.	Person-Environment-Occupation Model	The environment defined as those contexts and situation outside the individual (social, political, economic, institutional, and cultural) elicit responses from the person
1997	Canadian Association of Occupational Therapists	Canadian Model of Occupational Performance	The environment includes the physical, institutional, cultural, and social factors. The environment forms the outer ring of a conceptual model that supports the person as he or she engages in occupation

Table 13-2

The NCMRR Model

Pathophysiology	*Impairment*	*Functional Limitation*	*Disability*	*Societal Limitation*
Interruption or interference of normal physiologial and developmental processes	Loss and/or abnormality of mental, emotional or physiological function; includes all losses or abnormalities not just those attributable to the initial pathophysiology, also includes pain	Restriction or lack of ability to perform an action or activity in the manner or within the range considered normal	Inability or limitation in performing socially defined activities and roles expected of individuals within a social and physical environment as a result of internal or external factors	Societal policy, attitudes, and actions, or lack of, that create physical, social, or financial barriers to access
Level of Reference				
Cells and tissues	Organs and organ systems	Organism—action or activity performance (consistent with the purpose or function of the organ or organ system)	Individual—task performance within the social and cultural context	Society

Modified from work initially developed by the Institute of Medicine and published in *Disability in America*, 1991.

ditions and how these can be improved to achieve a productive, fulfilling life). The ICF takes into account the social aspects of disability and provides a mechanism to document the impact of the social and physical environment on a person's functioning.

The goal for the revision was to provide a unified and standard language and framework for the description of human functioning and disability as an important component of health. The classification evolved to cover disturbances in functional states associated with health conditions, the body, the individual, and society level and included two dimensions. The first dimension includes the functioning and disability factors and is divided into two sections. The body structure and function component includes the anatomical and physiological functions of the human body, while the activities and participation component covers the complete range of activities performed by an individual and describes areas of life in which an individual is involved. The second section includes the environmental and personal factors. The entire model is presented here; however, the environmental aspects of the model will be discussed later in the chapter (Figure 13-2).

Models of Person-Environment Interaction

Environmental theory has been developed, studied, and presented in the environment behavior (EB) studies literature. These theories support the PEOP model and provide the operational definitions and theoretical assumptions necessary to understand how environment can influence behavior (or occupational performance). There is a rich history of important models that OT can explore and study. In this section, we will introduce EB theories, discuss their relevance to OT model and theory development using examples from the EB literature, and review four theories that provide a basis for understanding

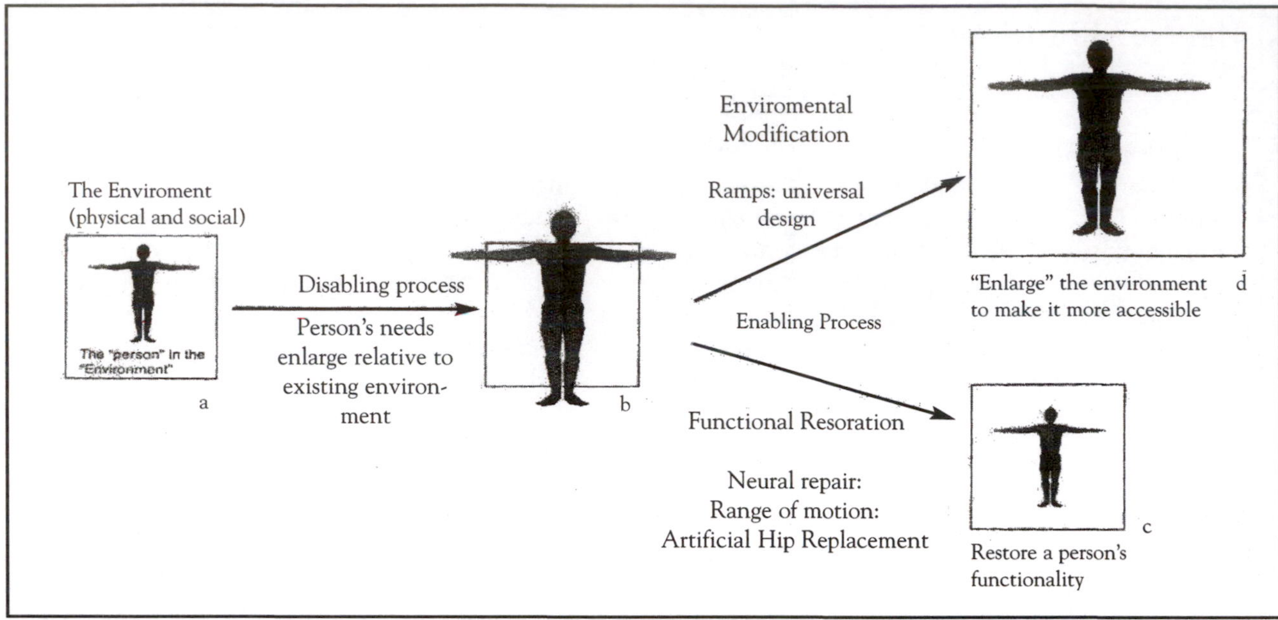

Figure 13-1. Conceptual overview of the enabling-disabling process. The environment, depicted as a square, represents both physical space and social structures (family, community, society). A person who does not manifest a disability (a) is fully integrated into society and "fits within the square." A person with potentially disabling conditions has increased needs (expressed by the size of the individual) and is dislocated from his or her prior integration into the environment (b) that is, it "doesn't fit in the square." The enabling (or rehabilitative) process attempts to rectify this displacement, either by restoring function in the individual (c) or by expanding access to the environment (d) (e.g., building ramps). (Reprinted with permission from [Enabling America: Assessing the Role of Rehabilitation Science and Engineering] © [1997] by the National Academy of Sciences, courtesy of the National Academies Press, Washington, D.C.)

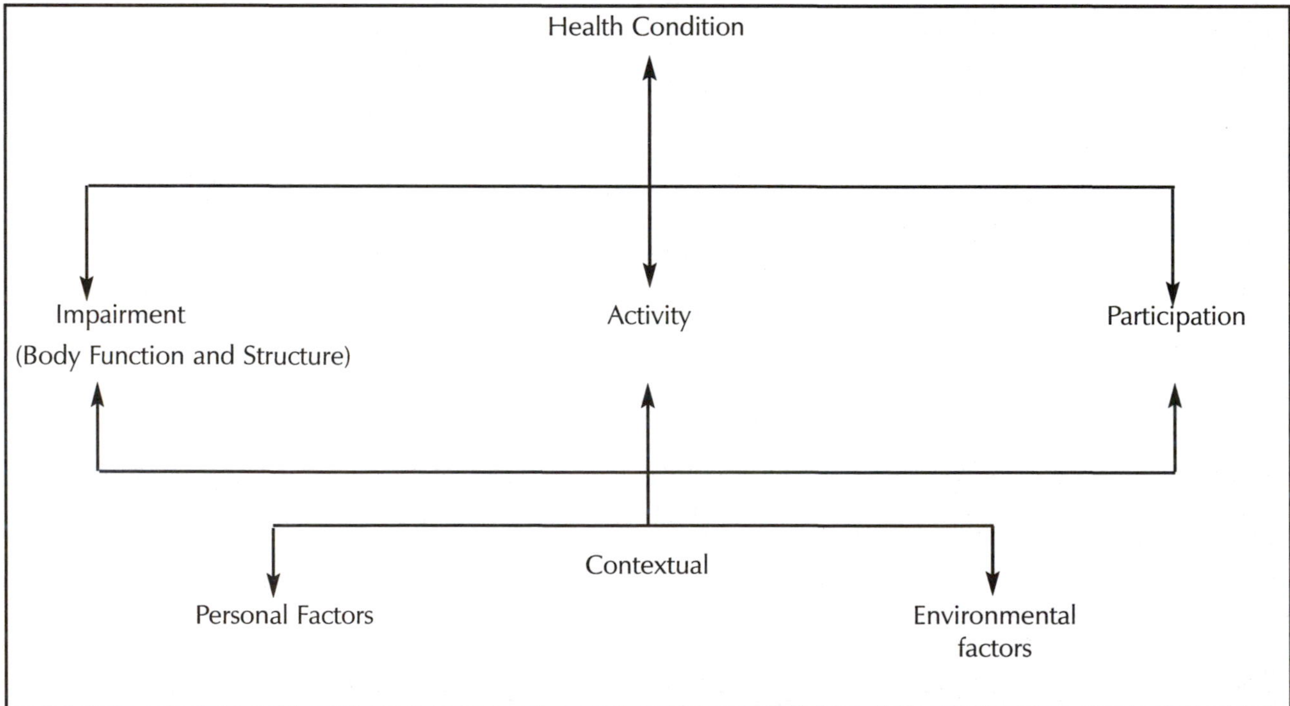

Figure 13-2. The International Classification of Function, Disability, and Health (ICF) model: Interaction between the components of ICF. (Reprinted with Permission of the World Health Organization, all rights reserved by the Organization. The International Classification of Function, Disability and Health, page 18 WHO, 2001 http://www.who.int/classification/ref.)

aspects of the environment that affect occupational performance.

Of the models that we will review in depth, the first three models focus primarily on person-environment interactions as predictors of occupational performance. The first model is a broad conceptualization of person-environment fit as defined by the transactional relationship between an individual's functional abilities and limitations and environmental factors, in general (French, Rodgers, & Cobb, 1974; Lewin, 1951). The second model defines the range of specific environmental elements and features that potentially interact with personal skills and impairment, although the two latter concepts are not specifically linked to the environment. The third model links impairment and specific environmental factors. In contrast to the first three models that predict performance, the fourth model is based on actual performance to individualize interventions. In addition, unlike the other models, this model focuses directly on the impact of specific characteristics and attributes of environments on occupational performance rather than on personal factors.

Person-Environment Fit: Environmental Press Model

Person-environment (PE) fit can be operationalized as the outcome of the transaction or interaction between the person and the environment (French et al., 1974). Optimal fit occurs when an individual's capacities are consistent with the demands and the opportunities within his or her environment. Conversely, when the demands of the environment exceed an individual's abilities, there is PE misfit.

The extent to which the environment affects an individual's ability to perform an activity was initially defined as environmental press by Murray in 1938 and was further explicated by Lawton and Nahemow's Ecological (Environmental Press) Model (1973). This model graphically illustrates the differential impact of the environment on behavior and performance as a function of an individual's competence. Most importantly for occupational therapists, the environmental press model supports the process of determining the types of environmental changes that must be made to match the abilities of an individual, a critical component to the occupational therapy treatment process (Figure 13-3).

Referring to Figure 13-1, the level of an individual's competencies (e.g., functional, cognitive, social, and behavioral skills and abilities) are represented on the Y axis of a graph, and the amount of press resulting from demands are represented on the X axis. Competence ranges from low to high, and environmental press ranges from weak to strong. The outcome of a transaction is depicted on the graph at the intersection of an individual's skill level and the strength of environmental demand. The central diagonal line or adaptation level represents the "average" or baseline environmental press for that person. This is the point at which there is optimal PE fit. At this point, an individual does not need to adapt his or her behavior, skills, or environment.

The ranges on either side of the baseline represent generally positive affect and successful performance of the person, as demands are in line with the skills of an individual. However, as an individual moves farther away from the baseline, performance outcomes decrease, either as a result of an environment that is too challenging (as represented by stronger demands) or one that is not sufficiently challenging (as represented by weaker demands). When demands are greater or less than an individual's skill level, negative outcomes or maladaptive behavior occurs, resulting in environmental interactions that are marked by poor occupational performance. For example, when a grab bar is located too far away (demand) for a frail older individual to reach (competency), he or she may lose balance, fall, or experience fear of falling. As a consequence, the individual may require assistance in toileting or may avoid the toilet altogether (maladaptive behavior) (Lawton & Nahemow, 1973).

Two general principles/hypotheses derived from the Environmental Press Model are important in understanding the impact of the environment on people with diminished skills. First, the "Environmental Docility Hypothesis" (Lawton, 1990; Lawton & Simon, 1968) proposes that people with diminished physical, cognitive, or psychological capacity are at a greater risk for influence by the environment. Thus, more impaired individuals are likely to be more susceptible to environmental demands than less impaired individuals. Second, excess disabilities occur when the environment is not responsive to an individual's capabilities. Thus, when there is a mismatch between environment and ability, observed levels of dependency would be greater than those expected given an individual's level of impairment.

The Environmental Press Model provides an explicit understanding of the transactional relationship between person and environment and establishes the basis from which outcomes of a supportive environment can be measured. Whereas the model provides a basic understanding of the transactional nature of PE fit, it does not identify specific environmental factors that can be targeted for intervention. Therefore, the next step is to break down the environment a little further and explore the specific environmental features that might impact the component skills and abilities of an individual.

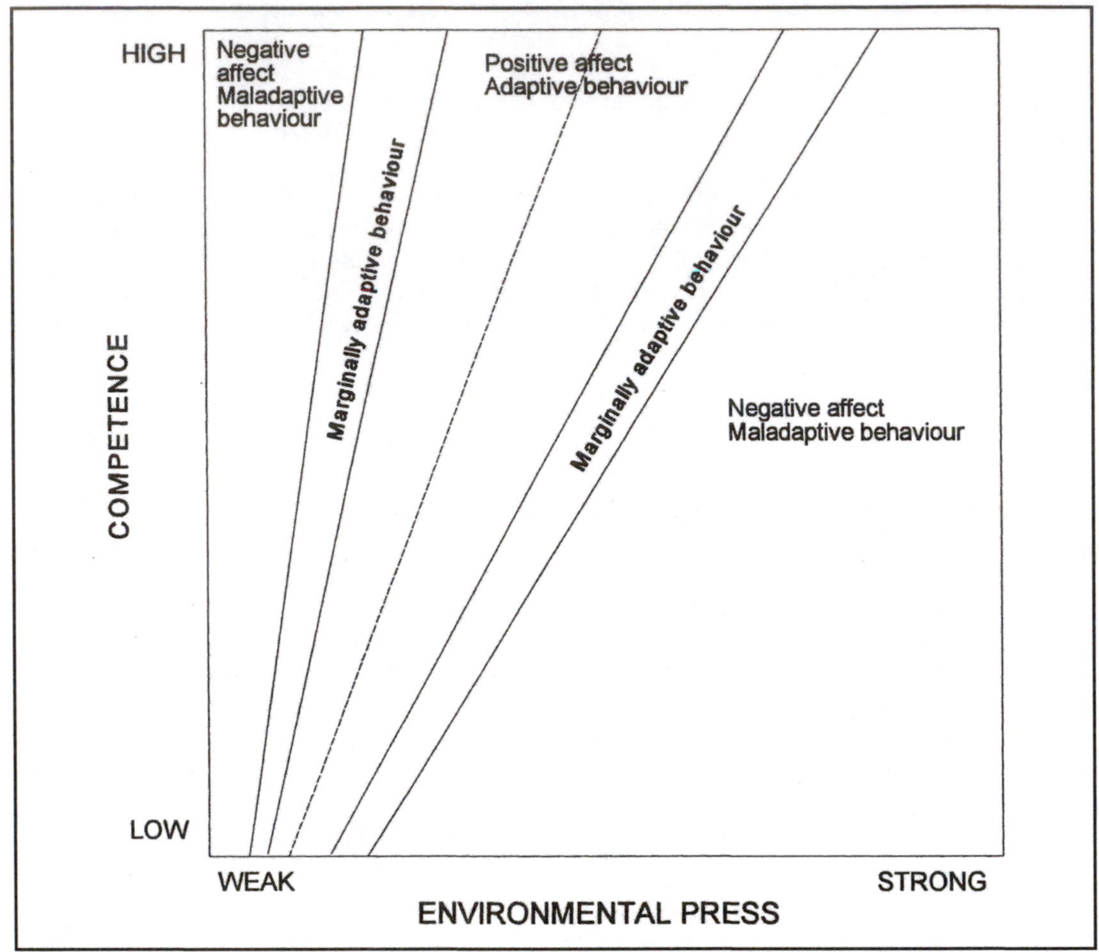

Figure 13-3. The Ecological model. (Adapted from Lawton, M. P., & Nahemow, L. (1973). Toward an ecological theory of adaptation and aging. In W. Preiser (Ed.), *Environmental design research* (pp. 24-32). Stroudsburg, PA: Dowden, Hutchinson, & Ross.)

A Model for Precontext of Performance: International Classification of Function Classification

Understanding and describing the range of environmental factors that impact the performance of individuals is difficult given the vast number of environments and different features associated with each. Moreover, for each individual, occupations occur within a context that is unique to their circumstance. Each human lives in a life space that is built on a system of environments. The environments include a mix of physical and social elements. Physical elements can include the built environment, objects within the environment, and the geographical and climactic features of the natural environment. Social elements can include people, including their attitudes and cultural values as well as social support offered by these people. Policies and services are also social elements in the environment that influence performance. The PEOP model extrinsic factors are made up of the physical dimensions of the environment including the built environment, the natural environment, and the social dimensions of the environment such as the cultural, societal, social support, and economic factors in an environment.

The PEOP model works well with the WHO's classification of the environment that is part of the ICF (WHO, 2001). Table 13-3 includes the ICF classification of environmental factors in terms of specific features and elements, including products and technology, natural and human changes to the environment, support and relationships, attitudes and services, and systems and policies. This classification system is being developed in conjunction with a broader classification index of disability and the precursors to disability (WHO, 2001). The development of the environmental classification index is still in its infancy; however, to date, it is the most comprehensive

Table 13-3

International Classification of Function Environmental Factors

Products and Technology

- Products or substances for personal consumption
- Products and technology for personal use in daily living
- Products and technology for personal indoor and outdoor mobility and transportation
- Products and technology for communication
- Products and technology for education
- Products and technology for employment
- Products and technology for culture, recreation, and sport
- Products and technology for the practice of religion and spirituality
- Design, construction, and building products and technology of buildings for public use
- Design, construction, and building products and technology of buildings for private use
- Products and technology of land development
- Assets
- Products and technology, other specified
- Products and technology, unspecified

Natural Environment and Human-Made Changes to the Environment

- Physical geography
- Population
- Flora and fauna
- Climate
- Natural events
- Human-caused events
- Light
- Time-related changes
- Sound
- Vibration
- Air quality
- Natural environment and human-made changes to environment, other specified
- Natural environment and human-made changes to environment, unspecified

Support and Relationships

- Immediate family
- Extended family
- Friends
- Acquaintances, peers, colleagues, neighbors, and community members
- People in positions of authority
- People in subordinate positions
- Personal care providers and personal assistants
- Strangers

(continued)

Table 13-3

- Domesticated animals
- Health professionals
- Health-related professionals
- Support and relationships, other specified
- Support and relationships, unspecified

Attitudes

- Individual attitudes of immediate family members
- Individual attitudes of extended family members
- Individual attitudes of friends
- Individual attitudes of acquaintances, peers, colleagues, neighbors, and community members
- Individual attitudes of people in positions of authority
- Individual attitudes of people in subordinate positions
- Individual attitudes of personal care providers and personal assistants
- Individual attitudes of strangers
- Individual attitudes of health professionals
- Individual attitudes of health-related professionals
- Societal attitudes
- Social norms, practices, and ideologies
- Attitudes, other specified
- Attitudes, unspecified

Services, Systems, and Policies

- Services, systems, and policies for the production of consumer goods
- Architecture and construction services, systems, and policies
- Open space planning services, systems, and policies
- Housing services, systems, and policies
- Utilities services, systems, and policies
- Communication services, systems, and policies
- Transportation services, systems, and policies
- Civil protection services, systems, and policies
- Legal services, systems, and policies
- Associations and organizational services, systems, and policies
- Media services, systems, and policies
- Economic services, systems, and policies
- Social security services, systems, and policies
- General social support services, systems, and policies
- Health services, systems, and policies
- Education and training services, systems, and policies
- Labor and employment services, systems, and policies
- Political services, systems, and policies
- Services, systems, and policies, other specified

description of environmental elements that contribute to the disablement process.

While the ICF classification provides a fairly complete list of all of the environmental features and elements that may influence performance, there is still no description of these features and elements from which a direct link between the environment and performance can be ascertained. For instance, a 30'-long, accessibility code-compliant, 1:12 (i.e., 1" rise for every 12" of run) ramp at a building entrance might facilitate entry to that building for a young individual who uses a wheelchair, but an older wheelchair user who also has diminished upper body strength might not be able to push him- or herself up the same ramp. In contrast, the same older individual might be able to use a 1:16 ramp or one that was only 20 feet long.

For example, the ramp is an environmental feature that falls into the ICF model, and removing it entirely would not help the older individual get into the building. Moreover, it is unlikely that bodybuilding to improve upper body strength will be of much help. On the other hand, changing specific characteristics of the ramp, such as slope and length that place too high a demand on the older wheelchair user, would facilitate that individual's access to the building. The following model begins to illustrate how impairment and environmental characteristics affect occupational performance.

Environmental Factors and Impairment: The Enabler

As the ramp example above illustrates, environmental features can either support (i.e., enablers) or hamper (i.e., barriers) performance. Whether an environmental feature is supportive or not depends on both the skills and abilities of an individual (competence) and the characteristics of the environment (press). The Enabler Matrix (Ivarsson, 1997; Steinfeld et al., 1979) begins to address these issues by linking competence defined by impairments to a limited set of press-producing environmental characteristics.

As described in Chapter Ten, each person has abilities regardless of impairment diagnosis. Each of these measurable and objective abilities exists on a continuum from personal capacity to disability. Within any environmental context, personal capacity (Lawton and Nahemow, 1973a, 1973b) can be viewed as the person's occupational performance potential, whereas disability can be viewed as diminished performance (Figure 13-4).

Based on the work of Murray (1938) and Lewin (1951), the Enabler model captures the broad spectrum of abilities for individuals with a variety of limitations. The Enabler explores the capacities of the person, including cognitive, sensory, internal body regulation, and motor capacities. The major contribution of this work to the current understanding of the PE interaction is the concept that a person with a disability is not simply "disabled," but has a unique set of abilities and limitations that are differentially impacted by various environmental factors.

The Enabler Matrix has specifically been used to assist in understanding accessibility in the physical environment (Steinfeld et al., 1979) and, more recently, to everyday occupations in the home (Ivarsson, 1997). To measure the impact of environmental factors on occupational tasks, Ivarsson has applied the Enabler Matrix to home activities as a method of evaluating environmental barriers to performance in the home. The evaluation tool is a helpful conceptualization of the home barriers. A list of 144 environmental barriers is provided (e.g., narrow paths, irregular walking surfaces, and unstable walking surfaces) for the home environment. The list is coded by the types of impairments that may encounter barriers if this environmental attribute is present. Each barrier is rated by severity by impairment, and a score has been assigned based on a four-point system. The potential of the barriers can be rated as 1) potential problem, 2) problem, 3) severe problem, and 4) impossibility. For example, if stairs are present in the home of an individual who depends on a wheelchair, a score of 4 will be tallied for that barrier.

The Enabler model clarifies, at the conceptual level, the relationship between impairment and a specific set of environmental factors. How do we know that the set of environmental factors included in Ivarsson's model covers all of the possible environmental factors that impact performance? Just as importantly, how can we be sure that functional abilities imbedded in generic descriptions of impairment truly represent the skills and abilities of all individuals with those particular impairments? To answer these questions, we need to look at the conceptual framework suggested by the fourth model that defines environmental characteristics by occupational tasks and links those characteristics to an individual's occupational performance, regardless of impairment.

Linking Environmental Characteristics and Performance: A Framework for Home Modification

As noted earlier in this chapter, environmental features and elements, in and of themselves, do not exert demands on individuals. Rather, the characteristics of those features, such as the length and slope of a ramp, the height and location of a toilet, the number of family members available to provide assistance and support, or the types of transportation services available, create demands that impact occupational performance.

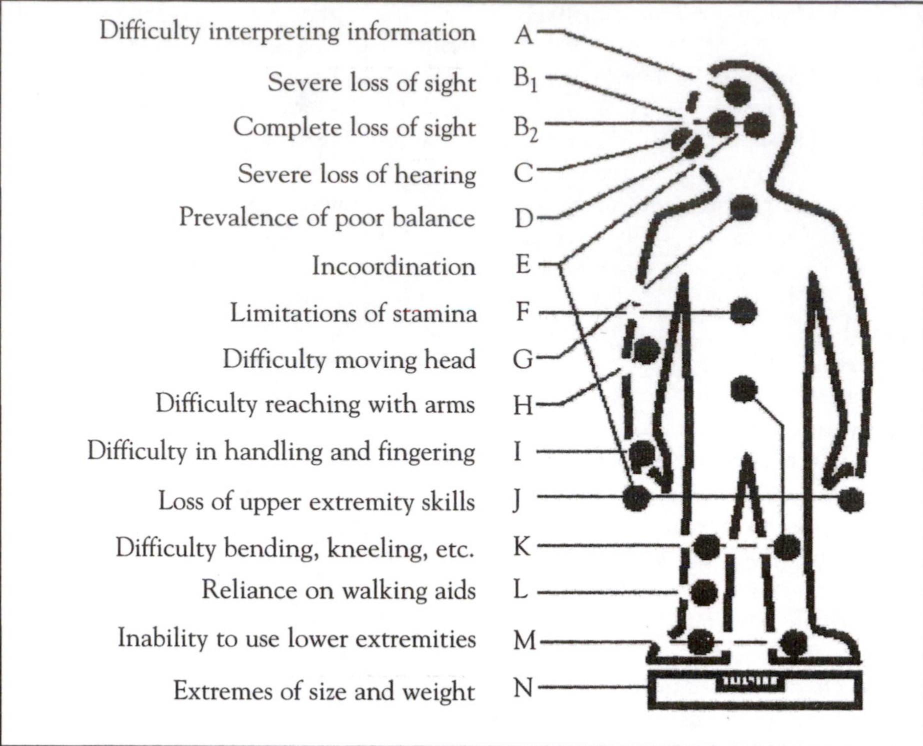

Figure 13-4. The Enabler.

Similarly, competence is defined by abilities and skills such as range of motion, not by impairments, such as low vision or difficulty bending. The issue then is to construct a model that describes who (i.e., ability and skill levels) is impacted by what (i.e., environmental characteristics) and when (i.e., occupational performance). To understand these relationships, a task analytic approach is useful. Such an approach relies on defining task-relevant environmental characteristics rather than ones that are impairment-related. As a result, occupational performance can be linked to environmental characteristics irrespective of personal factors, including impairment, skills, and abilities. Unlike the prospective approach of the first three models, this model is retrospective, based on actual performance of what an individual can or cannot do in a real environment.

One application of this approach is the conceptual framework to guide the process of developing home modification (Connell & Sanford, 1997; Sanford & Jones, 2001). The conceptual framework (see Figure 13-2) links occupational performance to the physical environment of the home and permits the assessment of occupational performance in the context of the environmental features and characteristics used in the conduct of each activity. Each activity is subdivided into its component and requisite tasks (e.g., turning on the water, regulating water temperature, getting in the tub, grabbing the soap). These tasks are linked to multiple characteristics of relevant environmental features. For example, bathing is dependent upon such task-related characteristics as the location of the tub relative to other fixtures in the bathroom and the type and location of faucet handles.

Specifically, the framework describes the major environmental features of the home, including spaces, products, hardware/controls, and the critical characteristics of these features that impact occupational performance for each task. These are briefly discussed below.

Spaces

The physical characteristics of rooms and other spaces place demands on people that can determine successful performance or require excess effort to complete a task. For example, the layout of the tub and toilet in a bathroom can determine if a lateral wheelchair-to-toilet transfer is possible, and light levels can determine if an individual with low vision can read the label on a medicine bottle. Specific spatial characteristics that create demands include the following:

- Size and spatial configuration/layout
- Entry dimensions (doorway width and threshold height)
- Systems locations (location of switches, outlets, fixtures, and appliances)
- Floor materials/finishes
- Ambient conditions (illumination and noise)

Products

The design of products, including fixtures, appliances, and other off-the-shelf items, also creates demands that impact occupational performance. For example, the location of controls at the rear of an electric range requires an individual in a wheelchair to reach across the burners to operate the appliance, or the weight of a pot may be too much for an individual with limited strength to pick up. Product characteristics of interest include the following:

- Type
- Size
- Force required to activate, engage, operate, lift, or move
- Materials/finishes (type, texture, and color contrast)
- Auditory/visual signals (intended to alert user to take some further action)

Hardware/Controls

Controls and hardware include a variety of user interfaces. They are either operable (such as a doorknob) or fixed (such as a drawer pull). Generally, their function is to operate products, although occasionally inoperable hardware, such as grab bars, serves its own independent function. Controls and hardware typically create demands that require the user to manipulate the environment using fine motor control to grasp, twist, rotate, push, or pull an object, although many interfaces also require the ability to attend to sensory feedback. For example, round doorknobs may be difficult for someone with arthritis to grasp, a black knob on a black appliance might not have sufficient color contrast for someone with a vision impairment to locate, or the sound of an oven control clicking into a heat setting may not be loud enough for an individual with a hearing impairment. Specific characteristics of hardware/controls that affect use include the following:

- Type of device (opener, dispenser, plumbing, lock, assist, receptacle, controls)
- Minimum approach distance and angle
- Hardware configuration
- Size
- Force of activation
- Operational characteristics (direction and distance to be moved, calibration, type of sensory feedback)
- Materials/finish (type, texture, and color contrast)

Although this conceptual framework was developed for linking physical characteristics to occupational performance in the home, it is relevant and adaptable to any setting. Moreover, using characteristics to describe environmental features is equally applicable to the social environment as it is to the physical environment.

Two additional models that lay a foundation for understanding developmental and social issues include Baker and Intagliata's quality of life model and Broffenbrenner's developmental model. Both models provide an understanding of the social dimensions of function and how they are influenced by contextual factors.

The Objective Versus Perceived Environment: The Biopsychosocial Model

Baker and Intagliata (1982) developed a model to identify factors that influence quality of life from the perspective of an individual with a long-term mental illness attempting to live in the community. The model was developed from a study of community-dwelling individuals. The model contains four foci, including the environmental system, the experienced environment, biopsycho system (individual's health status), and the behavior of the individual (coping, satisfaction). Briefly, the environmental system or objective environment contains the physical, social, economic, political, and cultural attributes of the environment. The experienced or subjective environment includes material (housing, food, and possessions), social (family and friends), and activity (work, leisure, and religious) constructs. These constructs represent the life conditions and events perceived by the individual, which are both an influence and are influenced by the biopsycho system. The biopsycho system includes the physical and mental status, need levels, knowledge, beliefs, and attitudes held by the individual. The interaction of the experienced environment and the biopsycho system as influenced by the environmental system results in the behavior of the individual. Behavior is operationally defined as the coping, adaptation, quality of life, or satisfaction of an individual. This model explicitly describes the relationships between the objective environment, the perceived or lived environment, and person factors and attributes the quality of life of an individual to each of these constructs. Thus, in this model, person and environment fit is expressed as quality of life. This was a significant contribution to the mental health literature, as comfort rather than cure became the priority for intervention in the population of individuals with chronic mental illness.

Environmental Influences Across the Lifespan: An Ecological Model

Urie Bronfenbrenner (1977, 1993) developed a model that is useful in understanding the influence of PE interactions that affect development. Bronfenbrenner assumed that development occurred within an environmental context when he developed the ecological paradigm that he said captures the context-specific PE interaction that "emerges as the most likely to exert influence on the course and content of subsequent psychological develop-

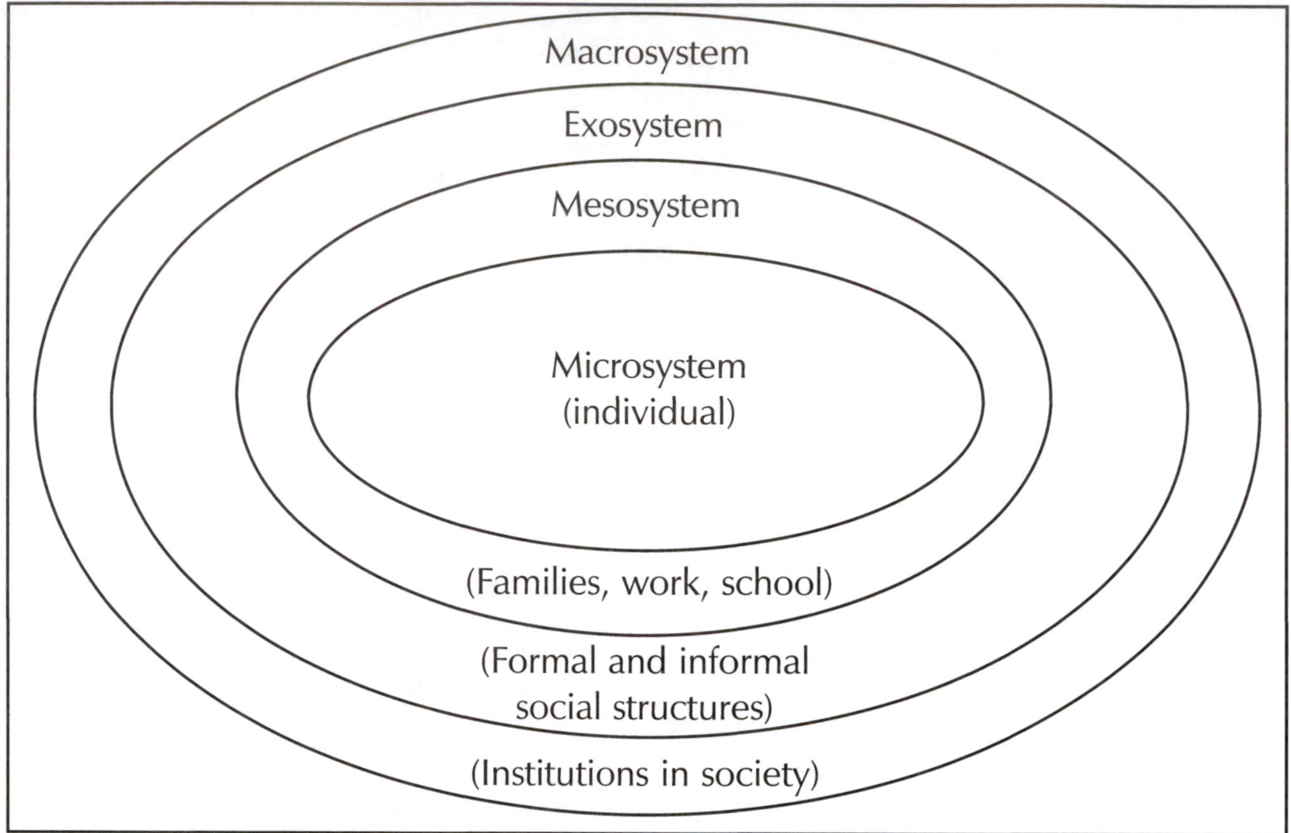

Figure 13-5. Bronfenbrenner's ecological systems model (1977).

ments in all spheres, including cognitive growth" (Bronfenbrenner, 1993, p. 10).

Bronfenbrenner rejected the common assumption of most of his contemporaries in psychology that developmental attributes could be examined out of the context of an individual's life. Instead, he identified individual spheres of environmental influence that influenced development and set out to explore development in context. Bronfenbrenner's (1977, 1993) Ecological Model consists of microsystems, mesosystems, exosystems, and macrosystems. These environmental spheres of performance describe the nested networks of interactions that create an individual's ecology (Figure 13-5). Bronfenbrenner assumes that this ecological network changes over time as an individual develops.

Briefly, there are four major spheres of influence within Bronfenbrenner's ecological model. The microsystem is a specific interaction that occurs between the developing person and one or more others. Parent-child interactions or parent-teacher interactions would occur within the microsystem. A mesosystem consists of interactions between and among two or more microsystems. An exosystem comprises an environment that has an impact on the developing individual but does not contain him or her. The community represents such a system. Finally, the macrosystem contains a person's entire micro-, meso-, and exosystems and involves the entire realm of developmental possibilities for him or her. Macrosystems are temporally and culturally specific to that individual and are dynamic rather than static. The macrosystem places the person in the context of his or her developmental ecology (see Figure 13-5).

The complex interactions within and between each system can inhibit or enhance development. For example, the possibility of developing an identity as a child with a disability is provided—or not provided—by the macrosystem of modern culture, but then an individual must also have micro-, meso- and exosystems that provide opportunities for that identity to develop.

Summary of Theoretical Models

The six theoretical models presented here provide a basic understanding of the key environmental influences on occupational performance. Lawton and Nahemow's Ecological Model assists us in understanding the balance between support and challenge that must be present in order for us to perform maximally our daily occupations. The Enabler provides us with a matrix to guide our thinking as we consider the various person factors that feel the influence of the environment. The types of environmental features that impact performance are understood using the ICF classification framework. Through this hierarchical organization of the environment from its broadest conceptualization as the context in which activity occurs to the link between specific characteristics and task performance, occupational performance can be understood, measured, and ultimately intervened upon by those interested in minimizing the impact of a disabling environment. The Baker and Intagliata and Bronfenbrenner models provide an important understanding of how the environment influences development and quality of life.

Aspects of the Environment That Affect Occupational Performance

In this section, the features of the environment that influence performance will be introduced. These features will be discussed in terms of their contribution to occupational performance and their potential to serve as supports or barriers. The physical and social features of the environment will be described in terms of how they can be modified to improve occupational performance. Physical interventions will be described in terms of adapted strategies, assistive technologies, adapted devices, and design changes. Social modifications that will be introduced include social support, personal assistance, and professional or programmatic support. These intervention strategies will be followed by a discussion of the environmental characteristics that must be taken into consideration during intervention (the natural environment, culture, economics, and social attitudes). The intervention strategies and considerations will be followed by a case study that demonstrates the outcome of an intervention using environmental modifications using the PEOP model.

Strategies to improve occupational performance at the level of the physical environment may include changes to the person (e.g., skill acquisition, adaptive strategies, prosthesis, or physical rehabilitation), occupation (e.g., replacing one activity with another), or the environment (e.g., assistive technologies, adaptive devices, design changes, caregiver support, or personal attendant services). In most instances, a combination of strategies is needed to promote successful occupational performance. In this section, we will focus on environmental modification strategies. Although strategies provided during occupational therapy are often focused on the home, work, school, and community, facilities are also potential areas where PE fit intervention strategies can help individuals with disabilities reach their occupational performance goals.

As noted in the previous section, the identification of environmental strategies is embedded in a detailed understanding of the specific environmental characteristics that affect occupational performance. However, a simple understanding of relevant characteristics does not ensure that a strategy will be successful. Rather, successful environmental modifications require matching the intervention to the situation. The PEOP model defines the situation.

The Physical Environment: Its Effect on Occupational Performance

The physical environment can be organized into three categories using the domains of the ICF. These include the built (or human made environment), products and technology (appliances, fixtures, and hardware/controls, including assistive technology), and the natural environment (WHO, 2001). These three organizing factors will be used in the following discussion of the built environment (Table 13-4).

Built Environment

There are two basic approaches to modifying the built environment. They include 1) restructuring, reorganizing, or addition of a built environment and 2) replacement, alteration, or addition of fixtures, appliances, or other environmental products and use of assistive technologies. Any or all of these approaches may be needed to accommodate a particular individual. Restructuring the built environment can be the most and the least expensive approach. Building an addition to a home or community space, moving walls to reconfigure interior space, or changing the topography by grading to reconfigure the natural landscape can be expensive but necessary in some instances. On the other hand, rearranging furniture in rooms, converting a downstairs study into a bedroom, and using the least demanding parts of the natural environment can be achieved at little or no cost. The second approach focuses on changing off-the-shelf products, such as a standard toilet with an elevated one or bathtub with a curbless/roll-in shower. Alternatively, products can be used to provide information about environmental demands for users to make informed decisions about their ability to perform a task successfully. Examples of successful modification interventions are well documented. For example, Connell and Sanford (2001) found that people with disabilities who modified their homes had little to moderate difficulty and dependence in the conduct of daily activities. Gitlin and colleagues (1993, 2001) concluded that home modifications slowed the rate of functional dependency and enhanced caregiver self-efficacy.

Table 13-4

Example of Physical Environmental Characteristics That Impact Bathing Performance

Space	*Product*	*Hardware/Controls*
Bathroom	**Tub/Shower**	**Faucet**
Entry: doorway width, threshold height Size Layout Systems locations: plumbing, electric lighting, ventilation Floor materials/finishes Ambient conditions	Type (description) Size/dimensions Hardware configuration (location of hardware) Lighting Materials/finishes	Type (description) Size Approach: distance and angle Force required Operational characteristics: direction, distance, calibration Materials/finishes

Mann and colleagues (1999) reported that the rate of decline in independence of older adults and costs for personal assistance and health care were reduced with an increased use of assistive technology and environmental interventions.

Products and Assistive Technology

Another important method of changing the environment is the provision of products or assistive technology (AT). Products can include the addition of adaptive hardware or modification to environmental controls. AT is defined as any product or system that is used to improve the functional capacity of people who have disabilities (Technology-Related Assistance for Individuals with Disabilities Act, 1988). This technology is designed to make the best use of an individual's abilities to overcome environmental barriers that may prevent the person from achieving maximal occupational performance (Seelman, 1993). There are numerous types of assistive devices and systems, including seating and mobility devices that can influence community access, computer access systems, augmentative communication devices, adapted driving devices, and environmental control units as well as pieces of adaptive equipment that make it possible to accomplish tasks such as dressing. When providing AT, the costs must be considered (O'Day & Corcoran, 1994), as much of AT available today is still costly and may not be funded by a health insurance program. The possibility of disuse or "abandonment" of AT by individuals for various reasons such as complexity of use or embarrassment related to using something different may occur (Gitlin, 1995). These factors may affect an individual's ability to maximize his or her independence.

Finally, changing hardware/controls might entail replacing an individual interface such as a light switch, faucet, or door handle; adding a variety of electronic controls (e.g., timers, photocells, or motion sensors) to automate tasks; or replacing an entire fixture such as an oven because the controls are too hard to reach or see.

Natural Environment

Often, the natural environment presents features that cannot be modified. For example, the terrain in San Francisco presents hills, the climate in Montana will offer snow and ice, and the climate in Florida may offer extreme heat and humidity. These aspects of the natural environment, including climate, atmospheric pressure, terrain, and even population density, may impact the performance of individuals with disabilities. Although these features themselves often can not be changed, modifications can be made to address the elements present in the natural environment. For example, providing a covered drop-off area in a driveway may allow someone who has a mobility impairment the time and protection they need from rain in the Seattle area. An older adult in Minnesota may benefit from a heated walkway that would melt snow and eliminate the need to shovel.

There may be policy or legal protections that are possible to improve occupational performance. For example, ensuring that accessible parking places, sidewalks, and curb cuts are free of snow or providing air conditioners for individuals at risk during extreme heat may make the difference between occupation and disablement. In some cases, natural terrain cannot be modified for individuals who have disabilities. For example, an accessible path from the top to the bottom of the Grand Canyon is not possible given the technology that is currently available. In this case, information may be the most important accommodation possible. A trail map that provides information about the terrain, rest areas, or alternative methods of accessing the trail (horseback) would be important information to allow an individual to choose which aspects of the trail he or she would like to experience.

Support, Relationships, and Their Effect on Occupational Performance

The use of social supports, both formal (programs and services) and informal (family and friends), are common strategies to compensate for environmental barriers. There are many definitions of social support. From a therapeutic perspective, social support for individuals with disabilities is often defined by determining whether they are cared for, loved, and able to count on others should the need arise (McColl & Friedland, 1989). Social support can include practical support, informational support, and emotional support (McColl, 1997). Practical support is generally considered tangible, physical support. Assistance with transfers, preparation of meals, or driving one to a doctor's appointment are examples of practical support. This support can be informal (provided by a family member or loved one) or formal (provided by a paid caregiver or personal care attendant). Informational support is generally considered advice or guidance. For example, providing one with a list of tips for saving energy, identifying a support group in the community, or advising a client on the type of equipment to purchase for bathing may be considered advice or information. Often, professionals or peers (i.e., individuals with the same or similar disability) provide this type of information, although family or friends can be a source of informational support. Emotional support is generally the provision of a sense of belonging or esteem. While professionals may provide this type of support, it is generally the role of family members and peer groups to provide everyday opportunities to be a member of a group or provide moral support during difficult times.

Social supports can improve the match between the person and the environment in the same way that physical changes can improve performance. For example, the occupation of eating a meal may be disrupted in the life of a person who is temporarily using a wheelchair for mobility. The person may be unable to move about his or her kitchen due to the environmental barriers that include narrow space in the kitchen, no turning area, cabinets that are out of reach, and the inability to see what is cooking on the stove. One strategy may be to modify the space by increasing the clear floor space, moving furniture to make more room, moving cabinets, and installing an angled mirror above the stove. An alternative would include teaching the individual to use a microwave and providing one at the height that can be reached from a wheelchair (Kondo, Mann, Tomita, & Ottenbacher, 1997).

A third solution may be to engage a home-delivered meal service (practical support formal). A fourth alternative would include engaging the individual's family or friends and asking them for help or assistance in preparing and providing meals (practical support informal). Although problems can be solved by providing these approaches, the outcome results are often negative when practical support has been offered as a solution to environmental barriers (McColl & Rosenthal, 1994; Weinberger, Tierney, Booher, & Hiner, 1990), while informational support (e.g., instruction in the use of a microwave) has been perceived as helpful when provided by professionals (Kondo et al., 1997). Emotional support has consistently been shown to demonstrate positive outcomes (Holicky & Charlifue, 1999), pointing out the importance of providing interventions that allow caregivers the opportunity to provide more support and less instrumental (practical) assistance. In some cases, the care of family members with disabilities in the home has been attributed to increased caregiver stress or burden (Zarit, Todd, & Zarit, 1986). In that case, the intervention plan that includes social support may be provided for the caregiver (Gallo, 1990). Often, changes in the physical environment can influence lives of caregivers. For example, Calkins and Namazi (1991) found that caregivers often made effective physical changes that increased safety, security, or comfort for their loved ones with Alzheimer's disease.

Socioeconomic and Political Aspects of the Environment That Influence Occupations

Other important extrinsic factors influence the performance of occupations in a society. Issues facing people with disabilities are a result of the misfit between impairments and practically every feature of the social, economic, physical, and political environment (Zola, 1989). Changes in housing, transportation, and employment policies would augment the quality of daily living for those with disabilities today and in the future. The culture of an individual and a society needs to be considered and understood and deserves mention in this text. Other important factors that influence occupational performance include policies, economic factors, and attitudes toward people with disabilities. These factors may change slowly based on scientific outcome research, political or social pressure, or shifts in attitudes, but they are present and deserve consideration in their present state during any modification. They are also important considerations for occupational therapists who should consider their role in influencing policy, laws, and economics for people with disabilities as well as understanding them. Culture, policies, laws, economics, and attitudes and beliefs—all features described in the ICF—will be discussed in light of the influence they have on the occupational performance of people with disabilities.

Culture

Culture includes the values, norms, customs, beliefs, behaviors, and perceptions that are shared by a group or society (Barris, Kielhofner, Levine, & Neville, 1985). Culture can be relevant at the level of the individual, organization, community, and society. Individually, culture can determine the level of independence that an individual desires. For example, it may be acceptable for an older adult to accept assistance during dressing from his or her spouse due to the cultural beliefs that the couple holds. Culture can also affect home modifications. For example, in Japan, an accepted cultural norm of removing one's shoes upon entering the home has shaped the design of houses. Typically, a landing that is higher than the floor surface inside the door is the area where the shoes are removed and stored until the wearer is ready to leave the home. This tradition makes wheelchair access more difficult to achieve, due to the lack of a level surface in the home and the important cultural meaning of the landing. Culture may be one of the most difficult aspects of the environment to understand, for as Barney (1991) describes, often, we do not realize what it is we do not know. Rather, recognizing that cultural values may influence what an individual is willing to do in order to achieve his or her goals, and determining what those cultural values are, is an important consideration.

Policies and Laws

Policies that direct the funding of programs to benefit individuals with disabilities may play a role in whether there is funding or services available. There are few countries (i.e., Sweden and Denmark) with policies that support home modifications for individuals with disabilities. Currently in the United States, there is no federal program to provide home modifications for individuals who have disabilities (Center for Universal Design, 1997). It is ironic that insurance programs will cover the cost of nursing home placement and home health aids but will not fund the provision of simple environmental modifications that would increase the independence of individuals who have disabling conditions so they could stay at home. This requires that individuals rely on local services and programs for environmental modification assistance while others fund the changes themselves. Often, however, individuals with disabilities do not have the resources to pay for costly home modifications. This economic reality may influence the types of modifications that are made for an individual. Often, social support is provided as a gap filler, not because it is the choice of the client but because it was the option that might be covered by insurance. The other alternative is that the family provides the instrumental support (such as transfers, bathing, and dressing). This option can lead to caregiver stress.

To a great extent, many practical programs and policy changes that influence the built environment have been put in place as a result of legislation. As an example, a series of legislative acts has shaped the policies of the United States since the Vocational Rehabilitation Act of 1920 (Table 13-5).

This series of legislative acts has shaped the programs and policies that influence participation and can, to a great extent, affect the occupational performance of individuals with disabilities. Legislation that impacts people with disabilities is important to consider when making modifications, as the law can influence funding and the types of modifications that may be possible. The Americans with Disabilities Act of 1990 (ADA), the Amendments to the Fair Housing Act in 1988, and the Individuals with Disabilities Education Act (IDEA) (formerly called P.L. 94-142 or the Education for all Handicapped Children Act of 1975) are just a few of the laws that influence environmental modifications (Peterson, 1998). These legislative acts reflect an interesting shift in public attitude toward people with disabilities. The recognition of the needs of individuals with disabilities has become more explicit with each successive legislative action. With the passage of the Americans with Disabilities Act of 1990 (Access Board, 2002), the focus of laws targeting people with disabilities has changed to a more comprehensive, broad-reaching approach focusing on protecting the civil rights of people who have disabilities.

Economics

People with disabilities receive less education and are much less likely to find a job than are nondisabled people (Neufeldt & Mathieson, 1995). In fact, in the latest Current Population Survey (CPS), 72.2% of people with health conditions or impairments that limit their ability to work did not have jobs (Kaye & Longmore, 1997). This lack of income, coupled with the increase in costs associated with living with a disability (medications, increased health care costs, home modifications), has resulted in a poverty rate that is 60% greater than in nondisabled counterparts (Kaye & Longmore, 1997). Even legislative mandates do not protect people with disabilities from being excluded in society. For example, the reasonable accommodation provision of the 1990 ADA directs employers to alter the workplace so that qualified workers with disabilities have equal employment opportunity. In interviews with 200 government employees who had requested reasonable accommodation, Harlan and Robert (1998) found that employers are reluctant to modify the

Table 13-5

Important Legislation That Affects Occupational Performance

Americans with Disabilities Act (ADA) 1990	The ADA prohibits discrimination on the basis of disability in employment, state and local government, public accommodations, commercial facilities, transportation, and telecommunications. It also applies to the United States Congress. To be protected by the ADA, one must have a disability or have a relationship or association with an individual with a disability. An individual with a disability is defined by the ADA as a person who has a physical or mental impairment that substantially limits one or more major life activities, a person who has a history or record of such an impairment, or a person who is perceived by others as having such an impairment. The ADA does not specifically name all of the impairments that are covered
Fair Housing Act 1988	The Fair Housing Act, as amended in 1988, prohibits housing discrimination on the basis of race, color, religion, sex, disability, familial status, and national origin. Its coverage includes private housing, housing that receives federal financial assistance, and state and local government housing. It is unlawful to discriminate in any aspect of selling or renting housing or to deny a dwelling to a buyer or renter because of the disability of that individual, an individual associated with the buyer or renter, or an individual who intends to live in the residence. Other covered activities include, for example, financing, zoning practices, new construction design, and advertising. The Fair Housing Act requires owners of housing facilities to make reasonable exceptions in their policies and operations to afford people with disabilities equal housing opportunities. For example, a landlord with a "no pets" policy may be required to grant an exception to this rule and allow an individual who is blind to keep a guide dog in the residence. The Fair Housing Act also requires landlords to allow tenants with disabilities to make reasonable access-related modifications to their private living space, as well as to common use spaces. (Note: The landlord is not required to pay for the changes.) The Act further requires that new multifamily housing with four or more units be designed and built to allow access for persons with disabilities. This includes accessible common use areas, doors that are wide enough for wheelchairs, kitchens and bathrooms that allow a person using a wheelchair to maneuver, and other adaptable features within the units
Air Carrier Access Act	The Air Carrier Access Act prohibits discrimination in air transportation by air carriers against qualified individuals with physical or mental impairments. It applies only to air carriers that provide regularly scheduled services for hire to the public. Requirements address a wide range of issues, including boarding assistance and certain accessibility features in newly built aircraft and new or altered airport facilities. People may enforce rights under the Air Carrier Access Act by filing a complaint with the U.S. Department of Transportation or by bringing a lawsuit in federal court
Civil Rights of Institutionalized Persons Act (CRIPA)	CRIPA authorizes the U.S. Attorney General to investigate conditions of confinement at state and local government institutions such as prisons, jails, pretrial detention centers, juvenile correctional facilities, publicly operated nursing homes, and institutions for people with psychiatric or developmental disabilities. Its purpose is to allow the Attorney General to uncover and correct widespread deficiencies that seriously jeopardize the health and safety of residents of institutions. The Attorney General does not have authority under CRIPA to investigate isolated incidents or to represent individual institutionalized persons

(continued)

Table 13-5

Individuals With Disabilities	IDEA (formerly called P.L. 94-142 or the Education for all Handicapped Children Education Act (IDEA) Act of 1975) requires public schools to make available to all eligible children with disabilities a free appropriate public education in the least restrictive environment appropriate to their individual needs. IDEA requires public school systems to develop appropriate Individualized Education Programs (IEPs) for each child. The specific special education and related services outlined in each IEP reflect the individualized needs of each student. IDEA also mandates that particular procedures be followed in the development of the IEP. Each student's IEP must be developed by a team of knowledgeable persons and must be at least reviewed annually. The team includes the child's teacher; the parents, subject to certain limited exceptions; the child, if determined appropriate; an agency representative who is qualified to provide or supervise the provision of special education; and other individuals at the parents' or agency's discretion
Rehabilitation Act	The Rehabilitation Act prohibits discrimination on the basis of disability in programs conducted by federal agencies, in programs receiving federal financial assistance, in federal employment, and in the employment practices of federal contractors. The standards for determining employment discrimination under the Rehabilitation Act are the same as those used in title I of the Americans with Disabilities Act
Architectural Barriers Act	ABA requires that buildings and facilities that are designed, constructed, or altered with Federal funds, or leased by a federal agency, comply with federal standards for physical accessibility. ABA requirements are limited to architectural standards in new and altered buildings and in newly leased facilities. They do not address the activities conducted in those buildings and facilities. The ABA covers facilities of the U.S. Postal Service

Adapted from Federal Citizen Information Center. (n.d.). A guide to disability rights laws. Retrieved June 29, 2004, from http://www.pueblo.gsa.gov/cic_text/misc/disability/disrits.htm#ADA.

social structure of work because of their perceived need to contain costs and maintain control of the work process. Harlan and Robert also report that employers often discourage employees with disabilities from making requests for accommodation, and they deny 33% of requests.

Attitudes and Beliefs

In addition to cultural beliefs, the attitudes toward and beliefs about people with disabilities can also influence their occupational performance. Where at one time disability was considered a condition inherent in a person, there is now acceptance that, in large measure, disability is a social construct with roots in societal attitudes (Gray & Hahn, 1997). Often, attitudes can be the most important extrinsic factor affecting the lives of people with disabilities, for the attitudes and beliefs of a society shape the laws, policies, and environments. Historically, discriminatory practices have occurred in the area of access to education, meaningful participation in the labor force (Neufeldt & Mathieson, 1995), and community accesses for the purposes of social participation as well as housing. Negative attitudes toward people with disabilities influence participation in all aspects of life. Even health care providers, generally believed to understand disability, have been identified as having negative attitudes and a general lack of awareness of the needs of patients with physical disability problems (Bailey, 1994), pointing out the need for attention to this important issue.

Promoting and protecting the rights and dignity of people with disabilities will require a combination of legal approaches, attention to the concrete realities of disability and societal barriers, and changes in the perception of and societal attitudes toward people with disabilities.

An Organizing Continuum for Understanding the Environmental Features That Influence Occupational Performance

Physical environmental changes require changes to the physical or natural environment to accommodate the individual who has a disabling condition. Social environmental changes include the provision of some type of support to accommodate for a disabling condition. These changes are made in a political, cultural, or economic context. How do we organize and think about the factors that determine how the changes will be made?

Individual characteristics in addition to other environmental factors must be considered when making decisions about environmental modification. One strategy to use when considering environmental issues is to envision the environment as hierarchically arranged, with those environments most frequently encountered in the center of a circle and those larger, more contextual environments surrounding the inner circle with progressively larger circles (Hagedorn, 2000; McColl, 1997). The environment can be conceptualized in a continuum from proximal to distal (Bronfenbrenner, 1977; Davidson & Whalley, 1991; Lawton, 1980) with the most proximal environments consisting of those most personal places that one uses most frequently and distal being the wider, more expanded layer of the environment that includes community. Each of these layers of the environment contains physical and social attributes that affect how an individual performs.

Concurrent with the need to understand the impact of the environmental attribute on the performance of an individual is the need to understand the impact of proximal versus distal environments. The personal environment is the environment most easily controlled by an individual. Thus, logically, the more personal or proximal an environment, the more likely it will support or inhibit performance.

The model posits an individual within his or her environment. A person can be viewed as the center of his or her own individual environment with the layer that immediately surrounds him or her consisting of the person's own personal spaces. Personal spaces can include the home in which a person lives or perhaps a place that he or she occupies and influences during primary occupations. These places could also include a dorm room or a personal car. Individuals' closest personal relationships occur in these places. These are the spaces that are likely to have the greatest influence on the performance of an individual and are most likely to be influenced by an individual. Personal spaces are most likely to be adapted or customized for use by their occupants. Examples of these types of environments include one's home, workstation or office, or even one's car. These are the spaces that are most likely to be personalized or adapted to meet our needs. For example, we can organize our toothbrush and toiletries in a manner that suits us best in our own homes, or we adjust the seat, mirrors, and items in our car that best facilitate our ability to drive.

The second layer of the environment includes the semipersonal spaces encountered by individuals during their occupations. Semipersonal environments include those spaces frequented by individuals during their daily occupations. These spaces can include workspaces or "offices," local stores visited often, a favorite restaurant, a club, or a religious facility. These spaces may or may not be customized to suit an individual's needs. Individuals are known and recognized in these environments. Occupations occur within these contexts and can be supported or impeded depending on the mix of social and physical influences. Semipersonal environments, or those public places that we pass through or experience frequently, typically surround proximal environments. Examples of public spaces can include a mall or a shopping center, library, or government building. These spaces may have adaptations that were made for the use of all individuals. These spaces may actually even have modifications made specifically for an individual. For example, a frequent patron of a coffee shop who uses a wheelchair may have influenced the proprietor to add an accessible bathroom, or the proprietor may allow the user to use his or her private bathroom because it is accessible. Generally, these spaces provide less accommodation than proximal or personal spaces.

The third layer or public sphere of performance includes those spaces that an individual may or may not travel to on a frequent basis. These are community spaces used by many individuals in a society. They can include community gathering places such as arenas, public services such as government facilities, and areas of public accommodation such as stores or restaurants. The social and physical features are least likely to be customized to an individual's needs in this environment. The environment is typically designed to adhere to general anthropomorphic guidelines or governmental procedures. The outer layer of the environment is the public area. These spaces are the public or community spaces that may or may not be used by individuals but they are part of the community within which the person operates (Table 13-6).

To better understand how the environment, made up of these physical and social influences, can have an effect on the performance of each individual, it is important to consider each element of the environment within the context that is relevant to that person. It is important to remember that while the elements can be explored individually, they continuously change and influence each other. While individuals are constantly changing

Table 13-6

Examples of Environmental Elements Found in Personal, Semipersonal, and Public Environments

	Personal Environment	*Semipersonal Environment*	*Public Environment*
Built environment	Home Dorm room	Places of employment Neighborhood places Day care	Community spaces (sporting arenas, grocery stores, city hall)
Products and technology	Assistive devices and technology designed or prescribed for an individual during self-care, leisure, or productive pursuits Food, drugs Clothing	Assistive devices and technology designed or prescribed for an individual during education or employment outside the home or during school such as augmentative communication devices or specialized software	Technology used in the community such as motorized carts at the grocery store Products used such as automatic teller machines
Transportation systems	Personal car Personal means of transportation (horse and buggy, bicycle)	Transportation systems belonging to friends or family	Public transportation including busses, cabs, airplanes
Natural environment	Geography Climate Flora and fauna Light, sound, and air quality	Geography Climate Flora and fauna Light, sound, and air quality	Geography Climate Flora and fauna Light, sound, and air quality
Cultural/societal factors	Personal values Tasks that must be accomplished by individual related to culture/religion	Culture of workplace Policy of organizations Religious practices in group settings Attitudes of a small group or individual toward disability	Belief system of a society Attitudes (of a society or group) toward disability Public service systems and policies Health care systems and policies
Social support	Close friends Family Partner	Casual friends Work colleagues Informational support Emotional support	Groups Institutions Professionals
Economic factors	Personal resources	Resources of community	Community wealth (tax base)

throughout the developmental process, the environment is also constantly changing as a result of physical, social, and economic factors. To conceptualize the environment of an individual, it is helpful to consider the person within the context of the world in which he or she lives.

The layers of the environment do not exist in isolation but are influenced by each other. For example, policy and services that are offered to individuals within a community may influence the type of housing that an individual can obtain. Thus, the public environment might greatly influence the personal environment of an individual.

These factors must be considered when determining modifications, as they may play a role in the success or failure of the person to do what he or she needs and wants to do. Does the client define independence by the level of assistance he or she needs from another human? Do the individual's cultural beliefs or family system determine the amount of informal family support the person desires? Is the person interested in technology, gadgets, and physical support? Is the person predisposed to using technology successfully, or will he or she abandon the expensive equipment in favor of assistance from his or her spouse (Bativa & Hammer, 1990; Scherer, 1994)?

Case Example Using the Person-Environment-Occupation-Performance Model

Modifying the environment has been a common strategy for supporting people who have limited capacities due to disabilities. It is the role of the occupational therapist to determine the environmental factors that are influencing an individual's performance, consider the context of the occupations of the client and family, and, with the clients, identify a plan to resolve those barriers. The following case provides an example of this intervention method. We will use Jen's story to illustrate how these theoretical constructs, intervention strategies, and the PEOP model support decisions to make environmental changes to improve the occupational performance of an individual with a disability.

Occupational History and Person Factors

Jen is a 12-year-old girl who has cerebral palsy. Jen is active in her school, which promotes inclusion, and she is interested in pursuing social relationships of a typical adolescent. Her long-term goal is to graduate from high school and consider post-high school education options. She wants to eventually live in her own apartment. Jen currently lives in a single-story home with her 15-year-old brother Frankie, her mother Rita, and her father Jim. Jim owns a small pest control business, and Rita, previously a stay-at-home mom, has become an administrative assistant for a parent advocacy group. Jen is bright and outgoing. She has tremendous support from her family and is well liked by her peers and teachers. She is interested in supporting her school's athletic teams by attending their games and has recently considered becoming a cheerleader. She also has always enjoyed attending her friend's parties and "hanging out" with her peers. Jen has no cognitive limitations but has significant neuromotor and communication difficulties. Her speech is disarthric, making it difficult for anyone who does not know her well to understand her. She has some movement of her right arm and hand but experiences choreoathetoid movements and has trouble gripping items. She is unable to walk or transfer independently. She relies on a power wheelchair for mobility, and her mom lifts her to the toilet, bathtub, and bed. Jen has self-concept scores that are lower than her nondisabled peers. She wishes that she could visit more of her friends and is beginning to feel left out of her group as her friends become more active in the community and begin to assert their independence.

What Has Happened?

Jen has become very tall. She is nearly 5 feet 10 inches tall and would tower over her petite mother if she were standing. Rita has recently hurt her back and is having tremendous problems transferring Jen. She has become concerned that with her new job she will need to travel and will not be at home to accommodate Jen's needs. She is interested in finding a means to enable Jen to become more independent.

Occupational Roles

Jen has many roles as a preteen. She is a daughter, friend, classmate, student, "included child," and person with a disability. Her mother, the primary caregiver to Jen (and also a client), has multiple roles as well. She is a mom, advocate for her daughter, spouse, advocate for people with disabilities, and community leader. She is also a friend and caregiver.

Client's Immediate Goals

Because both Jen and Rita are involved, it is important to consider the goals of each client. Jen has immediate goals of being able to fix her own hair and wash her own hands. She would like to be able to get into the bathroom without bumping into everything. Rita is interested in transfers that are safer and put less strain on her back.

Long-Term Goals

Jen is interested in graduating and considering college or vocational educational opportunities. She is interested in becoming independent and living in and managing her own home some day. Rita has the same long-term goals for her daughter.

Environmental Enablers: Environment

Currently, Jen has the enablers of a supportive family, economic resources, policy support from her state (programs to assist funding the changes her family may wish to make to the environment), and a great belief in her abilities and success. Jen's parents have instilled a belief in her that she is a valuable person with contributions to make in life. Jen looks forward to making a contribution to society, to working, and to having a satisfying life. Jen's family perceives these environmental modifications as an important learning opportunity for Jen. They want her to understand that the environment can be a support and that asking for modifications will be an important part of how she will be able to participate in society. Jen believes that she will achieve her goals and seeks the assistance of an occupational therapist to bridge her current situation to her goals by providing environmental support. The local school system has coordinated efforts with the family. For example, they have made sure that the equipment they provide for Jen to enhance her learning (computer) fit within the home context so that she can study. The family has also applied for and been granted tax credits to assist in paying for the changes to their home.

Environmental Barriers

Jen and her family face several environmental barriers. Most of the barriers are in the built environment (her home, the context of this intervention). Her home has a small bathroom with a typical bathtub. She is currently unable to manipulate the handles of the bathroom faucet and is unable to see herself in the bathroom mirror because it is located at a height that she cannot use in a seated position (from her wheelchair). She is unable to transfer into the bathtub without maximum assistance from her mother. She is required to make a three-point turn to get into the bathroom because of the narrow hallway and the configuration of the space. It is difficult to maneuver Jen's chair to the tub for transfers due to the limited space.

Evaluation

First, using the Enabler (Ivarsson, 1997) to guide the organization of Jen's capabilities and constraints to her performance, the occupational therapist would begin to think about the environment in terms of the capacity that Jen currently has as well as the potential changes in her performance that may be expected given the prognosis of her diagnosis and her expected development. Using the Enabler as a guide, the therapist begins to think about the assessment results and begins to place them in the framework to consider the potential person and environment relationships that may be preventing Jen from reaching her desired goals. Jen has problems with mobility, reaching, grasping, and manipulating. She uses a wheelchair for mobility. The Enabler helps the therapist identify potential barriers in the home. These can then be verified by standardized measures that are based on observation of performance.

Evidence

The evidence that has been presented thus far suggests that modification of the environment can increase the performance of individuals who have limited functional abilities. For example, as you recall from the beginning of this chapter, Connell and Sanford (2001) found that people with disabilities who modified their homes had little to moderate difficulty and dependence in the conduct of daily activities. Gitlin and colleagues (1993, 2001) concluded that home modifications slowed the rate of functional dependency and enhanced caregiver self-efficacy. Mann and colleagues (1999) reported that the rate of decline in independence of older adults and costs for personal assistance and health care were reduced through increased use of assistive technology and environmental interventions. These are critical pieces of evidence that, when coupled with the theories presented, suggest that environmental modifications are an appropriate intervention for Jen and her family.

Client-Centered Intervention Plan: Options and Choices

With a set of tools to provide environmental modification, the therapist will continue to use the theory and models presented in this chapter to develop an intervention plan for Jen. When considering the potential opportunities for modification, the therapist can rely on the ICF environmental chapter to organize his or her thinking about the potential environmental strategies that are possible. The framework by Connell and Sanford (1997) can guide the therapist in his or her decisions about the characteristics of the environment that would support the occupational performance of the client. In the present case, the plan was developed by the therapist, the clients, and the contractor and included modification of the existing bathroom. The changes included enlarging the room by breaking through a wall to use the space offered by a spare bedroom to provide a larger area with a 6-foot circle of clear space in the middle of the room. This additional space accommodated Jen's power chair and a caregiver at the same time.

Jen and her mom also opted for an overhead lift system to make transfers to the bath or toilet easier for her mom and to give Jen more independence. They chose the overhead lift system instead of the option of a roll-in shower because Jen enjoyed relaxing in the bathtub. A special seating system was included in the tub so Jen could sit in the tub independently. The mirror over the sink was lowered to a height of 36 inches so Jen could easily check her appearance. The sink included a lever-type faucet and clear knee space so Jen could roll under.

Outcomes: Revisiting Occupational Performance Goals

Upon re-evaluation and observation of Jen in her bathroom, the short-term goals that Jen and her mom had for safer, easier transfers and increased independence in using a mirror and sink were achieved by using environmental modifications. Jen's mom reports decreased stress on her back, and Jen is delighted to see herself in the mirror. Her mom reports that Jen often rolls into the bathroom to check her appearance.

Although the intervention in Jen's case was in the home, there were other issues that Jen's occupational therapist asked Jen about. The context of Jen's other occupations, the school she attends, and the community in which she lives were other potential places for environmental barriers. By revisiting Jen's goals and considering her new occupational performance priorities, Jen decided to address her desire to spend time with her friends. She was currently facing many problems accessing the community center and the movie theater.

Jen and her occupational therapist have developed an educational program that Jen presented to the Chamber of Commerce about living with disabilities. As a result of her presentation, several local business have been working with the local Americans with Disabilities Act Technical Assistance Center to improve the physical accessibility of the community. Jen and her family look forward to her development as a teenager and feel that the control that Jen can exhibit over her environment truly helps her feel like a valued and important citizen.

Summary

A fundamental shift in how disability is defined has occurred within the past decade. No longer is the individual "disabled" based on functional capacity, but rather that he or she can become disabled by an environment that prevents optimum performance. This new definition requires new intervention strategies by occupational therapists.

This chapter has provided some important concepts to use in understanding the role of the environment in the performance of occupations. We have summarized five important models that describe the person-environment-occupational performance relationship that is inherent in the PEOP model. These theories included Lawton and Nahemow's Ecological Model, the International Classification of Function Environmental Factors list by the World Health Organization, The Enabler by Steinfeld and colleagues, and The Conceptual Framework to Guide the Process of Developing Home Modification by Connell and Sanford. These theories were used to explore the interventions possible in the physical and social environment. The environmental context in which these changes occur was examined, and a discussion of the contextual features that need to be considered when making environmental modifications was presented. Finally, a case study was presented to illustrate how the PEOP model could be applied to a real case.

The occupational therapy process as defined by the PEOP model explicitly defines the role of environmental modifications as improving the occupational performance of individuals who have limited capacity. The use of these theories and intervention strategies is central to the process of eliminating a "disabling" environment and maximizing occupational performance for the individual and society.

Acknowledgements

The authors wish to gratefully acknowledge the contribution of Carolyn Baum, PhD, to the discussion of the evolution of environment in occupational therapy and rehabilitative models. Dr. Baum personally influenced the IOM and WHO models and her experience is appreciated in the development of this section.

Evidence Worksheet

Author	*Year*	*Topic*	*Method*	*Conclusions*
Calkins & Namazi	1991	Effects of home environmental modifications on occupational performance (people with dementia)	Interviews with caregivers	Modifications made by caregivers to homes of people with dementia primarily focus on increasing safety or autonomy of person with dementia
Connell & Sanford	1997	Effects of home environmental modifications on occupational performance (older adults with disabilities)	Case study observations	Diagnosing an individual's housing needs as a basis for identifying the most appropriate interventions will result in more positive rehab outcomes
Connell & Sanford	2001	Effects of home environmental modifications on occupational performance (older adults with disabilities)	Mailed survey of people with disabilities	Home modifications make a positive impact on difficulty and dependence experienced by people with mobility impairment in conducting routine household tasks and impact varies as a function of level of disability
Gitlin & Corchran	1993	Effects of home environmental modifications on occupational performance (caregivers of people with dementia)	Observation of caregiver interventions	Caregivers develop effective environmental solutions on their own and accept solutions more readily for bathing than incontinence
Gitlin et al.	2001	Effects of home environmental modifications on occupational performance (caregivers of people with dementia)	Randomized control trial	An environmental intervention program has a modest effect on IADL dependence of people with Alzheimer's disease
Mann et al.	1999	Effects of home assistive technologies on occupational performance (older adults)	Randomized control trial	Individuals who received assistive technology spent less on medical and other in-home assistance services, and long-term nursing home costs
Holicky & Charlifue	1999	Effects of spousal support on psychological well-being and quality of life (QoL) (people aging with SCI)	Physical, functional, and diagnostic evaluations; and psychosocial evaluations for stress, depression, life satisfaction, QoL, and community integration	Married individuals have less depression, greater life satisfaction and psychological well being, and better perceived QoL

REFERENCES

Access Board. (2002). Laws concerning the access board. Retrieved June 16, 2004, from http://www.access-board.gov/publications/Laws/A12.html.

Bailey, A. (1994). A handicap of negative attitudes and lack of choice: Caring for inpatients with disabilities. *Professional Nurse, 9*, 786-788.

Baker, F., & Intagliata, J. (1982). Quality of life in the evaluation of community support systems. *Evaluation and Program Planning, 5*, 69-79.

Barney, K. (1991). From Ellis Island to assisted living: Meeting the needs of older adults from diverse cultures. *American Journal of Occupational Therapy, 45*, 586-593.

Barris, R. (1982). Environmental interactions: An extension of the model of occupation. *American Journal of Occupational Therapy, 36*(10), 637-644.

Barris, R., Keilhofner, G., Levine, R., & Neville, A. (1985). Occupation as an interaction with the environment. In G. Kielhofner (Ed.), *A model of human occupation: Theory and application* (pp. 42-62). Baltimore, MD: Williams and Wilkins.

Bass Haugen, J. B., & Mathiowetz, V. (1995). Contemporary task oriented approach. In C.A. Trombly (Ed.), *Occupational therapy for physical dysfunction* (4th ed.). Baltimore: Williams and Wilken.

Bativa, A. E., & Hammer, G. S. (1990). Toward the development of consumer-based criteria for evaluation of assistive devices. *Journal of Rehabilitation Research and Development, 27*(4), 425-436.

Brandt, E. N., & Pope, A. M. (1997). Executive summary. In E. N. Brandt & A. M. Pope. (Eds.), *Enabling America: Assessing the role of rehabilitation science and engineering* (pp. 1-23). Washington, DC: National Academy Press.

Bronfenbrenner, U. (1977) Toward an experimental ecology of human development. *American Psychologist, 32*, 513-531

Bronfenbrenner, U. (1993). The ecology of cognitive development: Research models and fugitive findings. In R. H. Wozniak & K. W. Fischer (Eds.), *Development in context: Acting and thinking in specific environments* (pp. 3-44). New York, NY: Erlbaum.

Calkins, M., & Namazi, K. (1991). Caregivers' perceptions of the effectiveness of home modifications for community living adults with dementia. *Journal of Alzheimer's Care and Related Disorder Research, 6*(1), 25-29.

Canadian Association of Occupational Therapists. (1997). *Enabling occupation: An occupational therapy perspective*. Ottawa: CAOT Publications ACE.

Carver, V., & Rhodda, M. (1978). *Disability and the environment*. London: Elek Books.

Center for Universal Design. (1997). *A blueprint for action: A resource for promoting home modifications*. Raleigh, NC: North Carolina State University, School of Design.

Christiansen, C., & Baum, C. (1991). *Occupational therapy: Overcoming human performance deficits*. Thorofare, NJ: SLACK Incorporated.

Christiansen, C., & Baum, C. (1997). *Occupational therapy: Enabling function and well-being* (2nd ed.). Thorofare, NJ: SLACK Incorporated.

Connell, B. R., & Sanford, J. (1997). Individualizing home modification recommendations to facilitate performance of routine activities. In S. Laspry & J. Hyde (Eds.), *Staying put, adapting the places to the people* (pp. 113-147). Amityville, NY: Baywood Publishing.

Connell, B. R., & Sanford, J. A. (2001). Difficulty, dependence, and housing accessibility for people aging with a disability. *Journal of Architecture and Planning Research, 18*(3), 234-242.

Davidson, J. W., & Whalley, D. B. (1991). A design environment for addressing architecture and compiler interactions. *Microprocessors and Microsystems, 15*, 459-472.

Dunn, W., Brown, C., & McGuigan, A. (1994). The ecology of human performance: A framework for considering the effect of context. *American Journal of Occupational Therapy, 48*(7), 595-607.

Dunn, W., Brown, C., McClain, L., & Westman, K. (1994). Ecology of human performance: A framework for thought and action. In C. B. Royeen (Ed.), *AOTA self study series: The practice of the future: Putting occupation back into therapy* (Lesson 1). Bethesda, MD: American Occupational Therapy Association.

Dunning, H. (1972). Environmental occupational therapy. *American Journal of Occupational Therapy, 26*(6), 292-298.

French, J. R., Rodgers, W., & Cobb, S. (1974). Adjustment as person-environment fit. In G. V. Coelho, D. A. Hamburg, & J. E. Adams (Eds.), *Coping and adaptation* (pp. 316-333). New York, NY: Basic Books, Inc.

Gallo, J. (1990). The effect of social support on depression in caregivers of the elderly. *Journal of Family Practice, 30*, 430-440.

Gitlin, L. (1995). Why older people accept or reject assistive technology. *Generations, 19*, 41-46.

Gitlin, L., & Corchran, M. (1993). Expanding caregiver ability to use environmental solutions for problems of bathing and incontinence in the elderly with dementia. *Technology and Disability, 2*(4), 12-21.

Gitlin, L. N., Corcoran, M., Winter, L., Boyce, A., & Hauck, W. W. (2001). A randomized controlled trial of a home environmental intervention: Effect of efficacy and use in caregivers and on daily function of person with dementia. *Gerontologist, 41*(1), 4-14.

Gray, D. B., & Hahn, H. (1997). Achieving occupational goals: The social effects of stigma. In C. H. Christiansen & C. M. Baum (Eds.), *Occupational therapy: Enabling function and well-being* (2nd ed.). Thorofare, NJ: SLACK Incorporated

Hagedorn, R. (1995). *Occupational therapy: Perspectives and processes*. Edinburgh: Churchill Livingstone.

Hagedorn, R. (2000). *Tools for practice in occupational therapy: A structured approach to core skills and processes*. Edinburgh: Churchill Livingstone.

Harlan, S., & Robert, P. (1998). The social construction of disability in organizations: Why employers resist reasonable accommodation. *Work and Occupations, 25*, 397-435.

Holicky, R., & Charlifue, S. (1999). Aging with a spinal cord injury: The impact of spousal support. *Disability and Rehabilitation, 21*, 250-257.

Howe, M. C., & Briggs, A. K. (1982). Ecological systems model for occupational therapy. *American Journal of Occupational Therapy, 36*, 322-327.

Ivarsson, S. (1997). *The enabler: A method for analyzing accessibility problems for housing*. Sweden: Lund University, Department of Community Health Services.

Kaye, H. S., & Longmore, P. K. (1997). *Disability watch: The status of people with disabilities in the United States*. Volcano, CA: Volcano Press, Inc.

Kielhofner, G. (1985). *A model of human occupation: Theory and application*. Baltimore: Williams & Wilkins.

Kielhofner, G. (1995). *A model of human occupation: Therapy and application* (2nd ed.). Baltimore: Williams & Wilkins.

Kiernat, J. M. (1972). Promoting community awareness of architectural barriers. *American Journal of Occupational Therapy*, 26(1), 10-12.

Kondo, T., Mann, W., Tomita, M., & Ottenbacher, K. (1997). The use of microwave ovens by elder persons with disabilities. *American Journal of Occupational Therapy, 51*(9), 739-747.

Law, M. (1991). 1991 Muriel Driver lecture. The environment: A focus for occupational therapy. *Canadian Journal of Occupational Therapy, 58*(4), 171-180.

Law, M., Cooper, B., Strong, S., Stewart, D., Rigby, P., & Letts, L. (1996). The person-environment-occupation model: A transactive approach to occupational performance. *Canadian Journal of Occupational Therapy, 63*(1), 9-23.

Lawton, M. P. (1980). *Environment and aging*. Monterey, CA: Brooks-Cole.

Lawton, M. P. (1990). Residential environment and self-directness among older people. *American Psychologist, 45*(5), 638-640.

Lawton, M. P., & Nahemow, L. (1973a). Ecology and the aging process. In C. L. Eisdorfer (Ed.), *Psychology of adult development and aging*. Washington, DC: American Psychological Association.

Lawton, M. P., & Nahemow, L. (1973b). Towards an ecological theory of adaptation and aging. In W. Preiser (Ed.), *Environmental design research* (pp 24-32). Stroudsburg, PA: Dowden, Hutchison & Ross

Lawton, M. P., & Simon, B. (1968). The ecology of social relationships in housing for the elderly. *Gerontologist, 8*, 108-115.

Lewin, K. (1951). *Field theory in social science*. New York, NY: Harper.

Mann, W. C., Ottenbacher, K. J., Fraas, L., Tomita, M., & Granger, C. V. (1999). Effectiveness of assistive technology and environmental interventions in maintaining independence and reducing home care costs for the frail elderly: A randomized controlled trial. *Archives of Family Medicine*, 8(3), 210-217.

McColl, M. A. (1997). Social support and occupational therapy. In C. H. Christiansen & C. M. Baum (Eds.), *Occupational therapy: Enabling function and well-being* (2nd ed.). Thorofare, NJ: SLACK Incorporated

McColl, M. A., & Friedland, J. (1989). Development of a multidimensional index for assessing social support in rehabilitation. *Occupational Therapy Journal of Research*, 9, 218-234.

McColl, M. A., & Rosenthal, C. (1994). A model of resource needs of aging spinal cord injured men. *Paraplegia, 32*, 261-270.

Meyer, A. (1922). The philosophy of occupation therapy. *Archives of Occupational Therapy, 1*(1), 1-10.

Murray, H. A. (1938). *Explorations in personality*. New York, NY: Oxford University Press.

Neufeldt, A., & Mathieson, R. (1995). Empirical dimensions of discrimination against disabled people. *Health and Human Rights, 1*(2), 174-189.

O'Day, B. L., & Corcoran, P. W. (1994). Assistive technology: Problems and policy alternatives. *Archives of Physical Medicine and Rehabilitation, 75*, 1065-1069.

Peterson, M. (1998). *Universal kitchen and bathroom planning: Design that adapts to people*. New York, NY: McGraw-Hill Companies.

Polatajko, H. J. (1992). Naming and framing occupational therapy: A lecture dedicated to the life of Nancy B. *Canadian Journal of Occupational Therapy*, 59(4), 189-200.

Reed, K. L., & Sanderson, S. R. (1980). *Concepts of occupational therapy*. Baltimore, MD: Williams & Wilkins.

Reed, K. L., & Sanderson, S. R. (1983). In K. L. Reed & S. R. Sanderson (Eds.), *Concepts of occupational therapy* (2nd ed.). Baltimore, MD: Williams & Wilkins.

Reed, K. L., & Sanderson, S. R. (1992). *Concepts of occupational therapy* (3rd ed.). Baltimore, MD: Williams & Wilkins.

Reilly, M. (1962). Occupational therapy can be one of the great ideas of 20th century medicine. *American Journal of Occupational Therapy, 16*, 300-308.

Sanford, J. A. and Jones, M. L. (2001). Home modifications and environmental controls. In *Clinician's guide to assistive technology* (pp. 405-423). Chicago: Mosby Inc.

Scherer, M. J. (1994). *Living in a state of stuck*. Cambridge, MA: Brookline Books.

Schkade, J. K., & Schultz, S. (1992). Occupational adaptation: Toward a holistic approach for contemporary practice, Part 1. *American Journal of Occupational Therapy*, 46(9), 829-837.

Seelman, K. (1993). Assistive technology policy: A road to independence for individuals with disabilities. *Journal of Social Issues*, 49(2), 115-136.

Steinfeld, E., Schroeder, S., Duncan, J., Faste, R., Chollet, D., Bishop, M., et al. (1979). *Access to the built environment: A review of literature*. Washington, DC: U.S. Government Printing Office.

Stewart, A. M. (1992). The Casson Memorial Lecture 1992: Always a little further. *British Journal of Occupational Therapy, 55*(8), 296-302.

Technology-Related Assistance for Individuals with Disabilities Act. (1988). Retrieved August 30, 2004, from http://www.resna.org/taproject/library/laws/techact94.htm.

Weinberger, M., Tierney, W. M., Booher, P., & Hiner, S. C. (1990). Social support, stress and functional status in patients with osteoarthritis. *Social Science and Medicine*, *30*, 503-508.

World Health Organization. (2001). *International classification of functioning, disability and health*. Geneva: Author.

Zarit, S. H., Todd, P. A., & Zarit, J. M. (1986). Subjective burden of husbands and wives as caregivers: A longitudinal study. *Gerontologist*, *26*(3), 260-266.

Zola, I. (1989). Toward the necessary universalizing of a disability policy. *Milbank Quarterly*, *67*(Suppl.), 401-428.

Chapter Thirteen: Environmental Enablers and Their Impact on Occupational Performance Reflections and Learning Activities

Julie Bass-Haugen, PhD, OTR/L, FAOTA

REFLECTIONS

This chapter addresses the environment factors that contribute to occupational performance. These factors have equal importance to person factors and must be considered in all occupational therapy interventions. However, it is only in the past several decades that we have come to understand the various dimensions of the environment and its influence on occupational performance.

Most of you were probably born after the enormous changes in federal policies designed to improve the lives of people with disabilities. I was born before these advances and lived in a seemingly progressive, medium-sized city in the Midwest. As a child of the 1960s, I saw very few people who used wheelchairs or walking aids outside of a nursing home. Children with disabilities were rarely seen in a regular school setting and people with physical, cognitive, psychological, or emotional impairments were often institutionalized in residential self-contained settings called state hospitals. There was an unspoken belief by many people that institutions were a "better place for those people to live." Many of these institutional environments were horrifying, and the lives of people living there were tragic. There was little attempt to determine if the home and community environment could support the societal participation of people with disabilities.

There had always been individuals who abhorred this terrible practice of institutionalization in the United States. They advocated for the rights of all people to be treated with dignity and respect. During the 1950s and 1960s, a wave of civil rights activity began that later resulted in legislation addressing the fit between people and their regular environments. During the 1970s and 1980s, enormous changes started to occur in the environment. These physical, attitudinal, and societal changes opened educational, employment, and community doors for many people with disabilities. There is still a long way to go, but at least we are headed in the right direction!

During the 1970s and 1980s, there was also a beginning recognition that if there was a problem in occupational performance and participation, the environment deserved examination along with the person. For example, when people could not get around their neighborhoods in wheelchairs, we finally recognized the problem was the curbs, not the impairment or the wheelchair. The impairment simply required a different way of doing things, and the wheelchair was a means for mobility not confinement. Similarly, when people could not work in regular employment settings or attend public schools, we began to look at the issues with the environment rather than the person. We found that modification of the physical, social, cultural, and attitudinal environment resulted in huge successes for people of all ages and abilities. None of this seems like rocket science now, but these changes represented huge advances in knowledge and ideas in the recent past.

In this chapter, we examined a number of practice models that include the environment as a key factor. We began by taking a historical look at occupational therapy and rehabilitation models. We saw that the evolution of environment in practice models paralleled changes occurring in society. There had been a few progressive thinkers in the earlier part of the century. However, primary recognition of the environment in practice models did not begin to occur until the 1970s.

A couple of key ideas were introduced during this time. One idea was that the environment includes more than just physical characteristics; it consists of psychobiological and societal factors as well. Another idea was that the degree of ability and disability is influenced in large part by the physical and social environment.

During the past several decades, several environmental behavior models have been introduced to examine the PE fit and its effect on occupational performance. Some of these models emphasized the physical (natural or built) environment. The Environmental Press Model looks at the match between the capabilities of the person and the demands of the environment. When the match is good, performance is good. When the match is poor, performance is poor. For example, pretend you are a typical ninth grader in a high school and you are being assigned to a mathematics class. If the mathematics class is advanced calculus or beginning arithmetic, the match between your capabilities and the demands of the classroom environment would be poor. You would either be totally confused or totally bored. In either case, the environmental press would be less than optimal for you. If the mathematics class is algebra or geometry, the classroom environment would more likely provide the "just-right" challenge for your current mathematics capabilities. This idea of PE fit is so important for occupational therapy practice. If we set up the environment to be too challenging or too easy for a person's current capabilities, we may see occupational performance deteriorate.

The ICF by the WHO is an impressive person-environment model. It clearly identifies environmental factors as important to a person's activities and participation in society and includes both physical and social components. ICF is an international, comprehensive PE approach that is helping us find a common language for our discussions on health and disability. There is an interesting thing to note in the figure depicting the interaction between the components of ICF. The arrows are bidirectional. What is the significance of this? This suggests clear recognition of the power of occupation. Our engagement in activities and participation in society has an impact on other aspects of our life: body functions and structures, health condition, person factors, and environment factors. This idea is supported in recent recommendations that engagement in an activity, like exercise, is important for people with a health condition, like osteoarthritis. We have come a long, long way in our understanding of the relationships between person, environment, and occupational performance.

Two PE models explore the nature of the relationship between specific impairments and specific environmental factors as it relates to occupational performance. The Enabler Model emphasizes the influence of a person's environment on the ability/disability status. A supportive environment strengthens a person's skills and abilities. An unsupportive environment does the opposite; it may result in disabilities. A Home Modification Framework is another example of an approach to link specific personal and environmental characteristics. It focuses on selecting physical modifications for the home (e.g., spaces, products, hardware/controls) to meet task requirements and specific personal abilities. Both of these models provide a foundation for specific strategies to improve the PE fit.

There are several other angles that may be taken to examine the PE fit with occupational performance. One question we might ask is, how can we measure the "fit" between the PE? For example, how could we measure the "fit" of well elders living in their neighborhood? Similarly, how could we measure the "fit" of children with special needs attending a neighborhood school? Quality of life has been proposed as one measure of "fit." If people report good quality of life, then the fit between personal capabilities and environmental characteristics must be optimal.

The Ecological Systems Model looks at PE fit from yet another angle. This model emphasizes the social aspects of our environment. The individual is the focus of the model, and the fit can be examined by looking at the layers of social connections. I might begin by asking myself, "What is my fit with the people closest to me—family, coworkers, closest friends?" Then, "what is my fit with other social structures—neighborhood, athletic club, volunteer organization?" Finally, "What is my fit with social institutions—government, church, school?" I can see by doing this exercise that, at any given point in time, my fit varies depending on a variety of recent circumstances and events.

When we work with an individual, we may use one of these specific models (or others) along with the PEOP model to guide our evaluation of and interventions for environmental factors. For example, the PEOP model introduces built environment/technology as an environmental factor. The ICF includes specific descriptions of similar physical domains: products and technology, natural and human-made changes. Let's look at an example related to the physical environment. Say you are working with someone who has begun to use a wheelchair for mobility. After taking an inventory of occupations having meaning and importance, you might begin to examine how the environment supports and limits performance using a wheelchair. What if you found there were three steps to the front door entrance of the home? What interventions would you consider? What if you found the eating area in the kitchen was a high counter with barstools? What interventions would you consider? What if you found a traditional bathroom was not working for toileting and hygiene? What interventions would you consider? Your ideas right now are probably consistent with the general interventions you would typically consider for the physical environment: modifying the current environment and using products and technology.

In this same example, it is also important to consider social support and relationships (social support mechanisms) as well as socioeconomic and political aspects of performance (cultural norms and values, social policies and values). What if you found this individual was recently divorced but had extended family living in the neighborhood? What interventions would you consider? What if you found this individual had limited economic means and there was a social service agency that provided low-cost equipment to people with needs? What interventions would you consider? What if you found this individual's community was seeking input on transportation issues for people with disabilities? What interventions would you consider? Your ideas right now likely include interventions that fit with the political, social, cultural, or economic environment. Some of these strategies might be targeted for a specific individual with specific needs. Other strategies might be targeted at the larger population of individuals with these types of needs. All of these strategies may result in improved occupational performance and a better PE fit.

Planning interventions for environmental factors requires prioritization. There are obviously many things that can be addressed related to the occupational performance issues of a person. Where do you begin? If you think about it, it is common sense that you would begin with the most immediate environments and progress to the environments that are frequented less often. For the person who now uses a wheelchair, issues in the home need to be addressed before the workplace and before the community theater. A continuum of environments like this (e.g., first, second, third layers) helps an occupational therapy practitioner develop priorities for interventions. The first layer would more likely require individual interventions, while the third layer would need population-based interventions. The second layer would likely need a mix of individual and population-based interventions. So you see, the nature of occupational therapy interventions for the environment will vary depending on the type of environment.

As you have seen in this chapter, environment factors are just as important and complex as person factors. As you continue your learning, you will acquire specific knowledge about environmental interventions designed to improve the PE fit and occupational performance. Your skills will be valued as you contribute to improved personal and public environments for people with special needs.

Journal Activities

1. Look up and write down a dictionary definition of environment and context. Highlight the component of the definitions that is most related to their descriptions in Chapter Thirteen.
2. Identify the most important new learning for you in this chapter.
3. Identify one question you have about Chapter Thirteen.
4. Observe a person performing an occupation for 30 minutes to 1 hour. (Note: You might find the learning activity more interesting if you choose an occupation that is not done alone). Take notes and reflect on observable characteristics and behaviors that give you information on environment factors. Use the PEOP environment factors and/or ICF environment classifications to record your observations. Write a summary of your conclusions about the environment factors for this individual doing the occupation.

Technology/Internet Learning Activities

1. Use a discussion database to share specific journal entries.
2. Use a good Internet search engine to find the *International Classification of Functioning, Disability and Health* (ICF) by the World Health Organization (WHO).
   - Enter the phrase "International Classification of Function WHO" in your search line.
   - Review the home page for the ICF.
   - Review the online version of the ICF.
   - Identify the main classifications (chapters) of environment in ICF.
     - ✧ Rank ICF body function classifications (chapters) that have the most and least relevance for occupational therapy (1 = primary relevance; 2 = secondary relevance)

Environment	*Rank*

✧ Examine subclassifications for one environment classification (chapter) of interest and relevance in occupational therapy. Identify one strategy for measuring or obtaining information on this subclassification for one person.

Environment	*Subclassification*	*Measurement/Information Strategy*
5 - Services, Systems, Policies	e535 Communication services, systems, and policies	Individual information—interview on current communication uses. Community information—local, regional governmental agency

- Scan the literature reviewed on environmental factors in the Web site.
- Identify three examples of literature that may be useful in your occupational therapy practice.

Topic/Section	*Reference*	*Brief Summary*

- Review the winners of the WHO Photo Contest on "Images of Health and Disability."
- Select one photo to examine in detail, and document the title of the photo.
- Write a summary on your perceptions of the environmental factors in the photo.

3. Use a good Internet search engine to find the Web site for "DisabilityInfo."
   - Enter the phrase "DisabilityInfo," "Disability government," or "Disability federal government" in your search line.
   - Review the Internet site.
   - What is the primary purpose of this site?
   - Identify the primary information areas on disability at this site.
   - Identify primary information areas that relate to environmental factors.
   - Search the site for useful information on the environment or access.
   - Give three examples of information on environmental factors useful in occupational therapy practice.
4. Use a good Internet search engine to find the Web site for the Minnesota State Council on Disability. Visit Internet sites for other state/province commissions and councils.
   - Enter the phrase "state council on disability Minnesota" in your search line.
   - Review the Web site.
   - Evaluate the quality of the Web site.
   - What resources are available on the site?
   - Review the "Building Access Survey" in the publications.
     - ✧ Identify the environmental characteristics that are included in this survey?
     - ✧ How might you use this resource in your practice?
   - Review the "Responding to Disability: A Question of Attitude" survey in the publications.
     - ✧ Reflect on the questions and your responses.
     - ✧ How are attitudes an environmental factor?

5. Use a good Internet search engine to find Internet sites on topics related to environmental factors. Enter the phrase in your search line.
   - "universal design"
   - "universal design file"
   - "assistive technology"
   - "assistive technology device"
   - "home modification"
   - "information technology access"
   - "disability access"
     - ✧ For each phrase, identify two to three Web sites with information on this topic.
     - ✧ Evaluate the quality of the Web sites.
     - ✧ Describe the information available on each Web site.
     - ✧ Evaluate the usefulness of the Web site as a resource in your practice.
     - ✧ Bookmark or document useful sites for future reference.

Applied Learning

Individual Learning Activity #1: Experiencing Environmental Influences of a Simulated Disability

Instructions:

- Create the strategies for simulating a disability, and schedule a 24-hour period of time when you will commit to experiencing the disability and its environmental influences (e.g., impairments in the lower extremities requiring use of wheelchair, impairments on one side of the body requiring use of only one side of the body for activities, visual impairments limiting overall clarity of vision or vision in one half of the visual field, hearing impairment).
- Explore the environmental influences on occupational performance for this simulated disability in a variety of private and public places (e.g., working on computer at library, making purchases in stores, using public transit, buying snacks/beverages from machines, making a meal, using private and public restrooms, attending a class, going to a restaurant, participating in a social activity).
- Analyze specific environmental factors for their effect on occupational performance. Identify specific characteristics that support (enablers) occupational performance and limit (barriers) occupational performance. Identify specific occupations that were supported and limited by these environmental factors. Summarize your information in the table provided. Put a * by the most significant barriers to performance.

Environmental Factors	*Enablers*	*Occupational Performance Area*	*Barriers*	*Occupational Performance Area*
Natural Environment				
Built Environment				
Cultural Norms and Values				
Social Supports				
Societal Policies and Attitudes				

- Write a brief summary of your experience and the feelings you had while living with a simulated disability.

Active Learning

Group Activity #1: Exploring the Influence of Environment on Occupational Performance Using a Simulated Disability

Preparation:

- Read Chapter Thirteen.
- Assign simulated disability to each member in the group.
- Talk about how you will enjoy the experience but remain respectful of the real disability.

Time:

- Session 1: 15 minutes, preparation for activity
- Session 2: individual time over 24 hours
- Session 3: 30 to 45 minutes, sharing and discussion

Materials: Simulated disability kit. Each kit includes a description of simulated disabilities that includes a limitation in mobility and a limitation in sensory, cognitive, or other person factors

Instructions:

- Individually:
  - ✧ Complete Individual Learning Activity #1.
- In small or large groups:
  - ✧ Share your experience of having a simulated disability with other members of the group.
  - ✧ Identify the occupational performance areas that were most affected by environmental barriers for most members of the group. What were the environmental barriers?
  - ✧ Identify the occupational performance areas that were relatively unaffected by the simulated disability or environmental factors for most members of the group.

Environmental Factors	*Enablers*	*Occupational Performance Area*	*Barriers*	*Occupational Performance Area*
Natural Environment				
Built Environment				
Cultural Norms and Values				
Social Supports				
Societal Policies and Attitudes				

Discussion:

- Discuss how your experiences were examples of PE fit for occupational performance. Where was the fit intact? How was the fit compromised?
- Discuss the effect of this experience on your person factors: energy, mood, thinking.
- Discuss how the experience of a real disability might be different from a simulated disability.
- Discuss your insights from this experience that will be useful in your occupational therapy practice.

Group Activity #2: Exploring Culture and Values Through One Occupation: Food

Preparation:

- Read Chapter Thirteen.
- Sign up the small group for a genuine food experience associated with one culture (e.g., Indian, Jewish, Chinese, Soul, Mexican, Vietnamese, Brazilian, Somalian, Cajun, etc.).
- If possible, identify a cultural guide for the food experience.

Time:

- Session 1: 15 minutes, preparation for activities
- Sessions 2 to 4: 1 to 3 hours each session for experiences (may be done over several weeks)
- Session 5: 30 minutes, organizing findings from small group work
- Session 6: 1 hour, culture and food fair

Materials:

- Notebook
- Camera
- Other materials to be determined related to specific activities

Instructions:

- In small groups:
  - Identify the individual and small group goals you have for exploring the food of another culture.
  - Select a culture to examine that is mostly unfamiliar for members of the small group.
  - Identify at least three specific activities that will help you to explore the cultural norms and values related to food and food preparation for the culture. If at all possible, identify a cultural guide from the community who will lead you through some of these activities. At least one of these activities should involve eating a meal or preparing a meal. Examples: create a menu for a special meal, shop for ingredients at an ethnic market, select recipes from an ethnic cookbook, observe a cook who understands the culture, eat at an ethnic restaurant, watch a cooking demonstration, eat a meal with someone who can provide background information on the culture, interview people who understand the culture.
  - Assign responsibilities/tasks for each group member and identify timelines for all components of the experience.
  - Keep a notebook on your experiences. You may want to include menus, history of dishes, occasions when dishes are served and why they are special, information on ethnic markets, essential/common ingredients, supplies/cooking equipment/dishes, recipes, typical/special meals, cooking instructions, cooking/eating practices and techniques, table arrangements, traditions at meals, photographs.
  - Discuss and document the information that you have obtained on the cultural norms and values through this food experience. What are the implications for occupational therapy practice?
  - Identify the information and food samples you will share with the large group at a culture and food fair.
- In large group:
  - Schedule a culture and food fair.
  - Set up a display that includes information and food samples from your small group experience.
  - Share your experience with the larger group.

Discussion:

- Discuss how your food experiences will help you plan assessments and interventions for people having cultural norms and values different from your own.
- Discuss strategies you can use to learn about other aspects of the culture.
- Discuss the cultures that are represented in your communities.
- Discuss cultural activities that will be important to include in your future professional development plans and strengthen your skills as a practitioner.

Group Activity #3: Exploring Environmental Factors in One Public Space

Preparation:

- Read Chapter Thirteen.
- Identify and obtain resources for evaluating public environments.

Time:

- Session 1: 15 minutes, preparation for activities
- Session 2: 1 to 2 hours, visit and evaluate a public space
- Session 3: 30 to 45 minutes, discuss summary of findings and prepare action plan
- Session 4: 30 to 45 minutes, share findings with large group

Materials: Camera, measuring tape, notebook. and resources on environmental assessment/evaluation

Instructions:

- In small groups:
  - ✧ Identify the individual and small group goals you have for exploring the environmental factors in one pubic space.
  - ✧ Select a public environment that the group would like to evaluate.
  - ✧ Identify at least five specific aspects of the environment that you will include in your evaluation.
  - ✧ Assign responsibilities/tasks for each group member, and identify timelines for all components of the experience.
  - ✧ Obtain specific resources that you will use to evaluate the environment.
  - ✧ Visit the public environment. Spend about 1 hour in the environment. Document your observations. Obtain permission to conduct any activities that would not be considered typical behavior in this environment (e.g., obtaining measurements, taking pictures, etc.).
  - ✧ Keep a notebook on your evaluation. Summarize both environmental enablers and barriers to performance in the table provided.

Environmental Factors	*Enablers*	*Occupational Performance Area*	*Barriers*	*Occupational Performance Area*
Natural Environment				
Built Environment/Technology				

  - ✧ After the visit, meet in your small group to discuss and summarize your findings. Identify environmental solutions for each barrier you identified. Propose inexpensive, creative solutions as well as major environmental modifications. Consider the likely budget of the public place for the solutions.
  - ✧ Develop an action plan to communicate an overview of your findings to a manager of the public place (e.g., a professional letter, a meeting). Remember to communicate the enablers as well as the barriers in the environment. Offer a variety of solutions for barriers in the environment. If you are a student, review your action plan with your instructor.
  - ✧ Implement your action plan and evaluate any results.
- In large group:
  - ✧ Prepare a poster or technology-based presentation of your environmental evaluation.
  - ✧ Identify the resources you used to evaluate the environment.
  - ✧ Include specific examples/evidence of the enablers and barriers in the environment.
  - ✧ Summarize the solutions you developed.
  - ✧ Discuss the action plan you developed and implemented.

Discussion:

- Discuss the prevalence of environmental enablers and barriers in public places.
- Discuss the strengths and limitations of resources you used to evaluate the environment.
- Discuss the challenges of evaluating a public environment and developing workable solutions.
- Discuss roles for occupational therapy practitioners as they relate to public environments.

Chapter Fourteen Objectives

The information in this chapter is intended to help the reader:

1. Describe the measurement process, what it does, what it involves, its importance, and its function in occupational therapy practice.
2. Describe how occupational performance assessment approaches support client-centered practice.
3. Understand the strategies that must be employed to use an occupational performance approach.
4. Describe the elements of clinical utility.
5. Describe reliability and the three types of reliability that must be considered in choosing measures.
6. Describe content and construct validity and its importance in choosing measures.
7. Describe the three phases for best-practice assessment and the factors that must be included in a measurement model that supports best practice.
8. Understand methods for gathering assessment data.
9. Become familiar with measures that enable the development of a client-centered plan to address the occupational performance issues of your clients.

Key Words

best practice assessment: The use of reliable and valid assessment strategies by occupational therapists to determine occupational performance issues from a client-centered perspective and to derive information to determine appropriate intervention.

clinical utility: The clinical usefulness of an assessment tool.

construct validity: The degree to which an assessment's findings fits with prior theoretical relationships among characteristics or individuals.

content validity: The comprehensiveness of an assessment tool; inclusion of all important aspects of the attribute that is being measured.

inter-rater reliability: Consistency of measurement between assessors.

intra-rater reliability: Consistency of measurement within one assessor.

occupational performance assessment: Evaluation of the performance and satisfaction of a person participating in everyday occupations.

test-retest reliability: Consistency of measurement over time.

The only man who behaved sensibly was my tailor;
he took my measurement anew every time he saw me,
while all the rest went on with their old measurements and expected them to fit me.
George Bernard Shaw

Chapter Fourteen

Occupational Performance Assessment

Mary Law, PhD, OT(C); Carolyn M. Baum, PhD, OTR/L, FAOTA; and Winnie Dunn, PhD, OTR, FAOTA

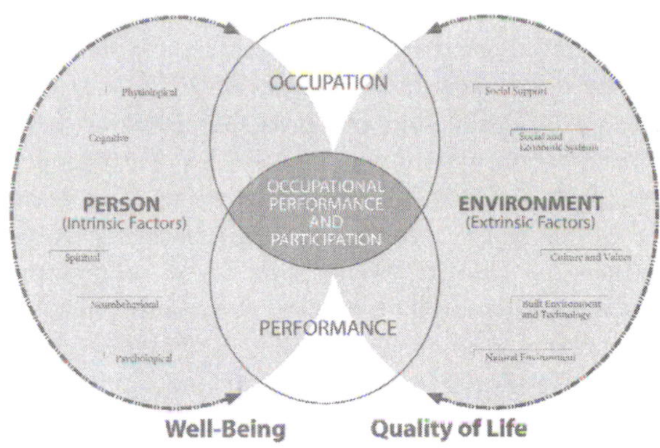

Setting the Stage

This chapter introduces the student or practitioner to concepts and tools that will facilitate understanding clients' needs, planning interventions, and documenting the effectiveness of services. The focus of occupational therapy is to enable people to carry out the occupations that support their tasks and roles in everyday living. The focus of measurement is to assess the occupational performance needs of an individual, an organization, or a community; to identify supports and barriers to occupational performance; and to document change in occupational performance over time and following intervention.

Don't miss the companion Web site to *Occupational Therapy: Performance, Participation, and Well-Being, Third Edition.* Please visit us at http://www.cb3e.slackbooks.com.

Law, M., Baum, C. M., & Dunn, W. (2005). Occupational performance assessment. In C. H. Christiansen, C. M. Baum, and J. Bass-Haugen (Eds.), Occupational therapy: Performance, participation, and well-being *(3rd ed.). Thorofare, NJ: SLACK Incorporated.*

Introduction

Occupational therapists work with people, groups, and organizations that are experiencing difficulties performing the occupations (self-care, work, voluntary activities, play, leisure) of life. The desired outcome of occupational therapy services is optimal occupational performance (i.e., the satisfactory experience of a person participating in everyday occupations).

Occupational therapists, as well as all other health care providers, strive to practice in a manner that is effective and efficient. Providing cost-effective, evidence-based care is the goal of every professional. One of the most important underpinnings of an evidence-based occupational therapy practice is the consistent use of outcome measures to evaluate occupational therapy service. Information from the application of outcome measurement enables therapists to make decisions about which programs are most effective, thus building evidence to support occupational therapy intervention.

There is a wealth of information in the occupational therapy literature and the broad health and social sciences literature that can be used by the occupational therapy practitioner to support occupational therapy measurement practices (Law, Baum, & Dunn, 2001; Van Deusen & Brunt, 1998). Using such information will enable occupational therapists to support their clinical observations and, indeed, will lend credibility to their day-to-day clinical observations. Occupations are complex, individualized, and essential for health and well-being. Evaluation of occupational performance (i.e., the outcomes of doing occupation) is enhanced by a broad measurement perspective.

What Is Measurement and Assessment?

Measurement is a process that involves an assessment, calculation, or judgment of the magnitude, quantity, or quality of a characteristic or attribute. In everyday living, we deal with measurements ranging from calculation of time, length, or weight to judgments of quality of life and satisfaction. It is helpful to think of measurement as an overall approach to gathering knowledge about an attribute. A measurement process organizes the way in which we learn about a person, his or her family, and the occupational performance issues that bring him or her to receive our services and the way that we evaluate the outcomes of those services. During measurement, we need to consider the purpose of gathering information, the context of measurement, and the specific methods to be used. Assessment refers to the overarching set of tasks of finding out about a person, while evaluation refers to specific procedures used in the assessment process. Assessment involves the collection of, appraisal of, and classification of information gathered in an organized manner. Such methods or tools for collecting information include naturalistic observation, interview, rating of task performance, and self-report (Christiansen & Baum, 1997). Assessment methods and specific assessment tools, whether qualitative or quantitative in nature, are developed and tested to ensure that they can be applied consistently and gather valid information.

Measurement in Occupational Therapy

Occupation is everything that we do in life, including actions, tasks, activities, thinking, and being. Engagement in occupation describes the interaction of the individual with his or her self-directed life activities. Occupational performance is the doing of occupation in order to satisfy life needs. Occupational therapy practice/assessment must place its focus on occupational performance, assisting our clients to become actively engaged in their life activities. Basic to an occupational performance approach are the skills of the therapist to analyze tasks, activities, and occupations and to propose and use learning or adaptive strategies to support the individual to perform meaningful occupations.

Measurement in occupational therapy serves multiple purposes. From an overall practice perspective, measurement is used to improve our decisions regarding specific clients or programs. As professionals, occupational therapists have an obligation to measure the need for service, design interventions based on knowledge gained from measurement, and evaluate the results of our interventions. Information gathered through measurement helps occupational therapists to design interventions for individuals or groups and to evaluate the outcomes of these programs. Management and policy makers use measurement information to make decisions about the continuance of funding for programs or the need to establish and/or evaluate new policy directions.

Measurement and Client-Centered Occupational Therapy Practice

During the past two decades, occupational therapists have described the need for a practice based on a client-centered approach to occupational therapy. Client-centered occupational therapy has been defined as "an approach to service [that] embraces a philosophy of respect for, and partnership with, people receiving services" (Law, Baptiste, & Mills, 1995, p. 253). The concepts of client-centered practice have the following implications for measurement of occupational performance:

- Occupational performance problems are identified by the client and his or her family, not by the therapist or team; if other issues, such as safety, are not identified, the therapist will communicate these concerns directly to the client and family.
- Evaluation of the outcome of therapy intervention will focus on change in occupational performance
- Measurement will reflect the individualized nature of people doing occupations.
- Measurement will focus on both the subjective experience and the observable qualities of occupational performance.
- Measurement of occupational performance involves assessment of self-care, work, other productive pursuits, play, and leisure.

Measuring Occupational Performance

Because of the importance of context for performance, we also discuss measurement of the environmental factors that influence performance. It includes the use of both quantitative and qualitative assessment approaches from the perspective of the client, his or her family or caregiver, and the occupational therapist. As occupational therapists develop an evidence-based practice, a valid measurement process is essential in providing evidence of the effectiveness and efficiency of our services. Our measurement practices need to fit within a client-centered practice in which people, their families, and therapists work in partnership to enhance occupational performance. Our clients expect, and have a right to know and receive, evidence of the outcomes of occupational therapy service provision.

The measurement of occupational performance requires the practitioner to employ three strategies:

1. What people do in their daily lives.
2. What motivates them.
3. How their personal characteristics combine with the environment in which occupations are undertaken to influence successful occupational performance.

Such an approach provides a framework for viewing human behavior that combines knowledge about the impairments (components) that impede performance; the environments that support performance; and the individual needs, preferences, styles, and goals (Christiansen & Baum, 1997; Law et al., 1996).

The purposes of assessment of occupational performance in occupational therapy practice include the following:

- Identifying client needs to perform specific occupations
- Gathering descriptive information about a client's current level of occupational performance and his or her satisfaction with performance
- Planning intervention
- Predicting occupational performance over time
- Evaluating the effects of occupational therapy intervention

Important Measurement Concepts

Clinical Utility

Occupational therapy practitioners require assessments of occupational performance that are clinically useful. It is important that such assessments not only provide information to assist their practice but are also efficient and effective in their everyday use. Aspects of clinical utility that are important for practitioners include the cost of an assessment, availability of a manual, ease of use, complexity of administration and scoring, time required to conduct an assessment, and requirements of the client during assessment process. When selecting occupational performance assessments, therapists should review clinical utility information because these characteristics will have an important impact on their ability to integrate the assessment into everyday practice.

Reliability

When measuring occupational performance, we must be concerned about whether the performance we observe and record is likely to be the same under various circumstances. Would the person perform the same in the morning or afternoon? Would various environments affect performance? Would persistence or endurance make a difference in what you measure and record?

Consistency of measurement is termed *reliability*. The important types of reliability to consider include reliability within an assessor (intrarater reliability), between assessors (inter-rater reliability), and over time (test-retest reliability). The level of reliability from studies is expressed using correlation coefficients from 0 to 1. Levels of reliability above 0.60 are considered to be good, while levels above 0.80 are considered to be excellent.

There are many times that professionals can control some of these factors and not others. It is less important to control all of the factors that may affect consistency. What is more important is to recognize what may affect the consistency of your findings. A simple way to handle consistency in daily practice is to be vigilant about recording factors that may affect consistency as part of measurement documentation. This way, if the team finds inconsistent performance, the related factors are available for comparison. When the team can discuss possible reasons for differences in performance, the team is more likely to increase its accuracy in understanding the person's difficulties and therefore design more effective interventions.

Validity

Another important consideration in the measurement process is the validity of the measurement (i.e., would everyone agree that you are measuring occupational performance?). There are formal methods for testing validity, and if professionals select standardized measures, it is important to review the validity features of the measure to be sure that the test is designed to offer the kind of information the professional desires.

Validity refers to the accuracy and comprehensiveness of an assessment in recording information about a specific attribute. The important types of validity to consider include content, criterion, and construct validity. Content validity is assessed by judging the comprehensiveness of the assessment and whether it includes all aspects of the particular attribute that are important to measure. In criterion validity, the agreement of the assessment with another more accurate assessment is judged. Construct validity focuses on the degree to which the assessment results fit with prior theoretical relationships among characteristics or individuals. Validity is established through a series of studies examining assessment results (Nunnally & Bernstein, 1994).

There may be situations in which standardized assessments are either unavailable or inappropriate. In these cases, qualitative measurement strategies such as interviews, skilled observations, and records reviews must be constructed with validity issues in mind. For occupational therapists, a skilled observation of a person in the kitchen would certainly appear to be a valid way to evaluate food preparation skills. But an occupational therapist could assess sensorimotor, cognitive, and psychosocial skills within this activity as well. When interpreting findings, the therapist would have to consider whether other team members would find it plausible that memory, sequencing, and dexterity could be measured in that activity via skilled observation. It is likely that team members would believe these connections, but would this therapist be free to go one step further and suggest that the person will have trouble with personal hygiene? Some team members would believe this step a "valid" extension of knowledge, while others might think this step was too big a leap and would be unwilling to consider personal hygiene rituals in the intervention plan.

What Is Best Practice Assessment?

Assessment is the process of systematically gathering information that enables people to understand the nature of a situation well enough to make initial hypotheses about what supports or creates barriers to desired outcomes.

Dunn (2000) outlines a three-phase process for best practice assessment. First, occupational therapy professionals are responsible for finding out what the person wants and needs to do. Secondly, we are responsible for determining where the person needs to perform the tasks of interest. After these two areas are addressed, then the professional conducts a person variable assessment to determine what role sensorimotor, cognitive, and psychosocial skills play in supporting or creating barriers to performance. Dunn (2000) points out that the primary focus of person variable assessment is deriving information from the person's actual performance; formal assessment of person variables only occurs when the therapist needs the data to establish eligibility or to verify hypotheses from other data sources.

When engaging in standard practice, assessment is more focused on person's skills and liabilities, with speculation about how these person variables are affecting performance (Dunn, 2000). Best practice assessment is centrally focused on occupational performance in everyday life; assessment strategies are only selected as they inform the therapists' understanding of the person's living issues.

Template for Best Practice Assessment

There are several factors to consider when designing a best practice assessment process. As occupational therapy professionals, our primary concern is everyday living, so the first factor to consider in best practice assessment is what the person wants and needs to do (Law et al., 1998). The second factor in best practice assessment is the environment in which performance takes place. The third factor we must consider are the person elements that are needed to engage in the desired performance. The therapist must also know the methods for gathering data for assessment. Table 14-1 provides a decision tool that includes all these factors to guide best practice assessment planning.

Table 14-1

Measuring Occupational Performance Outcomes—A Decision-Making Process

Stage in the Measurement Process	*Key Questions*
I. Identification of occupational performance issues by the person	• How will I enable the person to identify the occupational performance issues that are the reasons for seeking occupational therapy services? • Is the client able to complete this assessment? If not, who has the best information about theses issues? (See Stage II) • What assessment method will I use? • Where will I do the assessment? • Why am I evaluating occupational performance—to identify that there are occupational performance issues or to describe the person's status in performing occupations that he or she needs to, wants to, or is expected to do? • Is the assessment method reliable and valid? • Is the assessment method clinically useful? • Is the assessment method valid for client(s) with this type of problem? • How will the results of this assessment of occupational performance issues guide decisions about further assessment and occupational therapy intervention?
II. Identification of occupational performance issues for this person by another individual or group	• Why has another person or group identified potential occupational performance issues? • Have I discussed this issue with the person and his or her family? • What assessment method will I use? • Why am I evaluating occupational performance—to screen for issues or to describe occupational performance status? • Is the assessment method reliable and valid? • Is the assessment method clinically useful? • Is the assessment method valid for use with client(s) with this type of problem? • How will the results of this assessment of occupational performance issues guide decisions about occupational therapy assessment and intervention?
III. Further assessment of specific occupational performance areas	• What specific occupational performance attribute(s) will I assess? • What assessment method will I use—individualized or standardized? Quantitative or qualitative? • Who will complete the assessment? • Where will the assessment occur? • What is the age of the person? • Is the assessment method reliable and valid? • Is the assessment method clinically useful? • How will I use the results of this assessment?
IV. Assessment of environmental conditions and performance components	• What specific aspects of the environment and performance components are potential barriers to performance and need further assessment? • Who will complete the assessment?

(continued)

Table 14-1

Stage in the Measurement Process	*Key Questions*
	• Where will the assessment occur? • Is the assessment method reliable and valid? • Is the assessment method clinically useful? • How will I use the results of this assessment to focus occupational therapy intervention?
V. Selection of outcome measures	• Where do I look to find measures to use? • Does this assessment fit with my theoretical approach to occupational therapy? • What is the purpose of this assessment—to describe a person's status, to predict future performance, to evaluate change in performance over time? • What is the cost of the assessment? • How long does it take to administer? • How much training do I require before I can administer the assessment in a reliable manner? • Is there a manual available to guide the assessment? • How easy is it to administer the assessment, score it, and interpret the results? • Does the assessment have evidence of reliability—over time, between raters? • Does the assessment have evidence of validity—content, criterion, and construct? • If I am using the assessment to evaluate change over time, does it have evidence of responsiveness?
VI. Carry out the assessment	• How do I ensure a contextually accurate assessment? • How do I ensure a reliable assessment?
VII. Interpret measurement results	• How do I involve my client in assessment interpretation? • Am I trained to interpret the assessment results? • Do I need assistance in analyzing trends in assessment data? • Who will receive the assessment results? • What will occur based on the assessment results?

Reprinted with permission from Law, M., Baum, C., & Dunn, W. (2001). *Measuring occupational performance: Supporting best practice in occupational therapy.* Thorofare, NJ: SLACK Incorporated.

Identifying Occupational Performance Issues

Identification of a client's occupational performance issues is the most important factor in best practice assessment and guides all subsequent assessment and intervention decisions. The most obvious way to obtain information about desired or needed performance areas is to ask the person, family, group, or agency you are serving. However, this is not always feasible or possible. Some people are unable to communicate; some groups do not have clarity about what they want or need. Because this step is critical to framing the rest of the assessment process, we must persist in determining wants and needs. Table 14-2 provides information about several assessments that can be used by occupational therapists to identify occupational performance issues.

When people cannot communicate with us, we use family, other care providers, friends, or documentation about the person to identify wants and needs. We are careful when wants and needs emerge from other people; sometimes, others want things for us that we do not want for ourselves. So when we gather these initial data from others, we also plan ways to check in with the person as the intervention process emerges.

Table 14-2

Occupational Performance Assessments

Name and Source	*Purpose/Focus*	*Clinical Utility*	*Reliability*	*Validity*
Canadian Occupational Performance Measure (COPM) (Law et al., 1998)	To assess self-perception of performance and satisfaction of daily occupations	Semistructured interview; administered by occupational therapist Takes an average of 30 to 40 minutes to complete	Inter-rater reliability not reported Test-retest reliability ranges from 0.75 to 0.89	The construct validity of the COPM as an evaluative measure is well supported Criterion validity studies have also been completed
Occupational Performance History Interview II (OPH-II) (Kielhofner et al., 1997)	To gather information about occupational history	Semistructured interview; administered by occupational therapist Takes an average of 7 minutes to complete	Inter-rater reliability ratings range from 0.38 to 0.73 Test-retest reliability, in the most recent studies, ranges from 0.80 to 0.89	The validity of the OPHI-II has been well supported by studies using RASCH analysis
Satisfaction with Performance Skilled Questionnaire (SPSQ) (Yerxa et al., 1988)	To measure satisfaction with home-based and community or social aspects of occupational performance	Pencil and paper format Completion time not reported	Inter-rater reliability not applicable because it is a self-administered questionnaire Test-retest reliability not reported	The SPSQ discriminates between people with or without spinal cord injury Criterion validity not reported
Occupational Self-Assessment (OSA) (Baron et al., 2001)	To measure self-rated occupational performance and environmental adaptation.	Two-part self-administered questionnaire. Time to complete is 10 to 20 minutes	Inter-rater reliability not applicable because it is a self-administered questionnaire Test-retest reliability not reported	The validity of the OSA has been supported by studies using RASCH analysis

References

Baron, K., Kielhofner, G., Iyenger, A., Goldhammer, V., & Wolenski, J. (2001). *The occupational self-assessment (OSA)* (Version 1.2). Chicago, IL: Model of Human Occupation Clearinghouse.

Kielhofner, G, Mallinson, T., Crawford, C., Nowak, M., Rigby, M., Henry, A., Walens, D. (1997). *A user's guide to the occupational performance history interview-II (OPHI_II)* (Version 2.0). Chicago, IL: Model of Human Occupation Clearinghouse.

Law, M., Baptiste, S., Carswell, A., McColl, M. A., Polatajko, H., & Pollock, N. (1998). *The canadian occupational performance measure* (3rd ed.). Toronto: CAOT Publications ACE.

Yerxa, E. J., Burnett-Beaulieu, S., Stocking, S., & Azen, S.P. (1988). Development of the satisfaction with performance scaled questionnaire (SPSQ). *American Journal of Occupational Therapy, 42*(4), 215-221.

When providing population-based services, it is important to gather data about wants and needs from several sources. Sometimes, people will have different perspectives about this fundamental issue, and when you don't take time to understand the scope of wants and needs, subsequent assessment and then intervention will be less effective.

Characterizing the Context for Living

Best practice assessment also requires that we both identify relevant environments for wants and needs and gather data about those environments. The ultimate goal of the occupational therapy process is living a more satisfying life. We must, therefore, take responsibility for where this living occurs. Individuals and groups may not understand how their environments support or create barriers to their living. We can help with this insight.

Inventories, ecological assessments, and skilled observations are the best strategies for collecting context data. Dunn (2000) and Law and colleagues (2001) provide examples of assessments for practice.

Assessing the Contribution of Person Factors

People bring sensorimotor, cognitive, and psychosocial skills and difficulties to their lives. We can assess these factors in two primary ways. First, we assess person factors by observing their actions within actual performance. When people are doing things, their cognitive, sensorimotor, and psychosocial resources manifest themselves. This is a valuable source of information, particularly because this form of data gathering informs us about what and how the person uses personal resources. Sometimes, we need formal data to verify a hypothesis about person variables, or issues of eligibility require that we administer formal assessments to characterize particular skills and difficulties with cognitive, sensorimotor, and psychosocial factors. Chapter Twelve in this book discusses assessment of person factors in more detail.

Methods for Gathering Assessment Data

There are six categories for data collection. Each represents a different way for collecting data about the person, tasks of interest, and the context for performance:

1. Records review is a process of gathering data from the files, from other professional assessments, or other materials the person, family, or agency provides for use.
2. Informal measures include tools designed for specific use, such as a checklist designed by a group of therapists, to characterize a particular situation or performance.
3. Interviews involve guided discussion with members of interest to derive their perspectives on the situation.
4. Ecological measures include strategies to characterize the environment and the person's performance within that environment (see Dunn, 2000 for an example).
5. Skilled observations involve using professional knowledge and expertise to watch performance in the actual contexts of interest and to make hypotheses about the meaning of those observations for meeting needs.
6. Norm-referenced measurement and criterion-referenced measurement includes administering and interpreting evaluation protocols. In the first case, the tests are standardized to provide a precise administration and scoring procedure, and comparisons are made to a representative sample of people. In the second case (i.e., criterion referenced), the procedures result in comparison to some standard of performance (e.g., a developmental milestone) to determine level of skill or knowledge.

Assessment of Occupational Performance

Once the client's occupational performance issues have been identified, therapists often conduct further assessment of specific areas of occupational performance. These areas include activities of daily living, instrumental activities of daily living, work, school, play, and leisure. Occupational therapists also consider a person's roles, social supports, and how to balance performance of occupations across time and space.

Activities of Daily Living Skills

Activities of daily living (ADL) skills include self-care, functional mobility, communication, and management of medication and health routines. There is variability in the terms used to describe ADL, including self-care, basic ADL, personal ADL, personal care, and function. Although there are differences in definitions, there is a common understanding of what we mean by ADL—those activities that a person does to take care of him- or herself on a day-to-day basis. What is less consistent is which components of ADL should be included in any instruments that attempt to measure a client's abilities in activities of daily living. Table 14-3 includes information on specific ADL assessments that have been shown to be useful for occupational therapy practice.

Table 14-3

Activities of Daily Living Assessments

Name and Source	*Purpose/Focus*	*Clinical Utility*	*Reliability*	*Validity*
Barthel Index (Mahoney & Barthel, 1965)	To measure changes in functional status for clients undergoing inpatient rehabilitation	Ten items (feeding, bathing, grooming, dressing, bowel control, bladder control, toilet transfers, chair/bed transfers, ambulation, and stair climbing) Scoring by therapist rater can be quick (2 to 5 minutes), but observation of the activities can require about 1 hour	Internal consistency and inter-rater reliability excellent (>0.90) Test-retest reliability not reported for original Barthel	The Barthel correlated highly with the brief FIM, between 0.86 and 0.90 with different raters The Barthel has been found to correlate significantly with age and can predict discharge location
Functional Independence Measure (FIM) and Functional Independence Measure for Children (WeeFIM) (Data Management Service of the Uniform Data System for Medical Rehabilitation)	The FIM and WeeFIM are part of the Uniform Data System for Medical Rehabilitation. It was designed to measure the degree of disability being experienced, changes over time, and the effectiveness of rehabilitation	Eighteen items in six areas: self-care, sphincter control mobility, locomotion, communication, and social cognition The instrument itself can be easily completed in approximately 15 minutes, but the observations required to complete the form may require more time	FIM: 89 medical rehabilitation facilities contributed data for n = 1018; ICC = 0.96 for total scores, and ranged from 0.89 to 0.94 for items WeeFIM: children with disabilities (n = 205); tested between raters with short and long delay; ICC for short was 0.97 and for long delay was 0.94. Test-retest reliability ranges from 0.83 to 0.99	Both measures have excellent content, criterion, and construct validity. The FIM has been shown to predict discharge status and location. The WeeFIM distinguishes between children with and without disabilities as well as different levels of severity of disability
Klein-Bell ADL Scale (University of Washington Medical School)	To measure basic ADL	170 questions, divided into six categories: dressing, elimination, mobility, hygiene, eating, emergency telephone communication Observation of the ADL tasks will vary and could take anywhere from 1 to 3 hours. Scoring takes approximately 15 minutes	92% agreement on all items on all patients between observers. For children, inter-rater reliability of 0.99, and test-retest reliability of 0.98	Excellent construct and criterion validity Predicts number of hours per week of assistance

(continued)

Table 14-3

Name and Source	*Purpose/Focus*	*Clinical Utility*	*Reliability*	*Validity*
Activity Scales for Kids (ASK) (Young, 2000)	Self-report measure of personal care for children with physical disability	Administration can be to a single child or a group of children Children under 9 years of age may need a parent to read the questions for them Takes approximately 30 minutes	Internal consistency reported to be 0.99 Children's scores were compared to those of their parents (n=28); ICCs were 0.96 (ASKp) and 0.98 (ASKc) Test-retest 0.97 for ASKp and 0.98 for ASKc	Content and construct validity well-supported Relationship between the children's self-report and clinicians' observational scores were high (Spearman's rho = 0.92)
Pediatric Evaluation of Disability Index (Haley et al., 1992)	To describe a child's functional status, evaluate programs, and monitor change in individuals or groups of children with functional disabilities.	Three measurement dimensions: functional skills, caregiver assistance, and modifications Completed by parents or professionals. 45 to 60 minutes by interviewing parents or 20 to 30 minutes if a professional is completing it based on previous observations of the child	The reliability of the PEDI is excellent Inter-rater ranges from ranged from 0.96 to 0.99. Test-retest ranges from more than 0.95 for total scores and above 0.80 for the three domains.	Correlations with other measures include the Battelle Developmental Inventory Screening Test (results ranged from 0.62 to 0.97), the WeeFIM (results ranged from 0.80 to 0.97), the Gross Motor Function Measure (0.75 to 0.85), and the Peabody Developmental Motor Scales (0.24 to 0.95) Scores increase with age and appear to be sensitive to change
Functional Autonomy Measurement System (Hebert et al., 1988)	The SMAF was designed to evaluate people's needs by measuring their levels of disability and handicap	Five sections: ADL (7 items), mobility (6 items), communication (3 items), mental functions (5 items), and IADL (8 items) Based on interview and observation, and takes 40 minutes	Inter-rater reliability ranged from 0.61 to 0.81 with a mean of 0.68; ADL items were 0.95 Test-retest reliability is 0.95 (ranging from 0.78 to 0.96) and 0.96 for ADL item .	Correlation of scores to the nursing time required for care was 0.88. Significant changes in SMAF scores were noted between admission and discharge home of 94 people on an acute rehabilitation unit

(continued)

Table 14-3

References

Data Management Service of the Uniform Data System for Medical Rehabilitation, State University of New York at Buffalo, 100 High Street, Buffalo, New York 14230.

Haley, S. M., Coster, W. J., Ludlow, L. H., Haltiwanger, J. T., & Andrellos, P. J. (1992). *Pediatric Evaluation of Disability Inventory (PEDI) Version 1.0: Development, standardization and administration manual.* Boston, MA: New England Medical Center Hospitals Inc.

Hebert, R., Carrier, R., & Bilodeau, A. (1988). The functional autonomy measurement system (SMAF): Description and validation of an instrument for the measurement of handicaps. *Age and Aging, 17*, 293-302.

Klein-Bell ADL Scale. University of Washington Medical School, Health Sciences learning Resource Center, Distribution, SB-56, Seattle, Washington 98195

Mahoney, S. I., & Barthel, D. W. (1965). Functional evaluation: The Barthel index. *Maryland State Medical Journal, 14*, 61-65.

Pediatric Evaluation of Disability (PEDI). PEDI Research Group, Dept. of Rehabilitation Medicine, New England Medical Center Hospital, #75 K/R, 750 Washington Street, Boston, MA, 02111-1901

Young, N.L. (2000). *The Activities Scale for Kids (ASK) manual*. Toronto, ON: The Hospital for Sick Children.

When assessing ADL, it is best to integrate assessment into the typical routine of a person. For example, assessment of dressing is best done in the morning, while assessment of functional mobility is best done in the context of performance of the task that the person completes during his or her day. ADL assessment may need to be completed over several occasions to prevent fatigue. When conducting ADL assessment, safety must be paramount, and clients should not be asked to perform activities that may put them at risk for injury.

Instrumental Activities of Daily Living

Whereas ADL refer to life-sustaining and basic self-care practices (e.g., feeding, dressing, bathing), Lawton and Brody (1969) suggested that instrumental activities of daily living (IADL) represented a secondary set of tasks essential to independent community living. They identified eight activities as reflecting the core of this construct: managing money, using the telephone, taking medication, traveling, shopping, preparing meals, doing laundry, and housekeeping. Today, the centrality of IADL to quality of life and general well-being of individuals with disability is widely recognized. There is, however, no consensus as to the specific activities that are necessary for independent community living. Thus, although the eight activities first identified by Lawton and Brody remain central to this construct, there is wide variation in the number and type of activities that are included in more recently developed IADL measures. In a review of functional measures, Barer and Nouri (1989) categorized IADL items as representing three types of activities: getting about (e.g., using transportation, walking outside, getting into/outside cars, driving), household-based activities (e.g., laundry, meal and snack preparation, housework), or other leisure-oriented activities (e.g., gardening driving). Table 14-4 includes information on specific IADL assessments that have been shown to be useful for occupational therapy practice.

IADL represent multistep activities that are complex to perform. Performance can occur either inside or outside the home and requires the use of objects that are external to the individual, such as a telephone or other special instruments or tools. Independent performance requires high-level social, physical, and mental skills such as judgment, initiation, sequencing, and problem solving.

The assessment of IADL status is important for people who are preparing to return to community-living (Rogers, Holm, Goldstein, McCue, & Nussbaum, 1994). Additionally, an IADL assessment provides meaningful information when working with individuals who experience a change in cognitive status. Research has shown that deficits in four IADL, in particular, are correlated with cognitive impairment. These performance areas include telephone use, transportation use, medication taking, and managing finances (Barberger-Gateau, et al., 1992). Consequently, assessing IADL status is critical for the provision of individualized, quality care for both young and old clinical populations with disability and for individuals in which a change in cognitive status is suspected.

Work

Work-based occupations provide an organizing foci to people's lives. Involvement in work-related occupations is one important way that the individual's "urge toward competence" (White, 1971) is expressed. Occupational performance as a worker is dependent on successful interaction among the person, the environment, and the work role. Assessments of work used in occupational therapy practice often address specific tasks that contribute to a person's occupational performance in the area of work. Table 14-5 includes information on specific work assessments for occupational therapy practice.

Occupational therapists also use resources developed by government in this area of assessment. One example, the O-NET, presents short narrative descriptions of occupations that are based on job analyses that, in turn, are based on analyses of tasks found in similar positions. Specific information is provided about how to assess the tasks. At the elemental level, task demands are considered in terms of five categories: exertion, posture, manipulation, sensory demand, and environmental demand.

School

Assessments on the ability of a child, adolescent, or young adult to function within an educational setting are important information to be gathered by an occupational therapist. Occupational therapists focus on students' performance of functional tasks that support their academic and other school-related activities.

For children and youth, a very important occupational therapy assessment for use in schools is the School Function Assessment (SFA) (Coster, Deeney, Haltwanger, & Haley, 1998). The SFA provides information about a child's participation in school activities, activity performance, and the supports used for the child. The assessment is completed by those familiar with the student's typical performance. While the SFA is time-consuming to complete, the information that is provided is very comprehensive. Test-retest reliability ranges from 0.80 to 0.99. Two studies of content validity have supported the comprehensiveness and relevance of the items on the SFA. For construct validity, Rasch, multiple regression, and other statistical analyses have indicated that the scales of the SFA have excellent predictive and discriminative characteristics.

Table 14-4

Instrumental Activities of Daily Living Assessments

Name and Source	*Purpose/Focus*	*Clinical Utility*	*Reliability*	*Validity*
Assessment of Motor and Process Skills (AMPS) (Fisher, 1995)	To assess IADL, including motor and process skills required for performance	Administered by an occupational therapist who must be trained and calibrated in the use of this assessment Based on direct observation 56 IADL tasks included Completion time varies by individual who must perform two to three IADL of his or her choice	Internal consistency ranges from r = 0.74 to r = 0.93. Test-retest reliability ranges from r = 0.70 to r = 0.91 depending on test conditions and use of Rasch analysis	A series of studies with people with a wide range of conditions and ages has confirmed the validity of the AMPS
Performance Assessment of Self-care Skills (PASS) (Holm & Rogers, 1999; Rogers et al., 1994, 2001)	To assess short-term functional change in mobility, ADL, and IADL in older adults	Using a dynamic assessment approach, people are observed by an occupational therapist engaging in 26 tasks of daily living behaviors Scores of performance independence, safety, and adequacy are generated	Test-retest reliability is 0.92 for independence; 89% agreement for safety; and 0.82 for performance adequacy. Inter-rater reliability ranges from 88% to 97% agreement between raters	Content validity well supported Construct validity supports the ability of the PASS to differentiate based on diagnosis and functional severity Further information regarding the responsiveness to change of the PASS is required
Kitchen Task Assessment (KTA) (Baum & Edwards, 1994)	To measure level of cognitive support required by a person with Alzheimer's disease to complete a cooking task successfully	Not reported	Internal consistency ranges from 0.87 to 0.96 Inter-rater reliability for the total score = 0.853, range was 0.632 for safety to 1.0 for initiation Test-retest reliability not reported	Relationship between person's performance on the KTA and standard neuropsychological measures highly significant Further information regarding the responsiveness to change of the KTA is required

(continued)

Table 14-4

Name and Source	*Purpose/Focus*	*Clinical Utility*	*Reliability*	*Validity*
Structured Assessment of Independent Living Skills (SAILS) (Mahurin et al., 1991)	To measure performance of daily activities	The SAILS is completed by a health professional in a clinical setting Fifty tasks, each criterion-referenced Completion time of about 1 hour	Inter-rater reliability of 0.99 Test-retest reliability was 0.81	The SAILS correlated significantly with the MMSE, the Global Deterioration Scale, and the WAIS-R Construct validity or responsiveness not reported
Direct Assessment of Functional Status (DAFS) (Lowenstein et al., 1989)	To assess functional status	Based on direct observation of a patient's performance within each of seven functional domains Completion time 30 to 35 minutes	Inter-rater reliability ranged from 0.911 to 1.000 Test-retest reliabilities ranged from 0.55 to 0.928	The DAFS was compared to reported functional status at home using the Blessed Dementia Rating Scale (BDRS) = -0.66

References

Baum, C., & Edwards, D. F. (1994). Cognitive performance in senile dementia of the Alzheimer's type: The kitchen task assessment. *American Journal of Occupational Therapy*, *47*, 431-436.

Fisher, A. G. (1995). *Assessment of motor and process skills*. Fort Collins, CO: Three Star Press.

Holm, M. B., & Rogers, J. C. (1999). Functional assessment: The Performance Assessment of Self-Care Skills (PASS). In B. J. Hemphill-Pearson (Ed.), *Assessments in occupational therapy mental health: An integrative approach* (pp. 117-124). Thorofare, NJ: SLACK Incorporated.

Loewenstein, D., Amigo, E., Duara, R., Guterman, A., Hurwitz, D., Berkowitz, N., et al. (1989). A new scale for the assessment of functional status in Alzheimer's disease and related disorders. *Journal of Gerontology: Psychological Sciences, 44*, 114-121.

Mahurin, R. K., DeBittignies, B. H. & Pirozzolo, F. J. (1991). Structured assessment of independent living skills: Preliminary report of a performance measure of functional abilities in dementia. *Journal of Gerontology: Psychological Sciences, 46*, 58-66.

Rogers, J. C., Holm, M. B., Beach, S., Schulz, R., & Starz, T. (2001). Task independence, safety, and adequacy among nondisabled and OAK-disabled older women. *Arthritis Care and Research, 45*, 410-418.

Rogers, J., Holm, M., Goldstein, G., McCue, M., & Nussbaum, P. (1994). Stability and change in functional assessment of patients with geropsychiatric disorders. *American Journal of Occupational Therapy, 48*, 914-918.

Table 14-5

Assessments of Work Function

Name and Source	*Purpose/Focus*	*Clinical Utility*	*Reliability*	*Validity*
Worker Role Interview (WRI) (Velozo et al., 1998)	To identify the psychosocial and environmental factors that may influence return to work	Uses a semistructured interview format to focus on six content areas: personal causation, values, interests, roles, habits, and environment Completion time is 30 to 60 minutes	Acceptable levels of inter-observer and test-retest reliability	Validated using Rasch analysis The WRI discriminated between clients on psychosocial capacity for work
Spinal Function Sort (Matheson & Matheson, 1989)	To evaluate self-perceived ability to perform frequently encountered physical work tasks	Fifty-item instrument organized, each item composed of a drawing of an adult of working age performing a work task The evaluee describes his or her ability to perform the task along a five-point scale from "able" to "unable" Completion time 6 to 12 minutes	Internal consistency was 0.98. Test-retest reliability for a 3-day interval was 0.85 for 126 adult men and 0.82 for 84 adult women	Statistically significant and meaningful relationships were found between SFS scores and performance in a physically demanding functional capacity evaluation, and an inverse relationship was found between reports of pain and SFS scores
Valpar Component Work Samples (VCWS)	To assess task performance on simulated work tasks The tasks have all been analyzed according to the *Dictionary of Occupational Titles*	Work samples that simulate task performance (e.g., repetitive assembly work). For each task, there is a complete analysis of the skills and attitudes required for a worker to complete that task Completion time ranges from 20 to 90 minutes	Test-retest reliability values of 0.70 to 0.99	Many studies have demonstrated high correspondence between items on the VALPAR Work Samples and required worker characteristics in the *Dictionary of Occupational Titles* The VALPAR Work Samples discriminate between workers who were employed or not employed in specific jobs

References

Matheson, L., & Matheson, M. (1989). *PACT spinal function sort*. Wildwood, MO: Employment Potential Improvement Corporation.

VALPAR International Corporation, PO Box 5767, Tucson, Arizona, USA, 85703-5767

Velozo, C., Kielhofner, G., & Fisher, G. (1998). *Worker role interview (WRI)*. Chicago, IL: Model of Human Occupation Clearinghouse.

Play

Play is the primary occupation of childhood and youth. There is little agreement and much ambiguity about virtually every aspect of play from its definition, to its purpose, to the ways in which it manifests itself (Sutton-Smith, 1997). The only thing clear about play is that it is a multifaceted phenomenon. For the purposes of assessment in occupational therapy, play is comprised of the following five factors:

1. What the player does.
2. Why the player enjoys chosen play activities.
3. How the player approaches play (and other activity).
4. The player's capacity to play.
5. The relative supportiveness of the environment.

When doing play assessment, occupational therapists must be aware of the factor(s) addressed by the assessment(s) they have chosen. Table 14-6 includes information on specific assessments of play that have been shown to be useful for occupational therapy practice.

There are fewer assessments of play than there are assessments of ADL. Perhaps, in part, because of the lack of valid and reliable tools, therapists often resort to informal assessment based on unstructured observation of a child's play. This approach may yield valuable information to the experienced examiner who is cognizant of play's many facets. However, as play is extremely complex, formal measures provide the structure needed by most examiners to conduct and interpret the results of assessment in the most thorough and efficient way possible. Optimal intervention depends on quality interpretation of assessment data.

Leisure

From a conceptual perspective, leisure is regarded as a nonobligatory activity that is freely chosen, is more playful in nature, and provides individuals with satisfaction. Leisure activities are intrinsically rewarding and provide pleasure for individuals (Stebbins, 1997). It is argued that to have an experience of leisure, an individual must believe that he or she is controlling events and is engaged in the activity as a result of his or her own free choice, rather than being controlled by events or features of his or her life that impact the ability to make choices (Godbey, 1994; Neulinger, 1974). Important concepts to consider in assessing leisure include perceived competence, perceived control, intrinsic motivation, and playfulness (Bundy, 2001; Witt & Ellis, 1984). Participation in leisure activities has been shown to provide a positive impact on health (Iso-Ahola, 1994; Law et al., 1998). Occupational therapists assess leisure activities to help determine person, task, and environmental factors that are influencing performance. Table 14-7 includes information on specific assessments of play that have been shown to be most useful for occupational therapy practice.

Case Examples

Imagine for a moment that something has limited your ability to do what you want and need to do. You have permanently lost the use of your dominant hand and will be nonweight-bearing due to a fractured left leg for 6 weeks after a terrible accident. You luckily sustained no cognitive deficit. What do you want those who will be treating you to know about you and the impact of the accident on your occupations and choices?

ADL	Are you having difficulty with your basic self-care, including feeding, dressing, and hygiene?
IADL	Are there self-management and household tasks that are difficult? How are you going to get to school?
Work/School	Can you do your job? How will you keep up with school?
Play	How is your play affected?
Leisure	What impact does your injury have on your leisure activities? Will this impact your well-being?
Family/Friends	How has your injury affected your family and/or friends?
Person Factors	What is the psychological, sensory, motor, and/or physiological impact?
Environmental Factors	Will your environment enable your occupations and participation?
Occupational Performance	What are your goals?

An occupational therapy plan will be constructed to meet your needs and goals. By using reliable and valid instruments, the occupational therapist will contribute knowledge of your occupational performance needs to the team and will have data to report the improvement that you will make. Your clients will have similar needs and are counting on the occupational therapist to address the important issues that they will face in their everyday lives.

Table 14-6

Play Assessments

Name and Source	*Purpose/Focus*	*Clinical Utility*	*Reliability*	*Validity*
The Play History (Bryze, 1997; Takata, 1974)	To assess a child's play experiences and opportunities through the eyes of a caregiver across development	Semistructured interview with a parent or another caregiver Completion time not specified	Using videotaped interviews, overall inter-rater reliability was reported to be 0.91 At 3-week intervals, test-retest reliability was 0.77 with category coefficients ranging from 0.41 to 0.78	Scores correlated with the Minnesota Child Development Inventory at 0.97 for children without disabilities and 0.70 for children with disabilities. The correlation between epoch scores and age was 0.85
The Pediatric Interest Profiles: Survey of Play for Children and Adolescents (Henry, 1998)	To gain a profile of a child's play interests	Child/adolescent responds to questions regarding interest, participation, enjoyment, etc., in age-appropriate leisure/play activities Completion time is 15 to 30 minutes	Internal consistency ranged from 0.59 to 0.80 for subscale scores and was 0.93 for total scores Test-retest reliabilities ranged from 0.45 to 0.91 for total scores	Level of enjoyment in activities was shown to discriminate among adolescents with and without disabilities
The Test of Playfulness (ToP) (Version 3) (Bundy, 1997)	To capture four elements of playfulness in children: intrinsic motivation, internal control, freedom from some constraints of reality, and framing (i.e. the ability to give and read cues)	The ToP is a 24-item observational assessment administered during 15- to 20-minute free play sessions Raters are urged to administer the ToP in more than one setting (e.g., indoors and outdoors) Completion time is 20 to 30 minutes (including scoring time) for each setting	For observer reliability 96% of raters (n=170) demonstrate goodness of fit to the Rasch model	Correlation with the Children's Playfulness Scale (Barnett, 1990) was 0.46 Using Rasch analysis, 23 of 24 items have acceptable goodness of fit statistics

(continued)

Table 14-6

Name and Source	*Purpose/Focus*	*Clinical Utility*	*Reliability*	*Validity*
Revised Knox Preschool Play Scale (PPS-R) (Knox, 1997)	To provide a developmental description of a child's underlying capacities for play	Child's behavior is observed as it reflects four play dimensions: space management, material management, imitation, and participation Two 30-minute observations are done, one indoors and one outdoors	Inter-rater coefficients ranged from r = 0.88 to 0.996. Test-retest reliability ranges from 0.91 to 0.96	PPS scores correlated with Lunzer's Scale of Organization of Play Behavior (0.59 to 0.64), Parten's Social Play Hierarchy (0.60 to 0.64), and chronological age (0.74 to 0.95)

References

Barnett, L. A. (1990). Playfulness: Definition, design, and measurement. *Play and Culture, 3*, 319-336.

Bundy, A. C. (1997). Play and playfulness: What to look for. In L. D. Parham & L. S. Fazio, (Eds.), *Play in occupational therapy for children* (pp. 52-66). St. Louis, MO: Mosby-Year Book.

Bryze, K. (1997). Narrative contributions to the Play History. In L. D. Parham & L. S. Fazio, (Eds.), *Play in occupational therapy for children* (pp. 23-34). St. Louis, MO: Mosby-Year Book.

Henry, A. D. (1998). Development of a measure of adolescent leisure interests. *American Journal of Occupational Therapy, 52,* 531-539.

Knox, S. (1997). Development and current use of the Knox Preschool Play Scale. In L. D. Parham & L. S. Fazio (Eds.), *Play in occupational therapy for children* (pp 35-51). St. Louis, MO: Mosby-Year Book.

Takata, N. (1974). Play as a prescription. In M. Reilly (Ed.), *Play as exploratory learning* (pp. 209-246). Beverly Hills, CA: Sage.

Table 14-7

Leisure Assessments

Name and Source	*Purpose/Focus*	*Clinical Utility*	*Reliability*	*Validity*
The Activity Card Sort (ACS) (Baum, 1995)	To document the individual's participation or lack of participation in instrumental, leisure, and social activities	The ACS uses a Q-Sort methodology to rank order photographs of activities. Average completion time is 20 minutes	Studies are currently being conducted	Individuals who remained active in occupations demonstrated fewer disturbing behaviors, required less help with basic self-care, and their caregivers experienced less stress The percent of meaningful activities regained since the stroke was a better predictor of quality of life as measured by the SF-36 than the Functional Impairment Measure (FIM)
Activity Index & Meaningfulness Scales of Activity (Gregory, 1983; Nystrom, 1974)	To assess degree of interest and participation in leisure activities	Measure includes 23 leisure activity items Completion time estimated at 30 to 40 minutes	Reliability over time of 0.70 for the Activity Index and 0.87 for the Meaningfulness Scales of Activity	Correlations (0.29 to 0.43) with a measure of life satisfaction Low correlation (0.11) with age and length of retirement (0.01)

(continued)

Table 14-7

Name and Source	*Purpose/Focus*	*Clinical Utility*	*Reliability*	*Validity*
Leisure Diagnostic Battery (LDB) (Witt & Ellis, 1984)	To assess an individual's perceptions of perceived leisure competence	Self-report measure Version A includes 95 items related to competence, control, needs depth, and playfulness; 24 items related to barriers; and 28 items related to knowledge Version B is a short form Version A takes 30 to 40 minutes, while Version B takes 10 to 15 minutes	Internal consistency of 0.83 to 0.94 for Version A and 0.89 to 0.94 for Version B Test-retest reliability of 0.72	Moderate correlations between LDB and measures of barriers and knowledge regarding leisure Correlation of 0.16 by gender Have been found to be sensitive to change after a therapeutic recreation program

References

Activity Card Sort, Dr. Carolyn Baum, Program in Occupational Therapy, Box 8505, Washington University School of Medicine, 4444 Forest Park Blvd., St. Louis, MO 63108

Baum, C. M. (1995). The contribution of occupation to function in persons with Alzheimer's disease. *Journal of Occupational Science, 2*, 55-67.

Gregory, M. D. (1983). Occupational behavior and life satisfaction among retirees. *American Journal of Occupational Therapy, 37*, 548-553.

Nystrom, E. P. (1974). Activity patterns and leisure concepts among the elderly. *American Journal of Occupational Therapy, 28*, 337-345.

Witt, P. A., & Ellis, G. D. (1984). The Leisure Diagnostic Battery: Measuring perceived freedom in leisure. *Society and Leisure, 7*, 109-124.

References

Barberger-Gateau, P., Commenges, D., Gagnon, M., Letenneur, L., Sauvel, C., & Dartigues, J-F. (1992). Instrumental activities of daily living as a screening tool for cognitive impairment and dementia in elderly community dwellers. *Journal of American Geriatrics Society, 40*, 1129-1134.

Barer, D., & Nouri, F. (1989). Measurement activities of daily living. *Clinical Rehabilitation, 3*, 179-187.

Barnett, L. A. (1990). Playfulness: Definition, design, and measurement. *Play and Culture, 3*, 319-336.

Baron, K., Kielhofner, G., Iyenger, A., Goldhammer, V., & Wolenski, J. (2001). *The Occupational Self-Assessment (OSA)* (Version 1.2). Chicago, IL: Model of Human Occupation Clearinghouse.

Baum, C. M. (1995). The contribution of occupation to function in persons with Alzheimer's disease. *Journal of Occupational Science, 2*, 55-67.

Baum, C., & Edwards, D. F. (1994). Cognitive performance in senile dementia of the Alzheimer's type: The kitchen task assessment. *American Journal of Occupational Therapy*, 431-436.

Bryze, K. (1997). Narrative contributions to the play history. In L. D. Parham & L. S. Fazio (Eds.), *Play in occupational therapy for children* (pp. 23-34). St. Louis, MO: Mosby.

Bundy, A. (2001). Measuring play performance. In M. Law, C. Baum, & W. Dunn (Eds.), *Measuring occupational performance: A guide to best practice*. Thorofare, NJ: SLACK Incorporated.

Bundy, A. C. (1997). Play and playfulness: What to look for. In L. D. Parham & L. S. Fazio (Eds.), *Play in occupational therapy for children* (pp. 52-66). St. Louis, MO: Mosby.

Christiansen, C. H., & Baum, C. M. (1997). *Occupational therapy: Enhancing function and well-being* (2nd ed.). Thorofare, NJ: SLACK Incorporated.

Coster, W., Deeney, T., Haltwanger, I., & Haley, S. (1998). *The School Function Assessment*. San Antonio, TX: The Psychological Corporation.

Dunn, W. (2000). *Best practice occupational therapy in community service with children and families*. Thorofare, NJ: SLACK Incorporated.

Fisher, A. G. (1995). *Assessment of motor and process skills*. Fort Collins, CO: Three Star Press.

Godbey, G. (1994). *Leisure in your life: An exploration* (4th ed.). State College, PA: Venture.

Gregory, M. D. (1983). Occupational behavior and life satisfaction among retirees. *American Journal of Occupational Therapy, 37*, 548-553.

Haley, S. M., Coster, W. J., Ludlow, L. H., Haltiwanger, J. T., & Andrellos, P. J. (1992). *Pediatric Evaluation of Disability Inventory (PEDI) Version 1.0: Development, standardization and administration manual*. Boston, MA: New England Medical Center Hospitals Inc.

Hebert, R., Carrier, R., & Bilodeau, A. (1988). The functional autonomy measurement system (SMAF): Description and validation of an instrument for the measurement of handicaps. *Age and Ageing, 17*, 293-302.

Henry, A. D. (1998). Development of a measure of adolescent leisure interests. *American Journal of Occupational Therapy, 52*, 531-539.

Holm, M. B., & Rogers, J. C. (1999). Functional assessment: The Performance Assessment of Self-Care Skills (PASS). In B. J. Hemphill-Pearson (Ed.), *Assessments in occupational therapy mental health: An integrative approach* (pp. 117-124). Thorofare, NJ: SLACK Incorporated.

Iso-Ahola, S. (1994). Leisure lifestyle and health. In D. Compton & S. Iso-Ahola (Eds.), *Leisure and mental health* (pp. 42-60). Park City, UT: Family Development Resources, Inc.

Kielhofner, G., Mallinson, T., Crawford, C., Nowak, M., Rigby, M., Henry, A., et al. (1997). *A user's guide to the occupational performance history interview II (OPHI_II) (Version 2.0)*. Chicago, IL: Model of Human Occupation Clearinghouse.

Knox, S. (1997). Development and current use of the Knox Preschool Play Scale. In L. D. Parham & L. S. Fazio (Eds.), *Play in occupational therapy for children* (pp. 35-51). St. Louis, MO: Mosby.

Law, M., Baptiste, S., & Mills, J. (1995). Client-centred practice: What does it mean and does it make a difference? *Canadian Journal of Occupational Therapy, 62*, 250-257.

Law, M., Baptiste, S., Carswell, A., McColl, M., Polatajko, H., & Pollock, N. (1998). *Canadian Occupational Performance Measure* (3rd ed.). Toronto: CAOT Publication.

Law, M., Baum, C., & Dunn, W. (2001). *Measuring occupational performance: A guide to best practice*. Thorofare, NJ: SLACK Incorporated.

Law, M., Cooper, B. A., Strong, S., Stewart, D., Rigby, P., & Letts, L. (1996). The person-environment-occupation model: A transactive approach to occupational performance. *Canadian Journal of Occupational Therapy, 63*, 9-23.

Lawton, M.P. & Brody, E.M. (1969). Assessment of older people: Self-maintaining and instrumental activities of daily living. *The Gerontologist, 9*, 179-186.

Lowenstein, D., Amigo, E., Duara, R., Guterman, A., Hurwitz, D., Berkowitz, N., et al. (1989). A new scale for the assessment of functional status in Alzheimer's disease and related disorders. *Journal of Gerontology: Psychological Sciences, 44*, 114-121.

Mahoney, S. I., & Barthel, D. W. (1965). Functional evaluation: The Barthel index. *Maryland State Medical Journal, 14*, 61-65.

Mahurin, R. K., DeBittignies, B. H., & Pirozzolo, F. J. (1991). Structured assessment of independent living skills: Preliminary report of a performance measure of functional abilities in dementia. *Journal of Gerontology: Psychological Sciences, 46*, 58-66.

Matheson, L., & Matheson, M. (1989). *PACT Spinal Function Sort*. Wildwood, MO: Employment Potential Improvement Corporation.

Matheson, L., Ogden, L., Violette, K., & Schultz, K. (1985). Work hardening: Occupational therapy in industrial rehabilitation. *American Journal of Occupational Therapy, 39*(5), 314-321.

Neulinger, J. (1974). *The psychology of leisure: Research approaches to the study of leisure*. Springfield, IL: Charles Thomas Publishers.

Nunnally, J. C., & Bernstein, I. H. (1994). *Psychometric theory*. New York, NY: McGraw-Hill.

Nystrom, E. P. (1974). Activity patterns and leisure concepts among the elderly. *American Journal of Occupational Therapy, 28*, 337-345.

Rogers, I. C., Holm, M. B., Goldstein, G., McCue, M., & Nussbaum, P. D. (1994). Stability and change in functional assessment of patients with geropsychiatric disorders. *American Journal of Occupational Therapy, 48*, 914-918.

Rogers, J. C., Holm, M. B., Beach, S., Schulz, R., & Starz, T. (2001). Task independence, safety, and adequacy among nondisabled and OAK-disabled older women. *Arthritis Care and Research, 45*, 410-418.

Stebbins, R. (1997). Casual leisure: A conceptual statement. *Leisure Studies, 16*(1), 17-25.

Sutton-Smith, B. (1997). *The ambiguity of play*. Cambridge, MA: Harvard.

Takata, N. (1974). Play as a prescription. In M. Reilly (Ed.). *Play as exploratory learning* (pp. 209-246). Beverly Hills, CA: Sage.

Van Deusen, I., & Brunt, D. (Eds.). (1998). *Assessment in occupational therapy and physical therapy*. Orlando, FL: W. B. Saunders.

Velozo, C., Kielhofner, G., & Fisher, G. (1998). *Worker Role interview (WRI)*. Chicago, IL: Model of Human Occupation Clearinghouse.

White, R. (1971). The urge towards competence. *American Journal of Occupational Therapy, 25*(6), 271-274.

Witt, P., & Ellis, G. (1984). The Leisure Diagnostic Battery: Measuring perceived freedom in leisure. *Society and Leisure, 7*(1), 109-124.

Yerxa, E. J., Burnett-Beaulieu, S., Stocking, S., & Azen, S. P. (1988). Development of the Satisfaction with Performance Scaled Questionnaire (SPSQ). *American Journal of Occupational Therapy, 42*(4), 215-221.

Young, N. L. (2000). *The Activities Scale for Kids (ASK) manual*. Toronto: The Hospital for Sick Children.

Chapter Fourteen: Occupational Performance Assessment Reflections and Learning Activities

Julie Bass-Haugen, PhD, OTR/L, FAOTA

Reflections

This chapter explored how you gather the critical information on your client that is necessary for effective occupational therapy services. Part of the information you gather will be from your client's perspective. This information will help you complete your client assessment. Part of the information you gather will be your professional assessment of the person, environment, and occupational performance.

Many words are used to describe assessment in occupational therapy practice. This chapter introduced definitions for the terms *measurement*, *assessment*, and *evaluation*. These definitions of the terms are fairly common in the literature. However, I must forewarn you that the definitions used in this chapter are not the only definitions. In fact, some literature will provide definitions that seem to be the exact opposite of these definitions. I recognize that this is very confusing. It is for me, too. Once again, it helps me if I recognize that these terms are used by alot of professions and professionals. When we use the terms in a specific way, we will need to explain the framework that was adopted. Regardless of the definitions used, measurement, assessment, and evaluation are critical components of the occupational therapy process. For the purpose of simplicity, I will mostly use the term *assessment* in this chapter summary.

Over the years, you have likely been subjected to many forms of assessment. In schools, you've had achievement tests and aptitude tests. In medical settings, you've been measured for pulse, blood pressure, and lab tests. In an early childhood center, you may have had developmental tests. In athletic programs, you may have had your motor ability and eye-hand coordination measured. In all of these situations, there was a purpose to the measurement (hopefully!), certain people who were targeted for assessment, qualifications for the administrator, and practical characteristics of the assessment. In many of these situations, each assessment also was evaluated for the quality of the measurement.

As occupational therapy practitioners, we have an enormous responsibility in assessment. It is essential to remember that human beings (not building dimensions, weather, lab samples) are measured in our assessments. Assessment results are used to characterize the person to others, make decisions having huge implications for a person's life, and demonstrate the outcomes of occupational therapy services. Have you (or people you know) ever been characterized or described in a way that was not true? Have you (or people you know) ever made erroneous decisions based on poor information? Have you ever known of an organization (or agency, business, or population) that has been unfairly treated because of inaccurate information? Most of us are familiar with situations like these when assessment was used to the detriment of an individual or group of individuals.

There are several ways you can improve the quality of the information you obtain through assessment. First, be clear on your assessment needs in a given situation and the professional skills you bring to the assessment. If you adopt "client-centered" and "occupational performance" as your overall framework and reason for assessment, you can feel secure that you will choose assessments that fit with the PEOP model and occupational therapy practice. Second, your assessment of a client is only as good as the assessment you use. If you use a poor assessment you will end up with poor information. If you use a good assessment (and use it appropriately), you will likely end up with good, useful information. Practitioners should critique the assessments they use, select assessments with the best measurement characteristics (e.g., reliability and validity), and acknowledge the limitations of an assessment. Third, best practice for assessment should be used in every situation. Factors of best practice for assessment include occupational issues identified by person, occupational issues identified by others, specific occupational performance issues, specific person and environment factors, selection of outcome measures, and implementation and interpretation of assessment.

Reliability and validity are important measurement characteristics in assessment. What is reliability and validity? You probably can define them at an academic level. Let's take it down to the level of a silly example: your intelligence as measured by IQ on a not-so-famous intelligence test. On this not-so-famous test, the average IQ is 100.

What is reliability? If this test has good test-retest reliability, you would get approximately the same score on the test every time you take it. That is, if you score in the brilliant range (e.g., 150) one time, you will likely score in the brilliant range every time you take it. And vice versa, I might add. If this test has very poor test-retest reliability, you might score in the brilliant range (e.g., 150) one time and then in the not-brilliant-at-all range (e.g., 80) the next time. When a test has poor test-retest reliability, you have to ask if it is wise to use the score from one administration of the test. I know I would have concern about use of an intelligence test score for me that would vary from not-brilliant-at-all to brilliant. Wouldn't you? Now take this silly example of test-retest reliability and explain inter-rater reliability and intra-rater reliability.

What is validity? If this test has good content, construct, and criterion validity, then this not-so-famous intelligence test is really measuring your intelligence. If you score in the brilliant range (and the test has good reliability), you can brag about being a genius and submit an application to the Mensa International Society. On the other hand, if you score in the not-so-brilliant range, you might want to reconsider any application to Mensa. If this test has poor content, construct, and/or criterion validity, then you will probably wonder what this test is really measuring. If you score in the brilliant range, maybe all the items are ridiculously simple, and the test is only measuring how good you are at staying inside the line of those little circles on the test. Maybe the test is only measuring some obscure knowledge you have that others don't (e.g., medical terminology). Each type of validity measures a different aspect of the degree to which a test measures what it is designed to measure. Content validity examines the specific content or items in a test. Construct validity examines the trait or construct that the test measures. Criterion validity examines the relationship between this test and another criterion or outcome. Each type of validity makes an important contribution to the measurement characteristics of the test.

Occupational therapy practitioners have a wide assortment of methods for conducting assessment. These methods include record reviews, informal measures, interviews, ecological measures, skilled observations, and norm or criterion referenced tests. In most cases, several methods are chosen to obtain a complete picture of the client information and plan interventions. For a given client with orthopedic injuries who is concerned about performing ADL after discharge from the hospital, I might 1) complete a review of the medical chart to understand injuries, 2) have the client rank order a checklist of activities of daily living having the greatest to least concern, 3) conduct an interview with the client and/or family to understand the occupational performance history, 4) visit the home to assess the environment, 5) observe the client performing simulated bathing activities in the rehabilitation unit bathroom, 6) describe current function using the Katz Index of Activities of Daily Living. For each client, the methods and results of assessment are documented in a narrative or structured format.

As you have seen in this chapter, assessment is an important part of the occupational therapy process. Good assessment requires practitioner skills in a number of areas. The knowledge you acquire through reading and the experience you gain through learning activities are helping you develop the necessary skills for assessment. Assessment will be an important building block for your occupational therapy practice.

Journal Activities

1. Look up and write down a dictionary definition of assessment, measurement, and evaluation. Highlight the components of the definitions that are most related to their descriptions in Chapter Fourteen.
2. Identify the most important new learning for you in this chapter.
3. Identify one question you have about Chapter Fourteen.
4. Reflect on an experience where you were being assessed or measured. What was being measured? How did it feel to be the client in an assessment? How was the assessment information used? What were the strengths and limitations of the assessment? Describe your perceptions of the credibility of the assessment. What would you recommend to improve the assessment process in this situation? How does this experience influence the strategies you will use in assessment?

Technology/Internet Learning Activities

1. Use a discussion database to share specific journal activities.
2. Use a good Internet search engine to find the Web site for the "American Psychological Association."
   - Enter the phrase "APA" or "American Psychological Association" in your search line.
   - Review the home page of the Web site.
   - Search the Internet site for "psychological testing" or "tests and assessments."
   - Review the information on the APA Science Directorate: Tests and Assessments.
   - Review the information on FAQ/Finding Information About Psychological Tests.
   - What are TIP, MMY, Tests, and Test Critique?
   - What is the Standards for Educational and Psychological Testing?

- What resources are available for unpublished assessments, Internet searches, and databases?
- How might you use these resources to strengthen an assessment?
- What are some of your responsibilities as a test user?

3. Use a good Internet search engine to find the Web site for "The Test Locator."
   - Enter the phrase "The Test Locator" in your search line.
   - Review the home page of the Web site.
   - What is the purpose of this Web site?
   - Who sponsors this Web site?
   - Identify three "Free Tests and Instruments" that relate to occupational performance, ADL, IADL, work, play, or leisure. What information is provided on these assessments?
4. Use a good Internet search engine to find the Web site for the "American Occupational Therapy Association" or "OTSearch" through your library.
   - Enter the phrase "AOTA" in your Internet search line or find "OTSearch" through your library (Note: OTSearch requires an individual or institutional subscription fee).
   - Enter the name of a specific assessment from Chapter Fourteen in the search line for OTSearch.
   - Review three articles that are available on this topic.
   - Summarize the information that you found on this topic.

Applied Learning

Individual Learning Activity #1: Evaluating Your Need for an Assessment in Occupational Therapy Practice

Instructions:

- Imagine that you are starting a new occupational therapy practice.
- You want to select assessments for your practice.
- Select a client characteristic or attribute that you will want to assess in your practice (e.g., occupational performance, ADL, IADL, work, play, leisure).
- Identify a hypothetical purpose, population, and clinical utility characteristics for an assessment.
- Summarize your hypothetical needs in the table on p. 364.

Evaluating Your Needs for an Assessment in Occupational Therapy Practice

General Need	*Specific Purpose*	*Your Needs*
Characteristic or Attribute	Occupational performance, person, environment	
General Purpose		
Description	Clients' needs	
	Current level of performance	
Decision Making	Planning interventions	
	Predicting future performance	
	Evaluating outcomes of therapy	
Theory Building	Research, constructs, etc.	
Population		
Age		
Background		
Special Populations		
Clinical Utility		
User Qualifications		
Budget		
Time		
Desirable Format		

Individual Learning Activity #2: Evaluating Assessments in Occupational Therapy Practice as They Relate to Your Needs

Instructions:

- Identify and obtain two (or more) assessments that measure the characteristic or attribute of interest.
- Review each assessment.
- Record the stated characteristic or attribute, purpose, population, and clinical utility characteristics for each assessment in the table on p. 365.
- Select one assessment that has the best match with your needs as described in Individual Learning Activity #1.
- Summarize the similarities and differences between the selected assessment and your hypothetical practice needs.

Evaluating Basic Characteristics of Assessments in Occupational Therapy Practice

Assessment	*Specific Purpose*	*Assessment #1*	*Assessment #2*
Title			
Author			
Publisher			
Publication Date			
Characteristic or Attribute	Occupational performance, person, environment factors		
General Purpose			
Description	Clients' needs		
	Current level of performance		
Decision Making	Planning interventions		
	Predicting future performance		
	Evaluating outcomes of therapy		
Theory Building	Research, constructs, etc.		
Population			
Age			
Background			
Special Populations			
Clinical Utility			
User Qualifications			
Budget			
Time			
Desirable Format			

Individual Learning Activity #3: Critiquing Assessments in Occupational Therapy Practice

Instructions:

- Conduct a basic critique of one assessment.
- Obtain and identify resources you will use for critique of the assessment (e.g., manual, formal critiques, research articles, textbooks, Internet information, etc.).
- Review the manual for the assessment. Is a manual available? Does it summarize the rationale and purpose of the assessment, recommended uses, development, administration, scores, scales, norms (if applicable), reliability estimates and studies, and validity estimates and studies? What comments do you or others have on the manual?
- Review the information available on development and administration. Are the development process, administration, standardization, and revisions described? What comments do you or others have on test development and administration?

- Review the information available on scores, scales, and norms. Are they described in sufficient detail? What comments do you or others have on scores, scales, and norms?
- Review the information available on reliability and reliability studies. Are they described in sufficient detail? What comments do you or others have on reliability or reliability studies?
- Review the information available on validity and validity studies. Are they described in sufficient detail? What comments do you or others have on validity or validity studies?
- Summarize the strengths and weaknesses of this assessment. How would you use this assessment in your practice? What cautions would you advise when using this assessment?

Conducting a Critique of One Assessment

General	*Specific Information*	*Information Available?*	*Comments*
Name of Assessment	Author, publisher, publication date		
Resources Used	Manual		
	Expert critique of assessment		
	Literature review		
	Other		
Manual	Available?		
	Stated rationale/purpose		
	Recommended uses and support for uses		
Development and Administration	Test development process-plan, lit review, domain, items		
	Administration, scoring, reporting		
	Standardization		
	Test revisions		
Scores, Scales	Scores and scales used		
Norms	Information on scales		
	Descriptions of norms (if applicable)		
Reliability and Errors of Measurement	Reliability estimates given		
	Intra-rater reliability		
	Inter-rater reliability		
	Test-retest reliability		
	Reliability studies explained		

(continued)

Validity	Validity evidence given for all recommended uses of test Content validity Construct validity Criterion validity Validity studies explained	
Summary		

Active Learning

Group Activity #1:Exploring the Assessment Process Through a Hypothetical Individual Client

Preparation:

- Read Chapter Fourteen and get into groups of three people.
- Select a hypothetical case from the options below and review the case.
- Select and obtain available occupational assessments for the hypothetical case (Note: The tables in Chapter Fourteen may provide examples of assessments to consider).
- Determine the number of assessments you will explore.
- For each assessment, assign a role to each group member.
  - ✧ Occupational therapy practitioner conducts the assessment.
  - ✧ Hypothetical client portrays a given case (see description of cases in materials).
  - ✧ Observer records notes on the assessment process (Note: The focus of this activity is to explore the assessment process through one assessment and one hypothetical individual client. It does not represent the entire assessment process or the process used for populations or organizations).

Time: 30 to 90 minutes (depending on number of assessments)

Materials:

- Assessments
- Tables and chairs arrangement conducive for assessment
- Props to help portray the case
- Hypothetical Cases:
  - ✧ Client 1: a) an 80-year-old man who lives alone in apartment, b) had a recent right hip fracture and surgery, c) is currently nonweight-bearing on his right side and is very restricted in hip movements, d) wants to go home as soon as possible but is concerned about how he will do ADL and IADL
  - ✧ Client 2: a) a 40-year-old woman who lives in a group home, b) is on a medication regimen for schizophrenia, c) has recently responded well to medication and has no current disturbances of thought, perception, and affect, d) wants to improve leisure and work occupations
  - ✧ Client 3: a) a 60-year-old woman who lives with husband in home, b) has lung cancer that has metastasized to other areas of the body, c) has tried various forms of treatment but has not responded, d) is currently feeling better, e) wants to maintain control of life and engage in meaningful ADLS, IADL, and leisure activities

- ✧ Client 4: a) a 50-year-old man who is a widower and lives with his college-age son, b) has had arthritis for 5 years, c) was recently laid off from job as a computer programmer, d) reports painful hand joints after some activities, e) wants to explore work occupations and IADL that have required excessive force or repetitive movements
- ✧ Client 5: a) a 9-year-old boy in third grade at a local elementary school, b) is receiving special education services in speech and language for speech articulation, c) was referred to occupational therapy for handwriting issues, d) has begun to work on cursive handwriting in the classroom

Instructions:

- Individually:
  - ✧ Review the assessment(s) prior to small group work.
  - ✧ Review the selected case(s). Imagine each situation.
  - ✧ Explore resources that might help you understand the case(s).
- In small groups:
  - ✧ Explore the initial assessment process through a hypothetical client.
  - ✧ The occupational therapy practitioner should make introductions, establish a client-centered professional relationship, explain the purpose of the assessment, explain the process of the assessment, and conduct the assessment.
  - ✧ The hypothetical client should engage in the assessment process, create specific responses/behaviors that fit the case, and portray the individual in the case.
  - ✧ The observer should record the steps in the assessment process, identify assessment strengths of the practitioner and areas to improve, critique the scenario presented by the hypothetical client, record responses and behaviors of the client, and summarize the results of the assessment.
  - ✧ Practice summarizing the results of your assessment for this case using both written and verbal communication.

Discussion:

- Discuss the information you obtained from this assessment. What information do you feel is complete? What information is missing?
- What evidence would you like to obtain on this assessment?
- Discuss the experience of being in the different roles. What was comfortable? What was awkward? What skills do you have? What skills would you like to develop?
- Discuss the results of the assessment. What components of the PEOP model were you able to fully or partially examine in this assessment?
- Discuss what you learned about the assessment process. Why is it important? How does it help develop a client-centered professional relationship?

Group Activity #2: Reviewing Critiques of Assessments

Preparation:

- Read Chapter Fourteen.
- Complete Individual Learning Activities #1 to #3.

Time: 30 to 45 minutes

Materials:

- Assessments
- Completed assignments for Individual Learning Activities #1 to #3

Instructions:

- Individually:
  - ✧ Review the critique you completed in Individual Learning Activities #1 to #3.
  - ✧ Prepare a summary of your critique.
- In small groups:
  - ✧ Share your critique with the small group.

  - ✧ Summarize your recommendations regarding the assessment.
- In large group (optional):
  - ✧ Schedule a poster presentation of the assessments reviewed.

Discussion:

- Discuss the process for conducting a critique of an assessment. What were the easy parts? What was a challenge?
- Discuss strategies for incorporating this process in occupational therapy practice.
- Discuss resources you found most helpful in this process.

Group Activity #3: Exploring Assessment of a Hypothetical Population or Organization

Preparation:

- Read Chapter Fourteen.
- Select a hypothetical case(s) from the options provided below (Note: The focus of this activity is to explore assessment for one hypothetical population or organization. It does not represent the entire assessment process. Also, this activity does not give you sufficient details to develop a complete, accurate assessment).

Time: 30 to 90 minutes (depending on number of cases)

Materials:

- Assessment resources: catalogs, journals, texts, home programs, practice guidelines, online resources
- Hypothetical cases:
  - ✧ Client 1: a) elders living in an assisted-living environment, b) limited support system, c) high incidence of depression, d) some medical issues
  - ✧ Client 2: a) elementary school-age children in your community, b) below national average academic achievement, c) high incidence of obesity, d) delayed gross and fine motor skills
  - ✧ Client 3: a) homeless men in your community, b) working minimum wage jobs, c) some chemical dependency and mental health problems, d) affordable housing issues
  - ✧ Client 4: a) caregivers of family with Alzheimer's, b) burn-out and stress reported, c) financial issues, d) limited resources in area

Instructions:

- Individually:
  - ✧ Review the case prior to small group work.
  - ✧ Explore resources that might help you understand the case(s) and plan assessments.
- In small groups:
  - ✧ Explore assessment of a hypothetical client.
  - ✧ Give examples of the client defined as a population or organization.
  - ✧ Develop supplemental information on your client to assist you in assessment.
  - ✧ Summarize your supplemental information.
  - ✧ Brainstorm assessment ideas that might be appropriate for this client.
  - ✧ Select three types of assessment to describe in more detail and summarize them in the table on p. 370.

Discussion:

- Discuss the assessments you used for this case. Why did you choose them?
- What evidence would you like to obtain on these assessments?
- How are the assessments for populations and organizations similar and different from those used with individuals?
- How would the assessment process for populations and organizations feel different from the process used with individuals?
- Discuss what you learned about assessments for populations and organizations. Why is it important?
- Discuss the skills you have and the skills you would like to develop related to assessment of populations and organizations

Client:
Population Example:
Organization Example:
Supplemental Information:

Assessment Area—What do you want to know or learn about this client?	*Type of Assessment—Records, Informal Measures, Interviews, Ecological measures, Skilled observations, Norm or Criterion referenced measures*	*Client Information/Assessment—What will this assessment tell you from the client's perspective?*	*Practitioner Evaluation/Assessment— ---Person ---Environment ---Occupation ---Performance What will this assessment tell you about PEOP?*

Chapter Fifteen Objectives

The information in this chapter is intended to help the reader:

1. Organize the person, occupation, and environmental factors that support the occupational performance of people, organizations, and communities.
2. Understand the elements that must go into a client-centered care plan.
3. Recognize how knowledge obtained throughout higher education can be tapped to build a client-centered plan that focuses on the occupational performance needs of the client.
4. Understand that the client's medical diagnosis may provide clues to the issues he or she will be facing but that it is the client's experience with the condition that frames his or her goals for occupational therapy intervention.
5. Understand how to use a situational analysis to incorporate key elements into the occupational therapy plan.

Key Words

client-centered intervention plan: A plan that focuses on the individuals goals and has been constructed using a situational analysis that integrates evidence, the client's occupational history, and that what the client wants and needs to do to foster participation in family, work, and community life.

client-centered practice: Practice is focused on the needs expressed by the client.

evidence: The basis for your decisions, the knowledge on which to base your treatment.

evidence-based practice: "Evidence-based clinical practice (EBCP) is an approach to health care practice in which the clinician is aware of the evidence that bears on [his or] her clinical practice, and the strength of that evidence" (http://hiru.mcmaster.ca/ebm/default.htm).

occupational history: The individual's current roles, responsibilities, future roles, lifestyle issues, routines, and necessary and chosen occupations.

occupational profile: The term adopted by the American Occupational Therapy Association to reflect the occupational history (see above).

self-efficacy: An estimate by an individual as to his or her ability to manage a situation; the likelihood of something occurring.

situational analysis: A process that involves the collection of information and the analysis of factors intrinsic and extrinsic to the individual, the organization, or the population to determine the occupational performance issues that will impact the ability to reach client-centered goals. The situational analysis will identify strengths, weaknesses, opportunities, and goals and will help the practitioner choose the appropriate evidenced-base intervention to help the client achieve his or her goals.

stakeholders: Those who are affected by an outcome or have an interest in an outcome; in the occupational therapist's terms, this would be family, teachers, policy makers, elected officials, managers, etc.

Information is a source of learning. But unless it is organized, processed, and available to the right people in a format for decision making, it is a burden, not a benefit.
William Pollard

Chapter Fifteen

Person-Environment-Occupation-Performance: A Model for Planning Interventions for Individuals and Organizations

Carolyn M. Baum, PhD, OTR/L, FAOTA; Julie Bass-Haugen, PhD, OTR/L, FAOTA; and Charles H. Christiansen, EdD, OTR, OT(C), FAOTA

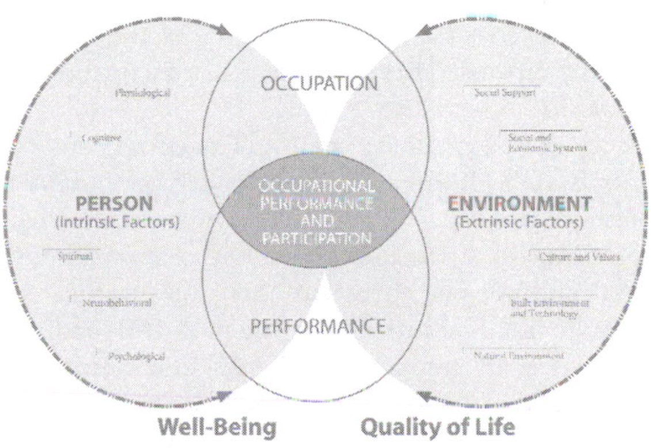

Setting the Stage

The Person-Environment-Occupation-Performance (PEOP) model provides a strong foundation to help practitioners conceptualize and organize the complex factors related to occupational performance, person, and environment. It helps us visualize the different levels of occupation, recognize the capabilities/constraints in the person, and identify enablers/barriers in the environment. The PEOP model is also an important tool for developing a framework for the occupational therapy process.

In this chapter, we introduce a framework for the occupational therapy process that incorporates the PEOP model, client-centered concepts, and evidence for the various decisions that are made during the process. The purpose of this framework is to give entry-level practitioners specific strategies to use for different components of the occupational therapy process.

Baum, C. M., Bass-Haugen, J., & Christiansen, C. H. (2005). *Person-environment-occupation-performance: A model for planning interventions for individuals and organizations.* In C. H. Christiansen, C. M. Baum, and J. Bass-Haugen (Eds.), Occupational therapy: Performance, participation, and well-being (3rd ed.). Thorofare, NJ: SLACK Incorporated.

Using the Person-Environment-Occupation-Performance Model in an Occupational Therapy Framework

Christiansen (2002) defines model as a device for organizing ideas or concepts to form an explanation. The PEOP model is the basis for an occupational therapy framework that practitioners may use in addressing problems that limit an individual's occupational performance. This chapter will explain how the PEOP model can serve as part of a framework to organize knowledge for practice for an individual, an organization, or a community population.

The PEOP model is designed to support the practitioner as he or she builds a collaborative plan with the client (i.e., the patient, the family, the physician, the social worker, the student, the architect, the employee, the organization, the employer, or the community) as the client seeks the knowledge and skills of the occupational therapist to address issues that impact occupational performance.

Mattingly and Fleming (1994) in their seminal work on clinical reasoning in occupational therapy made a statement that captures the essence of the occupational therapy process. They said that what occupational therapists do appears so simple, but it is so complex. Occupational therapists are problem solvers and consultants. Meyer (1922) said, "We provide opportunities, not prescriptions" (p. 7). The problems of clients have to be solved in the context of the client's life or the organization's culture. The client's internal and external resources must be mobilized to address the problems, and the resolution has to capture the client's motivation and also occur in the client's time frame. The practitioner is an agent of change, bringing to the situation knowledge of interventions that can enable clients to meet their goals.

Before we start planning treatment for someone else, let's think about occupational performance from your perspective. Imagine that you were riding your bike in the park (an occupation). You came up over a hill going at a pretty fast clip, and someone had left a tricycle in the path (natural/built environment). You fall off your bike, and the next thing you know you are in the hospital in a great deal of pain (person, psychological, physiological). You learn that you have broken your shoulder and pelvis (physiological) and have a mild head injury (neurobehavioral and cognitive). If that is not enough, you touch the bandages on your face and find that you have some serious abrasions on your face that will require plastic surgery (physiological, psychological). You don't have time for this. You have to study for your finals. You are in a friend's wedding in 3 weeks, and your family lives more than 1,000 miles away (environmental—social and cultural).

As you begin to comprehend what has happened, you think, "I can't do what I did before but I need to get back to my life as soon as possible." You want to go home but you wonder how it is going to work (occupation). You live on the third floor with no elevator (built environment). You live alone, and all of your good friends are at colleges all over the country (social support). You realize you are weak (physiological), your vision is not clear (neurobehavioral), you can't remember your new phone number (cognitive), and you wonder how you will pay for this (economical).

To provide the most appropriate care for you, your providers need to know who you are and what you need. What do you want people to know about you and your previous activities and roles? Do you want them to know what you need and want to do? How would it be to turn control over to someone else? Should you? In walks your occupational therapist. The story is really just beginning, and you can use your imagination regarding the scenarios that follow.

In your role as an occupational therapist, people won't always choose to be your client—a series of events has created the occupational performance issue that requires your service. Clients come to you because you have the knowledge and skills to help them build and execute a plan to accomplish what they want and need to do for themselves. It becomes your task to identify how impairments or problems have limited their activities and to identify how barriers are limiting their participation and to do this in a client-centered context.

Client-Centered Practice and Its Principles

This section will serve as a brief introduction to client-centered practice. It will highlight why a client-centered approach is central to the occupational therapy process. A client-centered approach requires the practitioner to facilitate the client's problem solving and goal achievement (McColl, 1997). It also requires the therapist to move beyond the therapist as the decision maker to one of a collaborator with the client. Asking clients to be partners in their own care requires the occupational therapist to explore the extent to which the client understands what has happened to him or her and whether or not he or she feels that the objectives can be accomplished.

Self-efficacy, or believing that a task or activity can be accomplished, allows one to feel competent, which in turn contributes to improved occupational performance and well-being (Gage & Polatajko, 1994). Self-efficacy is at the core of client-centered care. By viewing clients as individuals with unique characteristics and roles and focusing the plan on the client's needs, the person can gain motivation from his or her own perceptions and emotional efforts.

A model of care can only be described as client-centered when the client explains the problems and defines his or her needs and experiences in an environment of understanding, trust, and acceptance (Gerteis et al., 1993). It also requires the client and therapist to work together to define the nature of the occupational performance problems, the focus and need for intervention, and the preferred outcome of therapy supported by evidence. Every client must be encouraged to participate in planning his or her care at his or her own level, depending on the capabilities, but all people are capable of making some choices about how treatment should be approached. The therapist must have a fundamental respect for the client's values and for his or her style of coping with the current situation.

To be considered a client-centered model, there are several key elements: 1) the model must consider the activities, tasks, and roles of the person, the organization, or the community (Christiansen & Baum, 1997); 2) services must be organized to support the individual as an active participant (Blank, Horowitz, & Matza, 1995); and 3) the practitioner must encourage a partnership that enables individuals to assume responsibility for their own care (Law et al., 1994).

The PEOP model considers the client central to the care planning process. In addition to focusing on the client's goals, the PEOP model is built on an occupational history; includes information about the client's perception of what has happened to him or her; and includes consideration of the client's roles, responsibilities, and/or mission and values. The assessment and planning phase of care is grounded in evidence. The clients should enter into the intervention phase with a clear understanding of the likely result of the outcome that will result with the effort exerted by both the practitioner and the client.

Using the Person-Environment-Occupation-Performance Model to Plan Care

A planning process needs to be built on capabilities and environmental resources that can support the client in the occupations that he or she wants and needs to do. The planning process for the PEOP model appears somewhat complex, but you either have, or at the completion of your educational program will have, the knowledge to enable the client's occupational performance using this model.

It is at the treatment planning process that all of the knowledge you have learned in your OT program, in your prerequisite courses, and in your educational preparation for college comes together. It is that knowledge applied to the occupational performance needs of your client that defines your professional role as an occupational therapist and differentiates you from other professionals. You will employ client-centered strategies that engage the individual to develop or use resources that enable successful occupational performance.

Table 15-1 is meant to help you recall how you have obtained the knowledge to employ the PEOP model.

All of these concepts are addressed in your measurement coursework, your practice classes, and your research classes and projects. Your fieldwork and, in many cases, your case studies provide you with opportunities to integrate these concepts as you interact with real people and real situations.

Assessment, planning, and treatment occur concurrently throughout the time you are with a client or clients. You will use some formal assessments to establish baseline information for the person, environment, and occupational factors, but much of the information you need to build a client-centered plan comes directly from your client(s) as you use conversation and observation to understand their issues and to have a clear picture of what it is they need and want to do.

The intervention planning process is dynamic. Chapter Sixteen discusses the general categories of interventions. For some problems identified in the plan, the intervention will focus on remediation. Others will use compensatory strategies, and yet others will focus on maintaining or helping the client to self-manage performance. All of these strategies may be in the same intervention plan, depending on the goals the client has identified.

It is important to point out that when the PEOP model is used with an individual, it is not pathogenic- or diagnostic-based. It is based on the occupational performance problems presented by the individual. As an occupational therapist, you have knowledge about the relationships of impairments to a diagnosis, and while this information will give you clues about problems that the person might be experiencing, relying only on what one expects to find based on an impairment or diagnosis does not give credit to the client's ability to share his or her experience with the problem or to your knowledge about occupational performance. To further explain the point, a person is not seen as having a hand injury, a stroke, autism, or a mental illness. The person is presented to you as an individual who is limited in his or her capacity to do that which he or she wants or needs to do. In the process of developing a plan, you will use a variety of strategies to help the person address the problems that are limiting his or her occupational performance. This is the defining characteristic of an occupational therapist.

Table 15-1

Person-Environment-Occupation-Performance Model

Person *Intrinsic Factors*	*Occupation*	*Environment* *Extrinsic Factors*
Psychological/emotional	Actions	Physical environment
Physiological		Natural environment
Cognitive	Tasks	Social environment
Neurobehavioral		Societal environment
Spiritual	Roles	Culture
Source of Knowledge		
Anatomy	Occupational science	Environmental theory
Physiology	Occupational therapy theory	Sociology
Neuroscience	Psychology	Anthropology
Medical lectures		Political science
Psychology		Geography
Ethics/religion		

It is very difficult to visually represent the dynamic nature of the intervention planning process as it involves humans engaged in solving real problems. However, the PEOP model has a number of constructs that must come together to support both the practitioner and the client in developing a realistic and sequenced plan. This process depends on the practitioner's skills in forming a relationship with the client, asking the right questions, and being able to access the knowledge to understand the issues and options presented by the client's occupational performance issues and goals. This process requires the skills of a professional. An individual who lacks the conceptual ability, knowledge, or access to resources cannot perform it.

The PEOP model is a top-down approach and, in addition to considering the client's roles, occupations, and goals, it requires the occupational therapist to address the personal performance capabilities/constraints and the environmental performance enabler/barriers that are concepts basic to the model through assessment, observation, and conversational inquiry.

Let's look at the parts of the planning process. To incorporate key elements of planning, the occupational therapist completes a situational analysis. This analysis seeks information from the client by interview and by employing assessments that give the practitioner a clear understanding of constraints and/or barriers that may limit the person's activity and participation. As well, the practitioner will gain insight into capacities and environmental enablers that will support the individual in doing the things he or she wants and needs to do.

There are a number of key elements of a plan of care in the PEOP model. These client-centered elements change depending on whether the client is a person, an organization, or the community as reflected in a population approach. Each will be discussed. This chapter is not meant to describe the details necessary to assess or plan interventions, as this information is distributed throughout the book. This chapter is designed to set the context for how information provided by the client, information collected by the practitioner from the client, and evidence gathered from the literature are used to develop interventions designed to influence the occupational performance of a client. That client may be an individual, an organization, or a population (a community).

The following situational analyses are designed to help the practitioner organize information to address the issues of individuals, organizations, and communities. The situational analysis format will become routine with practice. The templates can be used as training or teaching tools to ensure that all necessary information is collected to support the clinician in the reasoning process as a client-centered intervention plan is developed and implemented.

You will notice that, in each situational analysis, evidence underpins the practitioner's decisions of what measures to include and which interventions to employ. All professionals are being held to a standard—that of competent practice using best-practice methods that have been determined to be effective. Evidence thus becomes the filter through which clinical decisions about the type of evaluation or assessment and the interventions that will support the client in achieving his or her goals will be made.

Traditionally, intervention decisions were made based primarily on experience and training. Students looked to their teachers and fieldwork supervisors, and new practitioners looked to more experienced colleagues to guide their approach to both assessment and intervention. Evidence-based practice takes into account the practitioner's experience and the unique needs of the client and adds to this evidence from relevant publications as decisions are made about interventions that will be effective (Baum & Law, 1998). You will note in this book that most chapters end with a table of research that supports the content of the chapter. This was done to integrate evidence into the basic learning process. It then becomes available for planning treatment that will be effective given the problems as presented by the client (Figure 15-1).

PLANNING PERSON-CENTERED INTERVENTIONS

The Collection of Client Information

The Occupational History

Except in an emergency situation, a physician does not begin to make decisions about a medical plan without a medical history. The occupational therapist should find it impossible to build a client-centered plan without an occupational history. It is during the process of obtaining a history that the practitioner learns what the person has done previously and how culture impacts his or her everyday life. An occupational history should include a description of leisure interests and social activities and should provide a clear understanding of the responsibilities the client has for work, self, and home management tasks. Such a history can be accomplished with an interview or an instrument like the Activity Card Sort (Baum & Edwards, 2001) or the Interest Checklist (Matsutsuyu, 1969).

Perception of What Has Happened

Another key element is the person's perception of what has happened to him or her. Every person has a different level of knowledge of his or her medical or health conditions, so it is important to know what the person thinks has happened, whether he or she thinks it is serious, and what he or she knows about the course of treatment. It is also important to learn the impact that the current situation is having on his or her life.

The Occupational Profile

It is important to form an occupational profile. The Role Checklist (Oakley, Kielhofner, Barris, & Richler, 1986) provides a valuable resource to the practitioner to determine the past, current, and future roles of the client. Especially important is to understand the client's roles and responsibilities that must be maintained during the time he or she is engaged in treatment. The profile should include a description of lifestyle issues and routines that enable daily occupations.

The Client's Immediate and Long-Term Goals

What are the client's goals? It is important to determine the client's long-term goals so that as discussions emerge about short-terms goals, the practitioner can help the client plan the steps to accomplish his or her goals. It is always easier to set goals if you have completed an occupational history. By knowing the person's interests, skills, roles, and culture, it is possible to help formulate goals that will not only be achievable, but also will be meaningful. The Canadian Occupational Performance Measure (Law et al., 1994) is an excellent tool to use in planning goals; it also detects change in a client's self-perception of his or her occupational performance over time.

Match Between the Client's Goals and Occupational Therapy

The final step in the client information section of the analysis is to determine the match between the person's goals and the occupational therapy approach. If there is not a match, the occupational therapist should make an appropriate referral to another professional or to other resources to address the client's goals. When there is a match, the practitioner should begin the second section of the situational analysis to determine the person's capabilities and enablers and to identify barriers and constraints that will need to be overcome.

Evaluation and Assessment of Intrinsic (Person) and Extrinsic (Environmental) Factors That Will Impact or Support Occupational Performance

Selection of Measures/Assessments to Understand the Intrinsic and Extrinsic Factors

The person factors (intrinsic) include physiological, psychological, cognitive, neurobehavioral, and spiritual. The environmental factors (extrinsic) include cultural, social, natural environment, built environment, and societal. Assessments are chosen that will allow the therapist to understand the person's capabilities and what might be

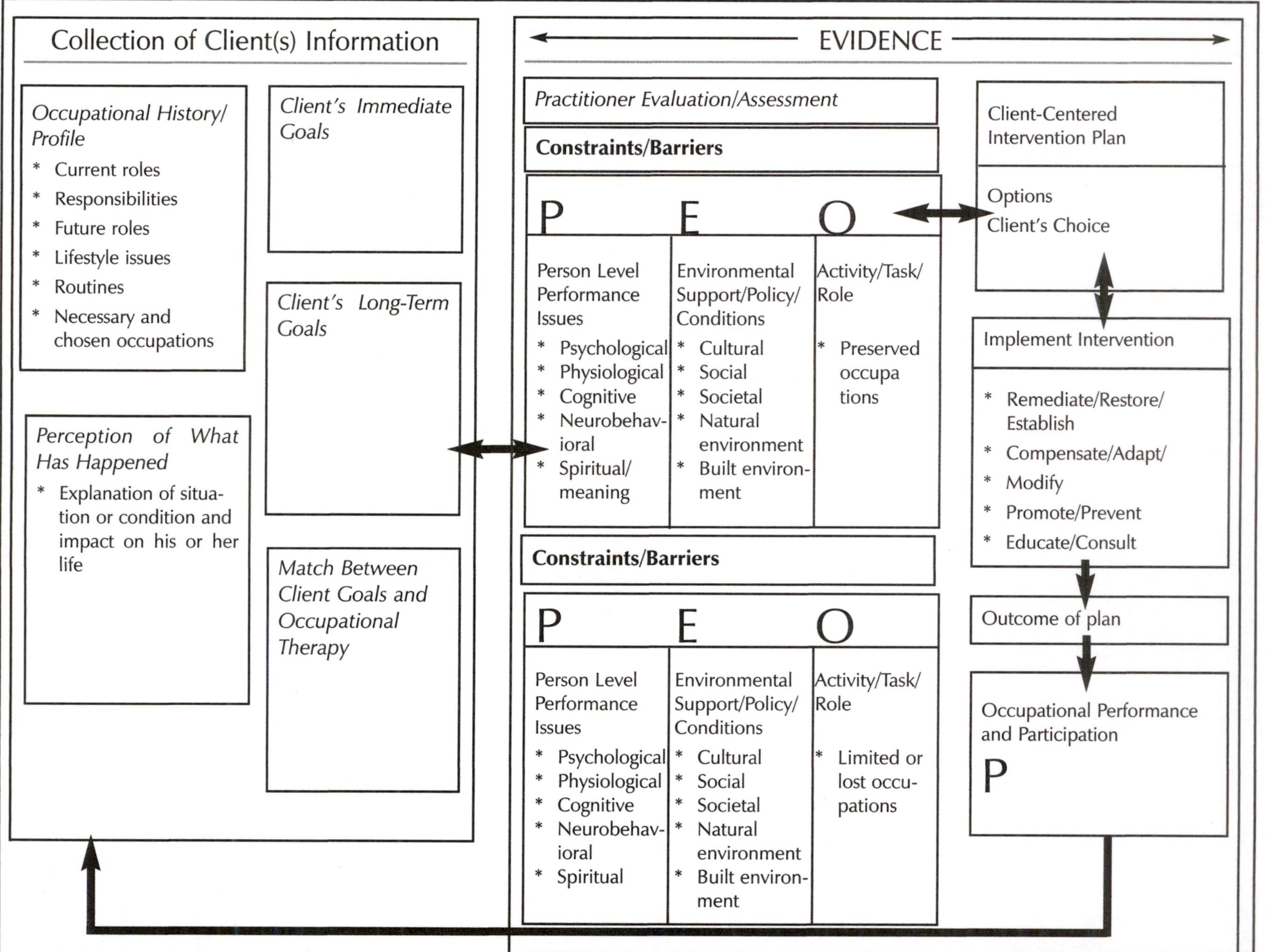

Figure 15-1. A situational analysis: using the PEOP model for planning person-centered interventions.

limiting his or her performance in activities, tasks, or occupations that are central to fulfilling his or her roles or expectations.

Client-Centered Intervention Plan

With the client's information and the practitioner's assessment of the client's capacity and constraints, a client-centered plan is constructed. The practitioner uses his or her skill to help the client understand what is possible and also helps the client understand the issues involved in helping him or her meet his or her goals. The client has the right and the practitioner has the responsibility to share the evidence that the interventions will be able to help the client achieve his or her goals.

Implement Intervention

Several interventions can and should be employed to meet the client's goals. These interventions range from remediation designed to restore function to compensation, including promoting health, preventing secondary problems, and educating the client and his or her support network to be able to self-manage the situation. One additional intervention is advocating for change to remove societal barriers that limit occupational performance. These interventions are discussed throughout the interventions section of the book.

Outcome of the Plan

Following the implementation of the plan, the client hopefully will be able to achieve his or her goals. Outcomes should be measured, not only to demonstrate the progress to the client, but also to demonstrate the effectiveness of the occupational therapy interventions to the referral source, to the payer, and to the public. The effectiveness of occupational therapy must be public to shape policies of institutions and payment sources.

Occupational Performance and Participation

The entire process leads to achieving the goals identified by the client and helping him or her return to the level of everyday life that meets his or her roles, responsibilities, and interests. Because many individuals have a chronic condition or a disability that requires a self-management strategy, part of the outcome should include the possibility of additional help from an occupational therapist if an occupational performance issue emerges in the future that could benefit from an occupational therapist's expertise.

Addressing the Occupational Performance Issues of Communities

The process described previously fits well when you, as the occupational therapist, are working with individuals or small groups of people like families. However, an emerging area of practice for occupational therapy is the occupational issues of populations and communities. Populations may be as large as all of the people in the world who fit some characteristic as described by an organization (e.g., people with AIDS, children who are homeless), or they may reflect a small group of people or a community with issues of concern in a given organization (e.g., mid-life women with family issues that affect their work for a company or seniors who have become isolated in your neighborhood because of transportation issues). You might guess that the situational analyses conducted will look different in these different situations. Population/community centered situational analyses may serve as the starting point for occupational therapists who are interested in improving the health of populations or communities in general or working with specific organizations.

Say you are an occupational therapist who has worked with older people in long-term care settings for several years and you wish to continue to work with older people but would like to work with well elders to prevent nursing home placement and improve quality of life. How do you begin? Do you already have the background and knowledge that will enable you to be successful in this new practice arena? Are you ready to jump in and promote your services to organizations that work with this population or in these communities? Perhaps, but not likely.

In this situation, a population/community situational analysis may better prepare you to understand the general characteristics and issues of the older population and the community in which they live and to develop interventions that will meet the needs and goals of specific organizations.

Let's follow this example through a situational analysis. Although you have worked with elders who have health conditions and diminished abilities in the long-term care setting, you don't have a clear understanding of well elders. You begin a population/community-centered situational analysis by acquiring general information and conducting a broad assessment. What things should you look at? (Figure 15-2).

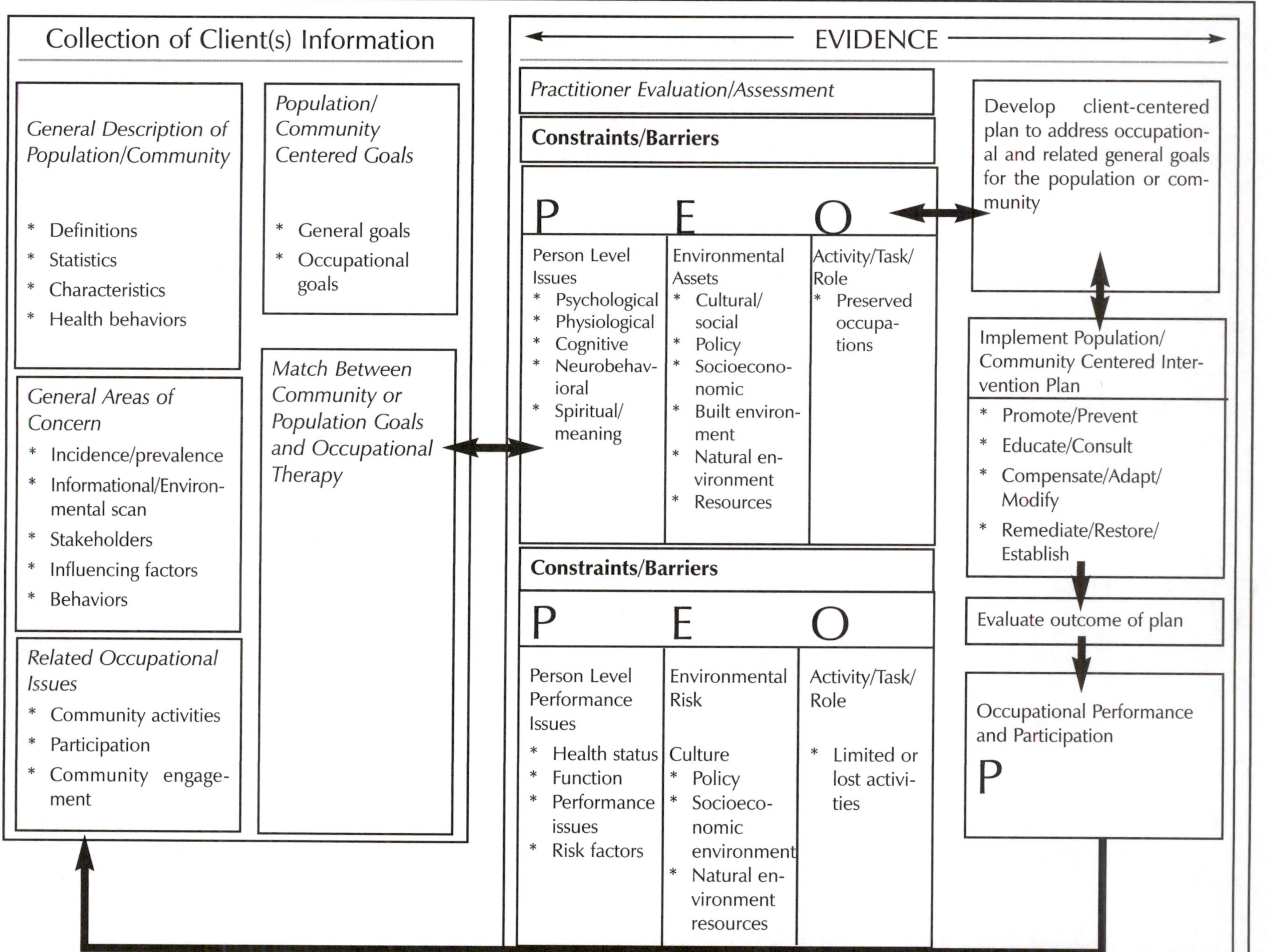

Figure 15-2. A situational analysis: using the PEOP model for planning population/community-centered interventions.

Planning Population of Community-Centered Interventions

The Collection of Client Information

A General Description of the Population/Community

This will help you define the population/community (e.g., age, gender, ethnicity, income, education, employment, religion, geographic area), obtain statistics of interest (e.g., risk factors), and identify characteristics that are associated with people who are part of this population/community (e.g., knowledge, attitudes, beliefs, habits, preferences, sensitivities). This exercise may also support some of your assumptions and/or dispel myths that are commonly held.

Identification of General Areas of Concern

Identification of general areas of concern for this population/community requires you to look outside of occupational therapy to gain a broader understanding of the array of critical issues (e.g., barriers, policy, supports, services, motivators for change). You will often find these areas identified by local, national, and international agencies and organizations, census information, and even in the popular press. In a sense, you are conducting an environmental/informational scan to learn more about the prioritized areas of concern for a population/community, the incidence/prevalence of the issues, and the major stakeholders (e.g., transportation has been identified as a major issue for seniors living in communities).

Related Occupational Issues

It is an important step to identify an occupational therapy role for this population/community. Some issues may not have significant occupational issues associated with them; others will. This step may require you to explore occupational therapy literature that can help you make this link, but more likely it will involve using strong critical thinking skills and your knowledge of factors that support occupational performance (e.g., transportation issues may limit engagement in all occupations that are typically done outside the home [i.e., shopping, financial matters, socialization, etc.]).

The Population/Community—General Goals

It is important to identify areas of concern. These goals may be broken into immediate goals and long-term goals, or they may be overall general objectives. Knowledge of these goals will help you in your communications with stakeholders for this population/community.

The Population/Community—Occupational Goals

These are developed from the identification of how the general health of the community is understood by the stakeholders.

Match Between the Community or Population Goals and Occupational Therapy

The final step in the client information section of the analysis is to determine the match between the community or population goals and the occupational therapy approach. If there is not a match, the occupational therapist should make an appropriate referral to another professional or to other resources to address the client's goals. When there is a match, the practitioner should begin the second section of the situational analysis to determine the person's capabilities and enablers and to identify barriers and constraints that will need to be overcome.

The Evaluation and Assessment of Intrinsic (Person) and Extrinsic (Environmental) Factors That Will Impact on or Support Occupational Performance

Selection of Measures/Assessments/Methodologies to Understand the Intrinsic and Extrinsic Factors

The occupational therapist selects appropriate tools to understand the intrinsic and extrinsic factors that are enabling as well as constraining the occupational performance of the community population. The person factors (intrinsic) include physiological, psychological, cognitive, neurobehavioral, and spiritual. The environmental factors (extrinsic) include cultural, social, natural environment, built environment, and societal. Clinical reasoning supports the occupational therapist in applying his or her knowledge of the person, environmental, and occupational factors to the activities and tasks that are central to the community roles. At the community level, many of the factors will be environmental (e.g., the lack of an accessible playground for children, inadequate public transportation to support older adult's community independence, poor or confusing signage at the health center). However, there are community problems that affect the person or intrinsic factors. Examples would be air quality and limited access to fresh food.

Develop a Client-Centered Plan to Address Occupational and Related General Goals for the Population or Community

With the client's information and the practitioner's assessment of the client's capacity, a client-centered plan can be constructed. The client has the right to know and the practitioner has the responsibility to share the evidence that the interventions will be able to help the client achieve his or her goals. Evidence will help you understand the approaches that have already been tried to meet general and/or occupational goals and the outcomes of these various interventions. This step is important in determining strategies that work for this population/community, discarding ideas that do not have evidence to support them, and identifying intervention plans that have not yet been evaluated in the literature. If an untried strategy will be used, it is important for the client to understand the principles on which you will base the intervention, and the client must agree to its use.

Implementing a Population/Community-Centered Intervention Plan

If your work entailed broad population/community initiatives and responsibilities (e.g., public health, labor, legislative), you may work with others to implement these strategies as part of an overall plan. If your work involved developing partnerships with organizations and agencies, these overall strategies may serve as the foundation for a new situational analysis designed for organization-centered interventions.

Outcome of the Plan

Following the implementation of the plan, the client hopefully will be able to achieve his or her goals. Outcomes should be measured, not only to demonstrate progress to the client, but also to demonstrate the effectiveness of the occupational therapy interventions to the referral source, to the payer, and to the public. The effectiveness of occupational therapy must be public in order to shape policies of institutions and payment sources.

Occupational Performance and Participation

The entire process leads to achieving the goals identified by the client and helping him or her achieve the goals that will improve the occupational performance of the population in his or her community. Because communities are facing new problems with an emerging population of older adults and those living with chronic diseases and disabling conditions, they need to provide the infrastructure to enable full participation of citizens in their communities. Part of the outcome should include the possibility of additional help from an occupational therapist if an occupational performance issue emerges in the future that could benefit from an occupational therapist's expertise (Figure 15-3).

Planning Organization-Centered Interventions

An organization situational analysis begins with a population situational analysis related to the types of clients served by the organization. This step in the process enables the occupational therapist to approach the organization with a level of credibility that will open doors of opportunity. After developing expertise with regard to a specific population, an occupational therapist may not need to do this step in an explicit manner. Rather, the knowledge base of the professional includes this foundational information. Entry-level practitioners, however, would likely need to begin with a population-centered analysis as a preliminary step and prior to any discussions with a specific organization.

The Collection of Client Information

Description of the Organization

Once there is an understanding of the population, its needs, its resources, and its goals, the next step in an organization situational analysis is to fully describe the organization. An understanding of the organization's mission, history, focus, values, activities, funding, clients, and stakeholders is essential for assessing their need and potential for occupational therapy services. Some of this information may be obtained in publications about the organization. Other information may be acquired through initial conversations with a contact person in the organization.

The Organization's Area of Concern

The occupational therapist begins to explore the organization's areas of concern and unmet needs for the clients they serve. Many of these concerns may be expressed in terms of general issues. For example, a community agency might be concerned about the adaptation of recent immigrants to the expectations of the larger culture. A school district may be concerned about the social and emotional health of some student groups. A corporation may be concerned about retention of workers who are mothers or caretakers. In this step, the occupational therapist also uses critical reasoning skills to identify and communicate the occupational issues that may be influencing the general areas of concern for the organization. For example, recent immigrants may have vocational backgrounds that are different from the work opportunities currently avail-

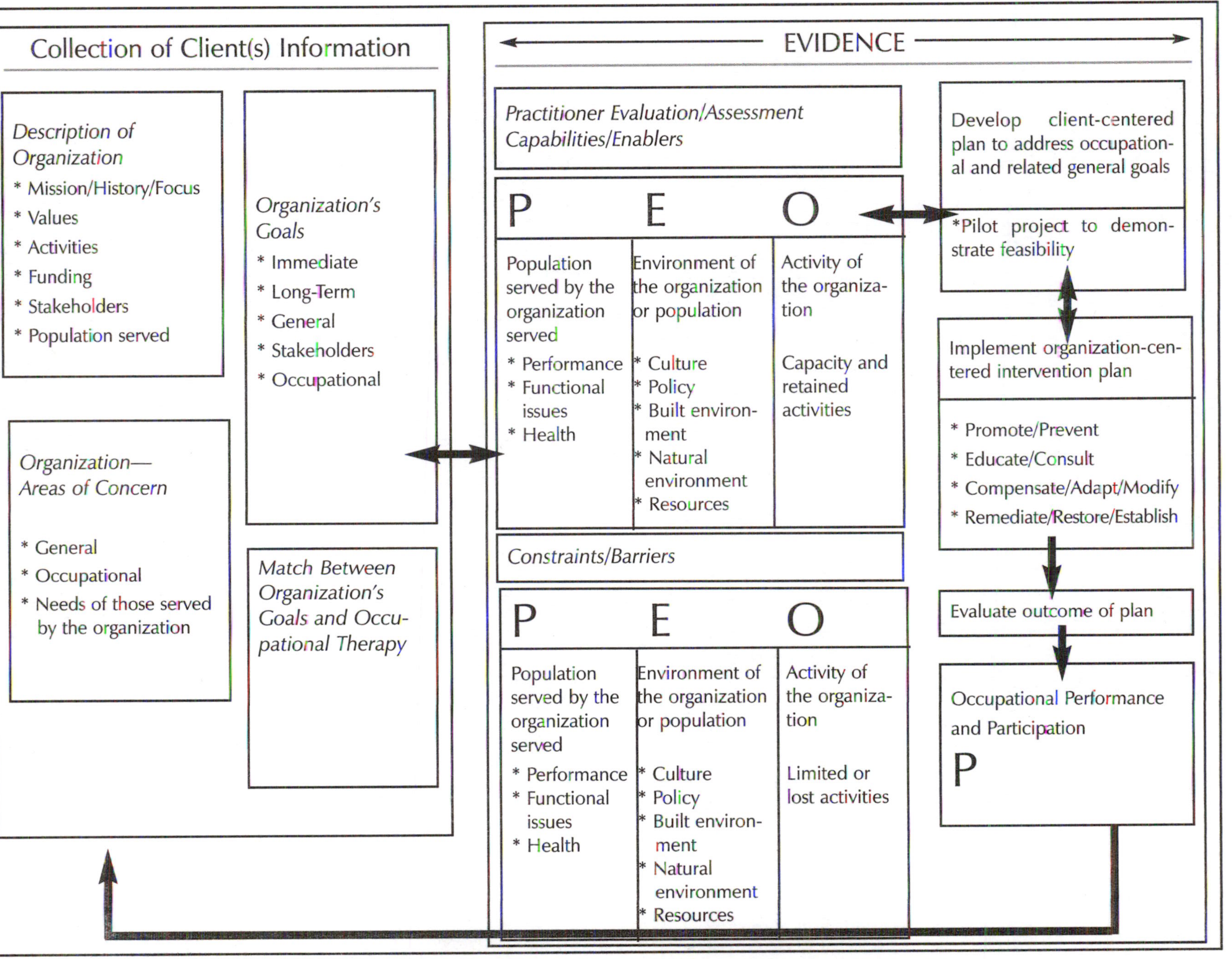

Figure 15-3. A situational analysis: using the PEOP model for planning organizational-centered interventions.

able, adolescents may only have access to extracurricular activities that are sports-related, and workers may not have sufficient support systems to solve parenting or care-taking problems as they arise.

The Organizational Goals

The goals of the organization and its stakeholders are considered next in the process. The occupational therapist inquires about the organization's immediate and long-term goals as they relate to general and occupational areas of concern. The practitioner also asks for information that will allow him or her to determine the organization's commitment and ability to achieve these goals.

The Match Between the Organization's Goals and Occupational Therapy

The final step in the first stage is to evaluate the match between the organization's goals and the occupational therapy services you can provide. You will use your population/community situational analysis, all the information you have gathered about the organization, and your discussions with people in the organization to decide whether to continue the process. At this point, your personal investment in the organization has been limited. However, if you continue the process, you and the organization may make a considerable commitment of personnel and resources for client assessment and interventions.

The Evaluation and Assessment of Intrinsic (Person) and Extrinsic (Environmental) Factors That Will Impact or Support Occupational Performance

Selection of Measures/Assessments/Methodologies to Understand the Intrinsic and Extrinsic Factors

The occupational therapist selects appropriate tools to understand the intrinsic and extrinsic factors that are enabling as well as constraining the occupational performance of the organization. The person factors (intrinsic) include physiological, psychological, cognitive, neurobehavioral, and spiritual. The environmental factors (extrinsic) include cultural, social, natural environment, built environment, and societal. Clinical reasoning supports the occupational therapist in applying his or her knowledge of the person and environmental and occupational factors to the activities and tasks that are central to the community roles. At the organization level, many of the factors will be environmental (e.g., the lack of training that fosters full participation of children in a mainstreamed classroom, managers who don't understand how to make accommodations for workers who wish to return to work after an accident or injury, or poor attendance related to lack of training of bus drivers). However, there are organizational problems that affect the person or intrinsic factors. Examples would be work practices that foster poor posture or repetitive motion injuries.

With the client's information and the practitioner assessment of the client's capacity, a client-centered plan can be constructed. The client has the right and the practitioner has the responsibility to share the evidence that the interventions will be able to help the client achieve his or her goals.

Implementing an Organization-Centered Plan

You are now ready to develop an organization-centered intervention plan that can help the organization achieve its general and occupational goals. You will want to consider your initial population/community-centered plan, variations of this plan that are appropriate for the organization, and the current evidence that is available. It also may be important to pilot any interventions, especially if this represents a new of area of occupational therapy practice. Pilot studies are a way to establish relationships with organizational clients, as initial outcomes can pave the way for additional work and funding. The organization will use the time to evaluate your capacity to help them achieve their goals. Implementation of your intervention plan may include any of the strategies identified in the person-centered situational analysis. However, promotion/prevention and education/consultation strategies are probably most common and effective when the target of the intervention is an organization and its clientele.

Evaluate the Outcome of the Plan

Your success with this organization can only be verified and documented if you conduct an evaluation of your interventions for their effectiveness in achieving goals. This step is important in helping you solidify your relationship with the organization and preparing you to work with other related organizations. Disseminating the outcomes of your interventions to the broader occupational therapy community is also essential for expanding practice into new arenas.

Occupational Performance and Participation

The entire process leads to achieving the goals identified by the client. Because organizations are facing new problems with an emerging population of older adults and those living with chronic diseases and disabling conditions, they need to provide the infrastructure to enable successful participation by clients in their organizations. Part of the outcome should include the possibility of additional help from an occupational therapist if an occupational performance issue emerges in the future that could benefit from an occupational therapist's expertise.

Summary

These three templates were outlined not to restrict the occupational therapist to the activities that are described, but to make explicit the activities that must come together to employ the PEOP model. Occupational therapists have always been known to "do good work." Because that work often employs common sense strategies, others may not know the thought process and knowledge that has gone into those recommendations. By using these templates, the practitioner is given the language to use in reports and recommendations that will make clear to others the complexity and the thoughtfulness that has gone into the plan to enable people, communities, and organizations to accomplish their goals when those goals are to improve the lives of those with or at risk for disabling conditions.

References

Baum, C. M., & Edwards, D. F. (2001). *The Washington University Activity Card Sort*. St. Louis, MO: Penultimate Publishing.

Baum, C. M., & Law, M. (1998). Community health: A responsibility, an opportunity, and a fit for occupational therapy. *American Journal of Occupational Therapy, 52*(1), 7-10.

Blank, A. E., Horowitz, S., & Matza, D. (1995) Quality with a human face? The Samuels Planetree model hospital unit. *Joint Commission Journal of Quality Improvement, 21*(6), 289-299.

Christiansen, C. (2002) Occupation and identity: Becoming who we are through what we do in. In C. H. Christiansen & E. A. Townsend (Eds.), *Introduction to occupation: The art and science of living*, Upper Saddle River, New Jersey: Prentice Hall.

Christiansen, C., & Baum, C. M. (Eds.). (1997). *Occupational therapy: Enabling function and well-being* (2nd ed.). Thorofare, NJ: SLACK Incorporated.

Gage, M., & Polatajko, H. (1994). Enhancing occupational performance through an understanding of perceived self-efficacy. *American Journal of Occupational Therapy, 48*(5), 452-462.

Gerteis, M., Edgman-Levitan, S., Walker, J. D., Stoke, D. M., Cleary, P. D., & Delbanco, T. L. (1993). What patients really want. *Health Management Quarterly 3rd Quarter, 15*(3), 2-6.

Law, M. C., Baptiste, S., Carswell, A., McColl, M. A., Polatajko, H., & Pollock, N. (1991). *The Canadian Occupational Performance Measure*. Toronto, Ontario: CAOT.

Law, M., Baptiste, S., Carswell, A., McColl, M.A., Polatajko, H., & Pollock, N. (1994). *Canadian Occupational Performance Measure* (2nd ed.) Toronto, Ontario: CAOT Publications ACE.

Matsutsuyu, J. S. (1969). The interest check list. *American Journal of Occupational Therapy, 23*(4), 323-328.

Mattingly, C., & Fleming, M. H. (1994). *Clinical reasoning: Forms of inquiry in a therapeutic practice*. Philadelphia, PA: F. A. Davis Co.

McColl, M. A. (1997). Social support and occupational therapy. In C. Christiansen & C. Baum (Eds.), *Occupational therapy: Enabling function and well-being* (2nd ed.). Thorofare, NJ: SLACK Incorporated.

Meyer, A. (1922). The philosophy of occupation therapy. *Archives of Occupational Therapy, 1*(1), 1-10.

Oakley, F., Kielhofner, G., Barris, R., & Richler, R. K. (1986). The role checklist: Development and empirical assessment of reliability. *Occupational Therapy Journal of Research*, 6, 157-169.

Chapter Fifteen: Person-Environment-Occupation-Performance Reflections and Learning Activities

Julie Bass-Haugen, PhD, OTR/L, FAOTA

REFLECTIONS

Over the years, I have talked with many students and practitioners about their motivations for choosing the profession of occupational therapy. Invariably, something in their answers relates to helping: "I want to help people have a better life. I want to make a difference in the lives of people. I want to be part of a helping profession." I suspect most of the readers of this text have this same motivation of helping.

What makes a good helper besides just motivation? I can remember times in my life when special people have really helped me in a tough situation. These people tried to understand me. They tried to respond to what I wanted or needed at a given point in time—even if it disagreed with what they wanted or needed. These helpers gathered important information before they gave suggestions—they wanted to know everything about me and my world. These people didn't just give suggestions off the top of their heads; they were thoughtful and proposed remedies that had been effective in similar situations. My helpers tried to help me in a variety of ways and somehow chose the right kinds of helping at the right time. They also checked back with me again and again to see if my situation had improved. As I reflect on their helping, I realize they used a framework for decision-making that is similar to one proposed in this chapter. It was client-centered and based on a process that resulted in the best possible outcome.

The individual situational analysis for decision-making in occupational therapy uses steps similar to the ones I depicted as the ideal helping in my own life. The practitioner begins by gathering as much information as possible from the client's perspective and analyzing the fit with occupational therapy services. This step requires the practitioner to have good questions, good observations, and good listening skills. The next step involves gathering specific information on the person, the environment, and occupations. Strong clinical reasoning skills, professional knowledge, and evidence are used to evaluate the key factors that support and hinder occupational performance for this person. Then, the most pertinent information from the client's perspective and practitioner's evaluation form the basis for developing, implementing, and evaluating interventions. Finally, the outcome of interventions is compared to the client's original perspective on occupational performance and participation.

Many students and practitioners begin their professional lives by only conceptualizing helping as one person helping one other person. This type of helping is a very important one in occupational therapy practice. A special interaction occurs between the practitioner and the client. The interaction is individualized, focused on the real needs of the client, based on an identified process, and designed to achieve specific outcomes that meet the unique goals of the client. It is a very gratifying type of helping because it involves a professional relationship between one practitioner and one client.

In occupational therapy, we have recently begun to explore other types of helping. We realize we need to use other types of helping for some people, in some settings, and in some situations. We know in health and human services there is an increasing emphasis on getting the "biggest bang out of the health care dollar." We are challenged to see how far we can stretch the influence of our helping beyond just one individual to populations and organizations. Helping focused on populations and organizations may in the end result in improved occupational performance and quality of life for all people, not just specific individuals who receive our services.

Initially, we may feel like we don't have the qualifications to recommend changes on a population or organization level. These are natural feelings, but over the ages there have been many unassuming people who made a huge difference in society through small actions. When Rosa Parks refused to sit in the back of a city bus, she contributed to a movement that forever changed the occupation of commuting for African Americans. Just think about the potential for change that is possible in populations and organizations when professionals with knowledge and commitment get involved.

If you decide to become an informed change agent for populations, a population situational analysis will guide you in the process. Perhaps you are already concerned about specific populations or communities. You may have a personal connection with a particular population/community or read about an issue of interest. If you want to get involved, where do you begin? First of all, you need more information. You need to immerse yourself in the population/community and the issue. Obtain facts and the personal perspectives of the population/community. Ask yourself, is there an occupational issue here? If yes, what are the occupational needs and goals? This step of the situational analysis need not take long. The next step requires more of an investment. You need to put on your evaluation hat and identify the attributes of people and their environments as well as their occupations. Some of this information may already be documented in the form of evidence. Other information may need to be gathered. From this evaluation of person, environment, and occupation, an intervention plan is developed. It is unlikely you will implement your plan independent of others. You will work with others to implement and evaluate the intervention strategies designed to make a difference. And how do you determine if you made a difference? As in the individual situational analysis, the outcome is compared to the original occupational needs and goals of the population/community.

If you decide to become a change agent for organizations, an organizational situational analysis will guide you in the process. This process is similar to a population situational analysis, but each step of an organizational analysis may be negotiated with the organization. When you work with an organization, you need to consider not only the needs of the population it serves but also key characteristics and goals of the organization itself. This first step in the process will help you determine if there is a match that supports an occupational therapy intervention. If there is, you may enter a consultant or contractual relationship with the organization to conduct a formal evaluation of capabilities and barriers for person, environment, and occupational factors. Your findings and recommendations will be discussed with the organization's key decision makers and may result in the adoption of an intervention plan. Implementation of an organizational intervention plan will require the full support of stakeholders. As in the other situational analyses, the outcome of your plan will be measured against the organization's original needs and goals.

Planning interventions for populations/communities and organizations will require some occupational therapy practitioners to do some risk taking. It may feel like this type of practice is outside our comfort zone. It may not be what we had in mind when we made a professional commitment to helping from an occupational therapy framework. I am convinced, however, that this type of professional practice is exactly what is needed at this point in time. If we do an inventory of critical needs in society and critical needs of the occupational therapy profession, I think we will see that interventions designed for the occupational needs of populations and organizations is an important addition to our practice.

As you have seen in all of these situational analyses, the overall process is the same. What were some of the key themes to note? First, the client (however it is defined) is a key part of the process. If we are unable to address the needs and goals of the client, then we have no occupational therapy role. Second, everything we do must have a tie to occupations. Our evaluations and our interventions must support improved occupational performance. Third, our analyses depend on the use of good evidence or information. If we fail to incorporate evidence in the process, we lose our credibility with the client. Fourth, our evaluation of the situation requires an examination of the capabilities and constraints for each component of the PEOP model. Fifth, there are a variety of intervention strategies that may help the client achieve occupational goals. Efficiency and effectiveness are two factors to consider in selecting strategies. Finally, it is essential that we contribute to the occupational therapy evidence by comparing intervention outcomes to initial occupational goals.

You now have a framework for helping individuals, populations/communities, and organizations that need your occupational therapy services. Hang on to your situational analyses for reference—and get ready, set, go!

Journal Activities

1. Look up and write down dictionary definitions of analysis and decision making. Highlight the components of the definitions that are most related to their descriptions in Chapter Fifteen.
2. Identify the most important new learning for you in this chapter.
3. Identify one question you have about Chapter Fifteen.
4. Reflect on an effective helping situation, one in which you helped or were helped. Briefly describe the situation. Draw your own model of the process (i.e., situational analysis) used for helping in that situation. Label the components of your analysis. Compare your model to one of the situational analyses in the chapter. Identify the similarities and the differences.

Technology/Internet Learning Activities

1. Use a discussion database to share specific journal entries.
2. Use a good Internet search engine to find the Web site for Agency for Healthcare Research and Quality (AHRQ).
   - Enter the phrase "AHRQ" or "Agency for Healthcare Research and Quality" in your search line.

- Review the Web site.
- What is the primary purpose of this site?
- Identify the primary resources areas for situational analyses at this site.
- Review the site for "clinical information" or "quality assessment."
- Give three examples of evidence that may be used in a situational analysis.

3. Use a good Internet search engine to find the Web site for International Development Research Centre—Science for Humanity.
   - Enter the phrase "International Development Research Centre" in your search line.
   - Review the Web site.
   - What is the primary purpose of this site?
   - Identify the primary resource areas for situational analyses at this site.
   - Review the clinical information on the site.
   - Review the site for "evaluation" or "technologies."
   - Give three examples of evidence that may be used in a situational analysis.
   - Identify three example areas to consider in organizational or institutional assessment.
   - How do your examples fit with the situational analyses?
4. Use a good Internet search engine to find the Web site for Trace Research and Development Center.
   - Enter the phrase "Trace Research and Development Center" in your search line.
   - Review the Web site.
   - What is the primary purpose of this site?
   - Identify the primary resource areas for situational analyses at this site.
   - Review the general concepts and information resources on the site.
   - Identify the general principles of universal design.
   - Identify three examples of information resources that may provide useful evidence in the future.

Applied Learning

Individual Learning Activity #1: Exploring the Person-Centered Situational Analysis

Instructions:

- Read the following statements adapted from the case study presented at the beginning of Chapter Fifteen.
- Place each statement in a section of the person-centered situational analysis.
- What general or specific information is missing from your person-centered situational analysis?
- Make up some details for the missing information.
- Is there a match between this client's goals and occupational therapy services? Why or why not?
- What evidence would you be interested in obtaining?
- Based on your hypothetical information, what interventions would you explore or consider for this client?
- How would you evaluate the outcome of your interventions?
  - ✧ Client (a 25-year-old woman in an occupational therapy program):

    Reports riding a bike over a hill at a fast clip and falling off after running into a tricycle
    Is in the hospital
    Reports a lot of pain
    Has a broken shoulder and pelvis
    Has a mild head injury
    Has bandages on her face
    Has serious face abrasions requiring plastic surgery

Reports she doesn't have time for this
Reports she wants to pass her finals in a couple of weeks
Reports she wants to be in her best friend's wedding in 3 weeks
Has family who lives 1,000 miles away
Is beginning to comprehend what has happened
Reports she can't do what she did before
Wants to get back to her life as soon as possible
Wants to go home
Wonders how it is going to work
Lives on third floor with no elevator
Lives alone
Has good friends at colleges all over the country
Is weak
Has unclear vision
Can't remember new phone number
Is concerned about costs of hospitalization

Individual Learning Activity #2: Exploring the Population-Centered Situational Analysis

Instructions:

- Read the following statements related to a specific population.
- Place each statement in a section of the population-centered situational analysis.
- What general or specific information is missing from your population-centered situational analysis?
- Make up some details for the missing information.
- Is there a match between this population's goals and occupational therapy services? Why or why not?
- What evidence would you be interested in obtaining?
- Based on your hypothetical information, what interventions would you explore or consider for this population?
- How would you evaluate the outcome of your interventions?
  - ✧ Client (a population of about 500 adolescents aged 12 to 18 years old):

Reports being totally bored outside of school hours
Reports there is "nothing to do" in the town
Some community members don't like the way the adolescents just hang out
Lives in a western rural town in the United States with a population less than 5,000
Some members leave small town for college or bigger city after turning 18 years old
Some members who leave for college/jobs after high school never return to small town as adults
Some members do not articulate any life goals
Some members have children while still adolescents and are single parents
Some members do not complete high school
Some members report "feeling down" alot of the time
Has behaviors of concern to some families
Sees no future in the area
Wants adventure and excitement
Wants to do something, be something
Lives in school district that has eliminated extracurricular programs due to budget cuts
Lives in town that is voting on planned merger of three school districts
Reports downtown stores and "hang-outs" are closing because of large store on the edge of town

May engage in risky behaviors (e.g., drinking alcohol, reckless driving, unprotected sex, etc.)
Most members drive as soon as they reach age 16
Some community members are concerned about recent vandalism
Some community members are fiscally conservative
Some community members don't want change
Some community members agree with adolescent's concerns
Lives where economic base of community is agriculture and nearby recreation areas
Has a high rate of sexually transmitted disease
Has a high rate of alcohol use and binge drinking
Has a high rate of obesity
Occasionally goes to community college and public library in nearby town
Has families that attend two churches with strong ties to community
States the town's baseball field is used for some activities

Individual Learning Activity #3: Exploring the Organization-Centered Situational Analysis

Instructions:

- Read the following statements related to a specific organization.
- Place each statement in a section of the organization-centered situational analysis.
- What general or specific information is missing from your organization-centered situational analysis?
- Make up some details for the missing information.
- Is there a match between this organization's goals and occupational therapy services? Why or why not?
- What evidence would you be interested in obtaining?
- Based on your hypothetical information, what interventions would you explore or consider for this organization?
- How would you evaluate the outcome of your interventions?
    - ✧ Client (a light manufacturing company with 500 employees):

Is a family-owned, midsize company located in the southern part of the United States
Has about 450 technical-level employees with specialized skills
Reports concern about employees' health, stresses, and excessive family commitments
Values employees and wants to retain them
Has many women employees who describe themselves as being in the "sandwich generation"
Is an older, established company with a stable, financial future
Reports concern about the current company policies and procedures and health of the workforce
Has had recent requests for leaves of absence, job-sharing, part-time work
Does not currently have much flexibility in job positions
Has a break room where employees may eat their cold lunch
Has a high percentage of loyal employees who have worked more than 10 years
Has mostly middle-aged work force
Has mostly female employees (80%) at technical level
Has female employees who report health changes due to stress and over-commitment
Has employees with average immediate family-size of three children and two adults
Has traditional hierarchical structure in other positions of the company
Has had three cases of repetitive motion injuries in the past 3 years
Has salary scale that is above average for this type of work
Is located six blocks from the elementary school and three blocks from a city park
Reports many female employees skip lunch to call home and meet family obligations

Has some concern about rising health care insurance costs
Has employees from European, African American, and Latino cultures
Has had gradual increase in sick days and personal leave days over the past 5 years
Has two work shifts currently: 8 AM to 4:30 PM and 5:00 PM to 1:30 AM
Is located in a city with a population of 30,000
Schedules 30 minute lunch break and two 15-minute breaks each day
Had employees complete a recent self-assessment of health and health needs
Has employees who report loyalty to the company
Has employees with extended families living in the same city

ACTIVE LEARNING

Group Activity #1: Exploring Situational Analyses as a Framework for Decision Making

Preparation:

- Read Chapter Fifteen.
- Complete Individual Learning Activities #1 to #3.

Time: 45 minutes to 1 hour

Instructions:

- Individually:
  - ✧ Review your situational analyses from Individual Learning Activities #1 to #3.
  - ✧ Be ready to present a summary of each situational analysis to your small group.
- In small groups:
  - ✧ Listen to the summary of the three situational analyses by each group member.
  - ✧ Discuss the variations in your summaries.
  - ✧ Come to consensus on where each piece of information belongs for each situation.

Discussion:

- Discuss the aspects of the situational analyses that were easiest and hardest. Why do you think this was the case?
- Discuss the aspects of the situational analyses where there was the most and least consistency by individual members. Why do think this was the case?
- Discuss the likely strategies for reimbursement of services in each situation.
- Discuss the specific evidence you would like to review for these situational analyses.
- Discuss the different intervention strategies you proposed. What strategies would you guess are the most effective and efficient in each situation?
- Discuss how you would determine if interventions worked.

Group Activity #2: Comparing the Situational Analyses to the *Guide to Occupational Therapy Practice* (1999) and the *Standards for Continuing Competence* (1999)

Preparation:

- Review Chapter Ten and this chapter.
- If possible, read the *Guide to Occupational Therapy Practice* and the *Standards for Continuing Competence* (Note: The references for these documents are found in Chapter Ten).
- Make a copy of the Person-Centered Situational Analysis.

Time: 30 to 45 minutes

Materials: Copy of the Person-Centered Situational Analysis
Instructions:
- Individually:
  - ✧ Review the components of the Situational Analysis.
  - ✧ Review the components of the *Guide to Occupational Therapy Practice* below
  - ✧ Review the components of the *Standards for Continuing Competence* below

Guide to Occupational Therapy Practice

Referral
- Referral sources
- Screening

Evaluation
- History...
- Occupations... that can and cannot be performed
- Needs, plans, and goals of the client
- Participation in meaningful and purposeful occupations
- Rehabilitation potential
- Underlying performance components causing... limitations
- Contextual factors affecting performance...

Intervention Plan
- Short-term
- Long-term

Intervention
- Remediation/restoration
- Compensation/adaptation
- Disability prevention
- Health promotion

Re-evaluation
Discharge/follow-up
Outcome measurement

Standards for Continuing Competence

Knowledge
Critical reasoning
Interpersonal abilities
Performance skills
Ethical reasoning

- In small groups:
  - ✧ For each component in the *Guide to Occupational Therapy Practice*:
    - Identify matched components in the Situational Analysis.
    - Identify any components in the *Guide* that have no match in the Situational Analysis.
    - Identify any components in the Situational Analysis that have no match in the *Guide*.
  - ✧ For each component in the *Standards for Continuing Competence*:
    - Identify where and how each standard may be used in the Situational Analysis.

Discussion:
- How do different representations of occupational therapy practice help your understanding of what you actually do as a practitioner?
- How do different representations of occupational therapy practice challenge your understanding of what you actually do as a practitioner?
- Why do you think there are different representations of occupational therapy practice?

Occupational Therapy Interventions: Individual, Organization, and Population Approaches

Section III

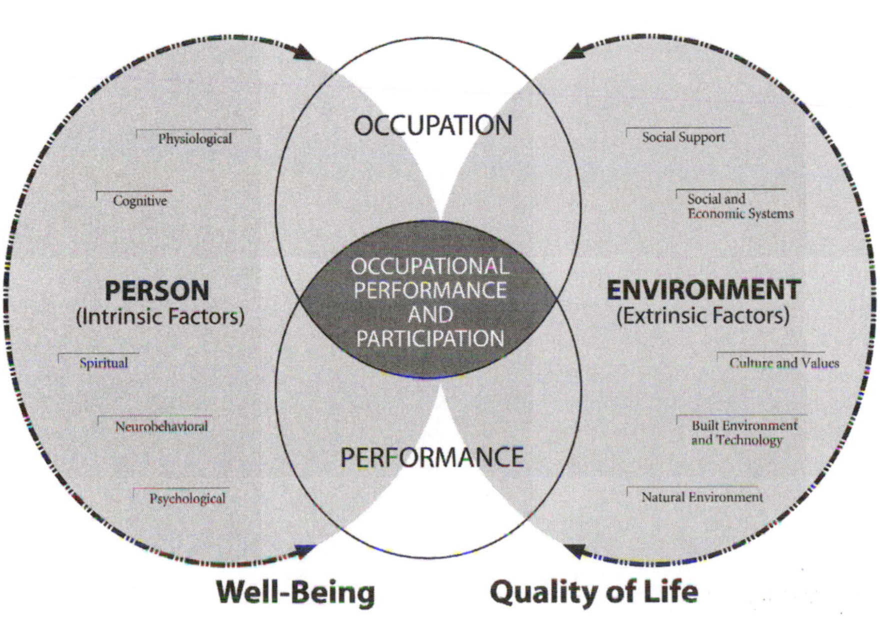

Chapter Sixteen Objectives

The information is this chapter is intended to help the reader:

1. Understand the purpose and outcomes of occupational therapy interventions.
2. Understand the basic principles that guide the intervention process.
3. Compare and contrast the various intervention approaches used by occupational therapists during the intervention process with individuals and populations.
4. Articulate the three broad goals of occupational therapy intervention—promoting, preventing, and resolving occupational performance problems.
5. Describe the types of intervention methods used by occupational therapists.

Key Words

compensation/adaptation/modification: Interventions aimed at diminishing personal constraints or eliminating environmental barriers. **compensation:** Use of environmental supports to avert occupational performance problems associated with a personal performance constraint. **adaptation/modification:** Reducing environmental barriers by changing the existing environment or the features of the task in which the client will engage.

intervention: The skilled process of effecting change in the client's occupational performance (AOTA, 2002).

making the best fit: Matching the capabilities of the person/population with the environment and/or task that is the most enabling.

prevent: Supporting occupational performance by anticipating problems and taking actions to avert problems that will impact occupational performance.

promote: Supporting occupational performance by focusing on enhancing well-being and quality of life.

remediation/restoration/establishment: Interventions aimed at enhancing personal performance capabilities and/or diminishing constraints. **remediation:** Correct the problem; **restoration:** Recover a skill that was lost; **establishment:** Attain a new skill.

resolve: Supporting occupational performance by identifying performance problems and taking action to correct them.

A problem is a chance for you to do your best.
Duke Ellington

Chapter Sixteen

Categories and Principles of Interventions

Mary Jane Youngstrom, MS, OTR/L, FAOTA and Catana Brown, PhD, MA, OTR, FAOTA

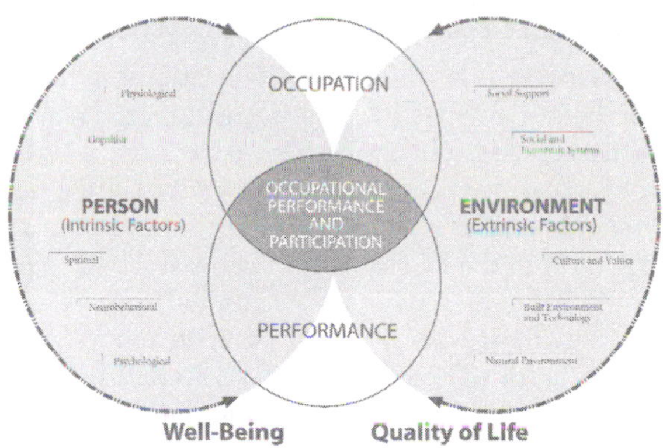

Setting the Stage

Intervention is the skilled process used by occupational therapy practitioners to effect change in the client's occupational performance leading to engagement in occupations that support participation in life. Occupational therapy practitioners center their interventions on an understanding of the clients' occupational performance needs and the client's priorities. In collaboration with the client, the practitioner uses clinical reasoning to choose one or more intervention approaches, goals, and specific therapeutic activities that will best achieve targeted client outcomes. Interventions are grounded in basic principles that guide the planning and implementation process.

As a backdrop for thinking about the principles and types of interventions, let us begin by understanding occupational therapy's overall purpose in providing interventions.

Youngstrom, M. J., & Brown, C. (2005). Categories and principles of interventions. In C. H. Christiansen, C. M. Baum, and J. Bass-Haugen (Eds.), Occupational therapy: Performance, participation, and well-being *(3rd ed.). Thorofare, NJ: SLACK Incorporated.*

PURPOSE OF INTERVENTIONS

Relationship to Health

Occupational therapy practitioners are dedicated to supporting the health of individuals, families, and communities. Occupational therapy interventions are aimed at promoting, preventing, and restoring health. Occupational therapy practitioners view health from a broad, multidimensional perspective that is convergent with the World Health Organization's (WHO) definition of health: "a state of complete physical, mental, and social well-being and not just the absence of disease or infirmity" (WHO, 1947, p. 29).

The profession's understanding of health focuses on the link between the individual's ability to engage in meaningful and productive everyday occupations in context and the person's state of physical, mental, and social well-being. This understanding of the importance of engaging in occupations and its relationship to health is the unique perspective that occupational therapy brings to health care. The profession's advocacy for and skill in supporting people in performing everyday life activities and occupations is occupational therapy's distinctive contribution to the health of our clients and communities.

As we consider how occupational therapy interventions are targeted to promote, prevent, and restore health, four beliefs need to be examined/considered:

1. Health is a multidimensional construct that includes the physical, mental, and social aspects of well-being. In evaluating performance and constructing interventions to support health, occupational therapy practitioners address all aspects of performance—sensory, motor, cognitive, and psychosocial.
2. Health is viewed as a positive, dynamic construct. It is more than the absence of illness/disease or disability. Occupational therapy practitioners believe that health is attained and maintained by active engagement in everyday life activities. Health is not a state that is "achieved," but is dynamically changing and evolving as individuals engage in everyday life activities.
3. Occupational therapy's understanding of health flows from the profession's understanding of the "occupational nature" of human beings (Wilcock, 1998). Humans are viewed as active beings who naturally seek to interact with their environments. Engaging in everyday activities is a natural response to human biological need and is needed to enable survival and health (Wilcock, 1998).
4. The contexts or environments in which everyday life activities occur influence health. Occupational therapy practitioners believe that the context(s) in which performance occurs is a primary factor that can support or inhibit performance and health.

Occupational therapy practitioners believe that health is disrupted or threatened when individuals are not able to access or participate in a variety of everyday life activities that have meaning and purpose for the person and/or the culture. Interventions are provided to support the person's ability to participate in desired and required life activities that bring satisfaction and support health.

Outcomes

Given the profession's understanding of the occupational nature of people and the importance of "doing" to health, the obvious overarching outcome toward which all occupational therapy intervention is targeted is engagement in occupation to support participation. Ultimately, no matter what the person's problems or the intervention's target, the overall aim of occupational therapy intervention is to facilitate the person's ability to engage in activities that are meaningful and productive and that support participation in daily life. Underlying the broad overarching outcome are more specific objective and subjective outcomes of occupational therapy intervention.

Objective outcomes achieved by occupational therapy intervention are most frequently described as changes in "occupational performance." *Occupational performance* is the unique term used by occupational therapy practitioners to describe the transaction between the person, the context, and the activity that results in the observable accomplishment of a selected activity (Law et al., 1996). Changes in occupational performance could include improved ability to perform an occupation (e.g., client is able to get dressed independently, client is able to return to work), enhanced ability to perform an occupation (e.g., client who did not know how to type learns to type, client learns how to ride a bicycle), or prevention of potential performance problems (e.g., client learns proper lifting techniques to prevent back injury, client balances work and play occupations to proactively manage stress). Another objective outcome that can be measured is participation in life situations. A change in participation (i.e., the types and numbers of life situations in which a person can participate) is a natural outcome of increased ability to engage in occupations.

Subjective outcomes influenced by occupational therapy intervention center around the client's perception of the effects of the intervention process on his or her ability to engage in daily occupations and participate in activities that fulfill roles. Subjective outcome measures of occupational therapy intervention include measures of life satisfaction and overall quality of life. Both of these measures tap into the individual's perception of change in his or her ability to participate in meaningful life activities.

PRINCIPLES OF INTERVENTION

Several basic principles guide the intervention planning and implementation process. These principles are illustrative of the profession's values and understanding of how engagement in occupations is best facilitated. Occupational therapy practitioners frequently provide intervention on a 1:1 basis, but they also may provide interventions for a group or population that may be at risk for or are experiencing problems with engaging in occupations to support participation. When providing interventions at the group or population level, the occupational performance needs and risks are evaluated as an aggregate, and intervention approaches, goals, and methods are directed at the entire group. Chapter Nineteen discusses these types of intervention in more depth. The principles that are outlined below are applicable to interventions applied to individuals, groups, and populations. When the term *client* is used, it refers to a client who may be an individual, a group of individuals, or a population.

Principle #1: Interventions Are Client-Centered

Client-centered practice applied during intervention planning and implementation is a continuation of a client-centered approach that began with the first contact and initial evaluation of the client. The client-centered approach is "an approach [that] embraces a philosophy of respect for, and partnership with, people receiving services" (Law, Baptiste, & Mills, 1995, p. 253). During the intervention planning and implementation phase of the occupational therapy process, the therapist demonstrates respect and value for the person by 1) basing interventions on the client's identified needs and priorities, 2) collaborating with the client to develop intervention approaches, 3) providing intervention options that are connected to occupations that are important and meaningful to the client, 4) offering opportunities for choice and control in intervention focus and activities, 5) supporting the client's decisions, and 6) providing supports for successes and risks. When providing interventions to groups or populations, these same approaches are used by considering the group's aggregate needs, priorities, and choices and by collaborating with the group as a whole.

Communication that occurs during intervention is also client-centered. Although the practitioner brings specialized knowledge and expertise to the process, the client is perceived as the expert in his or her life; he or she ultimately knows whether the intervention is meeting his or her needs and is useful, practical, and motivating. In a client-centered approach, the practitioner and client partner. They must collaborate and work together to address the client's skills and abilities in performing the daily life occupations. The very nature of occupational therapy intervention necessitates the use of a collaborative approach and respect for the client's choices and decisions. The occupational therapy practitioner who is providing occupational therapy services is very limited in what can be done "to" the client. Occupational therapy intervention requires that the client be actively engaged in the personal act of carrying out daily life activities.

Principle #2: Interventions Are Context Driven

Occupational therapy practitioners recognize that context impacts performance and consider it as a factor that must be assessed when evaluating performance. Context also is an important factor to consider during the intervention implementation process. During intervention, context will influence the client's learning and trials at performance and will also influence the practitioner's decisions about the types of interventions that can be implemented. For example, the client's ability to successfully attend to and complete a task in a noisy classroom may be very different from the client's ability to complete the same task in a quiet room.

When providing interventions at the group or population level, the context is often a primary feature that is addressed during the intervention. The context surrounds performance for all members of the group or population and can be changed to effectively influence performance for all members of the group or population.

Each context in which client performance occurs offers unique supports and barriers to performance. Often, performance is "simulated" in clinical medical settings such as hospitals or nursing homes. However, safe and effective performance in these settings does not always equate to safe and effective performance in the client's real life natural setting. The physical arrangement, sizes, and types of objects, although similar, will be different. The social supports offered by health care providers during intervention trials will not be the same as the support offered by natural social contexts. Differences in temporal context (e.g., normal time of day in which engagement in occupation occurs) and cultural contexts (e.g., expectations of practitioner as compared to spouse) also vary. Practitioners need to recognize the impact these differences will have on performance and to consider them as they interpret the outcomes and effectiveness of intervention. Best practice approach to intervention supports the implementation of intervention within natural environments (i.e., the context in which the client will actually be performing). Evidence suggests that skills learned in unnatural environments are often not effectively transferred or used in natural settings (Ma, Trombly, & Robinson-Podolski, 1999). On the other hand, the implementation of intervention in natural settings is not always feasible or practical. Practitioners need to recognize the constraints and supports offered by each context and use them to the client's advantage. For example, a client who is currently a patient in a nursing home will benefit from initially learning toilet transfers in the nursing home even though the arrangement of the toilet in the nursing home is not the same as in his or her own bathroom. When he or she is discharged, he or she will have to adapt the approach learned in a new physical and social context.

The occupational therapy practitioner operates within a context also. The practitioner's context provides certain resources that are available for use during intervention and also sets certain expectations based on the service delivery model being used. For example, a client may need to practice food preparation, but a kitchen and food supplies may not be available. A practitioner may be working in a setting that limits the amount of time available to provide service to a client. This limitation, an expectation of the practitioner's context, requires that the types of interventions used be carefully selected to maximize outcomes within the time available.

Principle #3: Interventions Are Occupation-Based

Interventions are occupation-based when they are directed at supporting the client to carry out his or her daily life occupations. Interventions should be targeted toward the client's real life. The client should be able to see how engagement in an activity is connected to performance in a life task that he or she finds meaningful and purposeful. Interventions are obviously occupation-based when they involve the client in the actual performance of the occupation that is of concern (e.g., cooking a meal) or in the activities and tasks that are the subsets of the occupation (e.g., planning the menu, slicing the tomatoes). These same premises apply to interventions directed toward populations or groups.

To ensure that interventions are occupation-based, practitioners should use occupations/activities that are centered on the client's interests, needs, and priorities. If the practitioner is employing a client-centered approach, this occurs easily. If the practitioner has been listening carefully to the client's story and narrative, it will help to identify the types of experiences and activities that are interesting to the client. Providing the client with some choices within the range of the client's interests and priorities helps to encourage motivation and offers the client a degree of control that supports self-efficacy.

Principle #4: Interventions Are Evidence-Based

In the past, treatment decisions have often been based on "expert" opinion (i.e., based on the practitioner's personal experience or those of others). Evidence-based practice is a systematic process of finding, evaluating, and applying research findings into practice. Research findings should be used to help occupational therapy practitioners make choices about the approach, methods, and techniques that will be most effective.

Although research data regarding occupational therapy interventions are not plentiful, practitioners need to stay updated on current research and apply the evidence that is available. In many situations, the occupational therapy practitioner can go to research from other disciplines to find evidence that is useful in making intervention decisions. For example, the education literature includes research on the effectiveness of particular teaching/learning strategies. Keeping up with the research literature can be a daunting task. Literature reviews, meta-analyses, and practice guidelines provide summaries of large bodies of research. Additionally, some practice guidelines useful to occupational therapy practitioners are available through AOTA and on the web at www.guidelines.gov and www.cochrane.org.

Principle #5: The Intervention Process is Dynamically Interrelated With Ongoing Assessment

Intervention is defined as the skilled process of effecting change in the client's occupational performance (AOTA, 2002). Although it is based on an initial evaluation and intervention plan, evaluation continues throughout the intervention implementation process. The practitioner assesses the client's response to intervention and makes adjustments as the client engages in intervention activities. Throughout the intervention process, the practitioner continues to gather data about client interests, values, and performance. As the client engages in activity, the practitioner makes note of the various aspects of the context, which support or hinder change. This newly gathered assessment information, gained during intervention implementation, is valuable and allows the practitioner to make needed adjustments in the intervention plan.

Intervention Approaches

For most occupational performance issues, there are several possible intervention approaches. In collaboration with the service recipient, the occupational therapy practitioner should consider all of the possible approaches in developing an intervention plan. The intervention options vary according to the target of change. Interventions that are directed at making changes in the person or population use approaches that remediate, restore, or establish skills. Alternatively, interventions may be directed at making changes in the environment or task. These intervention approaches are typically identified as compensatory or adaptive strategies. Finally, some intervention approaches do not make changes in people, environments, or tasks, but are designed to match people with environments or tasks. These approaches involve making the best person-environment fit. All three approaches can be considered for the same occupational performance goal.

For example, the occupational performance goal of independent dressing might be addressed through the following approaches:

- Targeting the person using occupations to restore fine motor skills.
- Targeting the environment or task by using a button hook.
- Making the best person-task-environment fit by purchasing pull-on pants with an elastic waist.

Remediation/Restoration/Establishment

Interventions designed to remediate, restore, or establish skills in people or populations have the goal of enhancing personal performance capabilities and/or diminishing constraints. *Remediation* is a general term that refers to fixing a problem or finding a remedy. Restore interventions remedy the problem by recovering a skill that was lost. In establish interventions, the problem is fixed through the attainment of a new skill. The skills addressed in the intervention may be personal performance capabilities in the realms of physiological, neurobehavioral, cognitive, or psychological skills. For example, interventions directed at enhancing problem solving, improving hand strength, or promoting self-efficacy would fall into the category of personal performance capabilities. Sensory integration is a type of occupational therapy intervention that targets personal performance capabilities and skills. In a meta-analysis of the use of sensory integration, when compared to no treatment, the greatest differences were found in the areas of psychoeducational skills and motor skills (Vargus & Camilli, 1999). Few differences were found in the attainment of skills when comparing sensory integration to other intervention approaches. These findings provide information on the use of interventions to facilitate the attainment of new skills.

In some cases, devices or technology are used in establish/restore interventions. For example, occupational therapy practitioners using orthoses to reduce contractures restored range of motion to individuals who experienced neurological or orthopedic conditions (Nuismer, Ekes, & Holm, 1997). In another example, Interactive Metronome Training was used to facilitate the development of the personal performance capacities of attention and motor control in boys with attention deficit hyperactivity disorder (Shaffer et al., 2001). In this intervention, new cognitive and motor skills were established. In occupational therapy, personal performance capabilities are enhanced to promote increased participation in daily life. For example, a program was implemented to improve visual motor skills for individuals after stroke who wanted to return to driving (Klavora et al., 1995).

In occupational therapy, typically, activities are used to develop personal performance capabilities. Sakemiller & Nelson (1998) used a favorite game to improve neck and back extension in children with cerebral palsy. In a functional model of cognitive rehabilitation, occupational therapists work to restore cognitive skills through the use of functional activities in natural contexts (Lee, Powell, & Esdaile, 2001). Activities are selected to meet the current skill level of the individual or population and then are graded to increase ability level. For example, craft activities used with children with psychiatric disorders were selected that progressively required higher demands on visuomotor skills. The result was an improvement in the visuomotor skills of the children treated (Kleinman & Stalcup, 1991).

In addition, the skills acquired in remediation/restoration/establishment interventions may be subskills of an occupation or activity. Interventions teaching how to read a bus map, fill out an employment application, or make reservations at a restaurant are examples of subskills of an occupation or activity. For example, a specific retraining protocol was developed to restore washing and dressing skills in adults with brain injury (Giles, Ridley, Dill, & Frye, 1997). An interdisciplinary team of occupational therapy, nursing, and psychology developed a grocery shopping intervention for people with psychiatric disabilities (Brown, Rempfer, & Hamera, 2002).

Remediation/restoration/establishment interventions need not only be applied to individuals, but can also be used for population interventions. In an assisted-living community, the occupational therapist may work with the activities director to provide programs that incorporate movement to enhance motor function for all of the residents in the assisted-living facility. An occupational therapy practitioner in a school setting may create anger management curricula for a newly developing after-school program. In a study of fine motor outcomes in a preschool, intervention included individual direct services to children with disabilities, but also involved consultation with teachers to incorporate fine motor activities in classroom activities that impacted the entire classroom population (Case-Smith, 1996).

Compensation/Adaptation/Modification

Interventions that change the environment or task can be directed at diminishing personal constraints or eliminating environmental barriers. The term *compensation* generally refers to the use of environmental supports to avert the occupational performance problems associated with a personal performance constraint. For example, an individual may compensate for limited range of motion by using a reacher. Assistive technology is often used in compensatory interventions. One study compared two different computer technologies for text entry that compensate for upper extremity paralysis (DeVries, Dietz, & Anson, 1998). One instrument used a head pointing system while the other used a mouth stick.

Other environmental interventions are directed at reducing environmental barriers by adapting or modifying the existing environment. A major barrier for many people with disabilities is social stigma. An intervention that adapts the environment to address this issue might include educational programs for work supervisors of people with disabilities. This intervention makes a change in the social environment of the workplace. A study of occupational therapy practice for individuals with intellectual disabilities living in the community found that a major role for practitioners was changing perceptions of others so that the clients could become more fully a part of their community (Tannous, Lehmann-Monck, Magoffin, Jackson, & Llewellyn, 1999). Curb cuts would be another example of an intervention targeting a population (wheelchair users) that adapts or modifies an environmental barrier.

When considering adaptations or modifications, occupational therapy practitioners often concentrate on the physical environment. However, it is important that a broader environmental view be considered, as other aspects of the environment may pose the greatest barrier or offer the most potential as an enabler. Therefore, interventions that adapt or modify social support systems, societal policies and attitudes, as well as cultural norms and values can play a bigger role in occupational therapy intervention. Kellegrew (1998) describes an intervention to promote self-care in children with special needs that focused on working with caregivers to restructure daily routines. By adapting the temporal environment, the children were provided with more opportunities to engage in self-care activities independently. A study of occupational practitioners' expectation in stroke recovery found practitioners were often dissatisfied when clients reached a plateau in recovery (Chang & Hasselkus, 1998). The researchers interpreted this dissatisfaction in relation to American cultural values of "personal autonomy, victory over disease, diligence and perseverance" (p. 636) and suggested that occupational therapy education may need to better prepare practitioners for realities of stroke recovery. This education would require an adaptation on the part of the cultural system of the practitioner.

Another target of adaptation/modification is the task. Occupational performance needs may best be met by changing features of the task. For example, a person's work responsibilities may be modified so that tasks requiring a great deal of endurance are spread out over the day rather than being done all at once. In another example, a student with difficulties related to the physical aspects of writing may take a test orally.

Making the Best Fit

Sometimes, interventions do not make changes in the person/population, environment, or task but match the capabilities of the person/population with the environment and/or task that is the most enabling. Occupational therapy practitioners sometimes find it difficult to recognize that they are providing an intervention when no change is being made. However, interventions that make the best fit require a great deal of sophisticated analysis of person, environment, and task factors. These interventions can also be the most efficient and relevant because they take advantage of the person's capabilities and naturally occurring environmental enablers. An example of making a good fit is provided by an intervention for elderly individuals with disabilities who found it unsafe or difficult to use a stove or oven. The intervention involved provision of and training in the use of a microwave oven (Kondo, Mann, Machiko, & Ottenbacher, 1997). Participants increased their participation in meal preparation and the number of food items prepared.

An obvious situation of making the best fit that is familiar to everyone is the person-environment-task interaction that occurs whenever people make employment decisions. A particular job placement will be most successful and satisfying when the person's capabilities and interests are matched with the work tasks and work environment. The same kind of thinking that goes into the employment decision-making process can be applied to all kinds of occupational performance situations. For example, occupational therapy practitioners working with children often help parents identify the particular characteristics of clothing, foods, toys, etc. that match the par-

Table 16-1

Examples of Interventions for the Three Intervention Approaches and the Three Intervention Goals

	Remediate/Establish/ Restore	*Adapt/Compensate/ Modify*	*Person-Environment-Task Match*
Promoting occupational performance	Teaching time management skills to college students to support development of balanced lifestyle	Contributing to policy change within county government to make more after-school activities available	Developing a grandparents program that matches elders and youth for purposes of teaching each other occupations (e.g., a youth might teach Internet skills, while an elder teaches sewing)
Preventing occupational performance problems	Teaching or providing information on lifting techniques to prevent back injuries at work	Adapting the computer workstations at a business to prevent repetitive motion injuries	Preventing isolation by identifying housing in a neighborhood that matches the person's ethnic background
Resolving occupational performance problems	Using computer games in cognitive rehabilitation	Sewing Velcro closures into clothing to make dressing easier	Adopting direct deposit and automatic rent and utility bill payment for someone having difficulty with money management

ticular sensory processing needs of the child. Furthermore, interventions typically focus on identifying play activities that are the best match for the child. In another situation, an occupational therapy practitioner may suggest alternative shopping methods (e.g., catalog, Internet) for someone who is cognitively overwhelmed by certain store environments.

Intervention Goals

Another consideration in the intervention planning process is the goal of intervention. As discussed earlier, all occupational therapy intervention is concerned with occupational performance. However, the intervention will differ as the purpose of the intervention differs. In some cases, the goal of the intervention is to promote occupational performance. In this case, a problem is not identified, but intervention is implemented to enhance occupational performance. In other situations, the goal is to resolve an occupational performance problem, while in still others, the goal is to prevent the problem before it occurs. With all goals, any of the aforementioned intervention approaches may be used. Table 16-1 provides examples of intervention approaches for each of the three types of intervention goals.

Promoting Occupational Performance

When the goal is promoting occupational performance, interventions are not directed toward a problem, but instead focus on enhancing well-being or quality of life. This is consistent with the first goal of *Healthy People 2010*, to increase quality and years of life (U.S. Department of Health and Human Services, 2000). *Healthy People 2010* states, "quality of life reflects a general sense of happiness and satisfaction with our lives and environment." Wilcock (1998) suggests that there are three overlapping individual components of well-being—physical, mental, and social—as well as community and ecological well-being. From an occupation perspective, goals of promotion would include interventions that enhance opportunities for engagement in occupation, give meaning to participation in daily life, and promote a balanced lifestyle.

Table 16-2

Levels of Prevention

Level	*Intervention Focus*	*Example*
Primary	Protection from risk factors or threats	Identifying and implementing reasonable accommodations for someone starting a new job
Secondary	Early detection	Screening new retirees to identify individuals having difficulty finding meaningful occupation, then providing interventions to increase occupational engagement
Tertiary	Limit consequences	Joint protection and energy conservation for someone with arthritis

Preventing Occupational Performance Problems

In prevention, a problem is anticipated, and the goal of intervention is to avert the problem. Prevention is often divided into three levels: primary, secondary, and tertiary. In primary prevention, the goal is protection from the problem by avoiding risk factors or threats. In secondary prevention, the problem is interrupted before it becomes significant and often involves early identification. In tertiary prevention, the goal is to limit the consequences of the problem and often involves prevention of complications. The Well Elderly Study is an example of primary prevention (Clark et al., 1997). The study indicated that engagement in occupation enhanced physical and mental health, occupational functioning, and life satisfaction for community-dwelling elders. In another example of primary prevention, mothers received information on child development techniques to enhance development (Parush & Hahn-Markowitz, 1997). Table 16-2 provides examples of occupational therapy interventions at all levels of prevention.

Resolving Occupational Performance Problems

Once a problem is identified, the goal for intervention is to resolve the problem. A performance problem may exist because of personal constraints, environmental barriers, or a lack of knowledge/experience related to a specific occupational performance issue. When determining the approach to resolving the problem, it is still essential to consider all options. It is not necessarily true that a personal performance constraint should be addressed by an intervention targeting the person, nor should all environmental barriers be best addressed by changing the environment. For example, an individual who has memory deficits is likely to receive more benefit from environmental adaptations such as calendars, labels, and cues than from activities to improve memory. Alternatively, a person with a controlling support system may gain more from developing assertiveness skills than from trying to find a new support system.

Intervention Methods

There are generally three types of intervention methods that are used in occupational therapy intervention. They are use of therapeutic activities/occupations, education, and consultation.

The practitioner specifically selects therapeutic activities and occupations based on their utility in meeting intervention goals. The selection process occurs in collaboration with the client, and selected activities are engaged by the client to reach specific goals. It is preferable if the client is offered a choice among activities that will allow the attainment of specified goals. Choice provides the client with a sense of control.

Therapeutic Activities/Occupations

Generally, therapeutic activities/occupations are selected and used to promote performance, prevent performance problems, or solve performance problems. Selected activities are used in two different ways: to improve performance when the client has the potential for improving his or her skills or capabilities and to compensate for performance problems that may or may not eventually improve by adapting the selected activity.

When selecting therapeutic activities to improve performance, practitioners choose activities that will gradually increase the demands placed on the performer for the specific level of skill required to support goal achievement. This method is frequently applied when the remediate/restore/establish approach is used. For example, when selecting an activity to improve reaching for an individual who is only able to reach 6 inches in front of his or her body, the practitioner would select an activity that required reaching for objects 6 to 8 inches away from his or her body. The practitioner would then "grade" the activity by making sequential changes within the activity that gradually increase the performance skill demand. In the example above, the practitioner might change the position of objects that are being reached for, gradually moving them farther away from the client and requiring a graduated increase in range of reach.

Practitioners can also select a series of activities that are "graded" to require increasing degrees of performance skill. In the case of a client whose goal is to increase pinch strength to be able to perform required job tasks, the practitioner may select a graded series of activities selected to gradually increase pinch strength. The intervention may begin by involving the client in a game of checkers that requires light pinch to pick up plastic checkers. Next, the client would become engaged in an activity requiring medium pinch strength, such as tearing construction paper into pieces to make a paper mosaic picture. Last, the client would be asked to lace a leather coin purse using a leather needle that required even stronger pinch to push the needle through the holes.

Activities may also be selected to grade for decreasing degrees of performance skill as well. This approach is used with individuals who are experiencing conditions that are progressive in nature and that lead to loss of ability (i.e., amyotrophic lateral sclerosis, Alzheimer's disease). Use of therapeutic activities in this manner will allow performance to continue in light of diminishing client capability.

When selected therapeutic activities are adapted to compensate for absent or lost performance capabilities, different aspects of the activity may be changed. These aspects may include one or more of the following: 1) the objects and materials used in the activity (i.e., a large ball or a small ball, thick paint or thin paint), 2) the process used to carry out the activity (i.e., number of steps, sequence, timing), and 3) the context in which activity takes place (e.g., physical environment, social context). To illustrate how an activity may be adapted, consider the many adaptations in the above three areas that may be made to the activity of cooking a meal for the person with decreased strength and poor endurance.

1. Objects and materials. The bowls used in preparing food may be changed from heavy ceramic bowls to lighter plastic bowls. Consideration may be given to selecting foods that offer less resistance when cutting. For example, potatoes can be boiled first and then peeled and sliced. Easier yet, purchasing canned potatoes that do not have to be peeled at all eliminates this problem.
2. The process. To compensate for lowered endurance, steps could be eliminated from the cooking process. Use of mixes or prepackaged entrees would eliminate steps, require less preparation, and save time and energy. The meal preparation process could also be paced, allowing for rest breaks. Use of a stool to sit on while preparing vegetables at the sink would also help to compensate for decreased endurance.
3. The context. The physical context can be adapted by arranging tools and equipment more closely together. For example, the seasoning used at the stove to flavor meats and vegetables should be stored near the stove to eliminate unnecessary steps. Frequently used equipment and supplies should be at waist level and within arms' reach to avoid bending and overhead reaching, which require more strength and endurance. The social context could also be adapted to include more people in the kitchen when meals are being prepared. The presence of others would allow certain tasks to be delegated to others—another way of decreasing the endurance demands of the task.

Therapeutic activities can also be specifically selected to allow the best fit between the person's capabilities and the demand of the environment or task. In this case, the therapeutic value of the activity is determined during the selection process when the performance demands of the occupation/activity are matched to the person's capabilities. For example, in selecting appropriate therapeutic activities for a person with poor social interaction skills, activities would be selected that require minimal or very structured social exchanges. A structured card game like UNO would be a better match than an activity like charades, which requires team interaction and self-initiated social exchanges.

Education

Education is another intervention method used by occupational therapy practitioners. This intervention method involves the transfer of specific knowledge to the client. For the education method to be "occupation based," the information needs to be related to the client's individual needs and priorities and must involve personal application. For example, general education about how to conserve energy during household tasks would not be occupation based unless it also included teaching and learning with the client about how this information could be applied while carrying out his or her own household tasks. Chapter Seventeen explores the use of education in intervention in more depth.

Consultation

Consultation is an intervention method whereby the practitioner uses his or her expertise to collaborate with a client to assist the client in addressing identified occupational issues. Jaffe (1992) defines a consultant "as a professional who provides an indirect service in a helping role" (p. 86). A practitioner who uses consultation as the method of intervention establishes a collaborative relationship with the client and works with the client to mutually define the problem, problem solve solutions, and develop intervention strategies. In this type of intervention, however, the actual implementation of the intervention strategies are the responsibility of the client. The client also has the choice to either accept or reject the advice and consultation that the practitioner offers. The consultation process seeks to enable the client to learn to solve his or her own problems. The practitioner's expertise and knowledge are used to define the occupational issues and performance problems and guide development of solutions.

Occupational therapy practitioners can use the consultation intervention approach in a variety of settings. Kemmis and Dunn (1996) reported on the efficacy of collaborative consultation in the public school setting. Cunninghis (1991) describes how consultation is used in a long-term care facility to facilitate appropriate activity programming to support engagement in meaningful everyday life activities, and Jacobs (1992) describes work-related injuries.

Methods of intervention may be used alone or in combination with one another. All methods may be used in conjunction with each of the intervention approaches and with each of the intervention goals previously outlined. Selecting an approach to an intervention assists the practitioner in focusing his or her attention on a specific intervention target (i.e., person, environment, making the fit between person and environment). Selecting an intervention goal defines for the practitioner the outcome toward which intervention is directed. The selection of a method (use of therapeutic activity, education, or consultation) tells the practitioner what he or she will be spending his or her time doing during the intervention. Table 16-3 provides examples of cases that demonstrate the application of intervention approaches, goals, and methods.

SUMMARY

The intervention process is based on key principles that guide thinking and selection of specific interventions. The five principles discussed in this chapter include 1) interventions are client-centered, 2) interventions are context-driven, 3) interventions are occupation-based, 4) interventions are evidence-based, and 5) the intervention process is dynamically interrelated with ongoing assessment.

The process of intervention requires a series of collaborative decisions made by the practitioner and consumer. Typically, the goal of intervention (promoting occupational performance, resolving occupational performance problems, or preventing occupational performance problems) is understood when the practitioner and person/population enter into a relationship. However, several different intervention approaches can be used to address the same intervention goal. These approaches can change the person/population, change the task/environment, or match people/populations with environment/tasks. The practitioner uses clinical reasoning, taking into account narrative, scientific, pragmatic, and ethical information (Schell, 1998) to identify relevant intervention approaches. The practitioner also identifies potential intervention methods (e.g., use of therapeutic activities/occupations, education, and/or consultation). Using client-centered principles, these intervention approaches and methods are presented to the client, and the client makes the decision as to which approach to follow.

REFERENCES

American Occupational Therapy Association. (2002). *Occupational therapy practice framework—Domain and process draft XVII*. Bethesda, MD: Author.

Brown, C., Rempfer, M., & Hamera, E. (2002). Teaching grocery shopping skills to people with schizophrenia. *Occupational Therapy Journal of Research, 22*(Supplement), 1-2.

Case-Smith, J. (1996). Fine motor outcomes in preschool children who receive occupational therapy services. *American Journal of Occupational Therapy, 50*, 52-61.

Chang, L., & Hasselkus, B. R. (1998). Occupational therapists' expectations in rehabilitation following stroke: Sources of satisfaction and dissatisfaction. *American Journal of Occupational Therapy, 52*, 629-637.

Clark, F., Azen, S. P., Zemke, R., Jackson, J., Carlson, M., Mandel, D., et al. (1997). Occupational therapy for independent-living older adults: A randomized controlled trial. *Journal of the American Medical Association, 278*, 1321-1326.

Cunninghis, R. N. (1991). Providing consultation to the long term care facility. In J. M. Kiernet (Ed.), *Occupational therapy and the older adult: A clinical manual* (pp. 260-274). Gaithersburg, MD: Aspen Publishers, Inc.

DeVries, R. E., Deitz, J., & Anson, D. (1998). A comparison of two computer access systems for functional text entry. *American Journal of Occupational Therapy, 52*, 656-665.

Table 16-3

Goals, Intervention Approaches, and Methods: Case Applications

Case	*Intervention Goal*	*Intervention Approach*	*Intervention Method*
Case #1: Fred is living with a roommate in an apartment. He receives social security income and a small income from a part-time job	**Resolving an Occupational Performance Problem** Fred would like to save up enough money to buy a car but has trouble saving money. He spends some money on lottery tickets every week	**Establish/Restore** Fred is given information on odds ratios in gambling to decrease the amount of money spent on lottery tickets	**Education**
		Adapt Therapist and Fred develop system of envelopes for dividing monthly expenses, including an envelope for savings	**Use of therapeutic activities**
		Alter Fred identifies and opens a savings account that best matches his needs for saving for a car	**Use of therapeutic activities**
Case #2: Opal is returning home after in-patient rehabilitation for stroke. She lives alone	**Preventing Occupational Performance Problems** Opal is very frightened of falling	**Adapt** Recommendations are made for removal of throw rugs and addition of grab bars, etc. at home	**Consult**
		Restore Occupational therapist meets with Opal and discusses leisure interests. Designs program that involves continuation of daily walks with neighbor and participation in household chores to restore endurance, flexibility, balance, and coordination.	**Use of therapeutic activities**
Case #3: After-care program for school-aged children	**Promoting Occupational Performance**	**Establish** Occupational therapist provides information on child development to day-care workers to design activities that are developmentally appropriate for children	**Education**

(continued)

Table 16-3

Case	Intervention Goal	Intervention Approach	Intervention Method
		Alter Occupational therapist provides list of community resources offering different activities for children. List is matched to developmental needs	**Consult**

Evidence Worksheet

Authors	*Year*	*Topic*	*Method*	*Conclusion*
Brown et al.	2002	Teaching grocery shopping skills to people with schizophrenia	Quasi-experimental (pre-test/post-test)	A skills training program for people with schizophrenia can improve grocery shopping accuracy and efficiency
Case-Smith	1996	Fine motor outcomes in preschool children who receive occupational therapy services	Quasi-experimental (pre-test/post-test)	Preschool children receiving occupational therapy showed improvements in fine motor skills, and these skills were associated with self-care and mobility function
Chang & Hasselkus	1998	Occupational therapists' expectations in rehabilitation following stroke: Sources of satisfaction and dissatisfaction	Qualitative	Therapists entered therapeutic relationships with expectations for recovery. Therapists were satisfied when expectations were met but became dissatisfied when clients reached a plateau stage
Clark et al.	1997	Occupational therapy for independent-living older adults: A randomized controlled trial	Experimental (RCT)	A preventive occupational therapy program resulted in improvements in physical function, occupational function, and life satisfaction
DeVries et al.	1998	A comparison of two computer access systems for functional text entry	Single-subject	Participants were able to use both systems successfully but were unable to achieve a rate of text entry sufficient for most employment situations

(continued)

Authors	*Year*	*Topic*	*Method*	*Conclusion*
Giles et al.	1997	A consecutive series of adults with brain injury treated with a washing and dressing retraining program	Single-subject	Three of four participants were able to achieve independence in washing and dressing following a specific protocol
Kellegrew	1998	Creating opportunities for occupation: An intervention to promote the self-care independence of young children with special needs	Single-subject	Two of three caregivers were able to create opportunities for their children to practice self-care skills after restructuring daily routines
Kemmis & Dunn	1996	Collaborative consultation: The efficacy of remedial and compensatory interventions in school contexts	Descriptive	The use of collaborative consultation facilitates positive intervention effects
Klavora et al.	1995	The effects of dynavision rehabilitation on behind-the-wheel driving ability and selected psychomotor abilities of people after stroke	Quasi-experimental (pre-test/post-test)	Participants receiving dynavision training had improvements in psychomotor variables and behind-the-wheel driving assessments
Kleinman & Stalcup	1991	The effect of graded craft activities on visuomotor integration in an inpatient child psychiatry population	Quasi-experimental (non-RCT)	Children in a graded crafts program demonstrated improvements in visuomotor skills
Kondo et al.	1997	The use of microwave ovens by elderly people with disabilities	Single subject	Participants who were provided a microwave oven and training in its use increased participation in meal preparation
Ma et al.	1999	The effect of context on skill acquisitions and transfer	Experimental	Motor learning that occurs in natural as opposed to simulated contexts facilitates improved acquisition of skill and ability to transfer skill
Nuismer et al.	1997	The use of low-load prolonged stretch devices in rehabilitation programs in the Pacific Northwest	Retrospective	People wearing low-load prolonged stretch devices had significant increases in range of motion and functional outcomes such as improvements in ADL

(continued)

Authors	*Year*	*Topic*	*Method*	*Conclusion*
Parush & Hahn-Markowitz	1997	The efficacy of an early prevention program facilitated by occupational therapists	Experimental (RCT)	Mothers in an early prevention program acquired greater knowledge, attitudes, and practices about child development than mothers in a control group
Sakemiller & Nelson	1998	Eliciting functional extension in prone through the use of a game	Single subject	When games were added to positioning interventions, children achieved better neck and back extension
Shaffer et al.	2001	Effect of interactive metronome training on children with ADHD	Experimental (RCT)	Children receiving the interactive metronome training exhibited improvements in attention, motor control, and selected academic skills greater than those in a control group
Tannous et al.	1999	Beyond good practice: Issues in working with people with intellectual disability and high support needs	Descriptive	The most positive effects were found from interventions that indirectly empower people with intellectual disability and that change others' perceptions
Vargus & Camilli	1999	A meta-analysis of research on sensory integration treatment	Meta-analysis	Sensory integrative treatment resulted in psychoeducational and motor performance improvements greater than no treatment groups but was not more effective when compared to other treatment approaches

Giles, G. M., Ridley, J. E., Dill, A., & Frye, S. (1997). A consecutive series of adults with brain injury treated with a washing and dressing retraining program. *American Journal of Occupational Therapy, 51*, 256-266.

Jaffe, E. (1992). Approaches to consultation. In E. G. Jaffe & C. F. Epstein (Eds.), *Occupational therapy consultation: Theory, principles, and practice* (pp. 86-117). St. Louis, MO: Mosby-Year Book.

Jacobs, K. (1992). Occupational therapy consultation in industrial settings. In E. G. Jaffe & C. F. Epstein (Eds.), *Occupational therapy consultation: Theory, principles, and practice* (pp. 434-444). St. Louis, MO: Mosby-Year Book.

Kellegrew, D. H. (1998). Creating opportunities for occupation: An intervention to promote the self-care independence of young children with special needs. *American Journal of Occupational Therapy, 52*, 457-465.

Kemmis, B. L., & Dunn, W. (1996). Collaborative consultation: The efficacy of remedial and compensatory interventions in school contexts. *American Journal of Occupational Therapy, 50*(9), 709-717.

Klavora, P., Gaskovski, P., Martin, K., Forsyth, R. D., Heslegrave, R. J., Young, M., et al. (1995). The effects of dynavision rehabilitation on behind-the-wheel driving ability and selected psychomotor abilities of persons after stroke. *American Journal of Occupational Therapy, 49*, 534-542.

Kleinman, B. L., & Stalcup, A. (1991). The effect of graded craft activities on visuomotor integration in an inpatient child psychiatry population. *American Journal of Occupational Therapy, 45*, 324-330.

Kondo, T., Mann, W. C., Machiko, T., & Ottenbacher, K. J. (1997). The use of microwave ovens by elderly persons with disabilities. *American Journal of Occupational Therapy, 51*, 739-747.

Law, M., Baptiste, S., & Mill, J. (1995). Client-centered practice: What does it mean and does it make a difference? *Canadian Journal of Occupational Therapy, 62*, 250-257.

Law, M., Cooper, B., Strong, S., Steward, D., Rigby, P., & Letts, L. (1996). Person-environment-occupation model: A transactive approach to occupational performance. *Canadian Journal of Occupation Therapy, 63*, 9-23.

Lee, S. S., Powell, N. J., & Esdaile, S. (2001). A functional model of cognitive rehabilitation in occupational therapy. *Canadian Journal of Occupational Therapy, 68*, 41-50.

Ma, H., Trombly, D. A., & Robinson-Podolski, C. (1999). The effect of context on skill acquisitions and transfer. *American Journal of Occupational Therapy, 53*(2), 138-144.

Nuismer, B. A., Ekes, A. M., & Holm, M. B. (1997). The use of low-load prolonged stretch devices in rehabilitation programs in the Pacific Northwest. *American Journal of Occupational Therapy, 51*, 538-543.

Parush, S., & Hahn-Markowitz, J. (1997). The efficacy of an early prevention program facilitated by occupational therapists: A follow-up study. *American Journal of Occupational Therapy, 51*, 247-251.

Sakemiller, L. M., & Nelson, D. L. (1998). Eliciting functional extension in prone through the use of a game. *American Journal of Occupational Therapy, 52*, 150-157.

Schell, B. B. (1998). Clinical reasoning: The basis of practice. In M. E. Neistadt & E. B. Crepeau (Eds.), *Willard and Spackman's occupational therapy* (4th ed., pp. 90-102). Philadelphia, PA: Lippincott-Raven Publishers.

Shaffer, R. J., Jacokes, L. E., Cassily, J. F., Greenspan, S. I., Tuchman, R. F., & Stemmer, P. J. (2001). Effective of interactive metronome training on children with ADHD. *American Journal of Occupational Therapy, 55*, 155-162.

Tannous, C., Lehmann-Monck, Magoffin, R., Jackson, O., & Llewellyn, G. (1999). Beyond good practice: Issues in working with people with intellectual disability and high support needs. *Australian Occupational Therapy Journal, 46*, 24-35.

U.S. Department of Health and Human Services. (2000). *Healthy People 2010:* (2nd ed.). Washington, DC: U.S. Government Printing Office.

Vargus, S., & Camilli, G. (1999). A meta-analysis of research on sensory integration treatment. *American Journal of Occupational Therapy, 53*, 189-198.

Wilcock, A. A. (1998). *An occupational perspective of health*. Thorofare, NJ: SLACK Incorporated.

World Health Organization. (1947). Constitution of the World Health Organization. *Chronicle of the World Health Organization, 1*(1), 29-40.

Chapter Sixteen: Categories and Principles of Interventions Reflections and Learning Activities

Julie Bass-Haugen, PhD, OTR/L, FAOTA

Reflections

In Chapters Ten and Fifteen, we received an overview of the entire occupational therapy process. This process included client information/assessment, practitioner evaluation/assessment, evidence, intervention planning and implementation, and evaluation of the outcome. This process was designed to fit clients who were individuals, populations, or organizations. In Chapter Fourteen, we examined assessment as a means to obtain the client's perspective and evaluate specific capabilities and constraints of the person, environment, and occupational performance. Once we summarize the results of the assessment, it is time to develop and implement an intervention plan. In this chapter, we reviewed the basic principles of intervention and our intervention options.

Because occupational therapy is such a broad profession, it is easy to lose track of the overall purpose of our interventions. Do we really have the same overall purpose when we work with a child with autism in a school setting, an adolescent with chemical dependency issues, a young adult who is emerging from a coma after a traumatic brain injury, a middle-aged adult who is recovering from a heart attack, and an older adult who has early signs of dementia? These are just examples of clients who are individuals! Do we have the same overall purpose in occupational therapy when we work with populations and organizations, too? If we look closely, we see two main themes in occupational therapy. First, we want our clients to be able to perform the occupations that are important and meaningful in their lives. Engagement in these occupations supports their participation in society and defines their lives. Second, we strongly believe that occupational performance supports overall health and well-being. If we can help clients realize their occupational goals, we believe we will also see improved physical, emotional, and mental health.

As you are planning interventions for all these different situations, there are only a few principles you need to keep in mind. Let's use a simple example to examine these principles. Let's say I have broken my right wrist and have just been referred to occupational therapy after having a cast removed. You are my occupational therapy practitioner. Aside from the assessments you will do, what principles should you use to guide your intervention plans? First, I need you to be client-centered. I, the client, am the only person who knows how this injury is affecting my life. I can tell you about the things that are now a "big deal" and the things that are "no big deal." I can tell you my needs and my priorities. Second, I need you to consider my usual environment and the context for my performance. My car, home, and office have some characteristics that support performance despite this injury (e.g., one-handle faucets, automatic transmission, a helpful family, supportive coworkers) and some characteristics that limit performance (e.g., few electric kitchen tools, a dog who is still frisky, family preference for home-cooked meals). Third, as soon as I leave your clinic, I have to figure out how I am going to do all the things I have to do. I need to learn how to open cans, style my hair, word-process, complete my wrist exercises, and tie my shoes—all of my two-handed occupations. Fourth, I need to know how and when I can use my injured arm again to do things. I expect that you will give me good information based on research and evidence related to this type of injury. Fifth, as things change, I want you to reassess my situation with me. I may need a different type of help at a different point in time. Now, these intervention principles are not so hard. In fact, they are common sense for the most part.

Based on what I tell you and what you determine about my situation, we might identify some goals requiring occupational therapy interventions. Each goal will include specific wording that depicts my unique situation and meets the documentation requirements for your work setting. Regardless of the wording in a specific goal, however, occupational therapy interventions are designed to promote occupational performance, resolve occupational performance problems, and/or prevent occupational performance problems. Let's go back to my little scenario. You, as my occupational therapy practitioner, understand the usual course of recovery from this type of fracture in the wrist. You know that it is important to follow a certain protocol to prevent occupational performance problems in the future. If this protocol is not followed, I may have limitations in or pain during movement. You also know that I will face occupational performance problems as soon as I return home, especially as I try to do things that typically require two hands. You will design interventions that are intended to help me resolve these problems. Finally, you recognize that an injury like this temporarily diminishes health, well-being, and quality of life. You may encourage my participation in a variety of activities during this recovery time to promote occupational performance and my sense of well-being.

Now that you know the principles and goals of intervention, what are the intervention approaches and methods you might use? A lot of terms have been introduced related to interventions. These terms are organized in the literature in different ways to give you a framework for intervention. In this chapter, the terms were organized by approach and method. The approaches were described as remediation/restoration/establishment and compensation/adaptation/modification. These two approaches were used to find the best person-environment fit. The methods were described as therapeutic activities, education, and consultation. It is proposed that these methods are used in combination with the approaches to meet occupational performance goals.

In most occupational therapy situations, you will choose more than one approach and more than one method to address each occupational therapy goal. In the simple scenario involving my broken wrist, you might use a specific protocol involving remediation/restoration/establishment to help me regain use of my injured arm. This approach might involve recommended exercises and activities as well as an orthosis or splint to restore optimal movement. Compensation/adaptation/modification approaches might also be appropriate. You might provide me with some assistive technology (e.g., elastic shoe laces, one-handed kitchen tools) and give me some ideas on how I can do things a different way until my wrist heals (e.g., stabilization techniques, temporary delegation of some household tasks). To implement these approaches, you might try several methods. You might give me some therapeutic activities to try, conduct an educational unit on one-handed techniques, and/or provide consultation to my family or employer regarding my needs during this temporary state.

These same intervention principles, goals, approaches, and methods apply to populations and organizations as well. Of course, the details of the interventions will change to meet the definition and needs of each client. You now have the basic tools to begin planning interventions for clients. As you acquire specific knowledge and experience, you will still find that your occupational therapy interventions fit these general principles and categories. Given the breadth of the occupational therapy profession, it is great that we can hang our hat on these ideas!

Journaling Activities

1. Look up and write down a dictionary definition of intervention, remediate, restore, establish, compensate, adapt, modify, promote, and consult. Highlight the component of the definitions that is most related to their descriptions in Chapter Sixteen.
2. Identify the most important new learning for you in this chapter.
3. Identify one question you have about Chapter Sixteen.
4. Reflect on a situation in which you, a friend, or family member needed interventions that were occupational in nature. It may or may not have involved formal occupational therapy services. Describe the occupational performance goals in the situation, the approaches, and the methods that were (or could have been) used (e.g., a grandparent moves from the family home to an apartment. A friend breaks a leg in a skiing accident. An aunt is on bedrest during the last month of her pregnancy).
5. After you do the Technology/Internet Learning Activities, reflect on the current level of evidence for occupational therapy interventions. If you were the director of research for an occupational therapy association, what strategic initiatives would you propose? Why do you think practice guidelines are important in a health care profession?

Technology/Internet Learning Activities

1. Use a discussion database to share specific journal activities.
2. Use a good Internet search engine to find the Web site for the National Guideline Clearinghouse.
    - Enter the phrase "National Guideline Clearinghouse" in your search line.
    - Review the home page of the Web site.
    - Evaluate the quality of this Web site. What are its strengths and limitations?
    - What is the purpose of this Web site?
    - What are practice guidelines?
    - Who sponsors this Web site?
    - Conduct a search on the phrase "occupational therapy."
        - Identify two to three guidelines that may have information on occupational therapy interventions.
        - Describe the goals, approaches, and methods for these interventions.

3. Use a good Internet search engine to find the Web site for the OTSeeker.
   - Enter the phrase "OTSeeker" in your search line.
   - Review the home page of the Web site.
   - Evaluate the quality of this Web site. What are its strengths and limitations?
   - What is the purpose of this Web site?
   - Who sponsors this Internet site?
   - Conduct a search on a specific condition (e.g., stroke, rheumatoid arthritis)
     - ✧ Identify two to three articles that have information on interventions. For each article:
       Describe the intervention and the likely client for this intervention.
       Propose general occupational performance goals consistent with this intervention.
       Identify the approach(es) consistent with this intervention.
       Identify the method(s) consistent with this intervention.
4. Use a good Internet search engine to find the Web site for the Cochrane Collaboration.
   - Enter the phrase "Cochrane Collaboration" in your search line.
   - Review the home page of the Web site.
   - Evaluate the quality of this Web site. What are its strengths and limitations?
   - What is the purpose of this Web site?
   - Who sponsors this Web site?
   - Conduct a search on several phrases related to "occupational therapy" and "rehabilitation."
     - ✧ Identify two to three abstracts that may have information on occupational therapy interventions.
     - ✧ Describe the goals, approaches, and methods for these interventions.
   - Conduct a search on a specific condition (e.g., Parkinson's disease, autism).
     - ✧ Identify two to three abstracts that may have information on interventions.
     - ✧ Describe the goals, approaches, and methods for these interventions.
   - Conduct a search for a specific intervention method (e.g., health promotion, education).
     - ✧ Identify two to three abstracts that may have information on interventions.
     - ✧ Describe the intervention.
5. Use a good Internet search engine to find the Web site for the McMaster Evidence-Based Practice Research Group.
   - Enter the phrase "McMaster Evidence-Based Practice" in your search line.
   - Review the home page of the Web site.
   - Evaluate the quality of this Web site. What are its strengths and limitations?
   - What is the purpose of this Web site?
   - Who sponsors this Internet site?
   - Identify two to three resources available at this site.
6. Use a good Internet search engine to find the Web site for the American Occupational Therapy Association and American Occupational Therapy Foundation.
   - Enter the phrase "AOTA" or "AOTF" in your search line (Note: AOTF may also be found on the AOTA Internet site).
   - Identify three to four resources available at AOTA related to interventions and practice guidelines.
   - Identify three to four resources available at AOTF related to interventions and evidence-based practice.

Applied Learning

Individual Learning Activity #1: Exploring Specific Occupational Therapy Interventions

Instructions:

- Gather and review a variety of resources on occupational therapy interventions (i.e., catalogs, journals, textbooks, home programs, practice guidelines).
- Select three to five specific interventions to examine in more detail.
- Summarize each intervention by type of client, description of client, goal(s), approach(es), and method(s).
- Describe the strengths and limitations of this intervention.

Description of Intervention	*Type of Client—* *Person* *Population* *Organization*	*Description of Client*	*Intervention Goal—* *Promote* *Prevent* *Resolve*	*Intervention Approach* *Remediate* *Restore* *Establish* *Compensate* *Adapt* *Modify*	*Intervention Method—* *Therapeutic Activity* *Education* *Consultation*
Wheelchair basketball in middle school	Population and organization	Children, ages 12 to 14, who have mobility impairments	Promote leisure Prevent health risk factors	Establish fitness Adapt or modify gym class activity	Therapeutic activity

Individual Learning Activity #2: Applying Occupational Therapy Intervention Principles to a Personal Situation

Instructions:

- Imagine this situation in your own life. You return from work or school and are shocked to find that your home has been totally destroyed by fire, tornado, or hurricane.
- Your family and close friends are not available.
- You are assigned a case worker who is an occupational therapy practitioner to help you on put your life back together.

- Close your eyes and imagine the ideal interaction between you and the case worker. Discuss how this case worker would use principles of occupational therapy intervention in working with you.
- Close your eyes again and imagine the worst-case scenario between you and the case worker. Discuss how this case worker would ignore principles of occupational therapy intervention in working with you.
  - ✧ Intervention Principles
    - Client-centered
    - Environment/context
    - Occupations
    - Evidence/research
    - Reassessment

ACTIVE LEARNING

Group Activity #1: Exploring Intervention Planning and Implementation Through a Hypothetical Individual Client

Preparation:

- Read Chapter Sixteen.
- Select or assign the hypothetical case(s) for each small group.
- For each case, assign a role to each group member.
  - ✧ Occupational therapy practitioner implements the intervention plan.
  - ✧ Hypothetical client portrays a given case (see description of cases in Materials).
  - ✧ Observer records notes on the occupational therapy intervention (Important Note: The focus of this activity is to explore intervention planning and implementation through one hypothetical individual client. It does not represent the entire intervention planning and implementation process. Also, this learning activity does not give you sufficient details to develop a complete, accurate intervention plan).

Time: 30 to 90 minutes (depending on number of cases)

Materials:

- Intervention resources (e.g., catalogs, journals, texts, home programs, practice guidelines)
- Tables and chairs arrangement conducive for interventions
- Props to help portray the case
- Hypothetical Cases:
  - ✧ Client 1: a) an 80-year-old man who lives alone in an apartment, b) had a recent right hip fracture and surgery, c) is currently nonweight-bearing on his right side and is on restrictions in hip movements, d) wants to go home as soon as possible but is concerned about how he will do activities of daily living and instrumental activities of daily living
  - ✧ Client 2: a) a 40-year-old woman who lives in a group home, b) is on a medication regimen for schizophrenia, c) has recently responded well to medication and has no current disturbances of thought, perception, and affect, d) wants to improve leisure and work occupations
  - ✧ Client 3: a) a 60-year-old woman who lives with her husband in a home, b) has lung cancer that has metastasized to other areas of the body, c) has tried various forms of treatment but has not responded, d) is currently feeling better, e) wants to maintain control of life and engage in meaningful activities of daily living, instrumental activities of daily living, and leisure activities
  - ✧ Client 4: a) a 50-year-old man who is a widower and lives with his college-age son, b) has had arthritis for 5 years, c) was recently laid off from job as a computer programmer, d) reports painful hand joints after some activities, e) wants to explore work occupations and instrumental activities of daily living require excessive force or repetitive movements

✧ Client 5: a) a 9-year-old boy in third grade at a local elementary school, b) is receiving special education services in speech and language for speech articulation, c) was referred to occupational therapy for handwriting issues, d) has begun to work on cursive handwriting in the classroom

Instructions:

- Individually:
  - ✧ Review the case prior to small group work.
  - ✧ Explore resources that might help you understand the case(s) and plan interventions.
  - ✧ Generate some intervention ideas.
- In small groups:
  - ✧ Explore the intervention planning and implementation through a hypothetical client.
  - ✧ Develop supplemental information on your client to assist you in intervention planning (e.g., history, occupational goals, assessment results).
  - ✧ Summarize your supplemental information.
  - ✧ Brainstorm intervention ideas that might be appropriate for this client.
  - ✧ Select three intervention ideas to describe in more detail and summarize them in the table.

Client:

Supplemental Information:

Description of Intervention	*Intervention Goal— Promote Prevent Resolve*	*Intervention Approach— Remediate Restore Establish Compensate Adapt Modify*	*Intervention Method— Therapeutic Activity Education Consultation*

✧ Select one intervention to role play:

The occupational therapy practitioner should introduce or establish a client-centered professional relationship, explain the intervention, implement the intervention, and evaluate the outcome.

The hypothetical client should participate in the intervention session, create specific responses/behaviors that fit the case, and portray the individual in the case.

The observer should record the steps in intervention session, identify intervention strengths of the practitioner and areas to improve, critique the scenario presented by the hypothetical client, record responses and behaviors of the client, and summarize the results of the intervention session.

✧ Practice summarizing the intervention session for this case using both written and verbal communication.

Discussion:

- Discuss the interventions you used for this case. Why did you choose them?
- What evidence would you like to obtain on these interventions?
- Discuss the experience of being in the different roles. What was comfortable? What was awkward? What skills do you have? What skills would you like to develop?
- Discuss the likely outcomes of this intervention. What components of the intervention planning and implementation were you able to fully or partially complete?
- Discuss what you learned about intervention planning and implementation. Why is it important?

Group Activity #2: Exploring Intervention Planning and Implementation for a Hypothetical Population or Organization

Preparation:

- Read Chapter Sixteen.
- Select or assign the hypothetical case(s) for each group (Important Note: The focus of this activity is to explore intervention planning and implementation for one hypothetical population or organization. It does not represent the entire intervention planning and implementation process. Also, this learning activity does not give you sufficient details to develop a complete, accurate intervention plan).

Time: 30 to 90 minutes (depending on number of cases)

Materials:

- Intervention resources (e.g., catalogs, journals, texts, home programs, practice guidelines, online resources)
- Hypothetical Cases:
  - ✧ Client 1: a) elders living in an assisted-living environment, b) limited support system, c) high incidence of depression, d) some medical issues
  - ✧ Client 2: a) elementary school-aged children in your community, b) below national average academic achievement, c) high incidence of obesity, d) delayed gross and fine motor skills
  - ✧ Client 3: a) homeless men in your community, b) working minimum wage jobs, c) some chemical dependency and mental health problems, d) affordable housing issues
  - ✧ Client 4: a) caregivers of family with Alzheimer's disease, b) burn-out and stress reported, c) financial issues, d) limited resources in area

Instructions:

- Individually:
  - ✧ Review the case prior to small group work.
  - ✧ Explore resources that might help you understand the case(s) and plan interventions.
  - ✧ Generate some intervention ideas.
- In small groups:
  - ✧ Explore intervention planning and implementation through a hypothetical client.
  - ✧ Give examples of the client defined as a population or organization.
  - ✧ Develop supplemental information on your client to assist you in intervention planning (e.g., history, occupational goals, assessment results).
  - ✧ Summarize your supplemental information.
  - ✧ Brainstorm intervention ideas that might be appropriate for this client.
  - ✧ Select three intervention ideas to describe in more detail and summarize them in the table on p. 419.

Client:

Supplemental Information:

Description of Intervention	*Intervention Goal—*	*Intervention Approach—*	*Intervention Method—*
	Promote	*Remediate*	*Therapeutic Activity*
	Prevent	*Restore*	*Education*
	Resolve	*Establish*	*Consultation*
		Compensate	
		Adapt	
		Modify	

Discussion:

- Discuss the interventions you used for this case. Why did you choose them?
- What evidence would you like to obtain on these interventions?
- Discuss the likely outcomes of these interventions. What components of the intervention planning and implementation were you able to fully or partially complete?
- Discuss what you learned about intervention planning and implementation. Why is it important?

Chapter Seventeen Objectives

The information in this chapter is intended to help the reader:

1. Identify and apply adult learning principles.
2. Analyze health behavior using models of client education.
3. Design client education plans using concepts from theoretical models.
4. Describe key terms used in adult education, models of client education, and learning theory.
5. Identify and explain the key components of designing an intervention plan based on learning principles.
6. Design practice and feedback schedules, tasks, and environments that will promote transfer and generalization of learning.
7. Describe specific treatment techniques for individuals with impaired learning abilities.
8. Describe the impact of the social and physical environment on learning.

Key Words

andragogy: The art and science of helping adults learn.

attentional focus: A term often used in motor tasks, relating to whether the focus of attention is internal (body alignment or movement) or external (environmental relationship or movement outcome).

attribution theory: Model of client education that focuses on the causal relationships a client attributes to events.

declarative knowledge: Knowledge of information or facts that can be named and recited.

errorless learning: A teaching technique in which individuals are not allowed to make errors during the acquisition of a skill.

explicit learning: Knowledge of information or facts that can be identified, like declarative knowledge.

generalization: Performing a variation of a task in a new environment.

health belief model: Client education model based on the client's perception of susceptibility to the consequences of a disease or set of behaviors.

implicit learning: Procedural knowledge, such as routines and habits, as well as automatic behaviors and motor skills, such as force generation and the development of skilled movement.

learning: "A set of processes… leading to relatively permanent changes in the capability for responding" (Schmidt, 1988, p. 346).

performance: Ability to complete a task after practice or cueing, may or may not indicate that learning has occurred.

procedural knowledge: Knowledge about how to do something; the sequences, habits, and routines used to perform operations.

scaffolding: A teaching technique in which a complex cognitive task is taught by breaking it down into a hierarchy of skills and building from the most basic to the complex.

self-monitoring: A metacognitive skill that involves a self-assessment of behavior (e.g., the self-assessment of the effectiveness of problem-solving strategies or self-assessment of the safeness and correctness of performance).

social cognitive theory: Analyzing behavior in terms of the person's characteristics, the behavior in question, and the intended context.

specificity of learning: The condition of learning exactly what is taught, including environmental variables.

theory of reasoned action: Theory of client education that highlights the client's net attitude toward the proposed behavioral change.

transfer of learning: Performing a previously learned task in a new environment

transtheoretical theory: Model of client education that frames the client's readiness for change into successive steps.

We learn by practice. Whether it means to learn to dance by practicing dancing or to learn to live by practicing living, the principles are the same.
Martha Graham

Chapter Seventeen

THERAPY AS LEARNING

Rondell Berkeland, EdD, OTR/L and Nancy Flinn, PhD, OTR/L

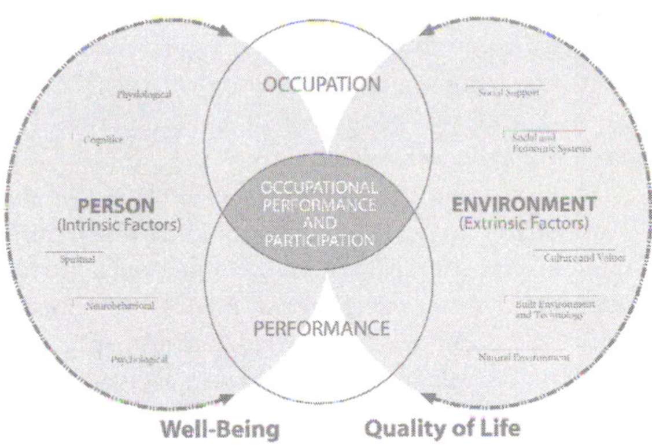

Setting the Stage

This chapter will discuss teaching and learning as key components of the occupational therapy process. Teaching and learning provide clients with new possibilities and capabilities for responding and engaging in occupations. Teaching roles are important in both traditional and emerging areas of occupational therapy practice. In designing teaching and learning experiences, practitioners consider models or frameworks for client education, principles of adult learning, and the mechanics of constructing educational programs. The skills and knowledge necessary for effective teaching are critical in almost all therapeutic interactions.

Berkeland, R., & Flinn, N. (2005). Therapy as learning. In C. H. Christiansen, C. M. Baum, and J. Bass-Haugen (Eds.), Occupational therapy: Performance, participation, and well-being *(3rd ed.). Thorofare, NJ: SLACK Incorporated.*

Current and Emerging Roles for Occupational Therapy as Teaching/Learning

While occupational therapy practitioners frequently speak of "caregiver education" or "skilled teaching" as if they were specific clinical events, a broader perspective on therapy would reveal that many of the interventions that practitioners plan would fall into the classification of teaching. One familiar definition of learning is that it is a "set of processes... leading to relatively permanent changes in the capability for responding" (Schmidt, 1988, p. 346). Given this definition, it becomes apparent that whether the practitioner is teaching dressing techniques, assertiveness techniques, or motor skills such as coordination or motor control, the goal of the process is to provide clients with new possibilities for response, and the principles of learning and teaching are involved. Because much of occupational therapy intervention is teaching, learning about the characteristics of the learner that influence learning and the principles of teaching would help to make this process more effective.

The approach to teaching taken in this chapter focuses primarily on the learner as an adult learner and as an occupational therapy client. The chapter is divided into three broad areas. First, several models or frameworks for client education are reviewed. Much like frames of reference, the models of client education each have strengths, they share components with the other models, and there are some client situations for which a given model may not be as appropriate as another. Second, principles of adult learning are discussed. The principles of adult learning are relevant for any model of client education and are not necessarily age constricted. Finally, the mechanics of constructing an educational program or event are discussed. The components, such as needs assessment, goal setting, method selection, and program evaluation, are reviewed.

Teaching roles for occupational therapy practitioners exist in both current and emerging practice areas. Traditionally, much of the teaching done by practitioners has been done with a client or caregiver, and the teaching has been done on a one-on-one basis (i.e., teaching a client and his or her caregiver a specific dressing or homemaking technique). However, many of the emerging practice areas for occupational therapy rely on teaching groups of clients, as in a well-elderly or other community setting. The use of group teaching in these situations can be very effective, and the participants can be encouraged to participate and reinforce teaching goals. These psychoeducational groups may be essentially supportive and focus on coping techniques or group support.

As we begin to speak of emerging practice areas, the role of the occupational therapy practitioner as a consultant creates new challenges as a teacher. In these new settings, the role of the practitioner is often primarily that of educator. Whether the practitioner is working in a senior high rise promoting health and wellness or working at an assembly plant teaching about injury prevention, the need to understand how individuals learn, to assess the learners and the learning environment, to set learning objectives, and to select an appropriate teaching approach is of paramount importance. The skills and knowledge necessary for effective teaching are critical in almost all therapeutic interactions.

Approaches to Client Education and Teaching/Learning Models

Approaches or models of health education can be used in the way occupational therapy practitioners use frames of reference or conceptual practice models (Kielhofner, 2004). Each model presents an explanation as to what motivates learning or behavior change, what the variables are that might affect learning, and a theoretical foundation for the model. Like frames of reference, some of the models of health education are more limited in application, while others are more global and have broader applications (e.g., transtheoretical model) (Prochaska, Redding, & Evers, 1997). Five models are discussed: the health belief model, attribution model, social cognitive theory, theory of reasoned action, and the transtheoretical model (readiness to change).

Health Belief Model

The health belief model (HBM) is based on an integration of an operant behavioral model and cognitive theory (Rosenstock, 1990). The HBM is based on several connected steps. First, the client perceives a threat. The threat, or perceived threat, is based on the combination of perceived susceptibility to a disease or consequence plus the belief that the consequence is serious.

Another component of the HBM model is the client's beliefs about the proposed education. First, what are the perceived benefits of the client education and adopting some new behavior? Second, what are the perceived barriers to engaging in the education and adopting the new set of health behaviors? The balance (i.e., the benefits versus the barriers) must be weighed and reconciled. Barriers might include cost, the degree of required change, changes in social life, changes in role, changes in self-concept, and the sheer effort involved. The final step is the client's belief in his or her efficacy to carry out the recommended actions for the identified health problem.

Is it perceived as realistic, from both technical and social constructs, to engage in the suggested new behavior?

One of the contemporary or popular education efforts that can be analyzed from a HBM perspective is the effort to curb driving while under the influence of alcohol. The consequences of driving and subsequently having an accident are realistically and dramatically evident by displaying crashed cars that have been associated with the death of a teenager who was drinking and driving. From an HBM perspective, the consequence is obviously serious, the behavior is clearly relatable to the intended audience, and the solutions are within the behavioral capability of most teenagers. Through educational efforts, peer support, and distribution of information, the target clients' efficacy can be strengthened to effectively carry out the desired behavior. Using the HBM as a theoretical model, these premises could be researched. The variables that comprise the model, severity of the threat, perceived benefits, barriers to change, and self-efficacy to change would be analyzed with respect to the client population's reported behavior.

Chen and colleagues (1999) used a similar approach to assess compliance with home exercise programs for clients with upper extremity impairments. They compared the HBM, the Model of Human Occupation (MOHO), and the Health Locus of Control. The element of the HBM that correlated with compliance to exercise programs was self-efficacy. In this study, the authors subsumed the HBM components into a MOHO framework. Hence, MOHO was reported as the model "partially supported as a framework for predicting compliance behavior with occupational therapy and physical therapy treatment" (p. 178).

The practitioner's intervention, from a health belief model, is to support the credibility of the threat, articulate the benefits of the new learning outcomes, acknowledge and realistically deal with the environmental barriers to carrying out the behaviors, and, finally, engage the client in a learning experience graded to provide a sense of self-efficacy for effectively applying the new learning.

Attribution Model

Attributions are the "causes individuals generate to make sense of their world" (Lewis & Daltroy, 1990, p. 92). Attributing or assigning causes to events can have both positive and negative effects. Positive effects include the ability to predict future events or behaviors, to maintain self-esteem, to reduce anxiety, to create feelings of control, to motivate, and to serve as a guide for intervention. Attributions can also negatively impact behavior and feelings. Depending on the focus of the attribution, they can facilitate feelings of hopelessness, loss of control, and anxiety, and they can feed into a self-fulfilling prophecy sequence of behavior and outcomes.

The overall goal of intervention from an attribution perspective is to reduce ambiguity about outcomes and increase individual control. This approach assumes people want to interpret, understand, and if possible be in control of their health and performance outcomes.

Attributions can be described or categorized according to four dimensions: locus of causation (internal or external), controllability, stability, and globality. For purposes of controlling events, the most desirable configuration is for the cause to have an internal locus of control, to be controllable by the individual, to be stable or consistent, and to be global. Global means the personal characteristic not only controls the specific behavior it was intended to, but it is a generally applicable trait. Being good in math, for example, is not as global as being intelligent. Having "test anxiety" is less of a global problem than school anxiety.

In a health-related example, a newly diagnosed diabetic was told that the reason she had the disease was that God was angry with her and she was a sinner. From an attribution frame, this explanation for the diagnosis presents a rather hopeless scenario. The cause for the client's problems was external (God), the client had no perceived control over God, her status as a sinner was stable (i.e., it was not a random, unlikely event), and God's influence was seen as rather global and all encompassing. The client was also diagnosed with depression.

The practitioner followed a series of steps designed to acknowledge the attributions the client had while trying to refocus the client's attention to more controllable attributes. The first step was developing a therapeutic relationship to provide support and empathy and to clearly understand the client's attribution system. The second step is to develop correct attributions. This is more complicated. The practitioner did not contradict the client's religious beliefs, but supported the alternate "hypothesis" given the client by the physician. The third step is to alter incorrect attributions. Once again, the practitioner simply supported an alternate explanation for the diagnosis. The fourth step is to alter the focus of attributions, in this case from what was uncontrollable to what was controllable—the daily management tasks of her diabetes. The fifth step was to attribute the daily management tasks to client characteristics (e.g., she is reliable and she understands the daily requirements). Finally, it is necessary to maintain a perception of personal efficacy. This is done through support, modifications of the maintenance routine, and teaching new skills.

Social Cognitive Theory

Social cognitive theory (Baranowski, Perry, & Parcel, 1997) (previously known as social learning theory) (Perry, Baranowski, & Parcel, 1990) is a familiar concept to occupational therapy practitioners. The organizing principle is that behavior, personal factors (including cognition), and environmental influences all interact (Baranowski et al., 1997). Each element is dynamic, changing, and responsive to each other. The basic questions surrounding intervention (teaching) include the following: What will be effective in the environment? Which behavior should be chosen? Can the person develop the behavioral capability to effectively perform the behavior? There are many side issues. How confident does the client feel using the new behavior? What are the social, attitudinal, normative, cultural, and geographic barriers in the environment toward the taught behavior? What behavior or behaviors are legitimate approaches to the client's performance issues?

An example illustrates the dangers of not thinking from the perspective of the person-behavior-environment triad. Shelly was a 45-year-old African American woman admitted to the outpatient mental health unit following an overnight admission to the emergency room and hospital. She had been beaten by her live-in boyfriend. This was a common occurrence, especially when the boyfriend and Shelly were drinking. They lived in a two-room apartment in the downtown area of a large city. Shelly was admitted to a day hospital program to explore options to her volatile living situation (which she was unwilling to leave) and relationship with her boyfriend. Shelly was first introduced to "assertiveness" training. The psychoeducational sessions used role playing, lecture, discussion, and simulation experiences to learn and apply the principles of assertiveness training. Midway through the third session, Shelly became angry and admonished the practitioner, saying, "Look, honey! I can't do this. If I do these things and talk like this, he'll kill me!" In retrospect, the approach was definitely a mismatch to the culture of the environment. In addition, the strategies of assertiveness training did not fit the culture and personality of the client. The approach for Shelly was individualized and a dual approach was implemented. First, Shelly was taught survival skills to avoid physical harm from her boyfriend and to not inflame the already dangerous situation. Shelly did learn several assertiveness "scripts," not for her personal relationships, but to use with the health care and social service systems. These systems supposedly are cultures that are familiar with and respond to this type of approach. It should be noted that assertive approaches were not entirely dismissed for Shelly's personal relationships. As time went on, Shelly began to incorporate these techniques into other areas of her life based on her assessment of her environment.

Social cognitive theory encompasses many principles inherent in occupational therapy groups: observational learning, learning coping responses for when the learned behaviors do not work, learning and practicing skills, developing confidence, and taking control of actions within unique environments.

Theory of Reasoned Action

The theory of reasoned action (TRA) is a framework for understanding behavior and the motivational intent to engage in a behavior. One of the key components of the TRA is that it links motivation and attitude with the proposed health behavior as opposed to the outcome of the behavior. Attitudes toward the behavior itself are a better predictor of engaging in the behavior than attitudes toward the object or outcome of the behavior (Carter, 1990; Montano, Karpryzk, & Taplin, 1997).

Assessing a person's likelihood of engaging in a health behavior is a two-part analysis. The first set of factors determines the client's attitude toward the behavior. The client's attitude consists of his or her beliefs toward the health behavior weighted against his or her beliefs about the outcome of the behavior. Together, these two factors yield an "attitude toward behavior" (Montano et al., 1997, p. 87). Working parallel to the client's own attitude toward the health behavior is the subjective norm regarding that behavior. The subjective norm is the client's perception of what important referents in his or her life think about the behavior weighted against the client's motivation to comply with the referents' beliefs. The client's attitude toward the health behavior combined with the subjective norm yield a behavioral intent, which, in turn, may or may not result in the behavior being carried out.

Using the TRA, it is possible to determine the likelihood of a given population carrying out a specific behavior. A combination of bipolar and unipolar questions are asked about the behavior in question, and then a numerical weighting is applied (-3, -2... +2, +3). Based on the overall ratings, a hypothesis can be developed as to whether or not a given population of clients or an individual client will engage in the proposed health behavior. Further analysis allows the educator to modify variables to increase the likelihood of the desired behaviors being viewed as positive by the client and thus leading to a positive behavioral intention.

One of the striking product advertisements that can be interpreted from a TRA perspective is the contemporary set of advertisements that show public figures, including politicians, athletes, and artists, drinking "milk." The effectiveness of the ads may be interpreted, in part, according to the global appeal of the public figures as referents and the subsequent motivation of the ad viewers to comply with the referents.

According to TRA, then, the client's attitude and perceived value of a given behavior is weighted against his or her perception of what referents think about the behavior as well as the client's motivation to comply with the referents' values. This model has been used as the fundamental theoretical construct for numerous questions, including health professionals' attitudes toward self-assessment (Fried, DeVore, & Dailey, 2001), predicting health behaviors such as "milk consumption" (Brewer, Blake, Rankin, & Douglass, 1999), examining alcohol use among young adults (O'Callaghan, Chant, Callan, & Baglioni, 1997), and studying smoking prevention efforts in preteen children (McGahee, Kemp, & Tingen, 2000). The TRA, either alone or in combination with other models, has been a sound framework to analyze health and social behavior.

Transtheoretical Model (Readiness to Change)

The transtheoretical model (TTM), also known as the readiness to change model, is a complex but functional way to analyze and predict change behavior. The TTM is defined by five stages of change, 10 processes within the stages of change, and three additional variables: the pros and cons of changing, self-efficacy with respect to the change, and temptation to return to the original behavior (Prochaska et al., 1997). The five stages of change are precontemplative, contemplative, preparation, action, and maintenance.

The precontemplative stage is when the client is not considering a change in health behavior in the next 6 months. Clients in this stage may have attempted to change in the past and are now demoralized or resistant to further change efforts. They may be uninformed or underinformed about the need for or benefits of change. The educators' approaches in this stage are to provide opportunities for awareness about the health condition, listen to the client's concerns and frustrations, and provide carefully timed behavior options and choices (Prochaska et al., 1997).

The second stage of change, contemplation, is characterized by considering the pros and cons of change. Typically, the client ambivalently considers the steps or actions involved in a behavioral change. An individual at this stage may be considered a procrastinator and may find him- or herself in a state of "chronic contemplation" (Prochaska et al., 1997, p. 61). At this stage, it is, once again, important to listen and to help the client articulate more specific barriers to and benefits of change. The educator could also provide more specific facts and information about the considered changes. Another approach that can be effective at this stage is values clarification (i.e., looking at what it means to be associated with the unhealthy behaviors as opposed to the healthy behavior [Health Partners, 1998]).

Four behavioral processes are associated with stages one and two, in particular moving from stage one to two. They are consciousness raising, dramatic relief, self-re-evaluation, and environmental re-evaluation. Consciousness raising is the process of becoming aware of new information related to increased benefits of changing one's behavior or increased risk of not changing. Dramatic relief is an affective response. It is a heightened emotional response, such as fear, worry, or anxiety, associated with the negative effects of not changing health behaviors. The impact of the emotional response is lessened if the appropriate health behavior actions are taken. Self- and environmental evaluation are similar processes, but with different targets. The process of self-evaluation causes the client to consider how comfortable he or she is with the image projected by the unhealthy behavior. For example, would one rather be an overweight, inactive person or a trim, active individual? The dissonance between one's values and current behavior may be such that a change would be considered. Environmental re-evaluation looks at the impact of one's current behavior on other people, the type of role model that the client has, and the potential cost of the unhealthy behavior.

The third stage is preparation. At this stage, the client is ready for and receptive to joining an action-oriented change program. The client has announced his or her intent to change within the next 30 days. Typically, he or she has investigated a change program, collected information, and perhaps purchased some of the supplies or paid the tuition to begin a program. Clients at this stage have usually tried to change the targeted behavior before and have been unsuccessful (Prochaska, DiClemente, & Norcross, 1992). This stage has previously been referred to as the decision stage. The client makes a commitment to begin a program or engage in a series of actions that define a significant behavior change. It is important, at this stage, to provide specific strategies for behavioral change. The client should be prepared as to the difficulty in actually making a change and to guard against trying to make too big of a change and then being discouraged when the task is unreasonable.

One of the change processes that may be evident during this stage is "self-liberation" (Prochaska et al., 1997, p. 69). Self-liberation is a public commitment to change. In the therapeutic context, this could take the form of goal setting, a behavioral contract, or a verbal pledge to significant others.

The fourth stage of change is action. At this stage, the client has engaged in the new behavior. Whatever criterion was set has been achieved. The action stage is classically defined as the first 6 months of a behavioral change. It is critical to note that displaying a behavior, such as what occurs during this stage, does not mean a change has occurred. The action stage is one of the steps in the process and, as such, depends on the preparatory stages as well as the subsequent maintenance stage. The health educator can assist the client by resolving problems related to barriers that threaten the change. Positive behaviors should be reinforced, and feelings related to the change can be discussed (Health Partners, 1998).

The maintenance stage is also an active process. This stage has variable lengths and may last a lifetime for certain addictive behaviors (Prochaska et al., 1992). Spanning the action and maintenance stages are four processes that facilitate continuation of the positive behavior: contingency management, helping relationships, counterconditioning, and stimulus control. Contingency management is working out a reward system in which the new behavior is rewarded and the discarded behavior is no longer rewarding. Helping relationships is using friends and significant others for support in maintaining the behavior change. Helping relationships take into account self-help groups, confiding in trustworthy friends, and sharing problems and concerns within a therapeutic alliance. Counterconditioning is replacing unhealthy behaviors with healthy behaviors (i.e., using relaxation techniques to deal with stress versus alcohol use). Finally, stimulus control is restructuring one's life and context to either deal with or remove those stimuli that previously led to the problem behaviors. An example would be to keep healthier foods at home and not have high-fat foods available as a stimulus for overeating.

In addition to the stages and processes within the stages, Prochaska and colleagues (1997) note three additional variables that impact the overall change process. The first is a simple decisional balance equation. That is, what are the overall pros and cons of implementing the change? The second variable is confidence. How confident is the client that he or she can deal with the temptations associated with relapse such as high-risk social situations? The third variable is the temptation itself. The intensity of the urges associated with various categories of temptation can lead to behavioral relapse. Confidence and temptation together are defined as self-efficacy within the TTM.

The TTM typifies the complexity of change and several important principles. One of the central issues is that the action taken by the health educator must match the client's stage of readiness. If the client is in one of the preparatory, reflective stages, an action-oriented approach will not be effective. Conversely, if the client has gone through the cognitive and affective preparation for change, he or she is, in fact, ready for a specific set of actions as opposed to tangential discussion. A second principle is that changes do not spontaneously occur across the stages. There is no inherent motivation to progress through the stages. Each stage is an active process that is facilitated by the appropriately matched actions and approaches. Third, for many behaviors, the TTM is a cyclical process. Clients may go through the stages several times before maintaining themselves at the new desired behavior. Finally, the underlying dynamic in stage-based interventions is to enhance the client's self-control.

The TTM has been heavily researched and used to analyze a wide variety of health problems. These include smoking (Prochaska, Velicer, DiClemente, & Fava, 1988), other addictive behaviors such as overeating and alcohol use (Prochaska et al., 1992), and general health issues such as engaging in exercise, getting mammograms, and using condoms (Prochaska, 1994).

The models of client education are rarely used in isolation. Like the occupational therapy frames of reference and conceptual practice models, successful components are often combined into an overall educational framework. Kretzer and Larson (1998, p. 251) propose a set of guidelines for combining elements of several practice models:

- Incorporate into interventions the constructs that have been shown consistently to be predictors of behavior or to have strong influences on behavior. These include beliefs, perceived health threat, cues, self-efficacy, attitude, subjective norms, perceived behavioral control, intention, and stages of change.
- Clearly define these variables. Consider the organizational context and include factors in the work environment most likely to maximize effectiveness. They would include communication, participation, active involvement of organizational leaders, fairness, mutuality, respect, and external and internal reinforces.
- Use the stages of change to assess individual and group readiness before selecting any interventions.
- Use a planning framework to track various components and processes in an ongoing evaluation of the effectiveness of interventions.
- Consider the complexity of individual and organizational factors when designing behavioral interventions, realizing that a multidimensional intervention will have a great impact on behavior.
- Avoid the use of words such as compliance. Replace them with descriptive phrases that promote a sense of active participation and internalization (e.g., enhancing practice).

These guidelines were constructed for a work setting to design a program to change the behavior of workers with regard to infection control practices. The guidelines are, however, equally applicable to a broad spectrum of "clients" and behavior change issues. As Kretzer and Larson (1998) note, a multifactorial approach has the greatest chance of success.

Given the range of theoretical models around which to construct the overall educational approach, the learner must also be considered. The learner, in most cases, will meet the criteria generally ascribed to the "adult learner" (Knowles, Holton, & Swanson, 1998). Regardless of the individual characteristics of the learner, there is a set of principles that apply to any adult learning situation.

Principles of Adult Education and Teaching/Learning

A number of years ago, Malcolm Knowles (1970, 1973, 1984) articulated the differences between pedagogy, the art of helping children learn, and andragogy, the art of helping adults learn. Regardless of the type of teaching, the content, or which approach to client education is chosen, the following basic principles are applicable to the adult.

Assumptions About the Adult Learner

Six basic principles that differentiate the traditional learner from the adult learner will be discussed. The first is the "need to know."

The Need to Know

Adults typically "need" to know why the learning is important (Knowles et al., 1998). "Why do I have to do this?" The first task in teaching adults is often selling the need (i.e., working with the learners to agree on the importance, usefulness, and personal benefit of learning the material, procedure, or task). In the case of client education surrounding a new set of health maintenance procedures, the learner may consciously or unconsciously resist the education as a way of denying the seriousness of or continued need for the health education. Caregivers may also minimize the need for education, claiming they will take care of the individual or he or she "will get better."

Self-Concept

The adult learner's self-concept is highly developed and ingrained. Adults generally consider themselves independent, self-directed, and responsible. These characteristics carry over to the learning experience. There is a conflict, however. Most adults have been educated in a pedagogical or traditional framework. There, the instructor has planned learning, and the learner has been told what to do, according to the instructor's timeframe. The adult learner, on the one hand, will expect to be taught in this way while at the same time resenting it. One of the challenging tasks of teaching adult learners is changing the process of teaching and learning. The instructor may need to facilitate a transition from dependent to more self-directed learning.

Learner Experience

Adults not only bring a "volume" of learning experience to the learning environment, but they bring a diverse and rich set of learning experiences. The richness of experience makes learning groups particularly effective, especially for ongoing disease management groups. Because adults bring general experience, the instructor has the luxury of using problem solving and application types of learning methods. The depth of experience also presents potential problems, however. The adult learner may have highly engrained ways of conducting a task. Not only might the adult have a fixed way of performing a task, his or her environment may expect this type and level of performance. Changing a personal environment (e.g., rearranging furniture or the rules for interacting with one's boss) may be akin to a paradigm shift dependent on past behavior.

Readiness to Learn

For the adult, learning is often associated with a significant lifestyle event decision. Events such as divorce, death, career change, job loss, or family role changes precipitate the active seeking of new learning. Readiness to learn then is not simply that the learning is offered at a particular time, such as a school schedule, but that the adult has encountered an experience in which the solution to dealing with the consequences of that event is perceived to be in new learning.

The learner can also be influenced to accept the timing for new learning. The practitioner can induce a readiness to learn by pointing out the gaps in the client's experience or skills that could be remedied by new learning and hence yield more desirable outcomes.

Orientation to Learning

For the classic student, from grade school through most college classes, the orientation to learning is subject centered. Students study a topic with the intent of someday being able to apply the content in an as yet unknown or unnamed environment. In an adult learning context, the learning is constructed for direct application to a problem the learner is experiencing. The orientation to learning is problem centered versus subject centered.

In most college environments, new learning paradigms have sought to integrate learner centered and applied learning phenomena into courses, hence crossing the boundaries from pedagogical to andragogical learning. The use of clinical experiences, service learning, and extended projects throughout occupational therapy education are examples of attempting to change the learning to more of a problem-centered orientation (Barr & Tagg, 1995; Campbell & Smith, 1997).

Motivation to Learn

Motivation for the adult learner is primarily internal. The reward is being able to deal with a new problem—to rectify the discrepancy within his or her self-concept of who he or she was and incorporating a new definition of health that comes with impairment or disability.

CHARACTERISTICS THAT AFFECT LEARNING

Thus far, some frameworks for learning have been discussed, including the health belief model, attribution theory, social cognitive theory, and the theory of reasoned action, and the transtheoretical model of readiness to change. These approaches to learning incorporate the principles of adult learning with varying emphasis. They are all based on some assumptions about adult learners: the focus on what the learner needs to know, the need for the teacher to be aware of the self-concept of the learner, the fact that the learner brings to the situation a wide range of learning experiences, a certain degree of readiness to learn, an orientation to learning, and some level of motivation to learn. All of these approaches focus on how to create changes in behavior, not just in some change in cognitive capacity. In other words, in occupational therapy, effective teaching usually results not just in increased cognitive content, but also in some change in behavior. In the same way, there are other characteristics that need to be considered.

The same characteristics that influence occupational behavior also affect learning. These would include the characteristics that the learner brings to the situation, including their physiological, cognitive, and psychological conditions. The environment also imposes structure and includes the social support for the individual and for the learning process, the societal policies and attitudes, cultural norms and values, and physical environment. Further, the task and its relationship to the roles of the individual also influence the learning possibilities of a given situation. To maximize learning within a situation, these parameters need to be addressed.

Person Characteristics

In addition to personal characteristics being included in the learning situation, it is important to remember that they may be present along a continuum, from typical to impairment, from optional to obligatory. For example, while some individuals might prefer active learning over a lecture format for class, most individuals can learn from either presentation. However, for someone with a learning disability, auditory presentation may be the only input from which he or she is able to benefit, and information must be presented in that format. In that circumstance, very individualized teaching must be done to accommodate the learner's requirement.

In clinical and community settings, the specific limitations of the audience will need to be included in the teaching plan to accommodate various learners' limitations. In individual teaching, the specific characteristics of the client can be addressed and incorporated into the teaching/learning session, but that is not always feasible. For example, in a presentation to a group of well-elderly people, it may not be feasible to assess each individual in the group. However, there are characteristics of an elderly population that need to be included in the design of the teaching program. Assumptions could be made about vision and hearing loss in that audience that would support presenting auditory information in a quiet environment, using large-print handouts, and using redundant delivery methods (i.e., repeating the same information in different ways to maximize the possibility that all individuals will be able to benefit).

Task Considerations

The most important component of designing a teaching situation is identifying the task to be learned. The task itself will often create constraints on possible teaching techniques and will help to define the approach. For example, if the task being taught is a motor task, then the approach will focus on motor behavior, and it would be inappropriate to address the task without a significant motor component. In the same way, if the task that is being taught is a behavioral response, then the teaching will emphasize initiation or practice of the behavior.

When defining the task, the practitioner must clearly define exactly what needs to be learned, so that the teaching plan can be organized around that task. Time is always an issue, and the goal is to teach the client the task as identified. This may require that the practitioner limit his or her objectives or defer other teaching to another setting or learning situation. Overestimating the client's ability to learn information can severely limit the effectiveness of a teaching situation. It is more appropriate for a client to learn a limited number of objectives thoroughly than to be overwhelmed by too much information and be unable to use any of it.

DIMENSIONS OF LEARNING

While in the past there has been a tendency to divide learning theory into motor learning theory and cognitive learning theory, there is increasing evidence that these interventions have the same mechanisms. While the research from these two areas has been approached from different directions and may use different language, there is increasing support for the concept that they are, in fact, the same process. Further, in most areas of occupational therapy, it would be difficult to find a task that is purely "motor" or purely "cognitive." Therefore, in this chapter, we will not be addressing these areas separately.

Specificity of Learning

One of the key things to remember when planning to teach a task is the issue of specificity of learning. Specificity of learning simply means that individuals learn what they are taught, but, more accurately, they learn exactly what they have been taught. The task is learned as taught, in the same sequence and exactly in the same environment (Zelazo, Zelazo, Cohen, & Zelazo, 1993). For many teaching situations, this presents a problem. For example, if a practitioner is teaching a client to cook a meal using a microwave oven in the clinic kitchen, even if the meal is the same as the client will be cooking at home after discharge, the environment will be very different. Further, the environment includes both the physical environment and the social environment. This means that the practitioner is included in the learning environment and becomes part of the context of the task. Therefore, clinicians must keep in mind the role they are planning in the teaching environment.

Transfer and Generalization of Learning

Two processes need to be taken into account in most learning situations to address the issue of specificity of learning. The first is transfer of training. Transfer of training occurs when the task itself remains the same and is performed in a new environment (Wulf & Schmidt, 1988). This occurs when the client is able to don a shirt in the hospital, and then puts on the same shirt at home. Transfer also needs to occur if the client dresses while sitting in a chair instead of sitting on the side of the bed. Most situations in which we ask clients to perform tasks require that they transfer the training from one environment to another.

Successful transfer of the task can be difficult for clients, in part because they may not recognize when the task should be performed without the environmental cues present at training (Godden & Baddeley, 1975). An example of the difficulty with task transfer occurs when teaching a client a skill such as assertiveness. The client may practice being assertive within the supportive environment of the teaching situation but may have difficulty identifying when to be assertive when no longer in that situation. One technique to help clients with transfer of training is to have the client practice in a variety of environments, so that he or she is able to recognize cues for performance (Wrisberg & Liu, 1991). This is why practicing tasks, whether they are cognitive or motor, within the performance environment is important.

Generalization is another major issue that needs to be considered to ensure that clients can continue to perform tasks after they leave the teaching situation. Generalization occurs when a client is asked to perform a task that is similar to, but not the same as, the learned task (Westling & Floyd, 1990). This occurs often in occupational therapy and can be very difficult for clients to resolve. An example of task generalization is asking a client to figure out how to put on a pullover shirt after he or she has been trained with a button-front shirt. The principles learned with the button-front shirt apply (weaker arm first), but the client needs to make adaptations and perform problem solving to perform the task. Many of the teaching situations that we encounter in OT require generalization of the task, and this must be included when designing the teaching situation.

One way to address the issue of specificity of learning and the challenges of transfer and generalization of learning is to systematically vary the task and the environment throughout the learning process (Neistadt, 1994; Toglia, 1991). This needs to be included in the original plan, as well as in any learning goals that are set. Issues of generalization and transfer of training must be addressed in order to plan effective teaching.

Procedural and Declarative Knowledge

Another factor closely related to specificity of learning is that of procedural and declarative knowledge. Procedural knowledge consists of knowing how to do something; a set of steps; a routine or operation that is performed, such as making a familiar meal or driving a familiar route (Katz, 1992). Declarative knowledge refers to knowing facts or information about objects or things (Katz, 1992). So, when designing a learning situation, it is important to determine whether the task you are teaching is primarily a procedural or a declarative task. For most activities in occupational therapy, the tasks will be procedural, such as dressing, cooking, or taking the bus. There is a routine that needs to be followed to complete a physical task. The issue of specificity of learning enters in here because there is poor evidence of transfer of training between procedural and declarative learning (Timmerman & Brouwer, 1999). For example, if an individual drives the same route to work everyday and the drive becomes routine, he or she may have difficulty writing down the steps that he or she takes. The person may not remember the names of the streets that he or she drives on or how many stoplights there are before a turn. However, they certainly know how to drive to work. Another example occurs in familiar cooking tasks. It is of limited value to ask a client to memorize the steps in making macaroni and cheese, but it is far more effective to have the person practice those steps as he or she makes the dish.

This distinction between declarative and procedural knowledge can become even more important with certain diagnostic groups. For example, some individuals with language or cognitive deficits may have extremely poor ability to access declarative knowledge but may be able to perform procedures that have become routine (Timmerman & Brouwer, 1999). They may not be able to explain how they do a task but are able to perform the task well. In this situation, focusing on declarative knowledge would be irrelevant to the task being taught and may lead to frustration.

Implicit and Explicit Learning

Implicit and explicit learning have many commonalities to procedural and declarative knowledge but are terms that are used in somewhat different ways. As was mentioned earlier, declarative and procedural memories are different in that they are different kinds of performance, with poor transfer of learning between them. Explicit knowledge is the same thing as declarative knowledge, meaning that it is information that can be found, named, and recited (Squire, 1994). However, implicit knowledge, while it includes procedural knowledge, also includes a number of other things. Specifically, implicit knowledge also includes skill-based learning that can only be demonstrated by the learner (Squire, 1994). Some examples of implicit knowledge are automatic behaviors in which behavior is set up by cues or the environment and may occur without a conscious decision to perform the activity. For example, people who have smoked for a long time and are trying to quit may find themselves smoking without thinking about it, the behavior triggered by the environment. In motor activities, force generation and the development of coordination or skill in movement are considered implicit knowledge. Individuals often are not consciously aware of how they have made these improvements and often cannot explain the process verbally, but, clearly, because behavior has changed, learning has occurred.

Designing a Teaching/Learning Session

Considering Learner Characteristics

As learners come to the learning situation, their current psychological state strongly influences their ability to learn. This state includes their personality, attitude toward learning the particular material, and current emotional state. Attention to this psychological readiness to learn will make the experience more successful. Furthermore, the learner also brings to the situation his or her past life experience, which can either facilitate or impede learning. It is critical to identify his or her attitude toward learning and his or her past learning experiences in order to develop an effective teaching situation. These factors will determine how well the person will be able to participate in learning at any given time. While the practitioner may not do a formal assessment of his or her current emotional state or attitudes toward learning, an informal assessment is included in the overall assessment that is performed prior to any teaching that occurs.

Identifying Learning Needs

One of the ongoing challenges of teaching is determining what "needs" to be taught in order to accomplish the desired outcomes. Setting the learning outcomes and conducting the needs assessment are reciprocal processes; it may be clear to the practitioner what the final outcome "should be," yet, the specific learning task needs to be set in response to a needs assessment. As the learning process continues, new information about the client may emerge, and the learning goals will change.

Robinson (1994) proposes three Rs of adult learning: relevancy, relationship, and responsibility. For the learning to be accepted, the content must be client centered (i.e., it must make sense to the learner, it must be related to the learner's perceived needs, and the learner must assume some level of responsibility for the learning). Robinson's three Rs are clearly consistent with the models of client education and the principles of adult learning previously discussed. The goal of the needs assessment is to determine what "needs" to be taught and to ensure that the learning is clearly focused on remediating a need, is meaningful to the client, and enhances self-efficacy.

Several sources or focuses of conducting a needs assessment will be briefly discussed: individual assessment, formal assessment or tests, group assessments, professional literature, and environmental analysis.

When preparing to teach a client information, the practitioner begins with an assessment of what is already known. This allows the teacher to target the content appropriately. This means that some type of evaluation is necessary as the session begins. This can be as simple as asking the client to perform a task and evaluating his or her performance, or asking the client what he or she already knows about the topic. In some settings, a formal pretest can be used to determine the prior level of knowledge. These assessments allow the teacher to assess any misinformation or assumptions that the client has made about the content area, as well as his or her attitude toward the material. It also identifies the level of information to provide and allows the teacher to make appropriate teaching goals.

In addition to a "content" assessment, it may be necessary to conduct an individual assessment to ascertain the client's problem-solving and other intellectual skills to properly plan teaching methods and to set realistic goals. It may be discerned that the client is not able to benefit from a client education session.

Another approach for conducting a needs assessment, especially in community settings, is through group discussion. A group of clients that share needs related to a universal condition (e.g., poverty, aging, a diagnostic condition) can serve as stimulants and clarifiers for each other in articulating needs as part of a planning process. In a transitional work setting where approximately six to nine marginalized workers were learning new work skills, a team of occupational therapy students were assigned to conduct weekly problem-solving groups. Given the setting and upon the advice of the program manager, the students decided to conduct a session on ergonomics and work safety. As the session started, the students noticed that they were getting little participation and interest in the topic. Finally, one of the students said, "Let's stop and talk about the session for a minute. What is going on?" One of the transitional workers timidly told the students that he or she had "had all of this material before." They have posters up all around the work area about safety tips. The students were resilient and immediately turned the session into a group needs assessment session: "What would you like to talk about in these problem-solving sessions?" The students asked the workers for ideas. What was on their minds? What were their concerns? They compiled a long and rich list of challenges to which a problem-solving approach could be applied. An additional benefit of conducting a group discussion is the elevated sense of commitment by publicly voicing a concern and having that concern reinforced by individuals in similar circumstances (Johnson & Johnson, 2000).

Although it is critical to be client-centered, the instructor must also teach content and use a teaching process that is evidence-based. That is, it is important to consult professional literature to ensure the various aspects of a condition. Approaches to teaching and variables important to success for change have been identified and included in the educational program.

Finally, the client's environment is critical in deciding what to teach. It really makes little difference how critical the learning might seem to the practitioner or how the literature supports the teaching. If the learned task cannot or will not be used in the client's environment, the teaching is likely going to be a waste of time. This is not to say one should give up in terms of attempting to change or add new behaviors to the client's repertoire; it simply means the client is not ready for an action-based program. The practitioner may need to evaluate the learning in terms of staged-based approaches, for example. The example noted earlier in the chapter (Shelly who wanted survival skills versus assertiveness training) demonstrates the necessity to include the client's anticipated environment in the needs assessment process.

Setting Learning Goals

Perhaps the first argument for taking the time to set explicit learning goals for the client is that goals are the measuring stick for the successfulness of the teaching/learning experience. Learning goals serve the same basic purposes as treatment goals and, like treatment goals, they must be relevant to the needs of the learner (McKeachie, 2002; Robinson, 1994).

One of the most common formats for expressing learning goals is the original version of Bloom's taxonomy. In this matrix, goals fall into three broad categories based on the type of learning: knowledge or cognitive, skill or psychomotor, and attitude or affective (Krathwohl, 1964; Robinson, 1994). The three types of objectives are important to differentiate because the teaching methods will vary depending on whether an attitude toward some action or behavior is being taught or the actual motor skill of carrying out the behavior. There are times when a complex skill includes objectives from more than one domain. For example, taking public transportation involves both cognitive planning and psychomotor skills.

In addition to the types of objectives there are three general levels of performance within each type of objective; the levels of performance are knowledge, application and problem solving. The knowledge level is an awareness and understanding of information level. The client, for example, may not necessarily apply the information to new situations and may only be able to mimic motor tasks. The application level includes using the learned information independently and in new, but related situations. From a values or attitude perspective, the client will act consistently when confronted with a situation that calls for value-based decision (e.g., stopping at red lights or taking turns in a food line). The problem-solving level allows the client to make independent decisions as to the appropriateness of a given action for a particular context. The client can invent new ways of carrying out a motor act, consistent with the overall goal when circumstances dictate (Krathwohl, 1964).

Bloom's taxonomy (Krathwohl, 2002) has recently undergone a revision and is expressed as a two by two matrix representing types of knowledge on one axis and cognitive processes on the alternate axis. The types of knowledge include factual knowledge, conceptual knowledge, procedural knowledge, and metacognitive knowledge. The most significant addition to types of knowledge was metacognitive. In the same way therapists place importance on a client being aware of his/her own ways of thinking and acting, it is important for the learner to be able to monitor her/her thinking and to be aware of what they do and do not know. The cognitive processes include familiar terms and additions to the original taxonomy previously described. The new categories of cognitive process are remember, understand, apply, analyze, evaluate, and create. Each of these categories is defined and subcategorized into explicit functions; apply, for example, includes "executing" and "implementing" (p. 215). Objectives, then can be analyzed and categorized by the type of knowledge required and the cognitive process being called for to achieve the outcome.

Once learning objectives have been written and analyzed, multiple key questions regarding the teaching/learning process are answered, what will be taught, what teaching processes should be used, what will be assessed, and how it will be assessed.

Selecting Methods for Teaching

Each individual has favored ways to learn information. For example, some individuals may be visual learners, while others benefit from audio presentation or from practice of the actual physical procedure. As mentioned earlier, these biases will range from preferred learning styles to obligatory learning styles. In many situations, presentation through a variety of modes, including auditory and visual presentation, as well as physical practice will help to address all of these learning styles. This is particularly important when presenting to groups of individuals whose learning styles will vary.

When using audiovisual presentations, such as videotapes, it is most effective to structure the session through the use of learning guides that focus attention on salient points or discussion of important information, either during the tape or at the end (Morgan & Salzberg, 1992; Rothstein & Arnold, 1976). Remember that a videotape is a teaching tool and needs the structure of a teacher to be most effective.

Assessing the Learning Environment

The general climate for adult learning will be humanistic in nature (Knowles et al., 1998). That is, the instructor should be prepared to construct a safe environment with a strong support system for the learner. Humanistic concepts such as positive regard, respect, and empathy all serve to free the learner to focus on the educational task. The conditions that have led to the learning experience for the adult learner are often stressful in nature; they could include poverty; recent trauma; new diagnosis; or losses such as death, divorce, or abandonment.

Barriers to Learning

Physiological

Physiological issues can also have a significant impact on learning. Clients who are uncomfortable, either physically or psychologically, are not in an optimal learning situation. These clients may need to have their learning needs addressed at a later time, for example, as an outpatient or through written or audiovisual material. Sometimes, this can be predicted, as in clients who are prepared for elective orthopedic procedures by learning the exercises and mobility techniques prior to surgery. This makes the overall teaching more effective, as the client needs only to review already learned material, rather than learn new information when he or she is recovering from surgery.

When individuals are unable to learn due to physiological issues, such as pain, level of alertness, or distress, and this could not be prepared for in advance, deferring teaching is one approach. However, there are times when that is not feasible. At those times, it is important to provide information that can be accessed by the client at a later time. Teaching a caregiver appropriate techniques and information is one approach, while providing written or audiovisual information is another. Again, multimodal presentation is best in this situation so that the individual will be more likely to be able to access the information later when it is needed.

When information is provided that may in itself be distressing to the client, providing a back-up form of this information is also helpful. This back up can be in the form of an audiotape of a family conference or clinic visit, a videotape of an exercise session, or a written progress note describing the session. In this way, the client is able to refer back to clarify and review content that he or she may not have been able to absorb at the time (Bruera, Pituskin, Calder, Neumann, & Hanson, 1999).

Social Environment

As noted earlier, the environment in which learning takes place is included in the learned content as the learning occurs. Because of this, the environment plays a significant role in any teaching that occurs. The environment referred to thus far has been the physical environment, but remember that environment includes not only the physical environment but the social environment including cultural norms and values. All of these factors influence how teaching occurs and how the individual client views teaching.

The most common goal of teaching in occupational therapy is to create a change in behavior. This applies whether the focus is cognitive or motor function. One of the social considerations in teaching has to do with the amount of support within the individual's social structure for the change in behavior that is being promoted. For example, in physical rehabilitation, there is often a great deal of peer support for the individual to improve and return to a previous level of function. However, in some cases, such as chemical dependency, there may be poor social support among the peers of a client to successfully change behavior. In that case, clients are often encouraged to create a new social support network, to create an atmosphere in which they are more likely to succeed. The health belief model, social cognitive theory, theory of reasoned action, and transtheoretical model all acknowledge the influence of the social environment on creating change in clients.

Some individuals may lack social support, living in an isolated social environment for a variety of reasons. For example, one problem for seniors is that, as they age, they may move into new environments and lose the support of their communities. These individuals often have difficulty developing support systems in their new environments, and part of the goal of occupational therapy programs for these groups is to help create new support structures in their current living situations.

Societal Policies and Attitudes

There are other social aspects to the learning situation. Policies and attitudes regarding teaching will influence how education is addressed. For example, much of the medical treatment provided for elderly Americans is funded by Medicare, which has policies about reimbursement of education in a health-care setting. Other third-party payers have also adopted these principles. Therefore, these policies have a profound impact on how this education is organized and provided. In this case, the term *skilled teaching* is used, and there are specific criteria that must be met in order to qualify (Berkeland, 1992).

Physical Environment

The physical environment can have a significant effect on how well individuals learn in another sense. Particularly for motor tasks, the meaning and purpose of the objects in the environment can influence how well clients move. For example, Mathiowetz and Wade (1995) demonstrated that the movement patterns of participants with multiple sclerosis and subjects with no central nervous system dysfunction depended on the type of props that were available to them. Eating applesauce with real objects (a bowl, a spoon, and applesauce) resulted in a different pattern of movement than pretending to eat applesauce with only a bowl and spoon, or pretending to eat applesauce with no physical props. This finding has also been found to be true for populations affected by stroke and brain injury as well (Nelson et al., 1996).

In other studies, it has been shown that the meaningfulness of a task can alter a client's tolerance for activity, tolerance for pain, and range of motion in ways that imaginary activities or rote activities do not (DeKuiper, Nelson, & White, 1993; Lin, Wu, Tickle-Degnen, & Coster, 1997). Also, when participants had some control over the task, such as choosing the task or when engaged in a game, they again had increased range of motion and endurance (LaMore & Nelson, 1993; Sietsema, Nelson, Mulder, Mervau-Sheidel, & White, 1993).

Applying Unique Learning Tools

Motor Learning

There are some special learning situations that have their own characteristics. One of these is the learning of motor tasks, although, as mentioned earlier, there is increasing evidence that these principles apply to all teaching. When teaching a motor task, a number of things must be planned. The first of these is the practice schedule or the organization of the tasks to be practiced. Then, the feedback schedule and format must be planned.

Practice schedules can be organized as blocked practice or as random practice. In blocked practice, individual tasks are repeated a number of times in succession, and then the next task is practiced in the same way (e.g., five repetitions of task A, then five repetitions of task B, then five repetitions of task C). In random practice, the tasks are ordered in a random order, practicing first task A, then B, then C, then B, and so on. Given the same number of repetitions of each task, the use of a blocked practice schedule results in faster acquisition of skill, but poorer retention; a random practice schedule results in slower acquisition of skill, but better retention of the tasks (Hanlon, 1996; Schmidt, 1988).

This discussion of acquisition and retention of tasks brings up the issue of performance and learning. Remembering our initial definition of learning as "a set of processes... leading to relatively permanent changes in the capability for responding" (Schmidt, 1988, p. 346), it is clear that any evidence of learning must be present at some time after the point of training. This means that if a client is able to perform a task after cues and practice, there is only evidence of performance. Evidence of learning must be evaluated at some point later (Schmidt, 1988). This is an important distinction; while it is important that clients be able to perform tasks, evidence of learning cannot be inferred from improved performance immediately after practice or cueing.

Appropriate feedback formats must also be identified for each task to be taught. For any activity, there is opportunity for internal and external feedback. After taking a test, students will have their own internal feedback about how they feel they did. External feedback is usually provided later after grading of the test has been completed. The accuracy of the internal feedback students provide themselves may be high or low, with students doing well on a test in which they anticipated a poor grade or performing poorly on a test they thought they aced. When working with clients, practitioners usually want to increase the accuracy of the internal feedback so that clients can accurately assess their own performance when no longer working with the practitioner (Schmidt, 1988).

Clinically, the most common form of external feedback is verbal feedback. However, verbal feedback can be a less effective feedback format for some types of tasks. For example, if a clinician is using verbal feedback for a motor task, the client may have difficulty interpreting the words used, such as "up," "down," "bend," or "straighten." For these types of tasks, video feedback can be more effective, allowing clients to make their own interpretations of the movement (Soderback, Bengtsson, Ginburg, & Ekholm, 1992; Tham & Tegner, 1997). Further, they can review the videotape as many times as they want to evaluate increased detail. Videotaped feedback can also be used to help clients identify impulsivity or other cognitive deficits (Guilmette & Kennedy, 1995). Other feedback formats include peer feedback or audio feedback. Again, these may be appropriate for specific situations.

Once the feedback format has been determined, the feedback schedule will need to be identified. Remember that it was stated earlier that context is included in information that is learned. This is particularly true of feedback schedules. Feedback schedules can be organized in a number of ways: constant feedback, summary feedback, or faded feedback (Schmidt, 1988). Constant feedback is feedback that is given after every trial. In this circumstance, the external feedback can become incorporated into the learning, and the learner becomes dependent on that external source of information and does not learn to provide his or her own internal analysis of the movement. The second type of feedback, summary feedback, is provided about each trial after a specific number of trials. For example, feedback will be given about each of five trials of a task after the fifth trial is completed. Using this type of feedback, individuals tend to analyze the tasks internally and use the external feedback to confirm or disconfirm their analysis. With this type of schedule, the teacher does not become as incorporated into the task that is learned. The third common type of external feedback schedule is faded feedback. In this case, feedback is given frequently as the practice is started and then is decreased over the practice session. In this case, the client gets more guidance as he or she begins the task and then learns to perform it without feedback at the end of the practice session (Schmidt, 1988; Weeks & Kordus, 1998).

One other type of feedback that has been discussed more recently is client-controlled feedback. In this case, the learner is responsible for requesting feedback when he or she wants it. The pattern of feedback that is typically requested is similar to faded feedback, with more frequent feedback initially and less feedback at the end of practice. Using this type of feedback allows clients to focus on the task and may make them more aware of the need to monitor their own performance and to attend to feedback when it is given (Janelle, Kim, & Singer, 1995; Janelle, Barba, Frehlich, Tennant, & Caurugh, 1997; McNevin, Wulf, & Carlson, 2000).

There are some concepts related to learning that have been studied recently that have clinical applications. These clinical applications include errorless learning, attentional focusing, scaffolding, and self-monitoring.

Errorless Learning

Errorless learning is a technique that is being used for primarily cognitive applications and was developed for individuals with significant cognitive deficits, including acquired brain injury, schizophrenia, and Alzheimer type dementia (Clare et al., 2000; O'Carroll, Russell, Lawrie, & Johnstone, 1999; Squires, Hunkin, & Parkin, 1997). When this technique is used, individuals are cued and directed as they learn a new skill, so that they do not make errors. This method is in direct contrast to the trial-and-error method often used in occupational therapy treatment. One justification for the errorless learning technique is that, for individuals who have impaired memory, it is difficult to identify when an error has been made and to then correct it. Therefore, the making of errors during learning for individuals with significant cognitive deficits is far more detrimental than for individuals with intact cognitive systems (Hunkin, Squires, Parkin, & Tidy, 1998).

The exact mechanism of errorless learning is somewhat unclear at this point, with current debate concerning whether it works because it uses implicit memory to compensate for lost explicit memory function, or whether prevention of errors during training simply limits interference of those errors on residual explicit memory. Nevertheless, particularly for those clients with memory deficits, the prevention of errors during the training process, through reverse chaining, or through the use of lists or other cues can have a significant positive impact on the ability to learn and retain new information (Evans et al., 2000).

When using errorless learning techniques, the task is clearly defined, and training is designed so that the client will make no errors during completion of the task. For example, the client might first complete the task with cues, and then, using a reverse chaining method, the clues are eliminated for the last step during the next practice. If an error is made, it is corrected immediately. Another technique used to prevent errors during practice is to have the client use a checklist during practice. However, there is some suggestion that checklists may promote more passive performance and may not require that the client be fully cognitively engaged with the task.

Attentional Focusing

Attentional focus is another special treatment approach that has primarily been addressed in motor tasks. The concept of attentional focus during motor performance is related to whether the focus of instruction and feedback is internal or external (Wulf, Höβ, & Prinz, 1998). Examples of internal focus are directions regarding force production, timing of muscle contractions, and body alignment. Examples of external focus include the effects of the movement and the rate or speed of an overall movement, such as focusing on the weight or movement of the golf club head or the location of the wheels in a simulated skiing machine.

In individuals with intact central nervous systems, it has been shown that internally focused information has a detrimental effect on the acquisition of complex motor skills and tends to make those skills more sensitive to breakdown with stress (Wulf & Weigelt, 1997). Furthermore, in several studies, control groups given no instructions for these complex motor tasks did better than those groups receiving internally focused instruction or feedback (Wulf & Weigelt, 1997; Wulf et al., 1998). Lastly, for individuals who were practicing complex motor tasks, internally focused information provided late in practice significantly degraded performance (Wulf & Weigelt, 1997; Wulf, Lautenbach, & Toole, 1999). While this research has not yet been replicated with individuals with central nervous system deficits, it does suggest that instructions and feedback regarding the performance of complex motor skills should be carefully planned.

Scaffolding

This is a technique that has emerged from the cognitive rehabilitation literature and has been applied primarily with clients who have significant cognitive deficits. This model of treatment breaks tasks down into a hierarchy of skills. The skills are then taught to the client, with each higher skill in the hierarchy building on and using the lower skill. Each skill that is learned serves as a platform for the new, higher level, more complex skill (Ben-Yishay & Diller, 1993). The strength of this type of training lies in accurately identifying the hierarchy of skills required for the functional task, so that the higher skills are well supported by the lower-level skills.

Self-Monitoring

The skill of self-monitoring is a metacognitive skill, which is necessary for individuals to be able to perform tasks independently. Without the ability to identify whether the task is being performed safely or correctly, the client will always require supervision. The issue of difficulty with self-monitoring arises in those clients with impaired self-awareness. As practitioners address treatment with clients, it is important to remember that there is no motivation to change or learn if individuals do not recognize that there is a problem. This fact explains why clients with brain injury who lack awareness of their deficits have significantly poorer outcomes than those individuals who have insight into their deficits (Guilmette & Kennedy, 1995).

The development of awareness of deficits is a prerequisite for developing compensation techniques, following the transtheoretical model of change, which was discussed earlier. Those individuals who are unaware of their deficits are in the precontemplative stage. Treatment directed at teaching these clients to compensate for their deficits will be frustrating for both the client and the practitioner because the client will view it as a waste of time because he or she is unaware that there is any reason to compensate. Treatment at this stage needs to be directed at helping the client become aware of the problem.

In an attempt to increase a client's awareness of the deficit, the practitioner can use questions to increase his or her awareness and control over his or her own thinking skills. The questions asked fit into several stages. The first stage is self-evaluation. The client is asked to estimate the difficulty of the task, time to complete the task, the number correct, and the amount of assistance he or she will need (Toglia, 1991). These questions begin to raise the client's awareness and provide a comparison point for discussion following the task. By following the task with the same kinds of questions, the practitioner is able to help the client compare them with the anticipated performance. Discrepancies between these two sets of answers provide the client with concrete, self-generated information about his or her deficit and his or her awareness of it (Guilmette & Kennedy, 1995; Toglia, 1991).

Other techniques to raise awareness include asking the client to assess someone else's performance (e.g., to identify errors in the practitioner's performance). This is followed by having the client ask him- or herself how he or she is doing during the task, to increase the chances for error detection and correction. The last step of this process is asking the client to evaluate the performance when it is completed. Is the work accurate? Is it completed? Did the client check for errors? How confident is he or she with the results (Toglia, 1991)? Through this process, the client is challenged to increase his or her awareness of his or her own performance.

Evaluation of Learning

The first place to look in evaluating the outcome of learning is the objectives. Evaluation methods should be planned at the beginning of the educational program to determine, first, if evaluation is possible or realistic and, second, to make the necessary preparations to evaluate. Two categories of evaluation include formative and summative. These terms have typically been applied to classroom settings, but they are equally applicable to adult learning and community settings. Formative evaluations take place during the educational program. They allow the instructor to change methods or the focus of the learning based on feedback. Formative evaluations look at what the client is learning, the level of thinking he or she is engaging, and his or her response to the learning environment. Angelo and Cross (1993) provide a rich set of examples and methods for designing formative evaluation techniques.

Summative evaluations come at the end of "formal" learning and classically evaluate whether or not the objectives have been achieved. Evaluation plans should have several steps (Robinson, 1994). First is a statement of the learning objectives. The objectives will be the primary focus of any evaluations conducted. Second, sources of evidence need to be identified. Who is likely to observe whether or not the learned behavior is consistently being used and how effectively is it being applied? In looking for change in a community mental health center client, for example, sources of evidence might be the client, the staff at the community drop-in center, the client's social worker, the client's family, and the apartment building caretaker where the client lives. The third step in the evaluation plan is deciding whom to evaluate (i.e., selecting the sample). It is possible that every client will be evaluated depending on the scope and type of program. If the educational program serves many clients, however, it may be more realistic to select a sample of clients representing a variety of objectives over time. Fourth is the method of data collection. How data are collected will depend on the type of objective being evaluated. Typical methods might include observation, tests, interviews, checklists, supervisor reports, questionnaires, or data review (e.g., recidivism). Finally, decisions must be made as to what to do with the data. These decisions should be made before the data are collected. The data will be analyzed with respect to the intended objectives and will be transformed into program recommendations.

Instructor Characteristics and Style

The concept of what makes a successful instructor is somewhat elusive and probably as contextual as what makes a successful practitioner. There are, however, some categories of behavior that seem to be associated with successful instructors and that seem to be noted as important behaviors in student evaluations of instructors (Chickering & Gamson, 1987; McKeachie, 2002; Smith & Waller, 1997). The categories include subject-related, intrinsic qualities; interpersonal skills; physical presence; and process characteristics.

Subject characteristics simply mean the instructor has a command of the subject or topic being taught. The instructor also has professional credibility to teach in the context of the learning.

Intrinsic qualities relate to the emotional characteristics of the instructor. The primary feature is that the instructor is emotionally stable and considered safe from the learner's perspective. Further characteristics in this category include patience, honesty, respect for the learner, empathy, warmth, accessibility to the instructor, having a positive attitude, openness, and basic intelligence.

Interpersonal skills important to the learning environment can be grouped into specific skills and a more global characterization of "counseling skills." Some of the noted specific skills include using humor, being enthusiastic, flexibility, and spontaneity. Counseling skills entail a mix of active listening, empathy, and effective verbal skills.

The effective teacher also projects a certain physical presence. The successful instructor projects confidence and comfort with him- or herself. The effective instructor has a positive affect and is aware of and in control of his or her gestures.

Finally, there is a set of process skills associated with being an effective teacher. Process skills include organization and respect for diverse talents and different ways of learning. Other instructional process skills include giving feedback; being objective; communicating high, but realistic expectations; and being goal directed. The successful instructor is student centered and encourages active learning.

A final note with respect to instructor style relates to the instructor's personality style or type. Most instructors teach with the same personality style(s) that they prefer learning from. This means that the learner may be experiencing a nonpreferred style of learning most of the time. In terms of learning styles, learners typically have preferred methods of taking in new information as well as preferred methods of analyzing and making decisions with respect to the perceived information (Myers, 1998;

Robinson, 1994). The challenge to the instructor is to present information in and to offer alternate analytical styles that reflect different styles of learning. Four learning styles include feelers, thinkers, doers, and intuiters. Doers, for example, prefer to learn by doing; they are more pragmatic and concrete and prefer to follow explicit directions. Intuiters, in contrast, tend to be creative, big-pictured, and future-oriented, and tend to seek possibilities. All learners are capable of learning from the perspective of different learning styles. It is the instructor's challenge, however, to maximize the students' possibilities by offering learning experiences that match their preferred learning styles. This requires variable approaches to learning, constant evaluation, and flexibility.

REFERENCES

Angelo, T. A., & Cross, K. P. (1993). *Classroom assessment techniques* (2nd ed.). San Francisco, CA: Jossey-Bass.

Baranowski, T., Perry, C. L., and Parcel, G. S. (1997). How individuals, environments, and health behavior interact. In K. Glanz, F. M. Lewis, & B. K. Timmer (Eds.), *Health behavior and health education, theory research and practice* (2nd ed.). (pp. 153-178). San Francisco: Jossey-Bass.

Barr, R. B., & Tagg, J. (1995). From teaching to learning: A new paradigm for undergraduate education. *Change, November-December*, 13-25.

Ben-Yishay, Y., & Diller, L. (1993). Cognitive remediation in traumatic brain injury: Update and issues. *Archives of Physical Medicine and Rehabilitation, 74*, 204-213.

Berkeland, R. S. (1992). A model of medical review consultation: Insurance criteria. In E. Jaffe & C. Epstein (Eds.), *Occupational therapy consultation* (pp. 519-532). St. Louis: Mosby.

Brewer, J. L., Blake, A. J., Rankin, S. A., & Douglass, L. W. (1999). Theory of reasoned action predicts mild consumption in women. *Journal of the American Dietetic Association, 99*, 39.

Bruera, E., Pituskin, E., Calder, K., Neumann, C. M., & Hanson, J. (1999). The addition of an audiocassette recording of a consultation to written recommendations for patients with advanced cancer: A randomized controlled trial. *Cancer, 86*, 2420-2425.

Campbell, W. E., & Smith, K. A. (Eds.). (1997). *New paradigms for college teaching*. Edina, MN: Interaction Book Company.

Carter, W. B. (1990). Health behavior as rational process: Theory of reasoned action and multiattribute utility theory. In K. Glanz, F. M. Lewis, & B. K. Timmer (Eds.), *Health behavior and health education, theory research and practice* (pp. 63-91). San Francisco, CA: Jossey-Bass.

Chen, C. Y., Neufeld, P. S., Feely, C. A., & Skinner, C. S. (1999). Factors influencing compliance with home exercise programs among patients with upper-extremity impairment. *American Journal of Occupational Therapy, 53*, 171-180.

Chickering, A. W., & Gamson, Z. F. (1987). Seven principles for good practice in undergraduate education. *The Wingspread Journal, 9*(2), special insert.

Clare, L., Wilson, B. A., Carter, G., Breen, K., Gosses, A., & Hodges, J. R. (2000). Intervening with everyday memory problems in dementia of Alzheimer type: An errorless learning approach. *Journal of Clinical and Experimental Neuropsychology, 22*, 132-146.

DeKuiper, W. P., Nelson, D. L., & White, B. E. (1993). Materials-based occupation versus imagery-based occupation versus rote exercise: A replication and extension. *The Occupational Therapy Journal of Research, 13*, 183-197.

Evans, J. J., Wilson, B. A., Schuri, U., Andrade, J., Baddeley, A., Bruna, O., et al. (2000). A comparison of "errorless" and "trial-and-error" learning methods for teaching individuals with acquired memory deficits. *Neuropsychological Rehabilitation, 120*, 67-101.

Fried, J. L., DeVore, L., & Dailey, J. (2001). A study of Maryland dental hygienists' perceptions regarding self-assessment. *Journal of Dental Hygiene, 75*, 121.

Godden, D. R., & Baddeley, A. D. (1975). Context-dependent memory in two natural environments: On land and underwater. *British Journal of Psychology, 66*, 325-331.

Guilmette, T. J., & Kennedy, M. L. (1995). Neurocognitive rehabilitation guidelines for therapists. *Topics in Stroke Rehabilitation, 2*, 32-43.

Hanlon, R. E. (1996). Motor learning following unilateral stroke. *Archives of Physical Medicine and Rehabilitation, 77*, 811-815.

Health Partners. (1998). Here's the secret to successful behavior change. *Discover*, 4-5.

Hunkin, N. M., Squires, E. J., Parkin, A. J., & Tidy, J. A. (1998). Are the benefits of errorless learning dependent on implicit memory? *Neuropsychologia, 36*, 25-36.

Janelle, C. M., Barba, D., Frehlich, S. G., Tennant, L. K., & Caurugh, J. H. (1997). Maximizing performance feedback effectiveness through videotape replay and a self-controlled learning environment. *Research Quarterly for Exercise and Sport, 68*, 269-279.

Janelle, C. M., Kim, J., & Singer, R. N. (1995). Subject-controlled performance feedback and learning of a closed motor skill. *Perceptual and Motor Skills, 81*, 627-634.

Johnson, D. W., & Johnson, F. P. (2000). *Joining together, group theory and skills*. Boston, MA: Allyn and Bacon.

Katz, N. (1992). *Cognitive rehabilitation: Models for intervention in occupational therapy*. Stoneham, MA: Andover Medical.

Kielhofner, G. (2004). *Conceptual foundations of occupational therapy* (3rd ed.). Philadelphia, PA: F. A. Davis.

Knowles, M. S. (1970). *The modern practice of adult education: Andragogy versus pedagogy*. New York, NY: Association Press.

Knowles, M. S. (1973). *The adult learner: A neglected species*. Houston, TX: Gulf.

Knowles, M. S. (1984). *Andragogy in action*. San Francisco, CA: Jossey-Bass.

Evidence Worksheet

Authors	*Year*	*Topic*	*Method*	*Conclusion*
Brewer et al.	1999	Theory of reasoned action used to predict milk consumption in women	CT	Theory of reasoned action demonstrated as a viable method for determining key decision factors
Bruera et al.	1999	The use of audiotapes to supplement written information	RCT	In situations of stress, redundant information improves recall and satisfaction of patients
Chen et al.	1999	Factors influencing compliance with home exercise programs	CT	Component of the HBM and MOHO, self-efficacy, was cited as contributing to prediction of compliance
Clare et al.	2000	Errorless learning in six clients with DAT	CT	The use of individualized training programs and errorless learning techniques resulted in improvement in daily memory performance in five participants, with retention at 6 months
DeKuiper et al.	1993	Comparing imagery-based materials and rote exercise	RCT	Participation in exercise using real materials elicited more repetitions than either of the other two conditions
Evans et al.	2000	Comparison of errorless and trial-and-error learning methods	RCT	In clients with TBI, errorless learning methods improved learning on implicit tasks, while it did not improve performance on explicit memory tasks
Fried et al.	2001	Application of the theory of reasoned action to self-assessment behavior of dental hygienists	RCT	Demonstrated that the model was a valid tool for analyzing future behavior. Discussed additional applications
Godden & Baddeley	1975	Transfer of learning between different environments	RCT	In a cognitive task, participants recalled information better in environment they trained in than in another environment
Hanlon	1996	Blocked and random practice in motor learning tasks	RCT	Random practice is more effective than blocked practice in teaching motor tasks
Hunkin et al.	1998	Errorless learning techniques with individuals with memory deficits	RCT	Errorless learning techniques are more effective than trial-and-error techniques in teaching individuals with memory deficits
Janelle et al.	1997	Self-controlled feedback while learning a motor skill	RCT	Learning of motor tasks is enhanced if the learner is allowed to control the feedback environment
Janelle et al.	1995	Schedules of feedback on motor performance	RCT	Participants who controlled their own feedback did significantly better than any other feedback condition

(continued)

Authors	*Year*	*Topic*	*Method*	*Conclusion*
Kretzer & Larson	1998	Addresses the need to combine elements of several theories of client education	Theory development	Presented a set of principles for a comprehensive approach to client education
LaMore & Nelson	1993	Effect of choice of activity on participation in patients with mental disabilities	RCT	The participants who had a choice of activity painted more than participants who did not have a choice of activity
Lin et al.	1997	Impact of occupational embedded exercise	Meta-analysis	In a broad variety of situations, exercise embedded in occupation is more effective than rote exercise
Mathiowetz & Wade	1995	Informational support and motor performance	RCT	The motor patterns elicited by three different levels of informational support were different from each other, indicating that the participants performed differently with different task demands
McGahee et al.	2000	Theory of reasoned action and social cognitive theory combined as a model to understand and impact smoking prevention efforts	Theory development	Developed a new theory combining elements of TRA and SCT
Morgan & Salzberg	1992	Use of videotape in training for adults with severe mental disabilities	CT	Videotape is effective in helping indviduals identify problematic behaviors, but specific training in appropriate behavior is then needed
Neistadt	1994	Effects of the type of practice activity on coordination scores	RCT	Participants practicing functional task of meal preparation made greater gains in coordination than those doing table top perceptual tasks
Nelson et al.	1996	Effect of activity selection on AROM	RCT	Greater AROM was elicited in patients with hemiplegia when exercise was embedded in occupation than when just exercise was performed
O'Carroll et al.	1999	Errorless learning in clients with memory impairments and schizophrenia	CT	Errorless learning was effective in improving learning in clients with memory problems and schizophrenia, while trial-and-error techniques resulted in poor performance
Prochaska	1994	Looking at factors influencing a change from the precontemplative to action stages of change	Cross-sectional analysis of multiple studies	Identified patterns of behavior change based on the strength of the pros and cons for the change
Prochaska et al.	1992	Investigation of how people change health behaviors	Descriptive analysis of studies	Described research supports a change process consistent with the stages of the transtheoretical model

(continued)

Authors	*Year*	*Topic*	*Method*	*Conclusion*
Schmidt & Wulf	1997	Effect of continuous feedback on motor skill learning	RCT	Continuous feedback interferes with learning of motor skills
Shea & Wulf	1999	Effect of externally focused instructions and feedback	RCT	Participants who were instructed to focus on environmental cues rather than body alignment cues were better able to generalize and retain motor tasks
Sietsema et al.	1993	Effect of activity on active ROM in people with TBI	RCT	Embedding exercise into an activity will elicit greater active ROM than rote exercise
Soderback et al.	1992	Use of videotape feedback with patient with left neglect	SCSD	Videotape can be an effective tool to increase awareness of left neglect in patients with deficits
Squires et al.	1997	Effectiveness of errorless learning in individuals with memory impairments	RCT	Learning using errorless techniques was more effective than trial-and-error in learning novel association tasks
Tham & Tegner	1997	Videotape feedback for individuals with unilateral neglect	RCT	The use of videotape feedback can be useful in improving performance in individuals with unilateral neglect
Timmerman & Brouwer	1999	Differences in recall of procedural and declarative information in individuals with brain injury	RCT	Individuals with memory deficits due to brain injury have better access to procedural memory than declarative memory
Weeks & Kordus	1998	Effects of feedback patterns on motor skill acquisition	CT	Feedback on one-third of the practice trials of a motor task was more effective for retention and transfer than constant feedback
Wrisberg & Liu	1991	Practice of tasks in a variety of contexts	RCT	Practice of tasks in a variety of contexts improves the performance of the tasks for retention and transfer
Wulf et al.	1998	The effect of focus of attention on motor learning	RCT	Directing learners to focus on contextual, or external, cues was more effective than directing them to focus on the body movement, internal focus
Wulf et al.	1999	The effect of focus of attention on motor learning	RCT	Using external cues to focus learners on the environment was more effective than internal cues directing them to focus on body movements themselves
Wulf & Weigelt	1997	Effect of instructions on the learning of a complex motor skill	RCT	Giving individuals instructions regarding the mechanics of a complex motor skill degrades learning
Zelazo et al.	1993	Specificity of learning in 6-week-old infants	RCT	Practice of specific motor tasks improved performance of only those motor tasks with poor transfer between tasks

Knowles, M. S., Holton III, E. F., & Swanson, R. A. (1998). *The adult learner* (5th ed.). Houston, TX: Butterworth-Heinemann.

Krathwohl, D. R. (1964). The taxonomy of educational objectives, its use in curriculum building. In C. M. Lindvall (Ed.), *Defining educational objectives*. Pittsburgh, PA: University of Pittsburgh.

Krathwohl, D.R. (2002). A revision of Bloom's taxonomy: An overview. *Theory Into Practice, 41*, 212-218.

Kretzer, E. K., & Larson, E. L. (1998). Behavioral interventions to improve infection control practice. *American Journal of Infection Control, 26*, 245-253.

LaMore, K. L., & Nelson, D. L. (1993). The effects of options on performance of an art project in adults with mental disabilities. *American Journal of Occupational Therapy, 47*, 397-401.

Lewis, F. M., & Daltroy, L. H. (1990). How causal explanations influence health behavior: Attribution theory. In K. Glanz, F. M. Lewis, & B. K. Timmer (Eds.), *Health behavior and health education, theory, research and practice* (pp. 92-114). San Francisco, CA: Jossey-Bass.

Lin, C., Wu, C., Tickle-Degnen, L., & Coster, W. (1997). Enhancing occupational performance through occupationally embedded exercise: A meta-analytic review. *Occupational Therapy Journal of Research, 17*, 25-47.

Mathiowetz, V., & Wade, M. G. (1995). Task constraints and functional motor performance of individuals with and without multiple sclerosis. *Ecological Psychology, 7*, 99-123.

McGahee, T. W., Kemp, V., & Tingen, M. (2000). A theoretical model for smoking prevention studies in preteen children. *Pediatric Nursing, 26*, 135.

McKeachie, W. J. (2002). *Teaching tips* (11th ed.). Boston, MA: Houghton Mifflin.

McNevin, N. H., Wulf, G., & Carlson, C. (2000). Effects of attentional focus, self-control, and dyad training on motor learning: Implications for physical rehabilitation. *Physical Therapy, 80*, 373-385.

Montano, D. E., Karprzyk, D., & Taplin, S. H. (1997). The theory of reasoned action and the theory of planned behavior. In K. Glanz, F. M. Lewis, & B. K. Timmer (Eds.), *Health behavior and health education, theory research and practice* (2nd ed., pp. 63-91). San Francisco, CA: Jossey-Bass.

Morgan, R. L., & Salzberg, C. S. (1992). Effects of video-assisted training on employment-related social skills of adults with severe mental retardation. *Journal of Applied Behavioral Analysis, 25*, 365-383.

Myers, I. B. (1998). *Introduction to type* (rev. ed.). Palo Alto, CA: Consulting Psychologists Press.

Neistadt, M. E. (1994). The effects of different treatment activities on functional fine motor coordination in adults with brain injury. *American Journal of Occupational Therapy, 48*, 878-882.

Nelson, D. L., Konosky, K., Fleherty, K., Webb, R., Newer, K., Hazboun, V. P., et al. (1996). *American Journal of Occupational Therapy, 50*, 639-646.

O'Callaghan, F. V., Chant, D. C., Callan, V. J., & Baglioni, A. (1997). Models of alcohol use by young adults: An examination of various attitude-behavior theories. *Journal of Studies on Alcohol, 58*, 502.

O'Carroll, R. E., Russell, H. H., Lawrie, S. M., & Johnstone, E. C. (1999). Errorless learning and the cognitive rehabilitation of memory-impaired schizophrenic patients. *Psychological Medicine, 29*, 105-112.

Perry, C. L., Baranowski, T., & Parcel, G. S. (1990). How individuals, environments, and health behavior interact: Social learning theory. In K. Glanz, F. M. Lewis, & B. K. Timmer (Eds.), *Health behavior and health education, theory, research and practice* (pp. 161-186). San Francisco, CA: Jossey-Bass.

Prochaska, J. O. (1994). Strong and weak principle for progressing from precontemplation to action on the basis of twelve problem behaviors. *Health Psychology, 13*, 47-51.

Prochaska, J. O., DiClemente, C. O., & Norcross, J. C. (1992). In search of how people change. *American Psychologist, 47*, 1102-1113.

Prochaska, J. O., Redding, C. A., & Evers, K. E. (1997). The transtheoretical model and stages of change. In K. Glanz, F. M. Lewis, & B. K. Timmer (Eds.), *Health behavior and health education, theory research and practice* (2nd ed., pp. 63-91). San Francisco, CA: Jossey-Bass.

Prochaska, J. O., Velicer, W. F., DiClemente, C. C., & Fava, J. (1988). Measuring processes of change: Applications to the cessation of smoking. *Journal of Consulting and Clinical Psychology*, 56, 520-528.

Robinson, R. D. (1994). *Helping adults learn and change* (rev. ed.). West Bend, WI: Omnibook.

Rosenstock, I. M. (1990). The health belief model: Explaining health behavior through expectancies. In K. Glanz, F. M. Lewis, & B. K. Timmer (Eds.), *Health behavior and health education, theory research and practice* (pp. 39-62). San Francisco, CA: Jossey-Bass.

Rothstein, A. L., & Arnold, R. K. (1976). Bridging the gap: Application of research on videotape feedback and bowling. *Motor Skills: Theory Into Practice, 1*, 35-55.

Schmidt, R. A. (1988). *Motor control and learning: A behavioral emphasis* (2nd ed.). Champaign, IL: Kinetic Publishers.

Schmidt, R. A., & Wulf, G. (1997). Continuous concurrent feedback degrades skill learning: Implications for training and simulation. *Human Factors, 39*, 509-525.

Shea, C. H., & Wulf, G. (1999). Enhancing motor learning through external-focus instructions and feedback. *Human Movement Science, 18*, 553-571.

Sietsema, J. M., Nelson, D. L., Mulder, R. M., Mervau-Sheidel, D., & White, B. E. (1993). The use of a game to promote arm reach in persons with traumatic brain injury. *American Journal of Occupational Therapy, 47*, 19-24.

Smith, K., & Waller, A. (1997). Afterword: New paradigms for college teaching. In W. E. Campbell & K. A. Smith (Eds.), *New paradigms for college teaching* (pp. 269-281). Edina, MN: Interaction Book Company.

Soderback, I., Bengtsson, I., Ginburg, E., & Ekholm, J. (1992). Video feedback in occupational therapy: Its effect in patients with neglect syndrome. *Archives of Physical Medicine and Rehabilitation, 73,* 1140-1146.

Squire, L. R. (1994). Declarative and nondeclarative memory: Multiple brain systems support learning and memory. In D. Schacter & E. Tulving (Eds.), *Memory Systems 1994.* Cambridge, MA: MIT Press.

Squires, E. J., Hunkin, N. M., & Parkin, A. J. (1997). Errorless learning of novel associations in amnesia. *Neuropsychologia, 35,* 1110-1111.

Tham, K., & Tegner, R. (1997). Video feedback in the rehabilitation of patients with unilateral neglect. *Archives of Physical Medicine and Rehabilitation, 78,* 410-413.

Timmerman, M. E., & Brouwer, W. H. (1999). Slow information processing after very severe closed head injury: Impaired access to declarative knowledge and intact application and acquisition of procedural knowledge. *Neuropsychologia, 37,* 467-478.

Toglia, J. P. (1991). Generalization of treatment: A multicontext approach to cognitive perceptual impairment in adults with brain injury. *American Journal of Occupational Therapy, 45,* 505-516.

Weeks, D. L., & Kordus, R. N. (1998). Relative frequency of knowledge of performance and motor skill learning. *Research Quarterly for Exercise and Sport, 69,* 224-230.

Westling, D. L., & Floyd, J. (1990). Generalization of community skills: How much training is necessary? *The Journal of Special Education, 23,* 386-406.

Wrisberg, C. A., & Liu, Z. (1991). The effect of contextual variety on the practice, retention, and transfer of an applied motor skill. *Research Quarterly for Exercise and Sport, 62,* 406-412.

Wulf, G., Höß, M., & Prinz, W. (1998). Instructions for motor learning: Differential effects of internal versus external focus of attention. *Journal of Motor Behavior, 30,* 169-179.

Wulf, G., Lauterbach, B., & Toole, T. (1999). The learning advantage of an external focus of attention in golf. *Research Quarterly for Exercise and Sport, 70,* 120-126.

Wulf, G., & Schmidt, R. A. (1988). Variability in practice: Facilitation in retention and transfer through schema formation or context effects? *Journal of Motor Behavior, 20,* 133-149.

Wulf, G., & Weigelt, C. (1997). Instructions about physical principles in learning a complex motor skill: To tell or not to tell… *Research Quarterly for Exercise and Sport, 68,* 362-367.

Zelazo, N. A., Zelazo, P. A., Cohen, K. M., & Zelazo, P. D. (1993). Specificity of practice effects on elementary neuromotor patterns. *Developmental Psychology, 29,* 686-691.

Chapter Seventeen: Therapy as Learning Reflections and Learning Activities

Julie Bass-Haugen, PhD, OTR/L, FAOTA

Reflections

What is occupational therapy all about? What happens in the therapeutic process? I think the answer to these two questions is "change." The purpose of occupational therapy is to facilitate change in occupational performance. Change in occupational performance occurs through learning. So, one of the roles of the occupational therapy practitioner is teacher.

Client education is a part of every interaction between the client and the occupational therapy practitioner. Sometimes, education is a smaller part of another type of intervention. For example, if a client is provided with adaptive equipment as part of a compensation intervention strategy, the practitioner uses educational strategies to introduce the client to the equipment. Sometimes, education is the primary intervention provided. For example, energy conservation principles are taught to many clients who have fatigue issues and limited endurance.

Let's look at the case of Brad who was diagnosed with multiple sclerosis (MS) 2 years ago. In this medical condition and others (e.g., myasthenia gravis, stroke), fatigue may be a significant physiological factor that constrains occupational performance and influences the course of the medical condition itself. Brad's physician has been concerned about the progression of the disease and has recommended that Brad re-evaluate his current priorities and lifestyle. Until now, Brad had maintained the same 60-hour-per-week work schedule he had prior to his diagnosis, is an officer in his local professional association, and plays basketball in pick-up games 5 days a week. Brad was referred to occupational therapy to examine the influence of fatigue on his performance and explore energy management strategies that might be employed in his daily life. The occupational therapy practitioner has adopted an education intervention as the method for addressing Brad's energy management and conservation needs. Let's explore different scenarios related to the four teaching/learning models as they apply to the case of Brad.

Health Belief Model

After visiting with his physician and doing some online research, Brad concluded his frequent bouts of extreme fatigue were likely influencing his condition. He was concerned that fatigue would have serious consequences for his future functioning if it was not brought under control. Brad had heard from members of his MS support group that they benefited from their participation in a health education program on energy conservation. They also felt the things they learned were easily implemented in their lives.

In occupational therapy, Brad was asked to complete a profile of his fatigue patterns, daily occupations and lifestyle, and his occurrences of problems associated with MS. The occupational therapy practitioner also presented evidence related to the effect of fatigue on MS and supported Brad's conclusion that control of fatigue was critical for the current and future management of his condition. An education program on energy conservation was designed to include description of the targeted health and performance outcomes, specific energy conservation strategies to implement in his daily life, and a success-oriented learning activity.

Attribution Theory

Brad and his occupational therapy practitioner explored the causes of his frequent bouts of extreme fatigue. After they reviewed his daily occupations and lifestyle, Brad concluded that he had not made any significant modifications in his routines to control fatigue and support management of his condition. He stated it was obvious that a good part of the fatigue issues could be addressed by making little changes in his life.

The occupational therapy practitioner supported Brad's conclusions about the cause of his fatigue and acknowledged that changing routines was difficult. They agreed that some aspects of Brad's work were not under his control (e.g., deadlines) but identified specific energy management strategies that could be built into his regular workday. Brad's therapist supported him in his selection of techniques to try at work, offered suggestions regarding their implementation, and provided a learning experience to pilot their use in a regular workday.

Theory of Reasoned Action

The occupational therapy practitioner asked Brad to describe his attitude toward routines and lifestyles that emphasized time management, balance, and self-monitoring of energy expenditures. Brad stated he admired people who seemed to handle all the commitments of their life with ease and energy to spare. These skills just did not come naturally for him.

The therapist concluded that Brad would like to live a different way but had not had the opportunity to develop the necessary skills. Brad viewed a motivational video to strengthen his positive feelings about this new lifestyle. They agreed he would benefit by linking up with a mentor or role model who could introduce specific strategies for time management and work simplification.

Transtheoretical Model

Brad and the occupational therapy practitioner reviewed the events that led up to this referral. Brad reported that fatigue had been an issue for at least a year even though he had periodically tried a few energy conservation techniques (e.g., precontemplative). During the past several months, he had considered the need for change but had delayed any appointment using one excuse after another (e.g., contemplative). After a particularly bad week recently, he decided he was tired of being tired. He wanted to commit to a change in his life by taking all the necessary steps to manage his energy (e.g., preparation). He had made this appointment because he wanted information on specific strategies.

The occupational therapy practitioner provided encouragement and prepared Brad for the action stage of change. They identified the problems he typically experienced in his workday and the barriers that would need to be addressed as part of the change. The therapist forewarned Brad of the processes that would be required to sustain the change over time as he entered the maintenance stage. They brainstormed ways to build in rewards, supports, healthy behaviors, and restructured stimuli.

Each of these models provides a framework for thinking about client education in a particular situation. Regardless of the model(s) chosen, the development and implementation of client education programs requires consideration of learning principles, characteristics having an effect on learning, dimensions of learning, design issues, and unique learning tools. Let's consider these concepts by continuing the example of Brad.

Principles and Characteristics

The occupational therapy practitioner needs to consider principles of adult education and Brad's characteristics in planning an education intervention. Brad will need to understand why energy management is important to learn. It is also not a given that Brad will agree to this intervention. The practitioner will need to consider what Brad brings to the education intervention, including his mature self-concept, prior experiences, readiness for learning, definition of the fatigue problem, and internal motivation for learning. An assessment of Brad's personal factors, environmental factors (social cognitive theory), and occupational performance will also influence the nature of the education intervention.

Dimensions of Learning

As specific energy management strategies are selected for the education program, the occupational therapy practitioner must consider specific dimensions of learning. When a work simplification strategy is introduced in the clinic setting, Brad's tendency will be to remember and apply the strategy in the exact same way it is taught (i.e., specificity of learning). If the work environment is quite different from the clinic, the practitioner can facilitate the transfer of learning from clinic to work and generalization of the strategy to other situations by introducing the work simplification strategy in a variety of occupations and environments. The therapist may also ask how this particular strategy is typically learned. Some strategies are learned by following procedures or steps (i.e., procedural knowledge) or by tapping into the personal skills of the learner (i.e., implicit learning), while other strategies are acquired through facts or information (i.e., declarative knowledge, explicit learning).

Design Issues and Unique Learning Tools

The design of an educational intervention involves the identification of the actual components of the learning session. An assessment of Brad can provide the basis for selection of the specific topics for inclusion in the session (i.e., the learner's needs). The topics then form the basis for learning goals targeted toward Brad's acquisition of knowledge, skills, or attitudes. The learning goals guide the selection of appropriate methods. Finally, physical, societal policies and attitudes, and social environment are constructed to provide the best possible climate for learning. Specific learning strategies may also be incorporated for unique motor or cognitive learning situations (e.g., practice, feedback, errorless learning, attentional focusing, scaffolding, and self-monitoring).

As you can see, teaching and learning in occupational therapy is just as complex as teaching and learning in a classroom. For education interventions to be effective, all of these teaching and learning qualities must be considered. How do you measure the outcomes of an education intervention? It is measured the same way as other interventions. The client's goals related to occupational performance and participation are the desired outcomes of the intervention. Now, you have a basic understanding of your role as a teacher in the therapy process.

Journal Activities

1. Look up and write down a dictionary definition of teaching, learning, and education. Highlight the components of the definitions that are most related to their descriptions in Chapter Seventeen.
2. Identify the most important new learning for you in this chapter.
3. Identify one question you have about Chapter Seventeen.
4. Reflect on the role of teaching and learning in occupational therapy practice. To what extent is it possible to provide occupational therapy interventions without a teaching/learning framework?
5. Reflect on one of the best teaching/learning environments you have experienced. Describe the characteristics of the environment that made it so positive. Reflect on one of the worst teaching/learning environments you have experienced. Describe the characteristics of the environment that made it so negative. What implications do these experiences have for your occupational therapy practice?

Technology/Internet Learning Activities

1. Use a discussion database to share specific journal activities.
2. Use a good Internet search engine to find the Web site for the National Commission for Health Education Credentialing.
    - Enter the phrase "nchec" in your search line.
    - Review the home page of the Web site.
    - Evaluate the quality of this Web site. What are its strengths and limitations?
    - What is the purpose of this Web site?
    - Who sponsors this Web site?
    - What are the responsibilities and competencies for a credentialed health educator?
3. Use a good Internet search engine to find several online health education programs.
    - Enter the phrases "American Heart Association," American Lung Association," and "American Cancer Society."
    - Document and review the home page for each Web site.
    - Evaluate the quality of this Web site. What are its strengths and weaknesses?
    - What is the overall purpose of this Web site?
    - Describe teaching/learning opportunities that are available on each site.
    - Identify health education models that are consistent with the learning activities on this site.
    - Identify teaching/learning opportunities that have the most personal appeal to you. Why?
    - Describe the benefits and limitations of online health education programs.

Applied Learning

Individual Learning Activity #1: Experiencing the Learning Challenge Associated With Changing Habits and Routines

Instructions:

- Describe a behavior you would like to change in your own life. This behavior could relate to a habit (e.g., smoking, biting nails, talking on a cell phone while driving, snacking) or a routine (e.g., exercise program, organization of papers, studying for a test) you want to change. What is your goal for this behavior?
- Learn about this behavior and the teaching/learning strategies that are recommended to change this behavior. Document the things you have learned.
- For 5 to 7 days, use teaching/learning strategies to change this behavior and work toward your goal.

- Keep a daily journal during this time. Include the following things in your daily journal:
  - What was your behavioral goal for the day?
  - What teaching/learning strategies did you use to work on your goal?
  - Describe the effectiveness of each teaching/learning strategy.
  - Analyze your learning for this day (Use the definition of learning from the chapter).
  - Describe the ease or challenge of meeting your behavioral goal on this day.
  - Describe the power of habit or routine on your behaviors on this day.
- Summarize your total experience of trying to change one behavior and the teaching/learning strategies you used.
- Describe three things you learned that have implications for your work with clients who need or want to make a change in their lives.

Individual Learning Activity #2: Experiencing the Learning Challenge Associated With Different Environments

Instructions:

- Select an unfamiliar recipe that requires a variety of ingredients, kitchen tools, appliances, and steps in the preparation process.
- Identify a friend who has a kitchen that is unfamiliar to you. Ask your friend if you can make the recipe in his or her kitchen.
- Purchase the required ingredients and ask your friend to store the ingredients in their usual location in the kitchen. You should not observe this location.
- Have your friend give you a 1-minute orientation to the kitchen.
- Make the recipe. Ask your friend questions about the kitchen only after you have tried to handle the situation on your own several times.
- If your recipe is a success, share the results with your friend.
- Document your experience.
  - What aspects of the experience went well?
  - What aspects of the experience were challenging?
  - How did this experience feel? What would have made it go better?
  - How would your experience be different if you had a specific impairment?
- Reflect on a hypothetical cooking activity for a client in a rehabilitation setting. Assume you have introduced some teaching/learning strategies in the rehabilitation kitchen.
- What are some of the challenges of transferring teaching/learning strategies from the rehabilitation kitchen to the home environment? Consider issues related to specificity of learning, transfer, and generalization. Give an example.
- Describe teaching/learning strategies you could use to facilitate application of strategies in the home environment?
- What characteristics of client behavior and performance would you see in the rehabilitation kitchen to support transfer and generalization in the home environment?

Active Learning

Group Activity #1: Developing Teaching/Learning Strategies for an At-Risk Population

Preparation:

- Read Chapter Seventeen.
- Select one at-risk population that has occupational issues of concern.

- Review information and resources on this population.
- Review theories of client education summarized in Chapter Seventeen.

Time: 1 to 1.5 hours, 2 to 3 sessions

Materials:

- Information and resources on the at-risk population
- Art supplies
- Computer and professional presentation software

Instructions:

- Individually:
  - ✧ Develop ideas for occupational goals for this population.
  - ✧ Develop ideas for teaching/learning activities for this population.
  - ✧ Prepare a summary of your ideas.
- In small groups:
  - ✧ Share individual ideas for goals and teaching/learning activities.
  - ✧ Select one occupational goal to address in the small group activity.
  - ✧ Identify two theories of client education you will use for this goal.
  - ✧ Develop a specific teaching/learning activity for each theory you chose.
  - ✧ Prepare a professional presentation of this activity.
- In large groups:
  - ✧ Share the outcome of your small group work with a larger group.
  - ✧ Provide a critique of the teaching/learning activities developed by other groups.

    What theories of client education are suggested by each activity?

    What are the strengths and limitations of each activity?

Discussion:

- Discuss your small group experience of creating a teaching/learning activity for an occupation-based goal. What were the enjoyable parts of the activity? What were the challenging parts of the activity?
- Discuss the skills of each group member. What additional skills would you like to develop related to teaching/learning activities?
- Discuss the challenges and rewards likely associated with a large scale client education project.

Group Activity #2: Examining Procedural and Declarative Teaching/Learning Strategies

Preparation:

- Read Chapter Seventeen.
- Review the information on procedural and declarative learning.

Time: 30 to 45 minutes

Materials: Textbook

Instructions:

- In small groups:
  - ✧ Identify three occupations (instrumental activities of daily living or leisure) that would benefit by a procedural approach to teaching/learning.

    Describe each occupation in detail.

    Identify your rationale for teaching these occupations from a procedural approach.

    Develop examples of teaching strategies for these occupations using a procedural approach.
  - ✧ Identify three occupations (instrumental activities of daily living or leisure) that would benefit by a declarative approach to teaching/learning.

    Describe each occupation in detail.

Identify your rationale for teaching these occupations using a declarative approach.

Develop examples of teaching strategies for these occupations using a declarative approach.

Discussion:

- Discuss the strengths and limitations of each approach in occupational therapy practice.
- Discuss situations in which you could not use the preferred approach for an occupation.
- Discuss the approach that seems the most natural to you.
- Discuss skills you have and skills you would like to develop for each of these approaches.

Chapter Eighteen Objectives

The information in this chapter is intended to help the reader:

1. Understand the history and assumptions underlying four models for providing occupational therapy within a rehabilitation setting: biomedical, client-centered, community-based, and independent living.
2. Compare and contrast each service model in terms of its advantages and disadvantages.
3. Identify circumstances where each service model may be most appropriate.
4. Identify, using case examples, how factors related to the person, the environment, and occupational performance influence the application of each model of rehabilitation service.

Key Words

biomedical rehabilitation: A team of rehabilitation professionals with recognized expertise, often headed by a physician, who collaborate to assess and diagnose functional problems of a patient, set goals and priorities, implement interventions to promote optimum functioning, assess progress, and discontinue services when an optimal level has been reached (Bakheit, 1995).

client-centered rehabilitation: A therapeutic orientation whereby clients engage the assistance and support of a therapist to facilitate their problem solving and the achievement of their own goals. It is influenced by client-centered practice as a non-directive approach to therapy (Rogers, 1942).

community-based rehabilitation: A community development approach that uses the combined efforts of people with disabilities, families, and communities, and health, education, vocational, and social services for the purposes of rehabilitation, equalization of opportunities, and social integration of people with disabilities (International Labour Organization et al., 1994).

independent living: An approach based on self-help and peer support, research and service development, and referral and advocacy aimed to ensure people with disabilities access to resources and full participation in society, including housing, health care, transportation, employment, education, and mobility (Canadian Association of Independent Living Centres [CAILC], 1989; Cole, 1979; DeJong, 1979; DeLoach, Wilkins, & Walker, 1983).

Whether or not we have a disability, we will never fully achieve our goals until we establish a culture that focuses the full force of science and democracy on the systematic empowerment of every person to live to his or her full potential.

Justin Dart

Chapter Eighteen

Occupational Therapy Interventions in a Rehabilitation Context

Mary Ann McColl, PhD, BSc

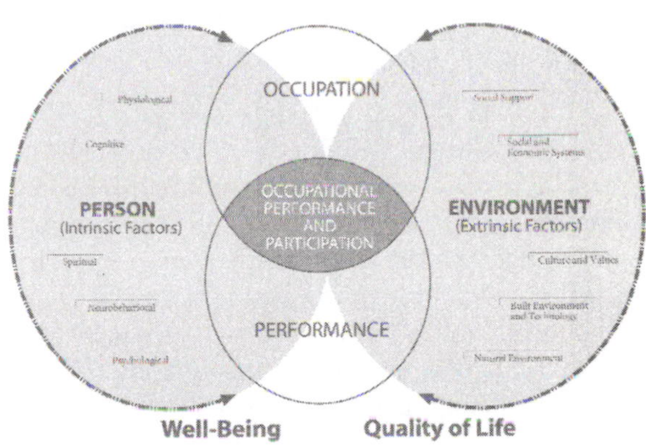

Setting the Stage

This chapter will introduce four models of rehabilitation: biomedical rehabilitation, client-centered rehabilitation, community-based rehabilitation, and independent living. Each model will be characterized by its assumptions, advantages, and limitations. Occupational therapy practitioners may work with people using these and other intervention models. Readers are challenged to develop a therapeutic repertoire to meet the unique person, environment, and occupational needs of individuals and populations.

McColl, M. A. *(2005). Occupational therapy interventions in a rehabilitation context. In* C. H. *Christiansen,* C. M. *Baum, and* J. *Bass-Haugen (Eds.)*, Occupational therapy: Performance, participation, and well-being *(3rd ed.). Thorofare, NJ: SLACK Incorporated.*

Introduction

Although new and exciting roles have developed for occupational therapy practitioners in the areas of primary prevention and health promotion, the majority of occupational therapy service continues to be delivered within the rehabilitation sector, in institutions, organizations, and the community. Rehabilitation has been defined by the United Nations (UN) as "a goal-oriented, time-limited process aimed at enabling an impaired person to reach an optimum mental, physical, and/or social level" (UN, 1983). Contained in this definition are a number of ideas that characterize rehabilitation:

- That it is a service directed toward people with disabilities
- That it is a finite process, with a beginning (referral), a middle (the rehabilitation process), and an end (goal achievement and discharge)
- That it addresses goals in a broad spectrum of areas of human functioning
- That its ultimate aim is to "enable"

In this chapter, I will discuss and compare four models for the delivery of rehabilitation service: biomedical rehabilitation, client-centered rehabilitation, community-based rehabilitation, and independent living. For each model, we will consider the assumptions underlying it, its advantages, and its limitations. For a summary, see Table 18-1. I will conclude with two examples that illustrate the utility of the four models at different times in the lives of two individuals.

Biomedical Rehabilitation

Historically, occupational therapy practitioners functioned exclusively within a biomedical rehabilitation model of service delivery. This view of rehabilitation arose in the early part of this century, as waves of veterans returned from World War I, many with permanent disabilities (Friedland, 1998; McColl, Law, & Stewart, 1993; Symington, 1994). It existed virtually unchallenged for the first 50 or 60 years of the profession's existence. Its dominance over the thinking of occupational therapy practitioners was strengthened in the 1950s and 1960s, as the status of professionals became enhanced by the scientific revolution (McColl et al., 1993).

In its modern iteration, biomedical rehabilitation is usually undertaken by a team of rehabilitation professionals, often headed by a physician (preferably a specialist in rehabilitation medicine). This team collaborates to assess and diagnose functional problems, set goals and priorities, implement interventions to promote optimum functioning, assess progress, and discontinue services when an optimal level has been reached (Bakheit, 1995). The recipient of services is usually referred to as a patient, denoting that he or she has limited responsibility in the therapeutic process, other than to simply be the object or recipient of service.

The biomedical model requires that patients and members of their support systems cooperate with the therapeutic team, primarily because of the recognized expertise of the team. The role of the patient and family is consistent with what Parsons (1975) described as the sick role. Within the sick role, the patient has two freedoms and two responsibilities: freedom from responsibility for the impairment, freedom from normal social roles for the duration of the impairment, responsibility to pursue optimal functioning, and responsibility to cooperate with service providers.

Assumptions

A number of assumptions underlie the biomedical approach to occupational therapy. First, it is assumed that the patient has an objective impairment that causes the disability (Bickenbach, 1992; Schlaff, 1993). The root of his or her difficulties lies within him- or herself and can be objectively detected and measured using biomedical technology.

A second assumption of the biomedical approach is that professionals have the information and skills necessary to understand the nature of the problems and to know what to do about them. A corollary to this is that patients themselves are ill-equipped to make decisions about the nature and course of rehabilitation because they lack this specialized expertise.

A third assumption of the biomedical model is that the problems associated with disability can be understood by reducing them to a series of subproblems associated with different body systems. These subproblems are best solved by a team of professionals, each working on a carefully defined area about which he or she has special expertise. The combination of efforts by an appropriately constituted team will result in the best possible outcomes for the patient.

Advantages

Although the traditional biomedical approach to rehabilitation has lost favor in some circles in recent years, it has a number of advantages, or it would surely not have prevailed for more than half a century. Although it is often portrayed in recent literature as authoritarian, one principal advantage of the biomedical approach is that it is primarily benevolent. Consistent with the Hippocratic Oath and other expressions of benevolent intent, the biomedical model aims to do good toward others. Beange

Table 18-1

Summary of Four Models of Practice for Occupational Therapy in a Rehabilitation Context

	Biomedical	*Client-centered*	*Community-Based*	*Independent Living*
Recipient of service	Patient	Client	Community	Consumer
Assumptions	1. Objective impairment is causing the disability 2. Professionals have knowledge and skill to solve problems 3. Problems can be analyzed into component parts and solved systematically	1. Clients know what they want and need from therapy 2. Professional dominance is counter-therapeutic 3. Therapist not the instrument of change, only the facilitator	1. People with disabilities seen in context of community 2. Communities can influence their own health 3. Small improvements for all preferable to maximum improvements for a few	1. People with disabilities are rational, informed consumers of service 2. Disablement stems from the environment, not the individual 3. Disability is a life-long personal issue, and a time-limited medical issue
Advantages	1. Benevolent intent of professionals 2. Professionals willing to assume responsibility	1. Empowering 2. Highly individualized 3. Opportunity for personal growth for therapist	1. Increases accessibility of service 2. Community members increase understanding of disability 3. Communities develop ability to solve problems 4. Sensitive to the context and culture	1. Promotes self-determination, mastery, and self-respect 2. Focuses on contributions that people with disabilities make 3. Focuses on equal participation in all aspects of daily life
Disadvantages	1. Disempowering/alienating 2. Time-limited in its relevance 3. Lacks expertise about living with a disability	1. Perception of less skilled, active role for therapist 2. Ambiguity about client-therapist relationship 3. Need for structural change to support client-centered practice 4. Based on therapist personality and beliefs	1. Applicable only to people living in the community 2. May take longer to achieve specific benefits 3. Vulnerable to changes in resources and attitudes of community 4. Rehabilitation professionals unprepared for community roles	1. Ambiguity around independence 2. Not applicable in some circumstances 3. Tension around role of professionals

(1987) refers to health professionals within a biomedical approach as *benevolent dictators*, recognizing their authority, but also acknowledging their benevolent intent.

Another advantage of the biomedical approach is the inherent willingness of professionals to shoulder responsibility for others in situations in which they may truly not be able to assume decision-making authority. For example, some people, in the wake of the onset of a disability, would be incapable of planning or decision making because of the magnitude of the medical and psychological issues. In such instances, professionals who function according to a biomedical model assume responsibility for determining the course of therapy that they believe will be most advantageous for the individual. In this way, precious weeks are not lost, and further complications are not incurred while waiting for the medical, psychological, and social situation to stabilize.

Disadvantages

There are also, however, several possible disadvantages to the use of the biomedical model. This very willingness of professionals to assume responsibility for decision making in therapy can be experienced as disempowering and alienating to individuals with disabilities who are capable of making their own decisions. At its extreme, this disempowerment is manifested as institutionalization, where individuals are rendered literally incapable of functioning outside of an institution because of their inability to make even the smallest of decisions.

Another disadvantage of the biomedical model is that its relevance is time limited. The freedoms and responsibilities associated with the patient role cannot become lifelong patterns, although the impairments or disabilities that initially invoked them may be lifelong. For example, individuals cannot be expected to make a career out of pursuing recovery, nor can they be allowed the freedom from social role obligations indefinitely. Thus, at some point, another model of service will be necessary for providers who have long-term relationships with people with disabilities, as many occupational therapy practitioners do.

The final, and perhaps most damning, disadvantage of the biomedical model is that it denies an essential area of expertise in the decision-making process. This expertise lies within the patient, and it pertains to the experience of living with a disability. To the extent that the disability is not merely an objective occurrence, as this model assumes, but also an experienced phenomenon, this phenomenological expertise is essential to good service.

Client-Centered Rehabilitation

In response to some of these disadvantages, occupational therapy practitioners have sought other models of service delivery to guide their interactions with consumers. One of these is the client-centered approach. Client-centered rehabilitation is a therapeutic orientation whereby clients engage the assistance and support of a practitioner to facilitate their problem solving and the achievement of their own goals. According to this model, clients seek a practitioner, explain their problems, and in an environment of understanding, trust, and acceptance, pursue change toward their goals (Burnard & Morrison, 1991). By its very name, it differentiates itself from the biomedical model by calling the recipients of service clients. Unlike a patient, a client seeks the advice of a professional in managing some aspect of his or her life (Herzberg, 1990; Patterson & Marks, 1992). Thus, the language implies that in a client-centered model, the client is in charge, is seeking from the relationship with the professional what he or she needs, and is discarding that which he or she does not feel is necessary at this time.

Client-centered practice was defined by its originator, Carl Rogers (1942), as a nondirective approach to therapy, where the therapist's role is to create an environment of trust and support, furnishing clients with the opportunity to use their own problem-solving capacities to realize their therapeutic goals. The client-centered approach has achieved considerable prominence in the past several years, yet the rhetoric associated with it often violates its intent. For example, we often hear about practitioners "allowing clients to make decisions" or "involving clients in the process of therapy" within a client-centered approach. Kerfoot and LeClair (1991) suggest that practitioners may even use client-centered rhetoric as a means of guiding or manipulating the therapeutic agenda. Client-centered practice is not simply a more respectful way to deliver a professionally dominated or biomedical rehabilitation. Rather, it is a different model of service delivery altogether, where the practitioner is engaged by the individual to assist with the achievement of personal goals in occupational performance.

Assumptions

There are a number of assumptions to the client-centered approach that may assist in differentiating it from other models. The first assumption of client-centered therapy is that clients know what they want from therapy and what they need to reach their optimum level of functional performance. This assumption is the ultimate extension of one of the most basic values of the occupational therapy practitioner: the belief in the uniqueness and worth of every individual (Clarke, Scot, & Krupa, 1993; Coring & Cook, 1999). This assumption also means that the only relevant frame of reference or vantage point for therapy is that of the client. While the practitioner may have knowledge and expertise about certain aspects of disability and therapy, he or she can never fully understand the values, beliefs, and experiences of the client and must, therefore, accept the client's reports as the most relevant source of information about the progress of therapy.

A second assumption of the client-centered approach is that the dominance of professionals in the process of therapy is counter-therapeutic (Goodall, 1992). Professional dominance creates dependency, disempowerment, and ultimately institutionalization (Rebeiro, 2000).

The third assumption of the client-centered approach is that the practitioner cannot actually promote change; he or she can only create an environment that facilitates change. This concept was first introduced to the occupational therapy literature by Meyer (1922) when occupational therapy first began. Change or new learning takes place only when an individual identifies it as necessary for the maintenance or development of the self (Rogers, 1965). Thus, any contention by the practitioner that he or she is the agent of change is misguided because the only agent of change can be the individual him- or herself, and the most potentially valuable role for the practitioner is to support the client through the change with information, ideas, suggestions, resources, and the communication of trust and belief in the ability of the client to succeed.

Advantages

This approach, like the others, has a number of advantages and disadvantages. Its main advantage is its tendency to enhance self-esteem, mastery, independence, resourcefulness, and empowerment among clients (Emener, 1991; Goodall, 1992). Because of this, service delivered according to a client-centered model is perceived by clients as excellent service (Kerfoot & LeClair, 1991).

A second advantage to the client-centered approach is the extent to which it supports a truly individualized or "tailored" approach to therapy (Brown, 1992). Because clients identify therapeutic goals and activities that are pertinent to their unique circumstances and context, no two occupational therapy programs can look exactly alike. Thus, practitioners are constantly challenged to use all three forms of clinical reasoning to understand the client's context (interactional), the details of the disability (procedural), and the effect of the disability on the client's life (conditional) (Mattingly & Fleming, 1994).

The third advantage of the client-centered approach is the opportunity that it presents for the practitioner's own personal and professional growth and development. Unlike the traditional model, where the practitioner is the expert and people are learning from him or her, in the client-centered model, the client is the expert. There is, thus, an opportunity for the practitioner to learn more about disability and its manifestations in people's lives, more about the multidimensional nature of human occupational performance, and more about him- or herself, both within the therapeutic role and more generally in human relationships.

Disadvantages

There are also a number of disadvantages to working from a client-centered perspective. Because the approach is essentially nondirective, some clients perceive the practitioner operating from this perspective as less skilled and less effective (Jaffe & Kipper, 1982; Schroeder & Bloom, 1979; Wanigaratne & Barker, 1995). The conventional perception of a health care practitioner is that of a person who will take charge and make things better. For those who hold to this view, there must be a certain amount of disappointment in a practitioner who asks how he or she can be of service.

A second disadvantage of the client-centered approach is the ambiguity around the nature of the therapeutic relationship. A number of authors in the occupational therapy literature have described it as a "partnership." While this definition is intuitively pleasing in that it invokes the image of two people working closely together toward a common purpose, the partnership idea falls down when we look more closely at the definition. A partnership can be described as a contractual arrangement whereby two or more individuals share in the liability for any losses and the benefits of any gains. This is clearly not the case in the relationship between a practitioner and a client; the losses and gains are both primarily incurred by the client. This ambiguity requires that the client-therapist relationship be negotiated on a case-by-case basis, to ensure clarity about who is responsible for what and what each might expect from the other.

A third disadvantage of the client-centered approach is the need for fairly significant technical and structural change in health care systems to accommodate this change in ideology away from the biomedical approach (Sumsion & Smyth, 2000). As an example, a number of reviews of the literature show that there are few occupational therapy assessments that are suitable for application in a client-centered practice (Pollock, 1993; Pollock et al., 1990; Trombly, 1993). Structural changes also will be required to allow systems to accommodate the needs and conveniences of clients, rather than of practitioners

(Brider, 1992; Carlisle, 1992; Holyoke & Elkan, 1995; Robinson, 1991). For example, outpatient service outside of regular business hours is uncommon in current systems, yet, for many people, therapy would be considerably more accessible if it were available evenings and weekends.

Finally, a disadvantage of the client-centered approach is that it may not be acceptable to all practitioners. Rogers (1965) himself admits that the success or failure of client-centered therapy is often a function of the practitioner's personality and his or her respect for others and belief in their resourcefulness and adaptiveness. Sumsion and Smyth (2000) found that the most significant barrier to client-centered practice was differing goals between client and therapist. To determine your own orientation toward client-centeredness, ask yourself whose interests, opinions, and goals should prevail when client and therapist disagree as to the appropriate course of action.

Community-Based Rehabilitation

Community-based rehabilitation (CBR) is a third model for the delivery of rehabilitation services to people with disabilities. CBR is defined as:

> ...a strategy within community development for the rehabilitation, equalization of opportunities, and social integration of all people with disabilities. CBR is implemented through the combined efforts of people with disabilities themselves, their families and communities, and the appropriate health, education, vocational, and social services. (International Labour Organization et al., 1994)

CBR emerged in developing countries, where traditional rehabilitation services that rely on highly trained professionals and well-equipped facilities could not adequately serve the needs of people with disabilities. In developed countries, interest in CBR was sparked by its apparent applicability to underserved populations, such as rural communities and minority groups, and by its emphasis on community participation, particularly of people with disabilities. CBR in the developed world includes home-based services, outreach services, and community development programs for issues related to disability. The definition of community in CBR may be geographical, referring to a particular area or locality, or it may be relational, referring to a group with shared interests and values, mutual obligations, a common history, or other affinity (Miles, 1994).

The roots of CBR lie jointly in the philosophies of community development and health promotion. Community development is defined as a process by which people work collectively to define common problems, discuss strategies for change, make decisions, and act on and evaluate their decisions. Implicit in the term is strong participation and ownership of the process by the community (Compton, 1971). Health promotion is defined as "the process of enabling people to increase control over the determinants of health" (Wallerstein, 1992).

The principle of individual and community self-determination is the common thread between health promotion and community development that underlies CBR when applied to the issues of people with disabilities. The essential difference between CBR and the two approaches to rehabilitation just discussed lies in CBR's emphasis on the social origins of issues relating to disability. CBR aims for a redistribution of community resources in favor of community members with disabilities. The whole community is the target of CBR programs, although people with disabilities themselves are the primary beneficiaries (Lysack & Kaufert, 1994).

CBR programs vary widely throughout the world due to the differences among communities in which they operate. However, most CBR programs have a number of features in common:

- Through community participation in social action, CBR programs assist communities to develop a greater awareness and understanding of community members who have disabilities.
- CBR programs help communities to work together to identify and overcome barriers that prevent people with disabilities from participating in the life of the community.
- Human and financial resources of the community form the basis of CBR.
- Simple rehabilitation techniques are taught by professionals to families and community members who carry them out with people with disabilities.
- Vocational skill development and income-generating activities are often included in CBR programs (Boyce & Johnston, 1998; Mitchell, 1999a, 1999b; O'Toole, 1991; Peat & Boyce, 1993).

Assumptions

A number of assumptions underlie CBR. First, people with disabilities are assumed not to exist in isolation; rather, they are seen as embedded in a web of family, kin, and community. The community both supports people with disabilities and benefits from their contributions to the economic and social environment. Rather than viewing disability as an individual matter, CBR views the issues of people with disabilities as the issues of the whole community. It builds on the family units and the norms of communal support to improve the lives of individuals and the community (Lysack & Kaufert, 1994).

A second assumption of CBR is that individuals and communities have at their disposal the resources to influence their own health. Through individual and collective learning, communities are empowered to assume mastery over aspects of the environment that affect their health. To this end, people with disabilities and their communities develop the capacity to identify the fundamental causes of disadvantage and to change the situation (Wallerstein, 1992).

Third, CBR assumes that it is more important (and more possible) to make small improvements to the quality of life of all people with disabilities in a community than to provide the highest standard of care for a privileged few (O'Toole, 1991). The lives of all people with disabilities are improved when communities view them as integral members and engage collaboratively in a process of community problem solving. This can be achieved by providing information and training to community members, providing basic aids and adaptations, and making simple, inexpensive accommodations, all of which benefit the majority of people with disabilities.

Advantages

There are a number of inherent advantages to the CBR approach to delivering services to people with disabilities. An important advantage is that CBR makes service accessible to a much larger number of people with disabilities and their families than traditional service models. Furthermore, this model of service delivery is not dependent on the availability of highly trained professionals and resource-intensive institutions. It is an extremely cost-effective approach to providing a basic level of service to a large number of individuals.

A second advantage of the CBR approach is that many community members, both disabled and nondisabled, increase their knowledge, skill, and understanding about disability. Through exchanges between people with disabilities and professionals and through participation in social action, individuals develop skills and competencies that are useful in many situations besides CBR. People with disabilities are seen as contributors to community life, while other community members learn to value the contributions that they can make when afforded the opportunity.

The third and perhaps most compelling advantage of CBR is the increase in competency that occurs in the community in which a CBR program resides. Through the process of community development, communities learn to listen to disadvantaged or marginalized groups, engage in collective problem solving, and marshal resources that were often previously unknown or underused. Reliance on the community's own people and resources reduces its dependence on external resources and helps to ensure that programs continue over the long term.

The final advantage of CBR is its inherent sensitivity to the social, economic, and cultural issues of the community. Because CBR is planned by the community to meet needs it defines, with professionals providing support where requested, programs tend to be technically, socially, and financially acceptable and may engender more commitment from the community. People with disabilities are also fully involved in the program; therefore, the systems developed by the community to encourage the integration of people with disabilities may be more holistic and comprehensive than those developed by professionals (Banerjee, 1992).

Disadvantages

On the other hand, there are also disadvantages to CBR. First, because CBR is delivered in the community, its applicability is restricted to issues of people living in the community (McColl, 1998; Mitchell, 1999a). Thus, it is of limited utility to people with newly acquired disabilities. Those individuals usually require one of the more resource-intensive models of service, at least in the initial phase. Also, for individuals living in the community with complex multiple disabilities, CBR may not be able to respond completely to their needs. For example, CBR is ill-equipped to provide highly technical or specialized service.

Another disadvantage of this approach is that it may take a long time to develop individual and community abilities to respond to the issues of community members with disabilities. Because the progress of the program may depend on changing community structures, the time frame may be longer than that for individual rehabilitation. This can be discouraging for people with pressing needs and can ultimately endanger the program's credibility and success. Further, success may be difficult to demonstrate. Indicators of community development and community competence are not well developed because research in this area is relatively young (Bichmann, Rifkin, & Shrestha, 1989; Hawe, 1994; Mitchell, 1999b).

A third disadvantage of CBR is that the continuity of the program can be threatened by changes in the community, such as turnover in CBR volunteers, changes in the interests of the community, and changes to the resources available for the program. Perhaps the most threatening of these is a change in the priority that a community assigns to issues of its members with disabilities. In a fiscal environment of scarce resources, CBR programs are vulnerable to shifting priorities away from issues of a minority disadvantaged group, such as people with disabilities.

The fourth and final disadvantage of the CBR approach is lack of preparedness of most rehabilitation professionals for community development and health promotion roles. While individual practitioners may be interested in this approach, they may not be certain how to intervene at the level of a community, instead of at the level of the individual. Because CBR programs are by definition "owned" by the community, the role of the professional is defined by the community (Boyce & Peat, 1995). Professionals may find the roles that communities and people with disabilities wish them to take in conflict with their own ideas. For example, professionals may want to control clinical aspects of programs, be involved in organizational aspects, and bow out of fund-raising. People with disabilities, on the other hand, may want to share control of clinical aspects, fully control organizational aspects, and delegate fund-raising to influential professionals (O'Toole, 1991).

Independent Living

Finally, independent living (IL) is a fourth model for the delivery of services to people with disabilities. This model differs significantly from biomedical, client-centered, and CBR models in that it developed out of a collective political movement of people with disabilities (DeJong, 1979; Driedger, 1989; Oliver, 1990). No longer willing to accept lifelong dependent relationships with professionals, people with disabilities asserted a political strategy in the 1960s and 1970s to promote a view of disability as a socially constructed phenomenon (Oliver, 1990). Independent living represents a new attitude, a new set of organizing principles, and a new approach to service delivery aimed to ensure people with disabilities access to housing, health care, transportation, employment, education, and mobility. These aims were achieved through self-help and peer support, research and service development, and referral and advocacy (CAILC, 1989; DeJong, 1979; DeLoach et al., 1983).

The primary goal of IL is to ensure access to resources and full participation for people with disabilities in society (Cole, 1979; CAILC, 1989). Although this goal may seem similar in many ways to that of traditional rehabilitation, IL's central distinction can be found in the way in which the goal is addressed. Unlike previously outlined models, in IL, the initiative for control of service rests with consumers or consumer groups themselves, rather than with programs, institutions, or professionals (Cole, 1979; DeLoach et al., 1983). Perhaps the greatest strength of the independent living approach is its commitment to placing in the hands of people with disabilities themselves control of the resources that affect their daily lives (Ben-Sira, 1983; DeJong, 1979).

Assumptions

A number of assumptions inform the IL model. First, the model understands people with disabilities as consumers of services, rather than as patients or clients. Consumers are seen as being in control of the resources that affect their lives and able to make informed choices about the disposition of those resources (Gadacz, 1994). This assumption requires a different view of people with disabilities and a different type of relationship between consumers and providers. Hierarchical relationships with professionals are incompatible with the view of consumers as autonomous and rationally driven (DeJong, 1979; Oliver, 1990).

A second assumption of the IL approach is that disability stems not from the individual him- or herself, but rather from the environment in which the individual lives (Driedger, 1989). This approach does not understand disabilities as deficits, but rather as conditions of life. IL advocates that individuals are disabled by inaccessible buildings, lack of access to education, unemployment, and hostile attitudes. Disablement lies not in the physical condition of the individual but in the construction of society (Brisenden, 1986). Therefore, the means to overcome disablement lies also in the environment and in greater access to resources, such as education, living arrangements, and mobility.

A third assumption of the IL approach is that the management of a medically stable disability is a personal matter first, and a medical matter second (DeJong, 1979). While acknowledging the need for rehabilitation in acute disabling episodes, the independent living approach sees this need as a strictly time-limited one. Once the medical condition stabilizes, proponents of the IL approach believe that people with disabilities are competent to assume responsibility over the resources that affect their lives and to make informed choices over their setting, context, and circumstances, whether medical or nonmedical (Gadacz, 1994).

Advantages

As in all previously outlined approaches, the IL model has a number of advantages and disadvantages. Its most important advantage is its commitment to providing people with disabilities with control over the resources that affect their daily lives, thereby enhancing their ability to act autonomously and achieve mastery and self-respect. For example, within an IL approach, people who require a personal attendant to assist with daily self-care would be provided with resources to directly hire, supervise, and fire personal attendants (whereas in traditional models, they would be referred by professionals to a program that would dictate to them the terms and conditions of attendant care that they were entitled to receive). The inherent increase in self-determination and participation associated with this approach represents increased independence and self-respect for people with disabilities (Boland & Alonso, 1982).

The second advantage of the IL approach is its focus on self-help and its recognition of the significant contributions that people with disabilities can make to the lives of others and to society as a whole. Similar to the personal and professional growth of the practitioner under the client-centered approach, independent living offers growth potential for individuals with disabilities themselves as well as for communities. People with disabilities are assisted, often by others with disabilities, to live independent lives in the community and to make significant and meaningful contributions. One example of self-help within the IL approach has been the development of Independent Living Resource Centres. These centers are community-based, consumer-controlled response centers aimed at addressing the needs of people with disabilities in the community and ensuring that these needs can be met in a non-institutional setting (CAILC, 1994).

The third advantage of the IL approach is its focus on citizenship, equality, and participation in society for people with disabilities. This holistic, nonmedical approach offers expression to the sociopolitical nature of people with disabilities, both individually and collectively (CAILC, 1994). It diverts the focus of service away from the impairment and disability and onto the real issues of day-to-day life, like employment, access, housing, and transportation. It offers a sociopolitical context for these issues and focuses on promoting change in social structures to enhance equity and participation of people with disabilities in all aspects of society (Oliver, 1990).

Disadvantages

Some disadvantages of the IL approach must also be outlined. First, there is still some ambiguity surrounding the term *independence*. Within an IL approach, the term *independence* is often replaced with the term *autonomy*, meaning freedom from domination by social structures, institutions, and professionals; control over the resources necessary for daily life; and expression of the sociopolitical nature of the individual (Brisenden, 1986; DeJong, 1979; Oliver, 1990). This concept of autonomy differs in many ways from the traditional definition of independence, meaning that an individual is capable of living alone in the community and doing activities of daily living without assistance. Research is underway that attempts to close this conceptual gap (Berrol, 1979; Boland & Alonso, 1982; Tamaru, 2004; Walton, Schwab, Cassatt-Dunn, & Wright, 1980).

A second disadvantage is that the strategies commonly used in the IL approach tend not to deal with the issues of people with newly acquired or exacerbated disabilities (Cole, 1979). Furthermore, the IL approach, like the community-based approach, is incompatible with inpatient or institutional service delivery. However, even in these instances, some of the principles of IL may be applied. For example, the use of peer counseling can be implemented even within an institutional setting, and by doing so, one acknowledges the autonomy and expertise that lies within the community of people with disabilities.

The third and final disadvantage is the difficulty in defining the role of professionals in the IL approach. The IL movement initially grew out of a desire among people with disabilities to be free of professionals, to limit the power of professionals in their lives, and to offer an alternative to traditional rehabilitation. Now, as a mature movement, proponents of IL see professionals as one of the resources that people with disabilities have at their disposal. However, there are often vestiges of the historical tension in the relationship, making both sides wary of the other. As successful models of collaboration between professionals and people with disabilities evolve, these tensions will surely dissolve, and this partnership will realize its full potential.

Applications of the Four Models of Service

Using the model presented in Chapter One, two applications are described of the four models of service discussed. In each, an effort has been made to identify how the four models of service are more or less applicable at different points along the continuum of rehabilitation and life with a disability.

Example 1: Steven

Steven is a 17-year-old who lives with his parents and two younger siblings. The family owns and operates a dairy farm and has lived in the same rural community for several generations. Steven was ready to enter his last year of high school when he was injured in a motor vehicle accident near his home. He sustained a C6-7 spinal fracture. At the time of his accident, Steven was taken by ambulance to the trauma center 40 minutes away. His fracture was surgically stabilized, and he was placed in a halo-traction vest until his spine was stable.

Biomedical Rehabilitation

Steven's first encounter with an occupational therapy practitioner was with Janet at the trauma center. The prevailing model of service in the trauma center was the biomedical model. Based on the assumption that Steven was not in a position to direct his own care at the acute stage, and given the knowledge and skill of the practitioners and doctors about the neurological condition, decisions about therapy were made by the team, in consultation with Steven's parents, and were communicated to Steven in a manner that was sensitive to the psychological and social issues at play. Treatments focused on the intrinsic factors underlying Steven's disability, including his physical, psychological, and neurological condition.

Initially, Janet came by daily to ensure that Steven was positioned appropriately in his bed to prevent contractures; that he was as comfortable as possible; that his skin was not breaking down at any of the pressure points; and that he was able to communicate with nursing staff, family, and friends. To meet these goals, she provided Steven with foot drop splints to maintain his ankle position and resting splints to protect his wrists. Janet performed several basic assessments of Steven's physical, psychological, and neurological functioning, including manual muscle testing, range of motion, sensation, tone, hand function, and functional independence. Janet also provided Steven with an adapted call bell that he could operate independently if he needed assistance from nursing or support staff and adaptive equipment for self-care and feeding. Finally, she organized with the evening staff to provide assistance to Steven in making telephone calls.

By the end of 4 weeks, Steven was able to sit up in a high back wheelchair for several hours at a time. At this point, the team conferred and determined that Steven's condition was medically stable, and it was appropriate that he be transferred to the rehabilitation hospital across the street.

Client-Centered Rehabilitation

Still wearing his halo-traction device, Steven was transferred to the rehabilitation center. On his second day at the center, Steven met Lloyd, his new occupational therapy practitioner. Lloyd, like many of his colleagues in the rehabilitation center, functioned from a client-centered model of service. Therefore, on his first meeting with Steven, Lloyd's first priority was to get to know Steven and to begin to develop an understanding of the meaning of this injury in Steven's life. Lloyd's primary objective was to communicate to Steven his desire to understand the situation from Steven's perspective and his commitment to help him solve his problems. Lloyd used a number of techniques and activities to learn more about Steven's life before his injury, his home and family, and his plans and hopes for the future. For example, Steven and Lloyd completed a detailed occupational history and a time use diary for a typical day. With Lloyd's help, Steven developed a social network diagram to describe his home and family and discussed the elements of the diagram with Lloyd as they went along. Lloyd also began to introduce the idea of the future by asking Steven to project the diagram forward in time. Steven realized that he was virtually unable to do this and began to tentatively explore various scenarios that might shed some light on the future. Lloyd and Steven made several attempts to use a narrative approach to raise issues about Steven's rehabilitation plans. They wrote a story about the accident, the rehabilitation process, and the next few chapters in Steven's life. Through the narrative, they began to set long- and short-term goals for rehabilitation. Steven identified a number of specific problems of occupational performance that he was concerned about: his inability to get around, the fact that he was missing school and falling behind, and the strained relationship with his girlfriend.

Steven's long-term goals were to walk again, to patch things up with his girlfriend, to finish high school, and to begin learning from his father about the operation of the farm. In the short term, he was quite amenable to the physical aspects of therapy, but resistant to learning daily living skills involving the wheelchair or other adaptive devices. Therefore, short-term goals were developed that focused strictly on developing strength, balance, and physical capabilities; getting around in the hospital; and looking after himself on the ward.

Steven participated actively in rehabilitation for 4 months, during which time he developed strength, tone, and balance, as well as a functional tenodesis grasp. He became independent in the basic elements of self-care and was able to propel the wheelchair independently. From time to time, assistive devices were introduced for the sake of expediency and were accepted as short-term solutions. However, Steven would not agree to order a wheelchair of his own, and he became angry when it was repeatedly suggested by team members and by family. He continued to use one of the center's chairs on a loan basis.

About 2 months into his rehabilitation, discussions began about the possibility that Steven might go home for a weekend. Reactions of family varied from fear and apprehension to excitement and anticipation. Steven himself experienced the same range of mixed feelings. To begin the process of adjusting to the idea of going home, and making the home environment ready for Steven, Lloyd and Steven did a number of visualization exercises, including detailed visualization of driving up to the farm, entering the house, eating dinner, and helping with the farm chores. Steven began to identify the feelings associated with going home, most prominent of which was his fear of failure and his embarrassment at being seen in the wheelchair. He also began to identify some of the barriers to accessibility and some of the adjustment issues that he might face on weekends home. Steven accompanied Lloyd on a home visit to assess for structural modifications but did not actually bring the wheelchair or get out of the car. Plans were developed for an exterior ramp, a downstairs bedroom, and an adapted main floor bathroom. Also, Steven's mother was taught to manage his bowel and bladder routine.

Steven's first weekend home pointed out some of the limitations of the loaner wheelchair, making future discussions possible about the selection of a more attractive and suitable wheelchair. Otherwise, the weekend was quite low-key, with no visitors, and was generally agreed by everyone to be a success. Subsequent weekends were used to identify problems in various aspects of home life and to begin the process of connecting with friends, neighbors, and community members. During the week, Lloyd and Steven sought solutions to each new issue as it arose.

Steven's visits home also raised issues in his mind about his ability to follow his original career path of taking over the farm; however, in the short term, everyone agreed that his first priority must be to complete high school. Steven was discharged home after 4 months of rehabilitation to his parents' partially renovated farmhouse, with plans to resume high school.

Several days after Steven returned home, he was visited by a community occupational therapy practitioner named Sylvie. Sylvie was hired by Steven's insurance company to assess Steven's needs for community living and to make recommendations about what was necessary to ensure Steven's return to school and preparation for gainful employment in the future. Using a traditional approach, Sylvie began by assessing Steven's ability to fulfill his self-care roles at home and to pursue his education.

On her second visit, Sylvie discovered that Steven and his family were managing very successfully and that they had effectively problem-solved most of the issues that had arisen. Steven, however, had not left the house, he was expressing some reluctance about returning to school, and family relationships were severely strained. Steven's mother revealed to Sylvie that a local service club was planning a fund-raising event in the community hall to raise money to help pay for an adapted van. Steven was expected to attend and was flatly stating that he would not.

Community-Based Rehabilitation

Recognizing that the issues faced by Steven and his family involved the whole community to some extent, Sylvie reconsidered her approach and began the process of community development that is central to community-based rehabilitation. She began by asking Steven and his family to identify the individuals and structures that comprised their community. They identified neighbors, Steven's friends, the church, the store, the school, and the service club, of which Steven's father was a member. Sylvie sought the family's and Steven's permission to talk to each of these people about how the community might participate in the process of facilitating Steven's re-engagement with the community, return to school, and plan for future productivity. Sylvie thus acted as a catalyst to a process whereby the community assumed ownership of some of the issues that Steven faced, assessed its resources to deal with these issues, and developed a sustainable plan to make changes.

She and Steven met first with the school principal, Steven's teacher, the student council president, and the school bus driver. They collectively problem-solved about adapting the bus with a lift and wheelchair tie-down; altering the pickup schedule to allow Steven time for his morning routine; making one entrance to the school fully accessible; ensuring that the entrance was kept clear of snow, bicycles, and other obstacles; altering the timetable and room allocations to accommodate Steven's schedule; and developing a rotation schedule for fellow students to provide peer assistance to Steven throughout the school day. Steven was furnished with a pager in case of emergencies, and three students were taught to assist with emptying Steven's leg bag when necessary.

Steven, however, continued to refuse to go to school, out of fear and embarrassment at the reactions of the other students. Members of Steven's homeroom took turns bringing notes and assignments to Steven at home. After 3 weeks, he had had a visit from virtually everyone and had overcome his fear of the "first day." Soon he was attending school on a part-time basis, with plans to graduate the following year.

The visits of his classmates and other community members also assisted with Steven's willingness to attend the community fund-raiser. He discovered at that time also that the store in the village had been rearranged to allow passage of his wheelchair and the single step at the front entrance had been ramped. The store had been a place where Steven and his friends had always convened informally. From time to time in the past, the storekeeper had shooed them away; however, this action sent a clear message that the teenagers were welcome patrons.

Steven finished high school in the spring, almost 2 years after his injury. He was 19 years old and anxious to be more independent of his family. He found the necessity of his mothers' help with personal care increasingly degrading. He recognized the growth that had taken place in his community to afford him the kinds of opportunities it had, but he still felt like a "charity case" and could not shake the feeling that deep down, people felt sorry for him and always would. They remembered him as an able-bodied teenager, and he saw the reflection of that image in their eyes. He felt he couldn't continue to live with reminders of the past in all his social relationships. Even his part-time job in the store offered little to his sense of self-sufficiency and self-respect.

Steven's family was horrified at the thought of his moving out. They had not a clue how to begin to assemble the resources needed for Steven to live alone. They called Sylvie for some advice. Sylvie was able to obtain authorization for two visits to help Steven secure appropriate housing and to assess the need for ongoing supports.

Independent Living

Recognizing the limits of her ability to help Steven with the challenges he faced and his need for self-determination and autonomy, Sylvie referred Steven to the Independent Living Resource Center (ILRC) in town and also encouraged him to contact his friend from the rehabilitation center who now lived independently in town. Sylvie advised that she would become more involved if requested, but that other services were more appropriate to help Steven with the issues he faced now.

Steven called his buddy Raymond, with whom he had been in touch by phone during the intervening year since leaving rehab, but had not seen for some time. Raymond's disability was slightly less severe than Steven's, but they shared an understanding that was largely unspoken. Steven told Raymond of his plans, and Raymond invited him into town to see his place. Steven arranged with his mother to take him into town, leave him alone for the day, and pick him up again about supper time. Steven also arranged a visit to the ILRC for the same day.

Steven returned home that evening exuberant at the possibilities for independent living. He had put his name on a waiting list for an accessible apartment, knowing that he might wait up to a year for a suitable place. In the meantime, his experience with Raymond had shown him that he had some work to do to be ready when his name came up. First and foremost, he needed to learn to drive. The ILRC recommended a driving instructor who specialized in teaching car transfers and hand-controlled driving. Steven was surprised to discover at his first lesson that the instructor also had a disability. Using his own van, that had been purchased jointly by his insurance company and the community, Steven got his driver's license before the end of the summer.

By fall, he was driving into town to attend community college, training to be a data systems analyst. On one of his free afternoons each week, he volunteered at the ILRC, answering phones, doing office work, and developing a computerized catalogue for the center's resource library. By the following spring, a suitable apartment had become available, and Steven prepared to move into town.

He contacted Sylvie again to make the first of her two authorized visits. Together, they assessed the apartment and identified the need for several minor adaptations. More importantly, however, they began to discuss the need for attendant care. Sylvie recommended to the insurance company that Steven be provided with 4 hours of attendant care a day, 2 hours each morning and evening. She further recommended that the resources to support this assistance be placed in a trust fund to be managed by Steven and accounted for on an annual basis.

The insurance company agreed to all of Sylvie's recommendations, except the last one, that Steven take responsibility for the management of his personal assistance. They insisted that Steven acquire attendant services through a program run by the rehabilitation center. In his haste to begin his new life, Steven accepted these conditions and moved into his apartment. However, after several months, Steven became dissatisfied with his attendant. When he complained to the program manager at the rehab center, he was told that there was no one else they could send. Therefore, he sought the support of the ILRC to advocate on his behalf with the insurance company to allow him to hire and manage his own personal assistance. Using information about the models used by other people to manage their own attendants, and the corporate assurance of accountability from the ILRC, the insurance company agreed to a pilot project whereby Steven would have sole authority over the resources to purchase his personal assistance. The ILRC would annually audit the accounts. Steven sought advice and information from the ILRC about how to advertise for, interview, hire, and train an attendant; how to supervise and give feedback to an attendant; and how to terminate a work relationship if necessary. Steven's first attendant was an occupational therapy student, who worked with Steven throughout the duration of his degree and, upon graduation, moved away but remained a close friend.

Example 2: Sandy

Sandy is a 35-year-old woman who has lived alone in a subsidized housing complex for much of her adult life and has little contact with her family or other members of her community. As a young woman, she was a good student and was enrolled in an engineering program at university. However, at the age of 19, she experienced her first episode of schizophrenia and was forced to drop out of school. Since then, she has made several attempts to take additional courses toward her degree, but has never been able to complete them. Sandy has been in and out of the hospital many times during the past 16 years. She has recently been hospitalized for another acute episode, where she discontinued her medication and quickly became delusional and paranoid.

Biomedical Rehabilitation

Sandy was admitted by ambulance to the emergency unit of the hospital in her area about 10:00 one night because voices were telling her that she was "a blight on society and didn't deserve to live." This had apparently been going on for 2 or 3 days, with increasing intensity, to the point where Sandy was afraid to leave her apartment and was afraid to go to sleep. She phoned a crisis help line and agreed to meet the counselor at the emergency department of the hospital. As an inpatient on a short-stay mental health unit, Sandy was initially stabilized on medication, and attention was directed at her general health and physical state.

Client-Centered Rehabilitation

After a couple of days, she met Janice, the occupational therapy practitioner. Janice practiced occupational therapy from a client-centered perspective, and, therefore, her first meeting with Sandy was spent finding out about her in her own words. Sandy told Janice about the night she came into hospital and characterized it as the logical culmination of her general inability to "make something of herself." She expressed profound disappointment in her life to date and pointed to normative social milestones that she had failed to achieve, such as career, marriage, and children. Janice guided the interview to find out more about specific problems that Sandy might experience in the areas of self-care, productivity, and leisure. Sandy specified her most pressing problems as having nothing to do all day, being lonely, and being afraid of another episode like the one that brought her here. Further, Sandy made clear that she did not wish to return to her apartment.

Over the course of a 10-day admission, Janice and Sandy explored a number of different long-term living options. With the cooperation of the psychiatrist and social worker, Sandy was assisted in securing a place in a community boarding home for people with mental illnesses.

Janice and Sandy also explored her use of time and the need for a balance in her daily activities. They did detailed time and occupation diaries, and identified temporal structures and patterns that could help Sandy to add meaning to her day-to-day life. Part of this process involved the identification of resources in Sandy's new community that might become part of her routine, such as a community clubhouse. However, to comfortably access these, Janice and Sandy had to work together to develop and rehearse strategies for making contact, attending initially, and sustaining participation. At the end of 10 days, Sandy was discharged to the boarding home, and Janice was authorized to provide outreach follow-up to Sandy for a transitional 6-week period.

Janice made her first visit to the boarding home the day after Sandy moved in. She found Sandy sitting on the bed in her room, with the door open a crack. She reported having her meals at the appointed times, but having met none of her neighbors. Mealtimes were brief and mostly silent. Sandy was very disappointed at how this was turning out.

Community-Based Rehabilitation

Janice saw in the boarding home a community with the capacity to provide a better quality of life for its members, through collective problem solving. Using a community-based rehabilitation approach, she began to identify stakeholders in this community, including the residents themselves, the boarding home owner, manager, and staff, several neighbors, the owner of a local coffee shop where residents commonly convened, staff of a day program Sandy was planning to attend, and the organizers of a community clubhouse run by former psychiatric patients. In her initial contact, she asked each of these people to identify problems or issues they might have, especially as they applied to the boarding home and its residents. Not surprisingly, issues diverged widely, and included everything from residents wandering the streets to inadequate finances. All were invited to an evening meeting to address these issues, held in the coffee shop.

Janice facilitated the meeting, attempting to ensure that everyone had an opportunity to raise their issues. By the end of the meeting, the group had tentatively and, in some cases, reluctantly agreed to several initiatives. The boarding home staff would review aspects of daily operation that could be assumed by residents; the boarding home operator and manager agreed to explore ways in which the residents could have more say in how the home ran, its rules, and regulations; Janice agreed to provide several informal information sessions to neighbors and local business people about mental illness and its consequences for individuals; residents agreed to form a planning council to plan at least one community social outing per week. Finally, the group had identified several resources and supports within the community that they could call on for help if they needed it.

Janice visited the home once or twice a week for the 6-week follow-up period. During that time, Sandy began to take a more active role in kitchen and laundry duties in the home, she participated in a couple of outings with other residents, she began volunteer work with a community newspaper, and she began to trust her next-door neighbor enough to tell her something about herself. Janice also witnessed the beginning of a process of development whereby individuals recognized their links and responsibilities to one another and their capacity to solve problems collaboratively with the resources available in the community.

Despite her improved relationship with her roommate, Sandy continued to feel that there were many issues about which she wished to talk to someone. She recognized that she needed to talk to someone who had experienced some of the things that she had experienced with her illness but did not wish to sacrifice her privacy within the boarding home.

Independent Living

She had heard about a support group for people with mental illness and decided to make some inquiries. In so doing, she discovered that the support group was part of a center, called the Survivors' Centre, that embraced an independent living philosophy, with individuals with mental illness helping and supporting others in similar circumstances. In addition to the weekly support group, the center offered peer support through telephone dyads, resource information, and referral to other services within the community, a weekly movie night, a monthly supper club, a public education committee, an emergency hotline, and a volunteer and vocational training program. In addition, the center ran several commercial enterprises, including a cafe, a dry-cleaning business, and a recycling center. After much thought, Sandy called and went down to the center for an orientation. Initially, she took the name of another woman whose circumstances were similar to her own, but who had just been discharged from hospital, and agreed to call her and see how she was doing. Bit by bit over the next few months, Sandy tried out more of the center's activities. Now, 2 years later, she is the manager of the recycling center. Her involvement with the center has resulted in her gaining confidence in her ability to contribute to her community, finding others with whom she shares important experiences relating to her illness, and broadening the scope of her daily life to include a more meaningful balance of activities.

Conclusion

The challenge of working with people with disabilities can be met in a variety of different ways. This chapter has outlined four different approaches to addressing occupational dysfunction through rehabilitation. Each of these approaches assists in the development of occupational functioning, but each requires different assumptions about the person, the environment, and the nature of occupation. Further, each has advantages and disadvantages that make it more or less applicable in different settings, at different times in the process of rehabilitation and community integration, and for different individuals.

For many years, occupational therapy practitioners have functioned primarily from only one model of service: the biomedical model. While this model of service has served some consumers of occupational therapy services well, it has apparently been counter-therapeutic for others. Occupational therapy practitioners need not be restricted to a single model of service delivery. The chapter describes three alternatives to the biomedical model, each based on a different belief system about the nature and origins of disability. As occupational therapy practitioners become more skilled in areas like phenomenology, community development, and sociopolitical analysis, the potential utility of other models of services increases. The occupational therapy practitioner who has in his or her therapeutic repertoire the ability to assess a situation and choose between models will undoubtedly be better prepared to meet the challenge of working with people with disabilities. He or she will be able to choose an approach to service that is based not simply on his or her own preferences, but on a multidimensional assessment of the person, environment, and occupational needs of people like Steven or Sandy.

Acknowledgment

The author gratefully acknowledges the two co-authors of the original chapter, Nancy Gerein and Fraser Valentine, which appeared in the first edition of this book.

REFERENCES

Bakheit, A. M. O. (1995). Delivery of rehabilitation services: An integrated hospital-community approach. *Clinical Rehabilitation*, *9*, 142-149.

Banerjee, R. (1992). CBR—*Is it an appropriate alternative? Sharing strengths—A workshop on community-based rehabilitation*. Bangalore, India: Seva-in-Action.

Beange, H. (1987). Our clients' health: Their responsibility or ours? *Australia and New Zealand Journal of Developmental Disabilities*, *13*, 175-177.

Ben-Sira, Z. (1983). Societal integration of the disabled: Power struggle or enhancement of individual coping capacities. *Social Science and Medicine*, *17*, 1011-1014.

Berrol, S. (1979). Independent living programs: The role of the able-bodied professional. *Archives of Physical Medicine and Rehabilitation*, *60*, 456-457.

Bichmann, W., Rifkin, S., & Shrestha, M. (1989). Toward the measurement of community participation. *World Health Forum*, *10*, 467-472.

Bickenbach, J. (1992). *Physical disability and social policy*. Toronto, Canada: University of Toronto Press.

Boland, J. M., & Alonso, G. (1982). A comparison: Independent living rehabilitation and vocational rehabilitation. *Journal of Rehabilitation*, *48*, 56-59.

Boyce, W., & Johnston, C. (1998). Collaboration in community based rehabilitation agencies. *International Journal of Rehabilitation Research*, *21*(1), 1-11.

Boyce, W., & Peat, M. (1995). A comprehensive approach to research in Community Based Rehabilitation. *Nytt om U-landshalsovard*, *9*(2), 15-18.

Brider, P. (1992). Patient-focused care. *American Journal of Nursing*, *9*, 27-33.

Brisenden, S. (1986). Independent living and the medical model of disability. *Disability, Handicap & Society*, *1*, 173-179.

Brown, S. J. (1992). Tailoring nursing care to the individual client: Empirical challenge of a theoretical concept. *Research in Nursing and Health*, *15*, 39-46.

Burnard, P., & Morrison, P. (1991). Client-centred counselling: A study of nurses' attitudes. *Nurse Education Today*, *11*, 104-109.

Canadian Association of Independent Living Centres. (1989). *Independent living promotion kit*. Ottawa, Canada: Author.

Canadian Association of Independent Living Centres. (1994). *A time for change, the time for choices*. Ottawa, Canada: Author.

Carlisle, D. (1992). Patients first. *Nursing Times*, 88(12), 16-17.

Clarke, C., Scott, E., & Krupa, T. (1993). Involving clients in program evaluation and research. *Canadian Journal of Occupational Therapy*, 60, 192-199.

Cole, J. A. (1979). What's new about independent living? *Archives of Physical Medicine and Rehabilitation*, 60, 458-461.

Compton, F. (1971). Community development theory and practice. In J. A. Draper (Ed.), *Citizen participation: Canada. A book of readings*. Toronto: New Press.

Coring, D. J., & Cook, J. V. (1999). Client-centred care means that I am a valued human being. *Canadian Journal of Occupational Therapy*, 66(2), 71-82.

DeJong, G. (1979). Independent living: From social movement to analytic paradigm. *Archives of Physical Medicine and Rehabilitation*, 60, 435-446.

DeLoach, C. P., Wilkins, R. D., & Walker, G. W. (1983). *Independent living: Philosophy, process and services*. Baltimore, MD: University Park Press.

Driedger, D. (1989). *The last civil rights movement: Disabled peoples' international*. New York, NY: St. Martin's Press.

Emener, W. G. (1991). Empowerment in rehabilitation: An empowerment philosophy for rehabilitation in the 20th century. *Journal of Rehabilitation*, *57*(4), 7-12.

Friedland, J. (1998) Occupational therapy and rehabilitation: An awkward alliance. *American Journal of Occupational Therapy*, *52*(5), 373-80.

Gadacz, R. (1994). *Rethinking disability: New structures, new relationships*. Edmonton, Canada: University of Alberta Press.

Goodall, C. (1992). Preserving dignity for disabled people. *Nursing Standard*, 6(35), 25-27.

Hawe, P. (1994). Capturing the meaning of "community" in community intervention evaluation: Some contributions from community psychology. *Health Promotion International*, 9(3), 199-210.

Herzberg, S. R. (1990). Client or patient: Which term is more appropriate for use in occupational therapy? *American Journal of Occupational Therapy*, *44*, 561-565.

Holyoke, P., & Elkan, L. (1995). *Rehabilitation services inventory and quality*. Toronto: Institute for Work and Health.

International Labour Organization, United Nations Educational, Scientific and Cultural Organization, World Health Organization. (1994). *Community-based rehabilitation for and with people with disabilities*. Geneva, Switzerland: WHO.

Jaffe, Y., & Kipper, D. A. (1982). Appeal of rational-emotive and client-centred therapies to first-year psychology and non-psychology students. *Psychological Reports*, 50, 781-782.

Kerfoot, K. M., & LeClair, C. (1991). Building a patient-focused unit: The nurse manager's challenge. *Nursing Economics*, 9, 441-443.

Lysack, C., & Kaufert, J. (1994). Comparing the origins and ideologies of the independent living movement and community based rehabilitation. *International Journal of Rehabilitation Research*, *17*, 231-240.

Mattingly, C., & Fleming, M. (1994). *Clinical reasoning: Forms of inquiry in a therapeutic practice*. Philadelphia, PA: F. A. Davis Co.

McColl, M. A. (1998). What we need to know to practice occupational therapy in the community. *American Journal of Occupational Therapy*, *52*(1), 11-18.

McColl, M. A., Law, M., & Stewart, D. (1993). *Theoretical basis of occupational therapy: An annotated bibliography*. Thorofare, NJ: SLACK Incorporated.

Meyer, A. (1922). The philosophy of occupational therapy. *Archives of Occupational Therapy, 1*, 1-10.

Miles, M. (1994). *CBR information accumulation and exchange: Research notes*. CBR Symposium, Bangalore, India.

Mitchell, R. (1999a). Community-based rehabilitation: The generalized model. *Disability & Rehabilitation, 21*(10-11), 522-528.

Mitchell, R. (1999b). The research base of community-based rehabilitation. *Disability & Rehabilitation, 21*(10-11), 459-468.

Oliver, M. (1990). *The politics of disablement*. London, England: MacMillan.

O'Toole, B. J. (1991). *Guide to community-based rehabilitation services. Guides for special education*. Paris, France: UNESCO.

Parsons, T. (1975). The sick role and the role of the physician reconsidered. *Health and Society, 25*, 258-278.

Patterson, J. B., & Marks, C. (1992). The client as customer: Achieving service quality and customer satisfaction in rehabilitation. *Journal of Rehabilitation*, 58(4), 16-20.

Peat, M., & Boyce, W. (1993). Canadian community rehabilitation services: Challenges for the future. *Canadian Journal of Rehabilitation*, 6, 281-289.

Pollock, N. (1993). Client-centred assessment. *American Journal of Occupational Therapy, 47*, 298-301.

Pollock, N., Baptiste, S., Law, M., McColl, M. A., Opzoomer, A., & Polatajko, H. (1990). Occupational performance measures: A review based on the Guidelines for Client-centred practice. *Canadian Journal of Occupational Therapy*, 57(2), 82-87.

Rebeiro, K. L. (2000). Client perspectives on occupational therapy practice: Are we truly client-centred? *Canadian Journal of Occupational Therapy-Revue Canadienne d Ergotherapie*, 67(1), 7-14.

Robinson, N. C. (1991). A patient-centred framework for restructuring care. *Journal of Organizational Nursing and Administration, 21*(9), 29-34.

Rogers, C. (1942). *Counselling and psychotherapy: Newer concepts in practice*. Boston, MA: Houghton-Mifflin Co.

Rogers, C. (1965). *Client-centred therapy: Its current practice, implications and theory*. Boston, MA: Houghton-Mifflin Co.

Schlaff, C. (1993). From dependency to self-advocacy: Redefining disability. *American Journal of Occupational Therapy, 47*, 943-948.

Schroeder, D. H., & Bloom, L. J. (1979). Attraction to therapy and therapist credibility as a function of therapy orientation. *Journal of Clinical Psychology, 35*, 683-686.

Sumsion, T., & Smyth, G. (2000). Barriers to client-centredness and their resolution. *Canadian Journal of Occupational Therapy*, 67(1), 15-21.

Symington, D. (1994). Megatrends in rehabilitation: A Canadian perspective. *International Journal of Rehabilitation Research, 17*, 1-14.

Tamaru, A. (2003). Understanding independence: Perspectives of Canadian and Japanese occupational therapists. Masters thesis. Queen's University, Kingston, Canada

Trombly, C. (1993). Anticipating the future: Assessment of occupational function. *American Journal of Occupational Therapy, 47*, 253-257.

United Nations. (1983). *World program of action concerning disabled persons*. New York, NY: Author.

Wallerstein, N. (1992). Powerlessness, empowerment, and health: Implications for health promotion programs. *American Journal of Health Promotion*, 6(3), 197-205.

Walton, K. M., Schwab, L. O., Cassatt-Dunn, M. A., & Wright, V. K. (1980). Techniques and concepts: Independent living. Perceptions by professionals in rehabilitation. *Journal of Rehabilitation*, 46(3), 57-63.

Wanigaratne, S., & Barker, C. (1995). Clients' preferences for styles of therapy. *British Journal of Clinical Psychology, 34*, 215-222.

Chapter Eighteen: Occupational Therapy Interventions in a Rehabilitation Context Reflections and Learning Activities

Julie Bass-Haugen, PhD, OTR/L, FAOTA

REFLECTION

Occupational therapy practitioners work in many different settings—each with a culture of its own. There are also many emerging areas of practice that require practitioners to work in entirely new models of service delivery. This chapter introduced four models of service delivery for rehabilitation: biomedical rehabilitation, client-centered rehabilitation, community-based rehabilitation and independent living.

As you saw in the description of each model and the case studies, the role of the occupational therapy practitioner, other professionals, and the individual receiving services varies depending on the service delivery framework. For example, in biomedical rehabilitation, the rehabilitation professionals have lead roles in planning and providing therapeutic interventions while in the independent living model occupational therapy practitioners may only serve as an occasional resource to individuals with disabilities. On the other hand, the individual receiving services has a more passive role in biomedical rehabilitation and a lead role in the independent living model. How would you characterize the roles of the occupational therapy practitioner and the individual receiving services in the other two models?

When I was reading this chapter, I noticed how the individual receiving services had different labels or names in each model. In the biomedical rehabilitation model, the recipient of services was referred to as a 'patient' while in client-centered rehabilitation the individual was a 'client.' In community-based rehabilitation, the 'community' was the focus of services but in the independent living model the focus was a 'consumer.' Words and labels are powerful tools of language that shape how we think about people and their life situation. It also shapes how people think about themselves and their ability to solve problems.

The assumptions supporting each model are also important to note. Each model has different assumptions about the nature of disability and the performance and participation problems associated with disability. In turn, these beliefs influence the focus areas for intervention. In the models, there were variations in whether the intervention priorities were placed on the individual or the community and on the person or the environment. Think about the array of intervention methods for occupational therapy. What methods would you likely choose for each model?

Finally, each model was examined for its advantages and disadvantages. You might have guessed before reading this chapter that one model was going to be recommended as the preferred model of service delivery for occupational therapy. As it turns out, there are trade-offs in each model. The challenge for the practitioner is to weigh the pros and cons of a given model and keep them in mind as services are provided. For example, if I am working in a biomedical rehabilitation model, I note that the intentions of the professionals are good when they care for patients and make medical decisions regarding interventions. At the same time, however, this model has the potential to make patients feel like they have lost total control of their lives and turned decision making over to others. Furthermore, the biomedical rehabilitation model is really only useful for a very limited period of time. What happens when patients are discharged from these types of services? Now take a look at the advantages and disadvantages of the other models. How would you describe the delicate balance between the advantages and disadvantages of each model?

As you have seen, specific rehabilitation models of service delivery are important for different settings and different stages of a person's life. The occupational therapy practitioner and the service delivery model are parts of the social support mechanisms and social policies and attitudes that either enable or constrain occupational performance. Thus, it is essential that the occupational therapy practitioner operate from the appropriate model at a given point in time. This is one of your challenges in occupational therapy practice.

JOURNAL ACTIVITIES

1. Look up and write down dictionary definitions of biomedical and rehabilitation. Highlight the component of the definitions that is most related to their descriptions in Chapter Eighteen.
2. Identify the most important new learning for you in this chapter.
3. Identify one question you have about Chapter Eighteen.
4. In the United States, occupational therapy has its primary roles in biomedical rehabilitation and client-centered rehabilitation. Reflect on why you think occupational therapy does not currently have a strong role in community-based rehabilitation and independent living centers. Propose a stronger role for occupational therapy in these models that is outside the traditional medical box.

5. Reflect on the role of occupational therapy in the school system. Does the school system fit in this rehabilitation framework or does it have its own framework? Justify your answer.

Technology/Internet Learning Activities

1. Use a discussion database to share specific journal activities.
2. Use a good Internet search engine to find the Web site for the National Rehabilitation Information Center.
   - Enter the phrase "NRIC" or "National Rehabilitation Information Center" in your search line.
   - Document and review the home page for each Web site.
   - Evaluate the quality of this Web site. What are its strengths and weaknesses?
   - What is the overall purpose of this Web site?
   - What resources are available on this site?
   - Use the Information Center to find information on one topic related to occupational therapy.
     - ✧ Document and summarize two to three abstracts on this topic.
   - Review the NIDRR Research Projects currently funded.
     - ✧ Document and summarize two to three projects that relate to occupational therapy.
3. Use a good Internet search engine to find the Web sites for the Office of Special Education and Rehabilitative Services (OSERS) and National Institute on Disability and Rehabilitation Research.
   - Enter the phrase "OSERS" and "NIDRR" in your search line.
   - Document and review the home page for each Web site.
   - Evaluate the quality of this Web site. What are its strengths and weaknesses?
   - What is the overall purpose of this Web site?
   - What resources are available on this site?
   - Examine the mission, plans, programs, and priorities of OSERS and NIDRR.
     - ✧ Document and summarize two to three priorities related to occupational therapy interventions.
4. Use a good Internet search engine to find the Web site for the classic article by Carl Rogers titled *Significant Aspects of Client-Centered Therapy*.
   - Enter the phrase "client-centered therapy" in your search line.
   - Skim the classic article by Carl Rogers.
   - Identify the conditions necessary for client-centered therapy.
   - Identify the results of client-centered therapy if these conditions are met.
5. Use a good Internet search engine to find Web sites on community-based rehabilitation.
   - Enter the phrase "community-based rehabilitation" or "world health organization community-based rehabilitation" in your search line.
   - Document and review the home page for each Web site.
   - Evaluate the quality of each Web site. What are its strengths and weaknesses?
   - What is the overall purpose of this Web site?
   - What resources are available on this site?
   - Identify resources available on community-based rehabilitation on the World Health Organization Web site.
     - ✧ Document and summarize two to three resources related to occupational therapy interventions.
6. Use a good Internet search engine to find the Web site for the National Council on Independent Living.
   - Enter the phrase "national council on independent living" in your search line.
   - Document and review the home page for each Web site.
   - Evaluate the quality of each Web site. What are its strengths and weaknesses?
   - What is the overall purpose of this Web site?
   - What resources are available on this site?

- Identify resources available on the Web site related to occupational therapy interventions.
  - ✧ Document and summarize two to three resources related to occupational therapy interventions.

Applied Learning

Individual Learning Activity #1: Exploring Biomedical Rehabilitation in Two Cases

Instructions:

- Steven
  - ✧ Read Steven's case on biomedical rehabilitation in Chapter Eighteen.
  - ✧ Gather and review some evidence and resources on acute care for spinal cord injury.
  - ✧ Identify two to three key medical issues in the acute care stage for spinal cord injury.
  - ✧ Review the interventions that are described in the case.
  - ✧ Summarize the characteristics of the interventions at this stage.
  - ✧ Are there other interventions you would consider for Steven at this stage?
  - ✧ Describe the feelings you would have during this stage as the client.
  - ✧ Describe how each of the interventions supports current or future occupations.

Description of Intervention	*Intervention Goal—* *Promote* *Prevent* *Resolve*	*Intervention Approach—* *Remediate* *Restore* *Establish* *Compensate* *Adapt* *Modify*	*Intervention Method—* *Therapeutic Activity* *Education* *Consultation*
Positioning			
Communication			
Foot drop splints			
Resting splints			
Call bell			
Adapted equipment			
Phone use			

- Sandy
  - ✧ Read Sandy's case on biomedical rehabilitation in Chapter Eighteen.
  - ✧ Gather and review some evidence and resources on acute care for schizophrenia.
  - ✧ Identify two to three key medical issues in the acute care stage for schizophrenia (Note: Chapter Eighteen does not describe any occupational therapy intervention for biomedical rehabilitation of schizophrenia).
  - ✧ Are there any occupational therapy interventions you would propose for this stage?
  - ✧ Describe the feelings you would have during this stage as the client.

Individual Learning Activity #2: Exploring Client-Centered Rehabilitation in Two Cases

Instructions:

- Steven
  - ✧ Read Steven's case on client-centered rehabilitation in Chapter Eighteen.
  - ✧ Gather and review some evidence and resources on rehabilitation for spinal cord injury.
  - ✧ Identify two to three key medical issues in this stage for spinal cord injury.
  - ✧ Review the interventions that are described in the case.
  - ✧ Summarize the characteristics of the interventions at this stage.
  - ✧ Are there other interventions you would consider for Steven at this stage?
  - ✧ Describe the feelings you would have during this stage as the client.
  - ✧ Describe how each of the interventions supports current or future occupations.

Description of Intervention	*Intervention Goal—* *Promote* *Prevent* *Resolve*	*Intervention Approach—* *Remediate* *Restore* *Establish* *Compensate* *Adapt* *Modify*	*Intervention Method—* *Therapeutic Activity* *Education* *Consultation*
Storying			
Strengthening and balance activities			
Tenodesis grasp			
Wheelchair mobility			
Self-care			
Visualization			
Home visit			
Home modification			
Bowel/bladder			
Discussion			
Wheelchair selection			

- Sandy
  - ✧ Read Sandy's case on client-centered rehabilitation in Chapter Eighteen.
  - ✧ Gather and review some evidence and resources on client-centered rehabilitation for schizophrenia.
  - ✧ Identify two to three key medical issues in this stage for schizophrenia.
  - ✧ Review the interventions that are described in the case.
  - ✧ Summarize the characteristics of the interventions at this stage.
  - ✧ Are there other interventions you would consider for Sandy at this stage?
  - ✧ Describe the feelings you would have during this stage as the client.
  - ✧ Describe how each of the interventions supports current or future occupations.

Description of Intervention	*Intervention Goal— Promote Prevent Resolve*	*Intervention Approach— Remediate Restore Establish Compensate Adapt Modify*	*Intervention Method— Therapeutic Activity Education· Consultation*
Guided discussion			
Residential planning			
Occupation diaries			
Resource planning			
Role playing			

Individual Learning Activity #3: Exploring Community-Based Rehabilitation in Two Cases

Instructions:

- Steven
  - ✧ Read Steven's case on community-based rehabilitation in Chapter Eighteen.
  - ✧ Gather and review some evidence and resources on community-based rehabilitation for spinal cord injury.
  - ✧ Identify two to three key issues in this stage for spinal cord injury.
  - ✧ Review the interventions that are described in the case.
  - ✧ Summarize the characteristics of the interventions at this stage.
  - ✧ Are there other interventions you would consider for Steven at this stage?
  - ✧ Describe the feelings you would have during this stage as the client.
  - ✧ Describe how each of the interventions supports current or future occupations.

Description of Intervention	*Intervention Goal— Promote Prevent Resolve*	*Intervention Approach— Remediate Restore Establish Compensate Adapt Modify*	*Intervention Method— Therapeutic Activity Education Consultation*
Advocacy			
School physical environment			
School social environment			
Peer training			
Housing arrangements			
Resource planning			

- Sandy
  - ✧ Read Sandy's case on community-based rehabilitation in Chapter Eighteen.
  - ✧ Gather and review some evidence and resources on community-based rehabilitation for schizophrenia.
  - ✧ Identify two to three key issues in this stage for schizophrenia.
  - ✧ Review the interventions that are described in the case.
  - ✧ Summarize the characteristics of the interventions at this stage.
  - ✧ Are there other interventions you would consider for Sandy at this stage?
  - ✧ Describe the feelings you would have during this stage as the client.
  - ✧ Describe how each of the interventions supports current or future occupations.

Description of Intervention	*Intervention Goal— Promote Prevent Resolve*	*Intervention Approach— Remediate Restore Establish Compensate Adapt Modify*	*Intervention Method— Therapeutic Activity Education Consultation*
Community organizing			
Problem-solving session			
Information sessions			
Resource identification			

Individual Learning Activity #4: Exploring Independent Living in Two Cases

Instructions:

- Steven
  - ✧ Read Steven's case on independent living in Chapter Eighteen.
  - ✧ Gather and review some evidence and resources on independent living for spinal cord injury.
  - ✧ Identify two to three key issues in this stage for spinal cord injury.
  - ✧ Review the interventions that are described in the case.
  - ✧ Summarize the characteristics of the interventions at this stage.
  - ✧ Are there other interventions you would consider for Steven at this stage?
  - ✧ Describe the feelings you would have during this stage as the client.
  - ✧ Describe how each of the interventions supports current or future occupations.

Description of Intervention	*Intervention Goal— Promote Prevent Resolve*	*Intervention Approach— Remediate Restore Establish Compensate Adapt Modify*	*Intervention Method— Therapeutic Activity Education Consultation*
Referral			
Home environment			
Personal care attendant planning			

- Sandy
  - ✧ Read Sandy's case on independent living in Chapter Eighteen.
  - ✧ Gather and review some evidence and resources on independent living for schizophrenia.
  - ✧ Identify two to three key issues in this stage for schizophrenia (Note: Chapter Eighteen does not describe any occupational therapy intervention for the independent living stage of schizophrenia).
  - ✧ Are there any occupational therapy interventions you would propose for this stage?
  - ✧ Describe the feelings you, as the client, would have during this stage.

Active Learning

Group Activity: Proposing New Roles for Occupational Therapy

Preparation:

- Read Chapter Eighteen.
- Complete the Technology/Internet Learning Activities.

Time: 45 minutes to 1 hour

Materials:

- Resources from Technology/Internet Learning Activities
- Flip chart, white board, or black board
- Art supplies

Instructions:

- Individually:
  - ✧ Review the four service delivery models in Chapter Eighteen.
- In small groups:
  - ✧ Examine community-based rehabilitation and independent living models in more detail.

Community-Based Rehabilitation

What are the assumptions, advantages, and disadvantages of this service delivery model?

What are the likely funding sources for this model?

What is the proper role of occupational therapy practitioners in this model?

Independent Living

What are the assumptions, advantages, and disadvantages of this service delivery model?

What are the likely funding sources for this model?

What is the proper role of occupational therapy practitioners in this model?

For the community-based rehabilitation and independent living models:

Brainstorm two new, creative employment positions for a person with an occupational therapy back ground for each model. Identify one position that is appropriate for a recent graduate of an occupation al therapy or occupational therapy assistant program. Identify one position that is appropriate for an occupational therapy practitioner with at least 5 years of experience. For each position:

What are the job responsibilities?

What skills are important?

Where does this person work?

Who is the client?

Who is the employer, supervisor, support staff?

How is this position funded?

Discussion:

- Discuss the rewards and challenges that you would associate with these positions.
- Discuss the likely job titles for these positions. Would it be "occupational therapy practitioner"?

- Discuss whether the essence of each of these jobs is occupational therapy.
- Discuss the advantages and disadvantages of developing these roles for occupational therapy.

Chapter Nineteen Objectives

The information in this chapter is intended to help the reader:

1. Be able to define community.
2. Understand the concept of community health from an occupational therapy perspective.
3. Identify the determinants of health in a community.
4. Define health from the perspective of the World Health Organization.
5. Understand what has guided the development of interventions at the community level.
6. Describe the relationship of poverty to chronic health conditions.
7. Understand the threats to the health of a community.
8. Describe how epidemiology uses health statistics to analyze health trends and evaluate community health interventions that will inform policy.
9. Describe community health promotion and the means of achieving it.
10. Understand the importance of coalitions and how they develop.
11. Describe occupational therapy's role in community level interventions.
12. Describe what occupational therapy practitioners need to do to prepare for community health practice.

Key Words

community: A collective of people identified by common values and mutual concern for the development and well-being of their group or geographical area (Green & Kreuter, 1991, p. 504).

community-based practice: Provision of services in community settings where people live, play, and work.

community capacity: "Combined assets that include a community's commitment, resources, and skills used to solve problems and strengthen the quality of life for its citizens" (2000 Joint Committee on Health Education and Promotion Terminology, 2001, p. 97).

community-centered interventions: Approach in which community members come together through partnerships and coalitions to identify common concerns and solve community problems.

community-level interventions: Population-based approaches that attempt to modify the sociocultural, political, economic, and environmental context of the community in order to achieve health goals.

community organization: "Process by which communities mobilize to identify common problems or goals, mobilize resources, and in other ways, develop and implement strategies for reaching the goals they have collectively set" (2000 Joint Committee on Health Education and Promotion Terminology, 2001, p. 97).

epidemiology: Study of the distribution, frequencies, and determinants of disease, injury, and disability in human populations and the application of this study to the control of health in populations (Last, 2001; MacMahon & Trichopoulos, 1996).

health promotion: Any planned combination of educational, political, regulatory, environmental, and organizational supports for actions and conditions of living conducive to the health of individuals, groups, or communities (Green & Kreuter, 1991).

health protection: "Any planned intervention or services designed to provide individuals and communities with resistance to health threats, often by modifying policy or the environment to decrease potentially harmful interactions" (2000 Joint Committee on Health Education and Promotion Terminology, 2001, p. 101).

health services: Interventions typically provided by organizations staffed with health care and medical professionals to improve access to quality health services by organizing and distributing resources more effectively.

incidence: Refers to the number of new cases of disease, injury, or disability within a specified time frame and measures how quickly a disease is spreading.

prevalence: Total number of cases of disease, injury, or disability that exist in a community at one point in time (Pickett & Hanlon, 1990).

risk factors: Those lifestyle behaviors or environmental conditions that, on the basis of scientific evidence or theory, are thought to influence susceptibility to a specific health problem (Turnock, 2001).

social ecology: Study of the effects of the physical and social environments on people.

threats to community health: Environmental, social, organizational, and political factors that interfere with the physical and mental health of individuals and families in a community.

In every community, there is work to be done.
In every nation, there are wounds to heal. In every heart, there is the power to do it.
Marianne Williamson

Chapter Nineteen

Occupational Therapy Interventions: Community Health Approaches

Marjorie E. Scaffa, PhD, OTR, FAOTA and Carol Brownson, MSPH, PHLC

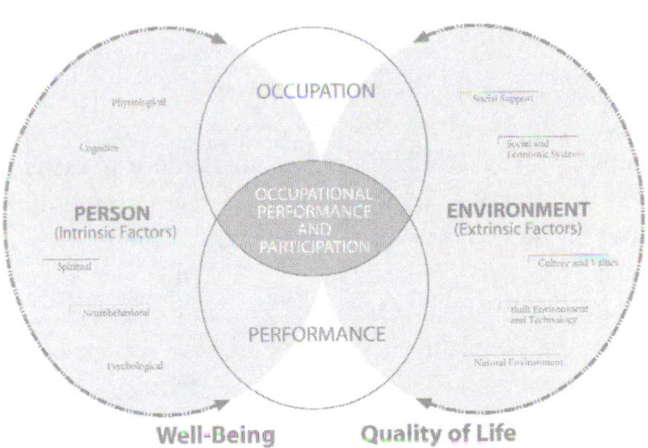

Setting the Stage

This chapter will introduce community health approaches for occupational therapy intervention. Community health interventions are intended to address the physical, mental, social, and spiritual health of communities. These emerging occupational therapy approaches are primarily targeted at the social and environmental determinants of health. At this time in history, occupational therapy practitioners have a unique opportunity to address the community health problems of the 21st century.

Scaffa, M. E., & Brownson, C. (2005). Occupational therapy interventions: Community health approaches. In C. H. Christiansen, C. M. Baum, and J. Bass-Haugen (Eds.), Occupational therapy: Performance, participation, and well-being *(3rd ed.). Thorofare, NJ: SLACK Incorporated.*

OVERVIEW OF COMMUNITY HEALTH

The definition of community varies across disciplines, although most definitions share the major concepts of place, shared interests, joint activities, and social relationship (MacQueen et al., 2001). Green and Kreuter (1991) define community as "a collective of people identified by common values and mutual concern for the development and well-being of their group or geographical area" (p. 504). Likewise, the concept of working "in the community" conjures up different images for different people. Occupational therapy practitioners fill a variety of roles outside the clinical setting. It might be useful to identify them first by the object of the intervention. For example, it is clear when one is working on bathing and dressing with a client during a home health visit that the desired outcome is improvement in functional ability for that individual; thus, the individual is the object or target of the intervention.

In contrast, if occupational therapy practitioners advocate successfully for ramps to replace curbs at intersections, the object of the intervention is the community's physical environment. In this instance, the change is at the community level; it changes the community itself, thereby improving access for many. Community health refers to both private and public efforts of individuals, groups, and organizations to promote, protect, and preserve the physical, mental, social, and spiritual health of those in the community (Aspen Reference Group, 2000; McKenzie & Smeltzer, 1997; Scaffa, Desmond, & Brownson, 2001). Unlike the individual or clinical approach, community health efforts attempt to affect whole populations or selected segments of the population in a community. These approaches emphasize the role of social and environmental determinants of health.

Figure 19-1 depicts a model of the determinants of health in a community. This complex set of interactions draws attention to a set of general factors that can influence the health of a community overall. Collectively, determinants of health include genetics, the physical and social environment, and the individual response. Prosperity, or the lack of it, affects both health outcomes and the physical and social environment. This model also provides a way of conceptualizing the influence of community on health. Communities contain the social environment (worksites, schools, friends, organizations, etc.) and comprise the physical environment. People are both agents and recipients of social influence and of the physical environment (Patrick & Wickizer, 1995). Consider, for example, the effects of air pollution on lung cancer, emphysema, and asthma.

The study of the effects of the physical and social environments on people is called *social ecology*. Socioecological approaches to improving health recognize the interdependence between people and their physical, social, cultural, economic, and political environments (Brownson, 2001; Stokols, 1992). In this framework, multiple factors in the larger environment explain and influence the health behavior of individuals. An ecological health promotion planning model that is similar in concept to Bronfenbrenner's Ecological Systems Model (Christiansen & Baum, 1997) describes five societal levels that affect individual health: individual, group, organizational, community, and policy (Simons-Morton, Greene, & Gottlieb, 1995).

At the individual level, health has been defined as a state of complete physical, mental, and social well-being and not merely the absence of disease or infirmity (World Health Organization [WHO], 1947). It is a resource for everyday life—largely culturally defined and multidimensional, emphasizing social and personal resources, as well as physical capacities (Turnock, 2001; WHO, 1986). The Healthy Cities/Healthy Communities program, begun in response to the World Health Organization's *Global Strategies for Health for All by the Year 2000*, was designed to involve communities in identifying and addressing the multiple factors affecting health at the community level (Norris, 1993). This initiative gave rise to the concept of healthy cities and communities, defined as "one that is continually creating and improving those physical and social environments and expanding those community resources which enable people to mutually support each other in performing all the functions of life and in developing to their maximum potential" (WHO, 1999). A healthy community, then, might have such features as:

- Access to affordable, high-quality health care
- Social and environmental supports for healthy lifestyles
- Clean air and water
- Adequate and affordable housing
- Access to affordable, high-quality schools
- Recreational facilities and opportunities for people of all abilities
- Opportunities to experience and express creative arts
- Safe and accessible work and community environments
- Religious freedom, etc.

Healthy communitu initiatives involve broad representation from the community in a collaborative process of visioning, planning, and implementing change strategies. The development of interventions at the community level has been guided by health promotion theory, research, and experience, from which the following lessons have been learned:

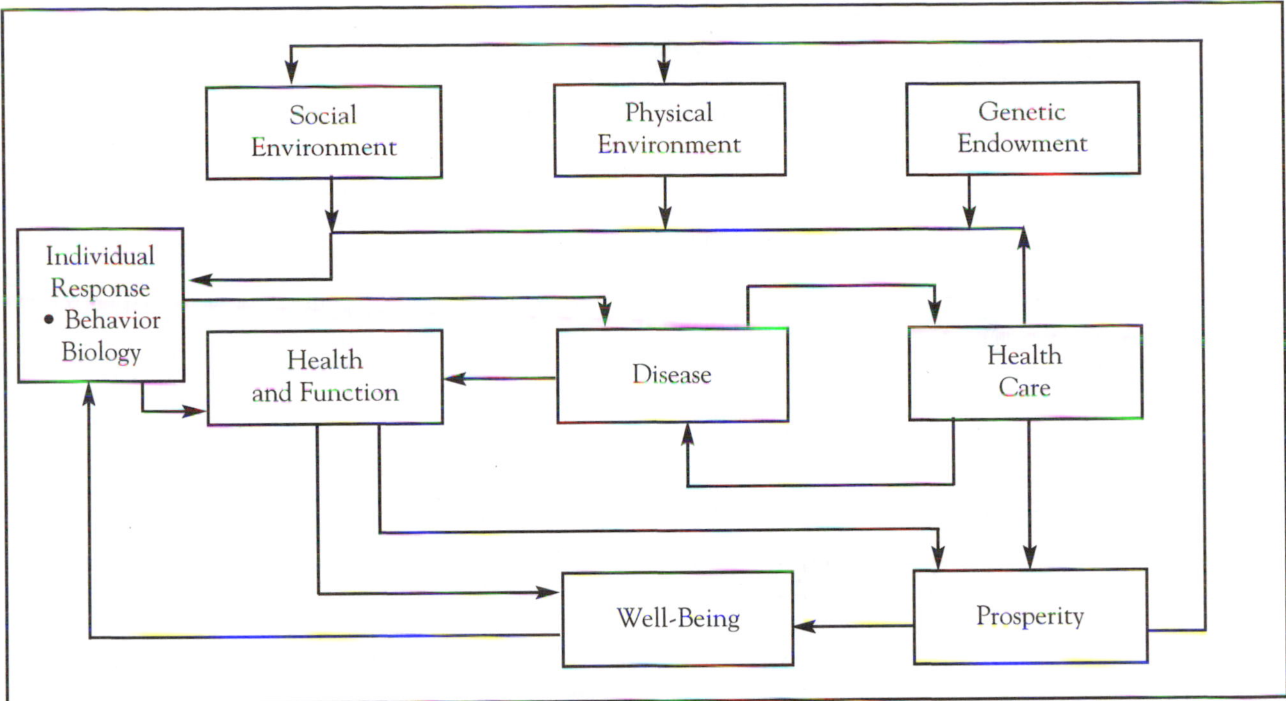

Figure 19-1. A causal model of the determinants of disease, health and function, and well-being (Evans and Stoddard, 1990).

- Comprehensive approaches that address economic, social, and political factors affecting health are more effective than traditional educational approaches.
- Changing community norms is an effective way to improve health.
- Community-level approaches will contribute more to reducing health risks and mortality than individual interventions alone.
- Programs are more effective if the at-risk community members and community organizations are actively involved in prioritizing, developing, and implementing intervention programs.
- Interventions are most successful if they build on traditional practices and cultural norms.
- Intervention strategies should be based on the needs and input of the community.
- Multiple strategies will enhance program effectiveness.
- Clearly defined and mutually agreed upon goals and objectives are essential for effective initiatives.
- Effective interventions also require ongoing evaluation and adjustment of strategies as needed (Davis, Schwartz, Wheeler, & Lancaster, 1998).

Disparities in Communities

It has long been recognized that disease, injury, and disability affect groups of people disproportionately. Population groups that have the highest poverty rates and least education have higher rates of most chronic conditions, including heart disease, diabetes, obesity, etc. Many ethnic groups are also disproportionately affected by diseases and disability, as are people who live in rural areas (U.S. Department of Health and Human Services, 2001). In general, lower socioeconomic status is associated with lower health status.

While, overall, the health of Americans has improved over the past 10 years, in some groups, health indicators have remained stable or declined. A disproportionate number of Americans in ethnic and racial minority groups lack access to preventive health services and, therefore, are more likely than whites to have poor health and die prematurely. For example, African American women are more likely to die of breast cancer than are women of any other racial or ethnic group. As compared to whites, the prevalence of diabetes is much higher in African Americans (70% higher), Hispanics (100% higher), and American Indians and Alaskan Natives (200%).

Although African Americans and Hispanics combined represented only 25% of the U.S. population in 1999, they accounted for approximately 55% of adult AIDS cases and 82% of pediatric AIDS cases of the total prevalence reported in that same year (National Center for Chronic Disease Prevention and Health Promotion, 2001). In addition, racial and ethnic minorities experience greater disability from mental illness than do whites. This is not due to higher rates of mental illness among minorities, as the prevalence and severity of mental disorders is comparable with whites, but rather to unequal access to mental health care. The social and economic environment of inequality that people of color experience has a significant negative impact on mental health (U.S. Department of Health and Human Services, 2001).

Healthy People 2010, the national health agenda, has two broad goals: (1) to increase the quality and years of healthy life and (2) to eliminate health disparities (U.S. Department of Health and Human Services, 2000). In an effort to address health disparities, the Centers for Disease Control and Prevention (CDC) has initiated a 5-year demonstration project titled Racial and Ethnic Approaches to Community Health (REACH) 2010 to eliminate racial and ethnic disparities in health. REACH 2010 has identified six priority areas to target: cardiovascular disease, immunizations, breast and cervical cancer, diabetes, HIV/AIDS, and infant mortality (National Center for Chronic Disease Prevention and Health Promotion, 2001).

Understanding Threats to Community Health

Threats to the health of a community include those environmental, social, organizational, and political factors that interfere with the physical and mental health of individuals and families in a community. Threats to community health may include disease, injury, disability, social isolation, low educational attainment, unemployment, poverty, overcrowding, violence, pollution, crime, racism, and discrimination.

Identifying health threats in any particular community or population is one of the functions of epidemiology. Epidemiology is the study of the distribution, frequencies, and determinants of disease, injury, and disability in human populations and the application of this study to the control of health in populations (Last, 2001; MacMahon & Trichopoulos, 1996). Epidemiology uses health statistics, including measures of incidence and prevalence, (1) to discover the factors that affect health; (2) to determine the relative importance of risk factors and courses of illness, disability, and death; (3) to identify high-risk populations; and (4) to evaluate the effectiveness of interventions (Terris, 1992). Epidemiological data provide indicators of the health status of a community and serve as the scientific foundation for prevention, health promotion, and community health interventions (Table 19-1). Health statistics are used to analyze health trends, plan and evaluate community health interventions, and make informed health policy decisions (Scaffa et al., 2001).

Incidence refers to the number of new cases of disease, injury, or disability within a specified time frame and measures how quickly a disease is spreading. Incidence rates are typically reported in terms of the number of new cases per year per 1,000 population (Green & Ottoson, 1999; Pickett & Hanlon, 1990). Prevalence refers to the total number of cases of disease, injury, or disability that exist in a community at one point in time (Pickett & Hanlon, 1990). According to Green and Ottoson (1999), "knowing statistically what the causes of disease, disability and death are most likely to be, the community can concentrate its efforts where they can have the greatest impact on health" (p. 88).

Interventions

Community health interventions are designed to decrease the incidence rates of disease, disability, and death through prevention activities and reduce the seriousness of the disease through early detection and treatment. Prevention, defined broadly, encompasses "actions and interventions designed to identify risks and reduce susceptibility or exposure to health threats prior to disease onset (primary prevention), detect and treat disease in early stages to prevent progress or recurrence (secondary prevention), and alleviate the effects of disease and injury (tertiary prevention)" (2000 Joint Committee on Health Education and Promotion Terminology, 2001, p. 101).

Community health initiatives include both public and private efforts of individuals, groups, and organizations to promote, protect, and preserve the physical, mental, social, and spiritual health of those in the community (McKenzie & Smeltzer, 1997; Scaffa et al., 2001). Community health strategies include health services, health promotion, and health protection (Figure 19-2). Health services are interventions typically provided by organizations staffed with health care and medical professionals. The goal is to improve access to quality health services by organizing and distributing resources more effectively. Health promotion is any planned combination of educational, political, regulatory, environmental, and organizational supports for actions and conditions of living conducive to the health of individuals, groups, or communities (Green & Kreuter, 1991). Health protection refers to "any planned intervention or services designed to

Table 19-1

Community Health Indicators

- Sociodemographic characteristics
- Health status
- Health risk factors
- Functional status
- Quality of life

Adapted from Durch, J. S., Bailey, L. A., & Stoto, M. A., (Eds.). (1997). *Improving health in the community: A role for performance monitoring.* Washington, DC: National Academy Press.

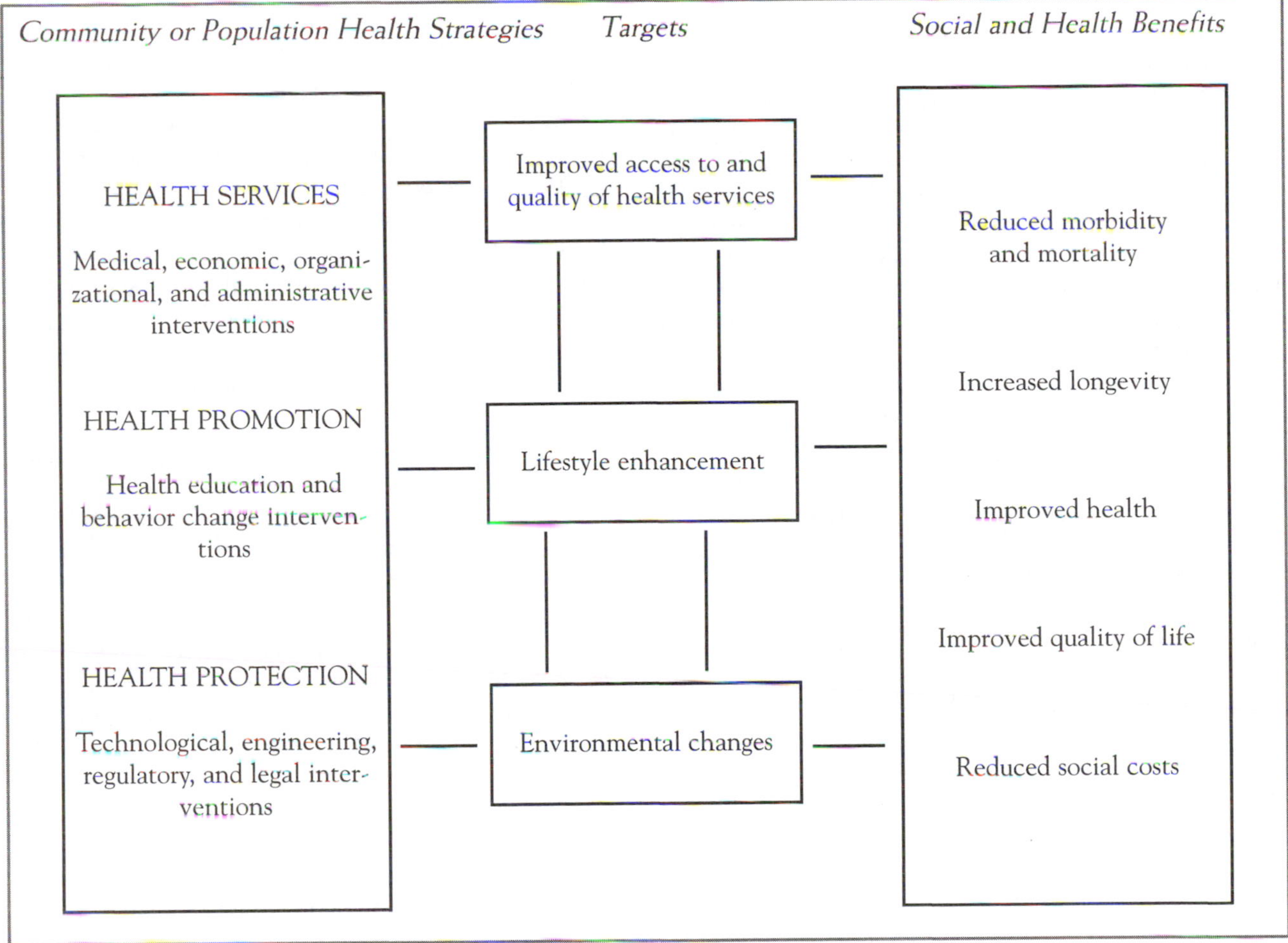

Figure 19-2. Community health strategies and outcomes. (Adapted from Green, L. W., & Ottoson, J. M. [1999]. *Community and population health* [8th ed.]. Boston, MA: WCB McGraw-Hill.)

provide individuals and communities with resistance to health threats, often by modifying policy or the environment to decrease potentially harmful interactions" (2000 Joint Committee on Health Education and Promotion Terminology, 2001, p. 101). The desired outcome of all of these community health strategies is reduced morbidity and mortality, increased longevity, improved health and quality of life, and reduced social costs (Green & Ottoson, 1999). Combining health promotion and health protection strategies with prevention and early detection produces the most comprehensive approach to community health.

Health promotion and health protection interventions often focus on reducing risk factors, those lifestyle behaviors or environmental conditions that, on the basis of scientific evidence or theory, are thought to influence susceptibility to a specific health problem (Turnock, 2001). For example, the well-known risk factors for cardiovascular disease include tobacco use, high blood pressure, obesity, diabetes, and a sedentary lifestyle. Risk factors for unintentional injury include safety belt noncompliance, alcohol/substance abuse, occupational hazards and stress, or fatigue (Green & Ottoson, 1999). Some risk factors are considered causal because the health problem cannot occur in the absence of the risk factor. Other risk factors are considered contributory because they interact with additional risk factors, leading to the development, exacerbation, or maintenance of disease, injury, or disability (Scaffa, 1998). Lifestyle risk factors (e.g., smoking and poor diet) account for approximately 50% of the years of life lost prematurely. Environmental factors account for 20%, genetic factors account for 20%, and lack of adequate medical treatment accounts for 10% of years of life lost prematurely (Green & Ottoson, 1999).

In addition to reducing risk factors, health promotion interventions attempt to increase resiliency or protective factors that contribute to overall health and well-being. Resiliency factors are those precursors that appear to increase an individual's or population's resistance to developing a disease or disability or sustaining an injury (Scaffa, 1998). For example, resiliency factors that appear to be protective for adolescent alcohol abuse include flexibility, adaptability and autonomy, good communication and problem-solving skills, social competence and opportunities for social participation, and a sense of purpose and high expectations for achievement (Scaffa, 1998).

The goal of community health promotion initiatives is change: individual behavior change and program and policy change. Community health promotion programs combine educational, social, and environmental interventions. Educational interventions, directed at high-risk individuals or populations, may be delivered through schools, workplaces, community organizations, the health care system, and the media. Social interventions include economic, political, legal, and organizational activities to improve the health of the community. Environmental interventions may involve physical, chemical, or biological modifications that reduce the risk of acquiring a disease, disability, or injury. The ultimate goal of community health is to enable every member of a community to experience a level of well-being that allows participation in, and enjoyment of, his or her chosen daily activities (Green & Anderson, 1982).

Community Organization and Development

To address the health needs of the entire community, including any existing health disparities, communities must organize around common goals. Some lifestyle changes individuals can do for themselves, but "many health benefits can only be attained through collective action or united community effort" (Green & Ottoson, 1999, p. 6). Community health initiatives use organized community action as a vehicle for change. Effective community development requires multi-sectorial involvement, decentralized authority, and participatory planning and implementation (Green & Ottoson, 1999).

There are a variety of successful strategies communities might use to improve health:

- Work to modify community conditions and norms. Community coalitions and the media are effective tools to empower individuals and groups to raise awareness about an issue and take action for change.
- Advocate for policies and regulations that promote health and safety. A vast array of policies and laws affect health, and efforts can occur at worksites, school, and community organizations as well as in the political system.
- Develop or ensure access to primary and secondary prevention programs in the community-early detection as well as health education programs and services that enhance knowledge and skills that support individual health (Davis et al., 1998).

Communities are systems. They are made up of individuals, groups, institutions, policies, shared values, interests, and norms. As in any system, if one component changes, a chain reaction of adaptations and adjustments is created in other parts of the system. Community health interventions can occur in any part of a system (e.g., political, economic, educational, social, religious, or health care) and can affect other parts of the system. No particular sector of a community is entirely responsible for the health of that community. However, change is most effective if it occurs at several levels simultaneously (individual, group, organizational, community, and governmental). This creates synergy, and change is reinforced and supported throughout the entire community.

Community organization is the "process by which communities mobilize to identify common problems or goals, mobilize resources, and in other ways, develop and implement strategies for reaching the goals they have collectively set" (2000 Joint Committee on Health Education and Promotion Terminology, 2001, p. 97). Ross (1967) describes several assumptions underlying community organization. These include the following:

- Communities can develop strategies to respond to their specific needs and problems.
- Community members should be involved in the change-making process.
- Changes that are internally motivated have more meaning and are more lasting than changes that are imposed from the outside.
- A "holistic" approach to change is more effective than a "fragmented" approach.
- Democracy requires the "cooperative participation and action" of community members and the requisite skills that make this possible.
- Communities may need assistance to effectively organize to meet their needs.

Participation in community organizing efforts can enhance the sense of community among participants, thereby improving their chances for success, which, in turn, can enhance the sense of community. The feeling of belonging, of making a difference, and of having a shared commitment can have a positive influence on the health of both the individuals involved and the community as a whole (Patrick & Wickizer, 1995).

Community Coalitions

Communities organize through the development of partnerships or coalitions. Partnerships and coalitions bring together members of various organizations and constituencies in the community to work together for a common purpose. Potential members of a coalition include health care organizations and associations, government agencies and programs, community organizations and neighborhood alliances, education-related groups and organizations, advocacy groups, business organizations and retail outlets, and the local media (Aspen Reference Group, 2000). Table 19-2 lists a variety of potential partners for community coalitions. The concept of partnership implies more than cooperation, more than collaboration. It reflects a synergism that multiplies the work done and thereby exponentially increases the benefit to the community. Each partner brings some resource, skill, or capacity that benefits the coalition, and the coalition provides some reciprocal value to the partner (True, 1995).

Coalitions afford an opportunity for community involvement in identifying and solving local health problems and can provide a vehicle for empowering and developing community capacity. Community capacity refers to "combined assets that include a community's commitment, resources, and skills used to solve problems and strengthen the quality of life for its citizens" (2000 Joint Committee on Health Education and Promotion Terminology, 2001, p. 97). Each community has a unique combination of assets, capacities, and resources. Coalitions also have the potential to reduce redundancy through better coordination of services and to make more efficient use of local resources (Parker et al., 1998).

Partnerships and coalitions develop in stages. Alter and Hage (1992) describe a framework with three stages: obligational network, promotional network, and systemic network. An obligational network is characterized by communication across groups and organizations that consist of simple information exchange among members of the coalition. The second stage, promotional network, is characterized by collaboration to identify common problems and potential solutions. Each organization or group retains its autonomy, and each fulfills a defined role. Members of the coalition relinquish a small degree of control by accepting the decisions and actions of the whole. In the systemic stage of development, the coalition has evolved to be able to address complex problems that require sharing of resources, joint decision making, and relinquishing organizational control for the greater good of the coalition. The stages in this model can also be thought of as levels of partnership. Depending on the purpose of the group and the community capacity, partnerships can occur at any of these three levels without necessarily progressing to the next.

In the spirit of the systemic network or stage, Florin and colleagues (1993) describe a six-stage process of coalition development including initial mobilization, establishing an organizational structure, building capacity and planning for action, implementation, evaluation, and institutionalization. Table 19-3 provides examples of tasks associated with each stage.

Much has been learned from both successful and unsuccessful community coalition efforts. In a cross-case analysis of four community health coalitions, Parker and colleagues (1998) identified six factors that contribute to coalition success. These factors appear to affect coalition functioning regardless of the stage of coalition development. The process of coalition building is positively affected by the following:

- Facilitating active participation of coalition members and the wider community.
- Ensuring a system for both formal and informal communication among organizational partners.
- Establishing a governance system and rules for operation as soon as possible.
- Clarifying division of labor between coalition members and staff.
- Identifying training needs and securing technical assistance and skills training for all coalition members, including staff.

Table 19-2 Potential Partners for Community Coalitions

Health Care

Visiting nurse associations, local and state medical societies, private practices, medical schools, walk-in clinics, managed care organizations, voluntary health agencies, pharmacies

Governmental

Child welfare agencies; local and state policymakers; local and state departments of health, social services, aging, transportation, labor and economic development; state department of motor vehicles; housing authority; area agencies on aging; head start; immigration offices

Community Organizations

Junior League, Red Cross, Rotary Club, Kiwanis, Lions, Elks, religious organizations, Salvation Army, Alcoholics Anonymous, United Way, YMCA/YWCA, March of Dimes, food banks, Little League, senior service programs, homeless organizations, parent-teacher organizations

Educational

Adult education programs, local and state Board of Education, fraternities/sororities, alumni organizations, day care centers, preschools, recreational facilities, trade schools, literacy volunteers, libraries, retired teachers associations, colleges, and universities

Advocacy

Children's Defense Fund, Urban League, American Association of Retired Persons (AARP)

Business

Airlines, beauty and barber shops, Chambers of Commerce, computer companies and stores, retail businesses, dairies, grocery stores, health clubs, insurance companies, bowling alleys, public transportation companies, video rental stores, second-hand stores, pharmaceutical companies, printing companies, local sports teams

Mass Media

Local television, radio, newspapers, cable providers

Table 19-3 Stages of Coalition Development

Stage of Coalition Development	*Tasks of Each Stage*
Initial mobilization	Identify important coalition members, stakeholders, and community agencies
Establish organizational structure	Determine organizational roles, group processes, and procedures
Build capacity and plan for action	Establish priorities and goals. Develop plan for intervention
Implementation	Implement all components of the intervention program
Evaluation	Evaluate intervention program and modify plan as needed
Institutionalization	Integrate intervention plan in the institution and evaluate outcomes of program

Adapted from Florin, P., Mitchell, R., & Stevenson, J. (1993). Identifying training and technical assistance needs in community coalitions: A developmental approach. *Health Education Research, 8*(3), 419 © 1993 Oxford University Press.

- Establishing mechanisms to anticipate and manage conflict (p. 36)

For coalitions to effectively address health disparities, every effort should be made to recruit a diverse membership that reflects the heterogeneity of the at-risk community.

Occupational Therapy's Unique Contribution to Community Health

Why should occupational therapy practitioners be concerned with communities? Communities are places where occupational therapy practitioners can intervene, and communities can have a direct impact on health. These two intervention approaches can be distinguished by the terms *community-based* and *community-level.*

Community-based practice, providing services located in community settings where people live, play, and work, is not a new concept in occupational therapy. Two founders of the profession, George Barton and Eleanor Clarke Slagle, developed community-based occupational therapy programs in the early 1900s. Barton, who was disabled by tuberculosis and a foot amputation, established Consolation House in New York in 1914. The program used occupations to enable convalescents to return to productive living. Eleanor Clarke Slagle was hired in 1915 to develop a program to provide people with mental or physical disabilities an opportunity to develop work skills and become self-sufficient. The program was located at Hull House in Chicago and served 77 people in its first year of operation (Scaffa, 2001).

Community-level interventions are not as familiar to occupational therapy practitioners. Community-level interventions are those that attempt to modify the sociocultural, political, economic, and environmental context of the community to achieve health goals. Community-level interventions are population-based approaches and are not focused on individual health behavior change, although this might be a by-product of the intervention. Community-level interventions may be initiated externally by health care organizations and government agencies or may be initiated and internally driven by the community itself through community organization. Community health can be viewed on a continuum from community-based to community-level to community-centered (Table 19-4). Community-centered interventions are those that are generated by the community itself using existing resources and generating new resources as the need arises. Community-centered interventions occur when community members come together through partnerships and coalitions to identify common concerns and solve community problems.

The community-centered concept is, in some ways, parallel to client-centered concept in occupational therapy practice. A client-centered approach "promotes participation, exchange of information, client decision-making and respect for choice" and "focuses on the issues which are most important to the person and his or her family" (Law, 1998, preface). Community-centered approaches adhere to these same principles. The key difference is that the "client" is the entire community. The role of the professional in such interventions is as a facilitator, educator, and mentor in the process. Occupational therapy practitioners can assist community coalitions with identifying occupational risk factors, engaging in problem solving, and proposing and implementing solutions that meet their community's unique needs. In a community-centered approach, community members are the experts. They have the power, they make decisions, and ultimately they are responsible for the outcomes.

Occupational therapy practice is based on the premise that participation in meaningful occupations can improve occupational performance and overall health. If one agrees that "occupation" is a determinant of health, then it is not difficult to perceive how occupational therapy practitioners might participate in community-level and community-centered occupation-based interventions. Wilcock (1998) provides some insight about the role of occupation as a determinant of health. She defines health from an occupational perspective as:

> The absence of illness, but not necessarily disability; a balance of physical, mental and social well-being attained through socially valued and individually meaningful occupation; enhancement of capacities and opportunity to strive for individual potential; community cohesion and opportunity; and social integration, support and justice, all within and as part of a sustainable ecology. (Wilcock, 1998, p. 110)

A variety of risk factors to health can result from less-than-optimal use, choice, opportunity, or balance in occupation. Risk factors for occupational dysfunction include occupational imbalance, deprivation, and alienation (Wilcock, 1998).

Occupational imbalance is a lack of balance among work, rest, self-care, and play/leisure that fails to meet an individual's unique physical, social, or mental health needs, thereby resulting in decreased health and well-being. Occupational deprivation includes circumstances or limitations that prevent a person from acquiring, using, or enjoying occupations. Conditions that lead to occupational deprivation may include poor health, disability, lack of transportation, isolation, poverty, and homelessness. Occupational alienation is a sense of estrangement and a lack of satisfaction in one's occupations. Tasks that

Table 19-4

Community Health Continuum

Community-Based Services/Interventions	*Community-Level Interventions*	*Community-Centered Interventions*
• Services provided in community locations • Interventions are contextually imbedded • Responsive to individual and family health needs • Professional is the expert and "visits" the community	• May be generated within community or by external agent • Loose partnerships and collaboration • Decisions made based on funding source (e.g., government or local agency) • Planning frequently done by "lead" agency • Professional is the expert and "leads" the community	• Generated by the community • Partnerships and coalitions • Community makes decisions, identifies needs and strategies • Participatory planning and evaluation • Self-governance • Professional is facilitator, educator, and mentor and serves at the discretion of the community

are perceived as stressful, meaningless, or boring may result in occupational alienation (Wilcock, 1998).

Traditionally, occupational therapy practitioners have viewed occupation as both the means and the ends of treatment. However, occupation can also be used to prevent occupational dysfunction. Preventive occupation can be characterized as the application of occupational science to prevent disease/disability and promote the health and well-being of people, families, and communities through meaningful engagement in occupation (Scaffa et al., 2001). The integration of occupation in community-level and community-centered interventions can enhance quality of life and promote wellness for all people.

The Person-Environment-Occupation-Performance (PEOP) model provides a framework for considering the role of occupational therapy in community health. The PEOP model is based on principles of social ecology and is therefore compatible with the philosophical foundations of community health. In the PEOP model, the environment is not only the context for occupational performance, but the characteristics of the environment also influence the nature and quality of occupational performance. Christiansen and Baum (1997) describe environmental enablers and barriers to occupational performance including social support mechanisms, societal policies and attitudes, cultural norms and values, and the built and natural environment. In addition to affecting occupational performance, all of these social ecological factors also affect community health.

To design occupation-based, community-level interventions or to participate effectively in community-centered coalitions, the occupational therapy practitioner must have a thorough understanding of the "community as client." A variety of individual and social ecological variables should be examined, including the following:

- Demographic information about the community (age, gender, ethnicity, income and education levels, types of employment, and religion)
- Risk factors and health behaviors of the people
- Health-related knowledge, attitudes, and beliefs
- Cultural habits, preferences, and sensitivities
- Environmental barriers to change
- Local and state policies that support or interfere with health
- Availability of social support and health-related services and patterns of use
- Effective motivators for change (Aspen Reference Group, 2000)

Occupational opportunities, choices, and balance also affect overall community health. Occupational therapy practitioners can provide this unique perspective in community health needs assessments and interventions. Finn (1972) suggested several issues that needed to be addressed for the profession to successfully move into community-based and health promotion service provision. A reinterpretation of her original work also applies today, as occupational therapy practitioners consider moving into population-based, community-level, and community-centered community health practice. To prepare for this transition, occupational therapy practitioners need to do the following:

- Become knowledgeable about community organizations and institutions and how they operate
- Acquire a thorough understanding of the unique perspectives and services they can offer in community health interventions and be able to communicate these clearly
- Develop strategies to translate knowledge into actual programs that are responsive to community needs
- Be willing to take risks when faced with challenges in unfamiliar environments
- Learn to relate to and communicate effectively with community members, leaders, and professionals from nonmedical disciplines
- Be secure in their professional identity, develop their role as health agent, and appreciate the opportunities for professional and personal growth in community health arenas (Scaffa, 2001, pp. 16-17)

At this time in history, occupational therapy practitioners have an opportunity to respond to and help resolve the community health problems of the 21st century, including poverty, joblessness, inadequate daycare and parenting skills, homelessness, substance abuse, mental illness, chronic disease and disability, unintentional injury, violence and abuse, and social discrimination (Baum & Law, 1998). With commitment, vision, and creativity, occupational therapy's contribution to community health is limitless.

References

Alter, C., & Hage, J. (1992). *Organizations working together: Coordination in interorganizational networks*. Newbury Park, CA: Sage Publications.

Aspen Reference Group. (2000). *Community health: Education and promotion manual*. Gaithersburg, MD: Aspen Publishers, Inc.

Baum, C., & Law, M. (1998). Community health: A responsibility, an opportunity, and a fit for occupational therapy. *American Journal of Occupational Therapy, 52*(1), 7-10.

Brownson, C. (2001). Program development for community health: Planning implementation, and evaluation strategies. In M. Scaffa (Ed.), *Occupational therapy in community-based practice settings* (pp. 95-118). Philadelphia, PA: F. A. Davis Company.

Christiansen, C., & Baum, C. (1997). *Occupational therapy: Enabling function and well-being*. Thorofare, NJ: SLACK Incorporated.

Davis, J. R., Schwartz, R., Wheeler, F., & Lancaster, B. (1998). Intervention methods for chronic disease control. In R. C. Brownson, P. L. Remington, and J. R. Davis (Eds.), *Chronic disease epidemiology and control* (2nd ed.). Washington, DC: American Public Health Association.

Evans, R. G., & Stoddard, G. L. (1990). Producing health, consuming health care. *Social Science and Medicine, 31*(12), 1347-1363.

Finn, G. L. (1972). The occupational therapist in prevention programs. *American Journal of Occupational Therapy, 26*, 59-66.

Florin, P., Mitchell, R., & Stevenson, J. (1993). Identifying training and technical assistance needs in community coalitions: A developmental approach. *Health Education Research, 8*(3), 417-432.

Green, L. W., & Anderson, C. L. (1982). *Community health*. St. Louis, MO: Mosby.

Green, L. W., & Kreuter, M. W. (1991). *Health promotion planning: An educational and environmental approach* (2nd ed.). Mountainview, CA: Mayfield.

Green, L. W., & Ottoson, J. M. (1999). *Community and population health* (8th ed.). Boston, MA: WCB McGraw-Hill.

Last, J. M. (Ed.). (2001). *A dictionary of epidemiology* (4th ed.). New York, NY: Oxford University Press.

Law, M. (1998). *Client-centered occupational therapy*. Thorofare, NJ: SLACK Incorporated.

MacMahon, B., & Trichopoulos, D. (1996). *Epidemiology principles and methods*. Boston, MA: Little, Brown.

McKenzie, J. F., & Smeltzer, J. L. (1997). *Planning, implementing, and evaluating health promotion programs: A primer* (2nd ed.). Boston, MA: Allyn and Bacon.

MacQueen, K. M., McLellan, E., Metzger, D. S., Kegeles, S., Strauss, R. P., Scotti, R., et al. (2001). What is community? An evidence-based definition for participatory public health. *American Journal of Public Health, 91*(12), 1929-1938.

National Center for Chronic Disease Prevention and Health Promotion. (2001). REACH 2010: Racial and ethnic approaches to community health. Retrieved March 1, 2002, from www.cdc.gov/reach2010/.

Norris, T. (1993). *The healthy communities handbook*. Denver, CO: The National Civic League.

Parker, E. A., Eng, E., Laraia, B., Ammerman, A., Dodds, J., Margolis, L., et al. (1998). Coalition building for prevention. *Journal of Public Health Management Practice, 4*(20), 25-36.

Patrick, D. L., & Wickizer, T. M. (1995). Community and health. In B. C. Amick, S. Levine, A. R. Tarlov, & D. C. Walsh (Eds.), *Society and health* (pp. 46-92). New York, NY: Oxford University Press.

Pickett, G., & Hanlon, J. J. (1990). *Public health: Administration and practice*. Bethesda, MD: American Occupational Therapy Association.

Ross, M. G. (1967). *Community organization: Theory, principles and practice*. New York, NY: Harper and Row.

Scaffa, M. E. (1998). Adolescents and alcohol use. In A. Henderson, S. Champlin, & W. Evashwick (Eds.), *Promoting teen health: Linking schools, health organizations and community*. Thousand Oaks, CA: Sage.

Scaffa, M. E. (2001). Community-based practice: Occupation in context. In M. Scaffa (Ed.), *Occupational therapy in community-based practice settings* (pp. 3-18). Philadelphia, PA: F. A. Davis Company.

Scaffa, M. E., Desmond, S., & Brownson, C. (2001). Public health, community health and occupational therapy. In M. Scaffa (Ed.), *Occupational therapy in community-based practice settings* (pp. 35-50). Philadelphia, PA: F. A. Davis Company.

Simons-Morton, B. G., Greene, W. H., & Gottlieb, N. H. (1995). *Introduction to health education and health promotion*. Prospect Heights, IL: Waveland Press, Inc.

Stokols, D. (1992). Establishing and maintaining healthy environments: Toward a social ecology of health promotion. *American Psychologist, 47*(1), 6-22.

Terris, M. (1992). The Society for Epidemiologic Research (SER) and the future of epidemiology. *American Journal of Epidemiology, 136*, 909-915.

True, S. J. (1995). Community-based breast health partnerships. *Journal of Public Health Management Practice, 1*(3), 67-72.

Turnock, B. J. (2001). *Public health: what it is and how it works*. Gaithersburg, MD: Aspen Publishers, Inc.

2000 Joint Committee on Health Education and Promotion Terminology. (2001). Report of the 2000 joint committee on health education and promotion terminology. *American Journal of Health Education, 32*(2), 90-103.

U.S. Department of Health and Human Services. (2000). *Healthy People 2010* (2nd ed.). Washington, DC: U.S. Government Printing Office.

U.S. Department of Health and Human Services. (2001). Mental health: Culture, race and ethnicity. Retrieved March 1, 2002, from www.surgeongeneral.gov/library/mentalhealth/cre.

Wilcock, A. A. (1998). *An occupational perspective of health*. Thorofare, NJ: SLACK Incorporated.

World Health Organization. (1947). Constitution of the World Health Organization. *Chronicle of the World Health Organization, 1*(1), 29-40.

World Health Organization. (1986). The Ottawa charter for health promotion. *Health Promotion, 1*, iii-v.

World Health Organization. (1999). Retrieved March 1, 2002, from www.who.int/hpr/archive/cities/what/html.

Chapter Nineteen: Occupational Therapy Interventions Reflections and Learning Activities

Julie Bass-Haugen, PhD, OTR/L, FAOTA

Reflections

Community health interventions are often described as a new and unfamiliar practice area for occupational therapy. In this chapter, we were reminded that the occupational therapy profession was started as a community-based practice. We also learned that community-level interventions are a nice fit with client-centered approaches and the PEOP model. So, involvement in community health should not be viewed as foreign to occupational therapy. Rather, attention to the person, environment, and occupation is central to optimal community health.

As you developed your knowledge about people, environments, and occupations, you began to appreciate the complexity of each of these factors. You also understood that each of these factors interact with the others. Different scholars have proposed different ideas about the nature of these interactions. In Figure 19-1, you examined one model of the determinants of disease, health and function, and well-being. As you studied the model, it likely took awhile to follow the arrows in all their directions and think about the effect of one factor on another. In this community health model, the social environment and physical environment had direct and indirect influences on most of the other factors. This makes sense when you think about health in terms of a population or group of people.

Social ecology is a discipline that examines the effects of environments on people. Five societal levels were identified as determinants of individual health: individual, group, organizational, community, and policy. It seems almost all community health issues have influences at these five levels. For example, driving under the influence or drunk driving is not just the dangerous behavior of a specific individual. It is supported (or not supported) by groups (e.g., families, friends), organizations (e.g., Mothers Against Drunk Driving, local bars and restaurants), communities (e.g., highway patrol, cultural norms, prevention programs), and policies (e.g., laws, judicial policies). Because each societal level has a potential effect on community health, each level must be considered in designing effective community health programs.

At times, it may seem that the idea of healthy communities is a better match for public health and international health organizations. However, the definition of a healthy community by the World Health Organization speaks to enabling performance and developing full potential of people. Thus, the outcome of efforts to build healthy communities is aimed at goals related to occupational performance.

So how do occupational therapy practitioners get a handle on the health of a community? It isn't practical, efficient, or effective to routinely conduct individual assessments to analyze a community's health. The measures of occupational performance and related factors will generally be at the population level (e.g., education levels, health behaviors, employment status, environmental characteristics) rather than at the individual level (e.g., activities of daily living). Many local, state, and federal agencies collect measures of community health indicators similar to those presented in the chapter.

As occupational therapy practitioners become more involved in community health initiatives, it will be important to design interventions using methods that have been successful in the past. These methods were outlined (e.g., change community norms), and some may seem pretty basic. However, many failed community health programs have ignored some of the wisdom in these lessons learned. Community health initiatives may include three approaches: health services, health promotion, and health protection. Occupational therapy may have a role in any of these approaches. Consider this example. Let's say a community is trying to improve the overall health of young children. A special concern might be child development and school readiness. Perhaps it was reported that regular health screening was not convenient for busy families, and, thus, at-risk children were not being identified prior to school. An occupational therapy practitioner might work with other health care and education professionals to improve the access to services in the neighborhood. As part of a community health assessment, it may be determined that the physical health and motor development of children was poor due to limited involvement in exercise and physical activity. The occupational therapy practitioner may coordinate a health promotion program that included educating parents on the importance of physical activity in child development and recreational opportunities to children. In coordinating the health promotion program, the occupational therapy practitioner may note that the neighborhood playground has safety and accessibility issues. Support from the city council might be needed to address the health protection needs of the children in the recreational program.

None of the community health approaches described above is possible without development of effective coalitions or partnerships. A single occupational therapy practitioner simply can't address all the needs to achieve a community health goal. Coalitions, partnerships, and networks are needed. There are various types of coalitions with different purposes and styles of working together. One community coalition may simply need to share information (e.g., obligational network) to keep abreast of changes or avoid redundancies. Another coalition may explore shared problems and possible solutions (e.g., promotional network). Finally, a coalition may decide it is in the community's best interest to work together rather than alone to solve complex problems (e.g., systematic network).

Occupational therapy is uniquely positioned and prepared to have a growing role in community health programs. Our knowledge of person, environment, and occupation and our commitment to client-centered practice is a perfect fit for collaborative efforts to improve the health of communities. This chapter provided you with the framework for engaging in this area of practice.

Journal Activities

1. Look up and write down a dictionary definition of community. Highlight the component of the definition that is most related to its descriptions in Chapter Nineteen.
2. Identify the most important new learning for you in this chapter.
3. Identify one question you have about Chapter Nineteen.
4. Review five to seven issues of a local newspaper or periodical. Identify two to three community health concerns identified in this publication. Describe the social or physical environment factors that contribute to this concern.
5. The chapter stated that the goal of health promotion initiatives was change in individual behavior, programs, or policies. We have all heard that "change is hard." Reflect on possible reasons that make change hard in behavior, programs, or policies.

Technology/Internet Learning Activities

1. Use a discussion database to share specific journal activities.
2. Use a good Internet search engine to find the Web site for the CDC Racial and Ethnic Approaches to Community Health (REACH) 2010.
   - Enter the phrase "CDC REACH" or "CDC REACH 2010" in your search line.
   - Review the home page of the Web site.
   - Evaluate the quality of this Web site. What are its strengths and weaknesses?
   - What is the overall purpose of this site?
   - What U. S. racial/ethnic groups are experiencing health disparities?
   - What agencies have a role in planning and coordinating initiatives?
   - What resources and links are available in this Web site?
3. Use a good Internet search engine to find the Web site for the American Public Health Association.
   - Enter the phrase "APHA" or "American Public Health Association" in your search line.
   - Review the home page of the Web site.
   - Evaluate the quality of this Web site. What are its strengths and weaknesses?
   - What is the overall purpose of this site?
   - Identify three to five legislation, advocacy, and policy priorities and activities of APHA that are related to occupational therapy.
4. Use a good Internet search engine to find the Web site for the *Healthy People 2010* Toolkit.
   - Enter the phrase "Healthy People 2010 Toolkit."
   - Review the home page of the Web site
   - Evaluate the quality of this Web site. What are its strengths and weaknesses?
   - What is the overall purpose of this site?
   - Identify the Action Areas for health planning and improvement efforts.

Applied Learning

Individual Learning Activity #1: Identifying Community Health Issues in Your Community

Instructions:

- Imagine that you have been hired to address community health issues from an occupational therapy perspective.
- Identify the community where you will provide services (Note: If other readers are doing this same activity, pick different communities).
- Gather and review resources that may help you learn about the community. This information may be obtained from pertinent Web sites or offices (e.g., mayor's office, chamber of commerce, school district, public health department, citizen/advocacy groups).
- Describe this community in terms of the features of a healthy community presented in this chapter.
- Identify the assets and community health issues for this community.
- Identify disparities in health for different groups in the community.
- Describe the health indicators you used to write your summary of this community.
- Identify possible occupational issues related to community health concerns.

Individual Learning Activity #2: Developing an Occupational Therapy Perspective on a Community Health Issue

Instructions:

- Select one community health issue to address from an occupational therapy perspective.
- Use the Population Situational Analysis from Chapter Fifteen to document client information and practitioner evaluation/assessment regarding this community health issue.
- Propose factors that influence this community health issue for all societal levels: individual, group, organization, community, policy.
- Propose occupational and related goals that may address the community health issue.
- What evidence would you want to obtain related to your goals?
- Identify the community health approach(es) you would use to reach your goals: services, promotion, protection.
- Identify the corresponding occupational therapy intervention approaches.
- How would you measure the outcome of your interventions?
- Describe the challenges and rewards you would likely experience from this occupational therapy role.

Active Learning

Group Activity: Addressing Issues From a Coalition Perspective

Preparation:

- Read Chapter Nineteen.
- Select a case from the list below to address from a coalition perspective
  - ✧ Membership in your national professional association has been declining for several years. You are concerned because you know that membership is important for the continued development of the underlying discipline and the profession. You also believe that your profession will begin to lose its influence in political arenas. You have been asked to address this issue.
  - ✧ You have been working in an emerging area of practice (e.g., health promotion, lifestyle coaching, prison rehabilitation programs, literacy programs) and realize that the stakeholders really do not understand occupa-

tional therapy. You know that an understanding of the profession will be essential to the development of this professional role. You have been asked to increase the visibility of occupational therapy in this area.

- ✧ There is a lot of public concern about a growing health problem in adolescents. It has been estimated that one out of four children in your community may be medically classified as obese. There is also a growing incidence of diabetes, high blood pressure, and other conditions associated with obesity. You have been asked to lead a community health initiative related to this issue.
- ✧ You have been working with your city council to develop plans for a changing community. There are goals to transform one neighborhood into a model community for both young families and older adults from diverse backgrounds. Your task is to make sure the needs of older adults are included in these plans.

Time: 45 minutes to 1 hour

Instructions:

- Individually:
  - ✧ Review the information on community coalitions in your chapter and other resources.
  - ✧ Generate specific ideas on the nature of the issue, the coalition members (i.e., both beneficiaries and stakeholders), your priorities for addressing the issue, and possible methods you would consider to address the issue.
- In small groups:
  - ✧ Share your individual ideas on the case.
  - ✧ Develop your ideas for three of the six stages of the coalition development process.

    Initial Mobilization

    Who would you invite to be coalition members? What are their skills?

    What members of the wider community would you consider as important stakeholders?

    What strategies would you use to encourage active participation?

    What formal and informal communication strategies would you use?

    Establishing an Organizational Structure

    How would you develop a framework for the coalition organization?

    Who, when, where, and how would decisions be made?

    What responsibilities would each coalition member have?

    What are the characteristics of your process for working together?

    What strategies would you use to anticipate and manage conflict?

    Building Capacity and Planning for Action

    What is the ideal outcome for this issue?

    What are three specific goals you could address in 6 months?

    For each goal, what are two to three methods you could use to achieve the goal?

    What additional information do you need on this issue?

    What general and specific training does the coalition need?

    What other skills and expertise might the coalition need to address the issue?

Discussion:

- Discuss the aspects of this case that interest or excite you.
- Discuss the opportunities or outcomes for occupational therapy in this issue.
- Discuss the challenges for occupational therapy in this issue.
- Discuss the importance of coalition building in occupational therapy.

Chapter Twenty Objectives

The information in this chapter is intended to help the reader:

1. Prompt self-reflection on enabling and reflection on enabling others.
2. Present enabling processes in client-centered, occupation-focused approaches.
3. Highlight enabling principles in client-centered, occupation-focused approaches.
4. Illustrate use of an enabling audit.
5. Consider strategies to develop enabling in practice situations.

Key Words

client-centered practice: Collaborative and partnership approaches used in enabling occupation with clients who may be individuals, groups, agencies, governments, corporations, or others; client-centered occupational therapists demonstrate respect for clients, involve clients in decision making, advocate with and for clients' needs, and otherwise recognize clients' experience and knowledge (Canadian Association of Occupational Therapists, 2002).

coaching: An enabling process to provide supportive comments, feedback, and input with the aim of enhancing physical or mental performance, insight, or growth in humans.

educating: An enabling process to facilitate learning in others using a variety of methods in various sites and times. While educators may facilitate learning, learning may or may not actually occur.

enabling occupation: Enabling people to choose, organize, and perform those occupations they find useful and meaningful in their environment (Canadian Association of Occupational Therapists, 2002).

encouraging: An enabling process of promoting hope through verbal support, compassion, practical help, advocacy, or the provision of resources to others.

facilitating: An enabling process that involves people as active participants in collaborative decision making and action toward identified goals.

guiding: An enabling process to offer directional clues to those who are seeking assistance in finding their way in thinking out an issue, deciding what to do, or developing an action plan. Those seeking assistance may or may not choose to follow the guidance of the enabler.

health: From an occupational perspective, health is a balance of physical, mental, and social well-being attained through socially valued and individually meaningful occupation, enhancement of capacities and opportunity to strive for individual potential, community cohesion and opportunity, and social integration, support, and justice, all within and as part of a sustainable ecology, beyond the absence of illness, but not necessarily beyond disability (Wilcock, 1998).

listening: An enabling process that requires full attention to another person to hear his or her words, watch his or her body language, consider the meaning behind his or her words and actions, and be aware of what is being communicated but not stated in words.

prompting: An enabling process of reminding others through supportive comments, written notes, organizational clues, or the use of time-sensitive technology, such as clocks or computer prompts. Prompting could be to remind a person to perform in a particular way to avoid pain; to increase effectiveness; or to refine the efficiency, power, or quality of performance. Prompting could also be to encourage a person or organization to follow through on intentions or plans.

reflecting: An enabling process of thinking to become more aware of one's self, of others, or of the surroundings for the purpose of contemplation or action.

> *You are not here merely to make a living. You are here in order to enable the world to live more amply, with greater vision, with a finer spirit of hope and achievement. You are here to enrich the world, and you impoverish yourself if you forget the errand.*
>
> Woodrow Wilson

Chapter Twenty

INTERVENTIONS IN A SOCIETAL CONTEXT: ENABLING PARTICIPATION

Elizabeth Townsend, PhD, MAdEd, OTReg(NS), OT(C), FCAOT and Jennifer Landry, PhD (Candidate), MSc, OTReg(Ont), OT(C)

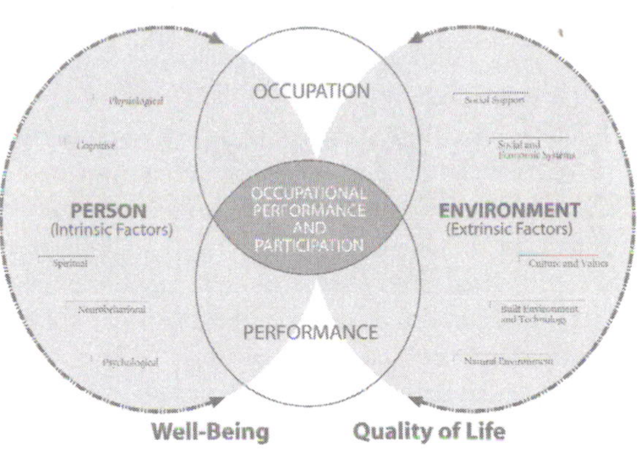

Setting the Stage

This chapter will introduce the idea of enabling as a key component of the occupational therapy process. Enabling in occupational therapy is intended to make possible the hopes, dreams, and achievements of others. Specifically, practitioners enable people to identify, choose, and engage in meaningful occupations for health and quality of life. Enabling processes, principles, and strategies are described for a client-centered, occupation-based occupational therapy practice. Readers are also invited to use reflection on self, others, and occupational therapy approaches to learn about enabling participation in occupations.

Townsend, E., & Landry, J. (2005). Interventions in a societal context: Enabling participation. In C. H. Christiansen, C. M. Baum, and J. Bass-Haugen (Eds.), Occupational therapy: Performance, participation, and well-being *(3rd ed.). Thorofare, NJ: SLACK Incorporated.*

Introduction

Enabling is the heartbeat of occupational therapy practice because enabling is the way in which occupational therapists work. The verb *enable* means to make it possible for somebody to do something and to make it possible for something to happen or exist by creating the necessary conditions (Oxford University Press, 2000). The aim of enabling is to make possible the hopes, dreams, and achievements of others. Moreover, enabling processes and principles are foundations for enabling empowerment and justice with people who are disempowered (Dunst & Trivette, 1989; Dunst, Trivette, Davis, & Cornwell, 1988; Dunst, Trivette, & Deal, 1998). Occupational therapists' aim is to enable people to identify, choose, and engage in meaningful occupations for health and quality of life. Of concern to this profession are people whose everyday occupations are constrained by potential or real challenges associated with aging, disability, or difficult social circumstances (Canadian Association of Occupational Therapists, 2002; Townsend, 2000).

The exploration of enabling in this chapter starts with an invitation for self-reflection, reflection on enabling others, and reflection on the implementation of enabling approaches in occupational therapy practice. Presented then are enabling processes and enabling principles. Three illustrations of enabling and an Enabling Audit Template are provided with reference to front-line practice. A final discussion offers strategies for enabling through client-centered, occupation-focused approaches. This exploration attends to the five objectives of the chapter.

Reflection: A Journey Toward Enabling

> Each of us must examine in our daily activities as occupational therapists by asking ourselves: Is what I'm doing—be it in my practice, my classroom, or my research laboratory—focused on occupation? Focused on enabling? If not, we must ask ourselves: How can I rename or reframe what I am doing to make the clear and powerful statement that occupational therapy enables a fundamental need—occupation! Occupational therapy named and framed in an enablement model, enables occupation—enables living. Thus, occupational therapy is: ENABLING LIVING! (Polatajko, 1992, pp. 197-198).

Reflection is subjective and personal and is a fundamental process for transforming the way people feel and act (do Rozario, 1994). It follows that self-reflection is an important place to start on the journey of learning to enable and to recognize occupational therapists' enabling as distinct from expert-driven professional approaches. Three forms of reflection are outlined to enhance your ability to personalize and experience enabling before, during, and after you read about enabling.

Before you read this chapter, you are encouraged to take a moment to reflect on enabling in your own life. Reflect alone, or gather a group to reflect on what is enabling or disabling you from realizing your goals today, during the past year, or during your life. Reflection tends to be easiest in a quiet, comfortable place without distractions of noise, interruptions, or discomfort. The most important point is that reflection takes time. Take time to look back and think about what is enabling you to live your life and what other enabling would be helpful (Table 20-1).

Now, as you read the chapter, consider Reflection on Enabling Others (Table 20-2). You are invited to think about someone you know and how that person is occupied. Then, choose two contrasting occupations in a typical day (e.g., driving and working in a machine shop, or playing baseball and doing laundry). Make two lists to consider what enables or does not enable that person to choose and participate in these occupations. Use Table 20-2 to develop your own checklist for reflection on enabling others.

Reflection (Table 20-3) may also help to draw attention to the issues and questions that need discussion in the implementation of a reflective, enabling occupational therapy practice (Schon, 1987). With occupational therapy students or colleagues, try the questions in Table 20-3. Among occupational therapists, the ideals of enabling are sometimes considered to be ivory tower concepts. Or enabling becomes such an innate way of practicing as an occupational therapist that it is taken for granted without questioning whether enabling is being done efficiently and effectively. To some, enabling seems out of reach in the realities of a busy practice in systems that are not set up to encourage or reward enabling approaches. Consider what societies lose without professions like occupational therapy that aim to use enabling approaches. Also, consider how occupational therapists will become more empowered to implement enabling with efficiency and effectiveness.

Enabling: A Conceptual Foundation in Occupational Therapy

Enabling is not a new concept in occupational therapy. Rather, the language and theory of enabling are emerging

Table 20-1

Self-Reflection on Enabling

We (the authors) began to examine the concept of enabling within the occupational therapy context by exploring our own definition of what enabling means and by briefly reflecting upon our experience of being enabled in our lives.

As a point of departure before reading the chapter, we encourage you to spend a few minutes alone or in a group jotting down a few thoughts about enabling. Think about three linked forces that enable you to live and learn with others: your personal qualities, your environment, and your occupations.

Personal Qualities

- What does enabling mean to you?
- Which personal qualities enable you to reach your goals? Which "disable" you?
- Consider your past or present mentors (family members, teachers, colleagues, or peers). How did your mentors enable you to learn and grow?
- What did enabling look like? Feel like?

Environment

- How does your environment enable you to learn and grow? How does it "disable" you?
- What cultural or social forces make life easy or difficult for you?
- How does the natural environment or the design of your rural or urban community help or hinder you?
- Are you aware of any policies or regulations that limit you in being healthy? Living the way you want to? Building the kind of community in which you would like to live?
- What does your environment look like or feel like to you?

Occupations

What do you experience or feel when an occupation

- provides a just right challenge, versus one that you feel is not challenging enough?
- fits well into your routines and habits, versus one that is at odds with your routines and habits?
- offers you lots of choice or control, versus very little choice or control?
- has purpose and meaning for you, versus being without any purpose or meaning for you?
- is something you want to do, versus something you have to do or need to do?
- enriches you so you can flourish, versus demeans you in the eyes of yourself or others?
- is readily at hand, versus being disrupted, taken away from you, or out of reach?
- gives you a sense of balance in life, versus making you feel overoccupied or underoccupied?
- contributes to a sense of identity and connection with others, versus feeling alienated?

Table 20-2 Reflection on Enabling Others

You are invited to think about someone you know and how that person is occupied. Choose two contrasting occupations in a typical day (e.g., for instance driving and working in a machine shop, or playing baseball and doing laundry). Then make two lists to consider what helps or does not help that person to choose and participate in these occupations.

- In general, what enables people to choose and participate in occupations that promote health and quality of life? What limits people?
- In particular, what enables the individual you are thinking about to choose and participate in his or her occupations? What personal characteristics would help or hinder the individual whom you are considering?
- What policies, physical conditions, cultural attitudes, laws, and funding arrangements enable this individual or groups of individuals you know to drive, work outside the home, play sports, or complete home-based occupations?
- What policies, physical conditions, cultural attitudes, laws, and funding arrangements undermine or "disable" this individual and others?
- What would enable greater choice and participation in the two occupations by the individual you are considering?
- How could an occupational therapist enable this individual and others to use the two occupations you identified to promote their health and quality of life?

Table 20-3 Reflection on Client-Centered, Occupation-Focused Enabling

- What distinguishes enabling approaches as being different from other approaches?
- What do enabling approaches look like or feel like? How does enabling look or feel that is different from the look or feel of doing things to or for others?
- Besides occupational therapists, do others use these different approaches?
- What knowledge, skills, and behaviors are needed to enable others to learn and grow?
- What support do enablers need to truly enable others to learn and grow through making choices and participating in everyday occupations?
- How can occupational therapists become more sophisticated in analyzing and more articulate in telling others about the complexity of what look like common-sense interactions in ordinary daily life events?
- What can be done to make enabling work in a highly prescriptive, managed environment where professional competence is measured against standardized criteria and protocols, or where professional fees depend on numbers of individuals treated in a limited time?
- If some approaches are enabling, what approaches are not enabling (i.e., disabling)?
- What distinguishes the enabling approaches of laypeople from professional enabling?
- What is gained by using enabling approaches? What is lost by doing things to or for others?
- Can society afford not to be enabling people who are alienated, dependent, vulnerable, unfulfilled, or otherwise disempowered?

Table 20-4

Conceptual Foundations of Enabling in Occupational Therapy
Educational Concept of Enabling
• Experiential learning
• Self-directed learning
• Cooperative or collaborative learning
• Joint decision making with professionals
• Holistic learning as a whole being
• Context-sensitive learning applicable to culture, social habits, physical space, policies
Policy Concept of Enabling
• Enabling policy development to support difference in communities and societies
• Enabling legislation to govern diverse forms of social inclusion without homogeneity
• Enabling funding for approaches that enable individuals and communities to flourish through choice and engagement in the occupations they decide are useful or meaningful in their context
• Enabling building codes for physical accessibility to private, public, built, and natural spaces
• Enabling management to develop accountability for enablement
• Enabling education and research to facilitate and research enablement

to describe occupational therapists' client-centered, occupation-focused approaches (Canadian Association of Occupational Therapists, 2002; Fearing & Clark, 2000; Polatajko, 1992). Enabling with individuals and groups is an educational concept, whereas enabling policy, legal, and other environmental change is a policy concept (Table 20-4).

The educational concept of enabling was embedded as an implicit rather than an explicit foundation of occupational therapy by educators who, with nurses, physicians, and social workers, were the early founders of occupational therapy in North America (Dunton, 1919; Meyer, 1922; Schwartz, 1992). Client-centered, occupation-focused practice involves people as participants in learning through experiences that relate to everyday occupations. It makes sense that early occupational therapists incorporated enabling approaches in their health practices. They drew on the ideas of educators, such as John Dewey and Eduard Lindeman, who were championing ideas about learning through practical experience at the time that the profession of occupational therapy was being formed (Brookfield, 1987; Dewey, 1922). Educational features that were adopted by occupational therapists, albeit without being fully articulated as such, are the profession's implementation of concepts such as experiential learning, self-directed learning, cooperative or collaborative learning in joint decision making with professionals, holistic learning as a whole being, and context-sensitive learning that looked at environmental as well as individual change.

The policy concept of enabling was also implicitly rather than explicitly incorporated in occupational therapy. Early occupational therapists, such as Eleanor Clark Slagle, enabled change in policies, legislation, and funding to open reconstruction training programs for soldiers and school programs for children with disabilities. Enabling inclusive environments for people with disabilities or other potentially disadvantaging situations is an historical as well as a contemporary part of occupational therapy practice (Grady, 1995).

Through myriad short- and long-term approaches, occupational therapists enable individuals or groups to learn how to shape a dream of possibility and then to develop experientially the habits, routines, attitudes, problem solving, performance, self-identity, and environment to make their dream come true in some form within the practical reality of their everyday occupations. Through consultation with advocacy groups and as professional advocates, occupational therapists enable policy, legal, and funding changes that, in turn, create enabling environments for individuals and groups. Enabling building codes, enabling management, and enabling education and research are all policy level approaches for creating an inclusive, accessible environment.

Enabling Processes: Client-Centered Practice, Occupation, and Empowerment

Enabling processes refer to ways of working with people and organizations. Occupational therapists often describe this profession as having different ways of working. Occupational therapy is aligned with collaborating, enabling professions in contrast to expert-driven professions that apply techniques to people who need to comply but not collaborate in decision making with them. Enabling approaches are based on participation, collaboration, holism in context, and empowerment as described under Enabling Principles on p. 504. The particular niche in the marketplace served by occupational therapy is in enabling occupation (Canadian Association of Occupational Therapists, 2002). Enabling occupation means engaging people in various ways to identify, choose, and participate in a variety of everyday occupations that they define as meaningful or useful in their environment. A broad view of occupations is taken to encompass everything people do to occupy life for various purposes, including to work, help others, look after the self, and enjoy life. Occupations occur within routines and habits that are interwoven throughout everyday experience to make daily life more than a series of defined physical tasks and activities. Occupational therapists' enabling approaches focus on occupations. A vision of possibility is combined with practical approaches to everyday challenges.

In enabling occupation, occupational therapists use complex professional reasoning (Mattingly & Fleming, 1994). Two examples are facilitating shopping by an elderly person who wants to live in her own home and coaching children with disabilities to play sports. The work of enabling occupation looks easy because it is located in ordinary, taken-for-granted occupations. Nevertheless, facilitating a shopping trip with clients is more than just shopping with friends. Facilitation may be for clients to risk establishing relationships with strangers during recovery from a mental illness, or occupational therapists may facilitate consumer groups to develop the skills and confidence to evaluate the physical accessibility of transportation and stores in a community. Coaching groups to create policies, for instance, to support housing or employment for people with disabilities is different from professionals writing policies. Coaching may be part of a larger skill development and community development program in which consumer groups are finding their voice to advocate for policies that take their needs into account. Coaching teachers, parents, and children to solve the challenges of including a child with a disability as a full participant in school is different from just building a ramp to the school door and hiring teachers' aids to give a child individual attention. Coaching may be a strategy to develop a school-based team of active participants whose collective perspectives on disability can change the school culture and routines to reduce stigma and increase opportunities for students with disabilities.

An awareness of enabling approaches has grown through explorations of client-centered practice. Guidelines for occupational therapy's client-centered practice were first developed in Canada in the early 1980s (Townsend, 1998a). Between 1983 and 1997, six Canadian guidelines texts outlined concepts, processes, implementation, outcome measurement considerations, issues in mental health services, and enabling occupation (Canadian Association of Occupational Therapists, 1991, 2002; Department of National Health and Welfare & Canadian Association of Occupational Therapists, 1983, 1986, 1987; Health Canada & Canadian Association of Occupational Therapists, 1993).

The language of client-centered practice in occupational therapy was inspired particularly by the work of American psychologist Carl Rogers (Milhollan & Forisha, 1972; Rogers, 1939, 1953, 1961, 1965, 1969, 1980). For occupational therapists, Rogers' idea of client-centered therapy offered an "ah-ha" moment of recognition. His description of working collaboratively with people, rather than doing things for them, fit well with what was (in the early 1980s) an implicit rather than an explicit philosophical foundation of occupational therapy (Kielhofner, 1983; Kielhofner & Burke, 1977; Reed & Sanderson, 1980).

Canada's 1997 guidelines for the client-centered practice of occupational therapy were called *Enabling Occupation: An Occupational Therapy Perspective*. Enabling was defined as:

> ...processes of facilitating, guiding, coaching, educating, prompting, listening, reflecting, encouraging, or otherwise collaborating with people so that individuals, groups, agencies, or organizations have the means and opportunity to be involved in solving their own problems; enabling is the basis of occupational therapy's client-centred practice and a foundation for client empowerment and justice; enabling is the most appropriate form of helping when the goal is occupational performance. (Canadian Association of Occupational Therapists, 2002, p. 180)

Furthermore, enabling occupation was described as fostering opportunities for individuals and groups to "participate in shaping their own lives" (p. 50).

Research with explicit reference to enabling and enablement in occupational therapy began to appear in the literature in the 1990s. In 1992, Polatajko illustrated the idea of naming and framing occupational therapy as a practice of enablement. She drew the concept from her critique of disablement in professional approaches that seem to limit rather than expand life opportunities for people with chronic illness or disability (Polatajko, 1992). Explicit interest in enabling and enablement seems to be growing, for instance, in research on an enabling occupational performance process for working with individuals (Fearing & Clark, 2000). The Occupational Performance Process is described as enabling people to participate in and shape their own occupational therapy services from the first naming and prioritizing of occupational performance issues to the final evaluation. Other examples of research focused on enabling include the identification of enabling characteristics of an affirming environment for people who live with severe and persistent mental illness (Rebeiro, 2001) and the analysis of processes and conditions for enabling empowerment and empowerment education in mental health services (Townsend, 1998b). With a focus on mental health services, both authors point to enabling processes in everyday situations and to policy, funding, and other conditions that would enable long-time users of these services to become more empowered.

Research on client-centered practice is also exploring enabling and enablement, although the concept of enabling is less explicitly defined and described than in the previously noted studies. Enabling processes are illustrated through case studies of occupational therapists working with people (Law, 1998; Sumison, 1999) and through assessment approaches that seek client perspectives of their occupational performance (Pollock, 1993; Watson, 1992). The organization of enabling approaches has been considered in research on the documentation of clients' own perceptions of their occupational performance (Watson, 1992). As well, enabling was at the core of an analysis of the integration of client experiential knowledge in occupational therapists' evidence-based practice (Egan, Dubouloz, von Zweck, & Vallerand, 1998). Questions about the meaning of client-centered practice and critiques about the possibilities for being client-centered all refer to the collaborative, power-sharing approaches that are characteristic of enabling practices.

Exploration of the theory and practice of enabling occupation is prompting new understandings about client-centered practice in occupational therapy. Captured in the phrase *enabling occupation* are two core concepts for being client-centered in this profession: enabling and occupation. A third implicit core concept, a vision of empowerment and justice, is embedded in enabling occupation. One becomes aware of this third core concept if one asks, "Why is enabling occupation important and what is the purpose of enabling occupation?" (Canadian Association of Occupational Therapists, 2002). Since the 1980s, occupational therapists have made considerable gains in making explicit the occupational focus of occupational therapy, and occupational therapists' interests in empowerment and justice are gradually being articulated.

Now, it is time to expand understanding of the enabling processes and principles for implementation of occupational therapy's client-centered, occupation-focused practice.

Enabling Processes

Enabling processes are discussed by considering occupational therapists' particular focus in enabling, by clarifying that enabling processes can be embedded in the management of a process of practice, and by highlighting the interconnectedness of enabling individuals (micro) and enabling environments (macro). A wide range of enabling processes is at the heart of occupational therapists' different ways of working with organizations as well as with people. Eight commonly used enabling processes are summarized (alphabetically, not in order of importance of frequency of use) in Table 20-5: coaching, educating, encouraging, facilitating, guiding, listening, prompting, and reflecting. Enabling processes are action verbs that are congruent with the enabling principles, summarized below, of participation, collaboration, holism in context, and empowerment and justice.

Three points frame consideration of enabling processes: occupational therapists are not the only professional enablers, enabling is not new in occupational therapy, and there are links between enabling individuals or groups to do something (micro enabling) and enabling something to happen or exist by creating the necessary conditions (macro enabling).

First, occupational therapists are not the only professional enablers. Education, psychology, social work, and other literature on "educating" or "helping" refer frequently to enabling. As in occupational therapy, the references in many fields point to processes or policies that aim to involve people in helping themselves or aim to create policies, legal, financial, and other conditions that enable people to do what they need or want to do (Deegan, 1997; Frank, 1992; Staral, 2000). Occupational therapists appear to distinguish themselves from other enabling practitioners in linking ideas on enabling with ideas on occupation and empowerment, even if this ideology is difficult to carry out in everyday practice.[1]

[1] The suggestion that occupational therapy is based on ideology will be controversial with some occupational therapists. Used here, the term *ideology* simply refers to a set of ideas, values, and beliefs that guide everyday practice. Some may prefer to refer to theory rather than to ideology, especially now that occupational therapists are becoming comfortable with naming assumptions, values, beliefs, and ideas that form the theoretical foundations of occupational therapy practice.

Table 20-5

Enabling Processes: An Alphabetical Overview

Coaching	Coaching is related to other enabling processes, but seems to warrant its own description because coaches enable people to set goals, prepare themselves to meet those goals, and perform in designated events. Occupational therapists coach people in many situations. Clients are invited to define goals, such as adolescents with schizophrenia being coached to set practical goals for seeking part-time work. Coaching would continue by providing feedback on adolescent role plays of interviews with prospective employers. The occupational therapist might arrange to meet the adolescent at a coffee shop after a real interview to listen and revise the coaching plan before the next "performance" in an interview
Educating	Educating is a broad term that covers many enabling processes. For occupational therapists, educating is an important distinction from treating people (i.e., doing things to or for them). Occupational therapists are often educating people to live differently, either to avoid unwanted change as for those with a degenerative disease or to learn to embrace change as for those who acquire a disability. Occupational therapy is an educational practice, drawing its educational foundations from the teachers who were occupational therapy's founding partners with physicians, nurses, and social workers
Encouraging	Encouraging is a process of enabling hope. Encouraging is central to occupational therapists' use of occupations as a medium for facilitating, guiding, reflecting, and other enabling processes. Where occupational therapists work from a vision of empowerment and justice, these ideas provide a compelling framework for encouraging people to hope. Occupational therapists might be involved in encouraging children with poor self-esteem to try again when they struggle to play games, encouraging families to organize respite care when their own caregiving energies are spent, or encouraging community agencies to seek funding to start a self-help group
Facilitating	Facilitating is an extremely important enabling process that is widely used in many fields by professionals and nonprofessionals who describe themselves as "facilitators." Typically, facilitators plan and implement participatory, sometimes called *experiential*, learning events, such as exercises, brainstorming, and discussion. Occupational therapists use facilitation extensively. A common example is when individuals or groups who are learning to live with a disability explore new approaches to occupations, such as cooking or driving a car. A brief introduction may precede an experiential session where real cooking and driving are done, followed by brainstorming on what worked and what didn't work, and what to try next. Occupational therapy consultants, managers, educators, and policy makers facilitate the development of enabling policies, enabling curricula, or enabling programs by leading brainstorming sessions, prompting the writing of drafts and revisions, and asking stakeholders to ensure that their perspective is included in policies
Guiding	Guiding is an enabling process of offering directions that may or may not be followed. Guiding is like mapping key points of information/interest for consideration along a journey. Occupational therapists guide clients, families, school teachers, government officials, and others by creating and holding information sessions with "maps" such as brochures and videotapes on topics such as injury or fall prevention, or by more personalized home programs, an example being to guide caregivers in ways of keeping a loved one at home

(continued)

Table 20-5

Listening	Listening is an essential enabling process for which there is a large amount of literature. In enabling occupation, listening is central in order to hear both the words and the unspoken intent of what individuals and groups need and want to do in their occupations. At the organizational level, listening tends to be through enabling processes such as thinking about whose perspectives and experiences are represented in documents or images
Prompting	Prompting is an enabling process that is distinct but also embedded in other enabling processes. Prompting is directed both at prodding memory and at prompting courage to risk what may seem fearful. Occupational therapists prompt people to remember steps, such as for using a computer with one hand following an amputation of the other hand. Prompting courage is a key enabling process in occupational therapy. Rather than talk about life and adaptations, occupational therapists involve people in occupations where they may risk failure. Prompting risk-taking and courage is related to encouraging. Prompting is an important process in enabling organizational change. For example, community members may be prompted to participate with occupational therapists. Then, together, they prompt policy and social change in communities, governments, or businesses
Reflecting	Reflecting is a process of looking at one's self or of helping others to "see" themselves figuratively as in a mirror. Reflecting involves raising awareness or consciousness raising, the aim being to generate insights. Occupational therapists enable others to reflect on their own lives by involving them in experiences of occupations. After participation in occupations, occupational therapists may invite reflections on the meaning, purpose, sense of accomplishment, sense of identity, perception of importance, or satisfaction with the occupation or occupational performance. Reflections then provide the basis for deciding what occupations to pursue with or without the occupational therapist. Occupational therapists may also provide a "lens" or "perspective" on organizational processes and the types of changes required to create more inclusive communities

Second, occupational therapists have a history of describing enabling within a process of practice. Descriptions of a process of practice identify stages or steps to manage occupational therapy assessment, planning, implementation, and evaluation (American Occupational Therapy Association, 1999; Canadian Association of Occupational Therapists, 2002; Fearing & Clark, 2000; Hagedorn, 1997; Reed & Sanderson, 1980, 1999). This managerial reference to "process" differs from the enabling processes described next. In the ideal practice, occupational therapists' enabling processes are embedded in their process of practice. Enabling works when principles of participation, collaboration, holism in context, and empowerment are embedded in the process of practice. The cornerstone of enabling is power sharing between those who want to enable others and those who choose to collaborate in being enabled to reach their goals.

In some practice situations, enabling may seem impossible because there are too many people to see in too little time, and the professional culture is one of expert-driven approaches, or management practices may favor standardized protocols that reduce flexibility in enabling. There is a need in these situations to redefine accountability criteria to identify the efficiency, effectiveness, and evidence for enabling approaches and to educate professional teams and families about enabling. Research is needed to compare other approaches with the efficiency and effectiveness of enabling processes, such as listening to client goals or facilitating change. Fearing and Clark (2000) describe an enabling occupational performance process of practice that they developed through pilot and demonstration projects in a major health sciences complex. They documented what they did and collaborated with management teams to redefine occupational therapy staffing patterns and resources to incorporate enabling approaches in their practice (Fearing & Clark, 2000).

Third, there are interconnections in enabling individuals (micro) and enabling environments (macro). Enabling processes can work in professional, helping relationships with individuals and groups. Enabling helping relationships would start ideally with micro-level concerns related to people and their occupations—with occupational performance issues identified from the perspective of the individuals or groups themselves. Enabling begins when occupational therapists ask clients for their own goals, rather than assuming to pursue goals that make sense from the therapist's perspective. Facilitating client goal setting is a process of enabling clients to give voice to their perspective and interests within a hierarchy where professional and management voices tend to dominate (Belenky, Bond, & Weinstock, 1997; Belenky, Clinchy, Goldberger, & Tarule, 1986).

In an enabling practice, client goal setting would be a point of departure for looking beyond individuals and groups to their environment. Family, coworkers, teachers, and others would need to be drawn into the problem solving and solution finding if clients are to realize their goals. Research on helping relationships in occupational therapy has raised insights on specific features, such as listening, reflection, and reasoning (Corring & Cook, 1999; Kinsella, 2001; Peloquin, 1993a, 1993b). However, there is a need to explore how facilitation, coaching, and other enabling processes could be more explicitly and fully incorporated in helping relationships.

While occupational therapists' enabling processes are often targeted at individuals or groups, enabling may also be targeted at the policy, legislation, and funding of communities, agencies, governments, and other organizations. Following the World Health Organization's publication in 1986 of the *Ottawa Charter for Health Promotion* (World Health Organization, 1986), occupational therapists' interest in enabling and empowering became more explicit. To give one example, Letts and colleagues reported on a Health Promotion project sponsored by the Canadian Association of Occupational Therapists. Based on their successful involvement in enabling individuals, families, and communities to participate in health promotion, they called for greater occupational therapy involvement in "enabling, mediating and advocating to build health public policy, creating supportive environments; strengthening community action; developing personal skills; and reorienting health services from within occupational therapy" (Letts, Fraser, Finlayson, & Walls, 1993, p. 10).

Organizational enabling would be through community development, management reform, and other approaches as long as they are participatory, collaborative, holistic, contextual, and empowerment-oriented. From a macro standpoint, the micro issues of individuals and groups would be given voice in order to ensure that buildings, policies, and plans are relevant to the populations they address. The interplay of macro and micro enabling approaches would ideally enable organizations to enable individuals and groups to become empowered to enhance their own health and quality of life.

Enabling Principles

Whereas enabling processes are ways of working with people and organizations, enabling principles are features and characteristics of those ways of working. Four principles are highlighted as fundamental to enabling occupation, and thus to occupational therapy's client-centered, occupation-focused practice. Participation, collaboration, holism in context, and empowerment (justice) are principles for guiding clients to take greater responsibility and for guiding professionals and managers to share power more equally with clients. Three illustrations of embedding these principles within enabling processes are provided in tables provided next.

The four principles point to the centrality of power in enabling and, thus, in occupational therapy practice. Power is organized differently in enabling, toward greater sharing of power in professional helping relationships and in the organization of the environment. The enabling processes described are all ones in which the professional recognizes the expertise of others, particularly the experiential knowledge of clients, and shares power in decision making. Enabling principles are actually features in the recognition, exercise, and acceptance of more equalized power relations between professionals and those seeking help. It seems that enabling processes and principles need to be discussed with reference to the power of occupational therapists to enable and the power of occupational therapy clients to be enabled. Enabling, in summary, represents different ways of working with people and organizations and also different ways of exercising power in which the hierarchical, expert use of professional power is replaced with collaborative power sharing.

The practical implementation of power sharing occurs most centrally in decision making with clients. The empowerment and justice principle underpins client-centered, occupation-focused enabling with individuals and members of social groups who are potentially disadvantaged because of age, disability, or social disadvantages. While occupational therapists work with well populations in health and wellness promotion, this profession's historical niche in society is with these three major groups. Within the profession's concerns for the occupational impacts of age, disability, and social disadvantages are concerns for differences that are experienced in everyday occupations because of such characteristics as culture, ethnicity, gender, race, rural/urban context, sexual orientation, or social class.

Participation

Occupational therapists sometimes refer to this profession's enabling principles through the saying:

Tell me, I forget
Show me, I see
Involve me, I understand

The enabling principle captured by this saying is participation. Enabling participation in occupations is done by working with people as active participants in helping themselves, rather than doing things to or for them.

The reason for naming participation as an enabling principle is that people are drawn to participate as autonomous, active agents (Metz, 2000; Sherwin, 1998). Recognition of human agency in enabling provides a fundamental point of contrast with the objectification of humans as cases that are managed through the coordination and control of standardized protocols, such as clinical pathways. Participation recognizes that active agents can be involved in action to help themselves. The power of people to participate makes enabling possible because people need to agree to be facilitated, coached, or encouraged. Participation is equated with approaches such as experiential learning, self-help, occupational engagement, and other action-oriented approaches (Borkman, 1999; Mader, 1998; McCaugherty, 1991; Wilson, 1999). Enabling can work through talking approaches, but if occupational therapists are enabling occupation, participation is through planning and action in the occupations that are relevant to those with occupational performance issues (Law, Baum, & Baptiste, 2002; Wilcock, 1998). To be timely, participation occurs in times and places that have been identified as appropriate to the goals of coaching, educating, or other enabling processes.

Collaboration

Collaboration is an enabling principle that is congruent with the principle of participation. Moreover, collaboration is fundamental to the power sharing that characterizes client-centered practice. It should be noted that power sharing sounds like a good idea, but the implementation is not straightforward. Professionals are historically allocated hierarchical authority over those who seek their help (Byrne, 1999; Coburn, 1993; Klein, 1995). The hierarchical structure of health services, schools, and other institutions gives professional expertise dominance over the experiential knowledge of clients. Even when people and organizations are asked for their perceptions or opinions, professional expertise will prevail in deciding what is best, unless policy or legal structures are put in place to require collaborative decision making with clients (Cohen, D'Onofrio, Larkin, Berkholder, & Fishman, 1999; Deegan, 1997; Redick, McClain, & Brown, 2000). Change toward power sharing begins in shared decision making about client goals in everyday practice. Change in systems needs to follow to enable shared decision making as a routine program or service requirement.

Occupational therapists worldwide who want to be more client-centered have raised questions about their own responsibility as a partner in therapy and about the power of the client to drive practice in directions that are not viewed by occupational therapists as being in a client's "best interests." At present, professional regulation and liability insurance hold professionals responsible for decisions about what is "best" for the client, not for collaborative decision making. Shared professional-client risk taking has not yet been written into most liability insurance clauses. Moreover, managers expect "best practices" to be efficient and effective from a management and professional perspective, not necessarily from a client perspective. Surveys of client satisfaction are taken into account, but the final decisions about health and other services are traditionally in the hands of professionals and managers.

Despite the difficulties in collaborating with clients, the commitment to make occupational therapy more client-centered is still strong (Sumison & Smyth, 2000; Wilkins, Pollock, Rochon, & Law, 2001). North American discussions about client-centered versus client-driven practice were captured in 1994 by Yerxa in the United States and Gage and Polatajko in Canada (Gage & Polatajko, 1995; Polatajko, 1994; Yerxa, 1994). Client-centered practice was described in this debate as an ideal view of practice that encourages occupational therapists to hold a client's "best interests" at heart. Gage and Polatajko contrast this with what they term *client-driven practice* to convey a practice in which a client drives the therapeutic process. Both terms recognize the central importance of collaboration, and both terms are seeking a language to recognize occupational therapists' responsibilities and liability for contributing expertise that clients can accept or reject. Whether practice is client-centered or client-driven, client participation in individualized or organizational enabling processes appears to foster greater collaboration and eventually fosters change in hierarchical structures toward greater power sharing between professionals and clients (Byrne, 1999; Lefley, 1998; Rebeiro, 2000; Redick et al., 2000).

Holism in Context

The principle of holism in context actually combines two components: holism and context (or environment). The emphasis on participation involves whole people in self-change or in organizational change. Even if practice is focused on a component of occupational performance (e.g., on a physical, mental, cognitive difficulty), an enabling, participatory, collaborative approach involves the whole person in deciding what is most relevant to work on (McColl, 1994; Peloquin, 1993b). A holistic approach to practice naturally involves people as active, collaborating participants in deciding whether or not it makes sense to enhance performance in, for example, homemaking occupations or community socializing occupations.

Practice that is "in context" attends to the context or may aim to actually change the context. Occupational therapists practice in a huge range of settings; for instance, members of this profession can be found in farm homes in rural communities or in specialized units in urban schools, hospitals, workplaces, or prisons. Client settings, culture, social class, policies, laws, and funding all constitute the client environment. Occupational therapists also live and practice in the context of their environment. The processes of enabling, then, are bound by or seek change in both the client and occupational therapy environment. Because enabling requires power sharing, occupational therapists might reflect on the reciprocal, mutual impacts on the client and the client's context as well as on the occupational therapist and the occupational therapist's context.

The environment is not a new focus for practice because early occupational therapists were active in adapting schools, designing sheltered workshops, and helping people with a disability live at home (Hopkins, 1988; Kidner, 1931). A refocus on the client environment and an interest in studying the context of occupational therapy practice is raising awareness of the importance of enabling environmental as well as individual change (Law, 1991; Townsend, 1996a). Moreover, this interest in the environment is captured in modern occupational therapy models (Canadian Association of Occupational Therapists, 2002; Chapparo & Ranka, 1998; Christiansen & Baum, 1991, 1997; Dunn, Brown, & McGuigan, 1994; Hagedorn, 1997; Kielhofner, 1995; Law et al., 1996).

The principle of "in context" is related to holism in that the whole person needs to participate in order to identify what enabling processes will work in a particular context. A common example of enabling holism in context is in the prescription of adaptive equipment. If an individual client, or a client group, experiences occupational deprivation because of a progressive disease, such as multiple sclerosis, a wheelchair may be prescribed. A professional who attends to the physical body without regard for the context would measure the body and prescribe a wheelchair. An enabling professional who is attending to the principle of holism in context would engage the whole person in considering potential uses of a wheelchair and assistance available in the particular places where wheelchair use will occur. Together, the occupational therapist and client would explore the personal meaning of using a wheelchair and any preferences the individual may have regarding cosmesis or the "look" of the chair. They would visit or look at information on the physical context: Are buildings and outdoor areas physically accessible? Is the community built on hills that are slippery in winter? They would consider the cultural and social context: Will the client's family and community encourage wheelchair independence or will everyone ridicule this as an unnecessary expense or a sign of weakness? The political and economic context would be considered: Is there any public support for establishing a wheelchair loan service for those who do not need their own chair or who are waiting for a new personal chair to arrive, and is a wheelchair the most effective piece of equipment if funds are limited? Participation and collaboration would draw in the whole person and require knowledge of context to determine what is possible and desirable and what is not. Enabling processes such as facilitation, listening, and reflection would be central in this approach.

It is unlikely that this full enabling approach would occur with each individual in a time-conscious practice where standard protocols would eliminate many of the steps described above. An enabling occupational therapist would move toward greater enabling through the strategies described in the final section of the chapter. In the situation just described, an occupational therapist might shift toward greater enabling by employing group approaches where possible to involve those with multiple sclerosis in developing community development skills. Within the management of services, the occupational therapist might convince funders of the importance of building in time to consult with self-help and consumer groups who, with help from some professional skills and support, would advance community cost-sharing with organizations to improve their community accessibility and appropriate wheelchair use (Mosher & Burti, 1992).

Empowerment and Justice

There are many definitions of empowerment and justice. As an enabling principle, empowerment and justice are introduced together because the aim in enabling versus profession-driven services is to enable clients to become empowered. Occupational therapists' interests in empowerment and justice have grown through awareness of the inequities and powerlessness in everyday occupations that may arise from age, disability, and social disadvantages (Redick et al., 2000). Occupational therapists who follow the enabling principles of participation, collaboration, and holism in context involve clients as decision-making partners whose holistic experience and environmental context are an acknowledged part of the process of practice. When these principles are followed with at-risk or disadvantaged populations, the empowerment of these groups has the impact of addressing potential or actual injustices.

Awareness of the need to shape environments to enhance occupational performance locates occupational therapists' practice implicitly and sometimes explicitly in the work of enabling empowerment and justice. Implicit empowerment and justice are embedded in home adjustments that enable elderly people to stay in their own homes when that is their wish or in skill development with children whose physical and mental development are slower than in other children in a community. Explicit empowerment and justice approaches are used by occupational therapists who develop policies to create flexible working conditions to accommodate people with a disability or who work with consumer groups who seek a stronger voice in local planning for housing and transportation (Kari & Michels, 1991; Pizzi, 1992; Townsend, 1996b).

To enable empowerment and justice is to enable hope with or without change actually occurring. Although empowerment and justice go beyond hope, hope is brought into the discussion as part of a vision of possibility for empowerment and justice (Kuyek, 1990). The link to justice is made because hope needs a direction. In enabling occupation, hope is directed toward increased opportunity for those whose opportunities for meaningful occupation are limited, or hope is directed toward the creation of equity and a more inclusive society. Hope may be directed toward the empowerment of those whose voices are subordinated or silent, as are the voices of populations with disability or other limitations with whom occupational therapists work (Borell, Lilja, Sviden, & Sadlo, 2001; Woodside, 1991). The concern is for occupational empowerment and occupational justice (i.e., for the enablement of opportunity and resources for all to flourish in health and quality of life in an occupationally just world) (Townsend & Wilcock, 2004a, 2004b; Wilcock & Townsend, 2000).

Enabling: Illustrations

Three illustrations are presented to explore what enabling might "look like" in occupational therapy practice. While each of the scenarios deals with front-line occupational therapy practice, the illustrations are relevant to occupational therapists who practice as consultants, managers, educators, or researchers. Remembering that micro front-line enabling processes are interconnected with macro organizational enabling processes, the difference between the two is primarily in the point of departure with people or with the environment. The illustrations are composite examples drawn from the authors' experiences of occupational therapy primarily in the United States and Canada. Included are features that are intended to spark the recognition of enabling processes and principles by occupational therapy practitioners who have differing perspectives and experiences based on gender, culture, ability/disability, context, or other sources of difference. Of note, the illustrations are extensions of the self-reflection invited at the beginning of the chapter.

Each illustration follows a slightly different format to encourage creative thinking, problem solving, and professional reasoning. The first illustration presents a typical work-related situation in which the reader is positioned as an occupational therapist and is asked to reflect on ways to engage in an enabling practice with a vision of empowerment and justice. The second illustration is of a school- and community-based practice in which an occupational therapist works as a consultant and highlights how an enabling approach leads to different outcomes. The third illustration focuses on transforming practice in the traditional institutional setting of a rehabilitation unit in a large teaching hospital so that practice more fully reflects enabling processes and principles.

Enabling Audit Template

An enabling audit template is presented with each of the three illustrations as a means for self-critique and the development of enabling practices. Following each illustration, the four enabling principles are explored by asking questions about possible enabling processes. Questions are raised to encourage further critical analysis of the different approaches to occupational therapy practice and the different ways of exercising power that enabling requires. The questions serve as samples only, not an exhaustive list. The enabling audit template can be used to consider which occupational therapy practices are enabling or disabling.[2]

Practice Illustration #1: Enabling Paid Work With George

As an occupational therapist, you have contracted your services out to a small private practice in a town with strong agricultural ties. Dr. Chung has referred George Perez for occupational therapy services. The referral requests that you "evaluate and treat as indicated" with

[2] Readers are encouraged to brainstorm other questions, to consider if there are other enabling processes and principles beyond those discussed in this chapter that would be helpful. While the idea of an Enabling Audit Template should be credited and referenced to the authors of this chapter, readers are encouraged to create their own Enabling Audit Templates for use in practice and for use in educating occupational therapy students and others about the different ways of working and different ways of exercising power that characterize enabling occupation.

Table 20-6

Enabling Audit #1: Enabling Paid Work With George

Participation

Which enabling processes would prompt greater participation by George in thinking about what to do and in taking action to "get things back on track"?

Who else in George's life needs to be coached to participate in getting him back to paid work?

How will you listen to gain George's trust before you can encourage him to participate in and take ownership of his own occupational restoration? How can you display respect for George's decisions about his participation and facilitate George's reflection?

Collaboration

What reflection would be useful to prompt George to make sure that the doctor's request for occupational therapy to "evaluate and treat as indicated" is actually relevant to George's occupational needs?

How will you educate the psychiatrist and the insurance company about your enabling occupation approach with George?

Holism in Context

What are the pitfalls of not prompting George to consider the impact or his injury not only on his own everyday occupations but also on the occupational wellness of his children or the family that owns the orchard?

What applications of financial, policy, and legal features of the environment do both the occupational therapist and George need to guide to ensure that George has a positive return to paid work?

Empowerment and Justice

How might the occupational therapist educate George, his coworkers, and his employer about changes that would prompt the creation of a safer working environment?

What social disadvantages associated with issues of age, rural/urban life, or disability may need reflection and guidance to increase George's chances of returning to work?

the goal of Mr. Perez returning to full-time paid employment, preferably in his former job. Mr. Perez's Disability Management Coordinator, Jeanette, is keen to get occupational therapy involved (Table 20-6).

From the file that Dr. Chung has provided, you are able to establish that George is a 42-year-old man who is employed by a small, family-run, fruit orchard business. In his job, he does a number of different tasks in a given day, and his job also varies depending upon the season. George fell off a ladder at work 6 weeks ago and sustained a soft tissue injury to his neck, shoulders, and lower back. You also note that he has also been referred to a psychiatrist, as George is reporting significant sleep disturbance, and Dr. Chung feels there is some evidence pointing to George experiencing a major depressive episode.

Other information gathered from your first meeting with George: George has been employed at the same job for 13 years and is pleased to describe his excellent work and attendance record. He notes that he is well liked by coworkers, employers, and the family that owns the orchards.

Within 3 hours of his fall, George received medical attention from his family physician. His medical records show no structural damage or neurological deficits. He was given a prescription for anti-inflammatory medication and was told to take it easy for 3 to 4 days. He had a follow-up appointment with the physician a week after his fall. He continues to experience significant pain, particularly in his low back, which has prevented him from returning to work. He is currently attending physical therapy approximately twice per week. George has never had a prior workers' compensation claim.

George noted that his wife died a year ago. He has four children: one teenage daughter and three very active children under the age of 8. His parents and siblings have been assisting him with childcare responsibilities, but George stated that he "has got to get things back on track so that I'm not depending so much on others."

Table 20-7

Enabling Audit #2: Sayed, the Occupational Therapist, Enabling Community Change

Participation

Who are the participants in Sayed's work with the school? Should Sayed facilitate and encourage the children's participation in developing solutions?

How will Sayed ensure that he encourages each of the stakeholders to listen to and carefully reflect upon the points of view and concerns of all involved in the participatory task force?

What enabling processes did Sayed use that were different ways of working from the architectural firm consultation?

Collaboration

How will Sayed educate himself and the Participatory Task Force about the hierarchical and collaborative power structures of the school system?

How did Sayed listen and prompt the school hierarchy to consider a more collaborative, community development approach for integrating children with different occupational needs in neighborhood schools?

Holism in Context

What coaching and guiding should Sayed do to make sure the children's situations are addressed holistically? With attention to the cultural and economic context of the occupations in this community?

What type of report (verbal, written, formal, informal) would educate the community about his holistic, context-sensitive approach and guide the community to continue after Sayed's contract has been completed?

Empowerment and Justice

How could Sayed educate the special education teachers and teacher assistants to prompt and guide them in ways of working with children with disabilities so that the children can participate in leisure and sports occupations with their classmates outside as well as inside the classroom?

How might Sayed coach the children and parents from the school to educate government officials of the benefits and challenges of creating a more inclusive classroom and school system?

Practice Illustration #2: Sayed, the Occupational Therapist, Enabling Community Change

Sayed works on salary with an occupational therapy consulting firm called Community Solutions For Everyday Living (CSFEL). Through his son's elementary school principal, Sayed has met the Chair of the School Board in his home community. On inquiring about school bus and school access for the four children in wheelchairs in his son's school, Sayed learned from the School Board Chair that an architectural firm was commissioned to design greater physical access to the five schools operated by the School Board (Table 20-7).

The architectural firm's report recommended extensive changes at a huge cost. The firm had used a typical, well-respected consulting process to look at the five schools under the Board's jurisdiction. The process used by the architectural firm included the following:

- Walk-about tour of the school and school bus
- Measurement of all key areas (bathrooms, entrances, turning spaces, stairs, elevator button heights, classroom space)
- Public meeting to which parents and teachers were invited to give input and to comment on draft ideas for change
- Draft report to the Board for input
- Final report submitted to the Board

Without ready funds, the School Board has filed the report for future budget consideration.

Sayed convinced the School Board Chair that a different approach could produce a different solution. Sayed signed a contract with the Board to use a process he called "Participatory Enabling" and to produce a report in

4 months on "Developing an Inclusive School." The contract was to focus on one school as a "case example" of the way "inclusion" and "exclusion" worked in the School Board district. The "Participatory Enabling" process outlined six steps to produce the report:

1. Collaborate with the Board to send a letter of explanation and support for Sayed's contract to all parents and children, teachers, and local community businesses near the school—a confectionary, recreation hall, and restaurant where the children and teachers often congregated outside classes.
2. Observe and record the daily routines and actions in four classes—the ones in which the four children in wheelchairs worked—for a full day each.
3. Meet with a "Participatory Task Force" to which he invited the four teachers, the parents of the four children, two parents from each of the four classes, and two Board members to ask questions to clarify how the school worked based on observations (e.g., Why were the students in wheelchairs carried to the school yard when there was a ramp at the back of the building? What were teacher assistants' duties, particularly with respect to the children in wheelchairs? Who paid for extra help if the children in wheelchairs went on school bus outings? Where did other School Boards find funds to include children in wheelchairs? What were the attitudes of local politicians to having the children in wheelchairs in the School system?)
4. Draft a report, and meet for a second time with the "Participatory Task Force" to make sure that he had not missed anything important in outlining "Strengths and Challenges for Developing an Inclusive School."
5. Final report submitted to the Board with copies to the Participatory Task Force.
6. Action Mapping meeting 3 months after the report was submitted to confirm actions regarding budgeting for the next fiscal year for changes, parental advocacy to the local politicians about funding for the School Board to address recommended changes, media releases with children, parents, and teachers telling their stories of being part of the Participatory Task Force.

The Participatory Task Force continued to advocate for change, using their report produced in collaboration with Sayed, and within a year, the funds were found and changes were made, monitored, and adjusted over the next 5 years by the community.

Practice Illustration #3: James, the Occupational Therapist, Enabling Rehabilitation Following Stoke

James works as an occupational therapist on a rehabilitation unit of a large teaching hospital in an urban center. Many of his clients are older adults who are experiencing occupational challenges due to stroke. On the unit, there are two teams. Each team consists of an occupational therapist, a physical therapist, a speech language pathologist, a recreation therapist, a social worker, a physiatrist, and three nurses (one for each shift). Other services, such as respiratory therapy, are available as required. James enjoys working with this team and finds the work environment to be very collaborative and supportive. Each profession is recognized as contributing a key element to the process of rehabilitation, and each member of the team has specific roles delineated. Occupational therapy is responsible for helping individuals improve their self-care and simple household management skills, as well as for collaborating on discharge planning with the social worker (Table 20-8).

The rehabilitation unit itself is a very structured, scheduled, and controlled environment. The daily schedule of events is clearly posted on the unit for everyone to see, and miscommunication about the timetable is rare. Upper management within the hospital and the accreditors have praised the rehabilitation unit for running like a "well-oiled machine."

Two of the traditional semiprivate hospital rooms on the rehabilitation unit have been converted into an "apartment," referred to as the "Transitional Living Centre" (TLC). The TLC is a living space that includes a bedroom, living room, kitchen, and bathroom and is designed to be a stepping stone between the institutional and the home environment. Individuals who stay in the TLC no longer require the amount of medical care and assistance that a wardroom provides, but are not quite ready to return home. The TLC is far less structured and supervised. Within certain guidelines including established times for meals and therapy, individuals are able to set their own schedules to reflect their personal preferences.

Mrs. Gamallo is a 68-year-old woman who was admitted to the hospital who had a stroke while attending church. Mrs. Gamallo is eager to prove to the team, her family, and herself that she is ready to return home and "start taking care of myself again." She views the TLC as the next step in the process that will get her back home. She and James have been working on improving her safety while performing occupations in the kitchen and bath-

Table 20-8

Enabling Audit #3: James, the Occupational Therapist, Enabling Rehabilitation Following Stoke

Participation

Mrs. Gamalla is keen to participate in helping herself, but how will James prompt her to reflect on her real abilities and limitations?

How can James coach and encourage participation by those like Mrs. Gamalla who are discharged from the Rehabilitation Center in self-help groups in the community?

How will James educate the social worker and two daughters about his expert opinion of Mrs. Gamalla's ability to participate in helping herself, while listening and reflecting carefully to their point of view and concerns?

Collaboration

What collaboration exists between the national heart and stroke association and the Rehabilitation Unit? With whom could James facilitate greater funding resources to facilitate the development of more extensive occupational therapy or other occupation-focused discharge and follow-up services?

Who is the "team" James needs to facilitate and guide in the collaborative approach you hope to achieve in your practice in this Rehabilitation Unit? How will James coach and encourage Mrs. Gamalla and her daughters to be collaborating decision makers on the "team"?

Holism in Context

In Mrs. Gamalla's community, what other available and affordable services such as help with household cleaning would prompt and encourage her to be safe in her everyday occupations at home?

What should James record to reflect his holistic, context-sensitive approach in enabling occupation when individual charts require progress only on key problem areas (pathology) as defined by the physician?

Empowerment and Justice

Whose rights prevail if Mrs. Gamalla wants to go home even if the occupational therapist and her family disagree? How can the occupational therapist enable a safe solution?

How long are people admitted to the specialized Rehabilitation Unit, and what educating and encouraging can James do as an occupational therapist to extend support beyond the hospital walls?

room. As Mrs. Gamallo frequently tells her family, she has a hard time "slowing down" and taking things one step at a time, and is just not as "steady on her feet" as she once was. She is concerned about falling, but feels that her family and the team working with her are being overprotective and overly cautious. James, the social worker, Mrs. Gamallo, and two of her adult daughters are in the midst of a planning meeting to discuss "where to go from here."

Strategies in Support of Enabling

The enabling processes and principles presented and illustrated in this chapter speak to an ideal practice. Since the advent of guidelines for client-centered, occupation-focused practice, occupational therapists have identified an array of opportunities and barriers (Hong, Pearce, & Withers, 2000; Lane, 2000; Sumison & Smyth, 2000; Townsend, 1999; Wilkins et al., 2001). The lists of barriers and questions about being client-centered may suggest that occupational therapists are victims of alien health, education, or other systems in which this profession has too little power for enabling occupation.

Four challenges and strategies in support of changing everyday practice and systems toward enabling are discussed briefly: occupational therapists' use of professional power, occupational therapists' focus on enabling occupation, enabling in managed systems, and enabling reconsideration of funding priorities.

Occupational Therapists' Use of Professional Power

The last challenge for enabling occupation raised here is about professional power (i.e., occupational therapy's power as a profession). Around the world, occupational therapy was founded by people who had been sufficiently educated for a profession. Western countries tended to establish occupational therapy as a profession following a war as a means of returning injured soldiers to the workforce (Hopkins, 1988; Low, 1992). Those available to work as occupational therapists were largely women. Occupational therapy does not appear to be women's work in that early practitioners were often the directors of rehabilitation workshops with heavy machinery. Yet, today's practice tends to focus on self-care and kitchen occupations, as one might expect of traditional women's work. Given the need for a university education, the class and race of occupational therapists tend to be those of the dominant groups in a society. Yet, a large part of occupational therapy's traditional clientele may be those from disadvantaged groups, such as nondominant races who need assistance in enabling occupation because they are elderly, living with a disability, or living in poverty without access to resources for organizing their lives without professional assistance.

Enabling requires professional power sharing. This is a difficult challenge for occupational therapy, a profession that is still exploring its own power now that there is decreasing sponsorship by medicine (Maxwell & Maxwell, 1983). Gender is a major question because the majority of occupational therapists in Western countries are women, while in Eastern countries, the majority of occupational therapists are men (Frank, 1992; Readman, 1992). The most urgent strategy for addressing challenges associated with professional power is to generate discussion and research on professional power.

Occupational Therapists' Focus on Enabling Occupation

There are significant challenges in enabling occupation toward the development of more inclusive communities with empowered citizens. A central challenge for occupational therapists is to educate communities about the broad range of occupations, including but going beyond jobs, that are required for health and quality of life. How will society learn about the occupational nature of humans, or the need for meaningful occupation from birth to death? Enabling occupation tends to be invisible, without expensive equipment or space. Client outcomes are the most visible impact of enabling, although outcomes are complicated to evaluate given the variety of forces that may influence outcomes. An important strategy would be to educate the public on enabling processes and principles and on enabling occupation, rather than on occupational therapy. Negative views of codependent enabling could be raised with examples of positive enabling that facilitate people to fulfill their potential. Rather than trying to explain what this profession is NOT about (not about components or body parts, not based on a medical model of practice, or not physiotherapy), the strategy of educating others would create an environment in which citizens would participate in enabling occupation.

Enabling in Managed Systems

Key challenges for occupational therapists also lie in enabling occupation within standardized management systems. Where quality and best practice are of concern to management, the challenge is to introduce evidence of accountability for efficient and effective enabling. Management systems were established to coordinate professional expertise in an era when the professional expert was idolized. Today, citizens around the world are challenging the "experts." Citizens need and want services that are efficient and accountable, but more than that, citizens want services that make a difference.

Occupational therapists can be ambassadors for enabling occupation with contacts both inside and outside systems. Enabling processes can draw citizens as participants in changing systems. Change in management systems depends on participatory solutions where diverse perspectives are brought together. Fiscally responsible partnerships could be developed between occupational therapists, other enablers, and citizens. This blend of professional and experiential expertise would greatly benefit planning to develop effective as well as efficient approaches to health, school, employment, housing, and other issues. With knowledge of enabling processes and occupation, it is imperative for occupational therapists to become more involved in changing systems rather than trying to get around them.

Enabling Reconsideration of Funding Priorities

There are also challenges to redirect funding. What can occupational therapy enabling do to change international funding systems? This is a tall order, but not impossible if this profession identifies allies who recognize the importance of enabling occupation. Occupational therapists work with powerful ideas in very practical ways. The development of human resources is a matter of universal interest at some level. Therefore, occupational therapy strategies are needed to create sufficient commitment to shift funding priorities toward enabling occupation. The competition is severe: national and international funding priorities are made by those who govern countries or corporations, not by community groups and small professions like occupational therapy. The World Bank, the International Monetary Fund, corporate financing, trade agreements, and other financial arrangements are all difficult to penetrate from the outside. However, there have been shifts over time when disgruntled populations make their needs known very publicly and in world venues.

Occupational therapists' enabling has been largely invisible to all but the individuals and groups with whom this profession comes into direct contact. Strategies for changing funding priorities are likely those already identified (i.e., to create greater public awareness of the importance of enabling occupation and to create practical approaches for people to participate as collaborating partners in making change within systems as well as in communities). The enabling here is not about what the profession thinks is best, but about enabling those who experience limited opportunity in daily occupations to voice their needs in the committees and board rooms where financial decisions are being made.

Conclusion

Enabling has been raised for occupational therapists and others to examine through self-reflection and through critique of the enabling processes and principles presented above. Also presented were three illustrations that raise questions about enabling through the format of an enabling audit template. Strategies were then outlined to develop and support client-centered, occupation-focused enabling. It has been illustrated here and argued elsewhere that enabling approaches are "the most appropriate forms of helping when the goal is occupational performance" (Canadian Association of Occupational Therapists, 2002, p. 180). Readers are encouraged to further explore approaches for enabling occupation by continuing to return to and reflect on the various questions posed throughout this chapter and by persisting to ask throughout their careers if what they are doing as students and practicing occupational therapists is consistent with occupation-focused, client-centered enabling.

The chapter paints a rather lofty picture of ideal enabling that is focused on occupation, empowerment, and justice. Readers may say "but real practice is not like that. There are few chances for enabling occupation in the real world." To these people, the authors encourage us all to enable them to generate a sense of hope. The illustrations are drawn from real practice where enabling was not fully achieved while some advances were made in making it possible for somebody to do something and making it possible for something to happen or exit by creating the necessary conditions (Oxford University Press, 2000). Most occupational therapists have experiences where clients have discovered and participated in meaningful occupations, recovering hope in themselves and their families. It seems worthwhile for this profession to learn how to enable more efficiently and effectively so that these moments are more frequent and forceful. When systems restructure their policies to support their clientele in meaningful occupation, then enabling comes alive for a whole community.

Acknowledgments

Acknowledgments are extended to Diane MacKenzie for her early research assistance on client-centred practice. The authors also extend thanks to two student occupational therapist reviewers at Dalhousie University, Nancy Boutcher and Bethany Lander. Their comments enabled the authors to refine the chapter as a learning tool.

References

American Occupational Therapy Association. (1999). The occupational therapy process. *American Journal of Occupational Therapy, 53*, 263-289.

Belenky, M. F., Bond, L. A., & Weinstock, S. (1997). *A tradition that has no name: Nurturing the development of people, families, and communities*. New York, NY: Basic Books.

Belenky, M. F., Clinchy, B. M., Goldberger, N. R., & Tarule, J. M. (1986). *Women's ways of knowing: The development of self, voice and mind*. New York, NY: Basic Books.

Borell, L., Lilja, M., Sviden, G. A., & Sadlo, G. (2001). Occupations and signs of reduced hope: An explorative study of older adults with functional impairments. *American Journal of Occupational Therapy, 55*(3), 311-316.

Borkman, T. J. (1999). *Understanding self-help/mutual aid: Experiential learning in the commons*. Piscataway, NJ: Rutgers University Press.

Brookfield, S. D. (1987). *Learning democracy: Eduard Lindeman on adult education and social change*. London, England: Croom Helm.

Byrne, C. (1999). Facilitating empowerment groups: Dismantling professional boundaries. *Issues in Mental Health Nursing, 20*, 55-71.

Canadian Association of Occupational Therapists. (1991). *Occupational therapy guidelines for client-centred practice*. Toronto, ON: CAOT Publications.

Canadian Association of Occupational Therapists. (2002). *Enabling occupation: A Canadian occupational therapy perspective*. Ottawa, ON: Author.

Chapparo, C., & Ranka, J. (1998). *Occupational Performance Model (Australia)*. Sydney, NSW: School of Occupation and Leisure Studies.

Evidence Worksheet

Author(s)	*Year*	*Topic*	*Method*	*Conclusion*
Byrne	1999	Explores facilitating as an enabling strategy. The focus is on facilitating empowerment groups with people with chronic and persistent mental illness and the process of dismantling of professional boundaries	Qualitative—participant observation via field notes. Grounded theory approach	The process of assisting in enabling (facilitating) empowerment requires the dismantling of professional boundaries between health professional and people with whom they are developing partnerships. Need to facilitate practitioners to confront/challenge existing ways of practicing. Working with as opposed to doing for as representative of a shift from traditional health care service provision to enabling
Corring & Cook	1999	Explores the perspectives of individuals with the experience of mental illness regarding the meaning of enabling in a client-centered approach to practice	Qualitative—focus groups. Modified participatory action	Central message from participants was related to what is wrong and what is needed in enabling positive everyday relationships between clients and service providers. Highlights need for individuals with mental illness to be viewed as valuable human beings and partners in therapy as a central value in enabling
Rebeiro	2001	Explores the meaning of enabling participation in occupation for women with mental illness. Addresses the influence on occupational performance of either enabling or disabling features of environment, specifically the social environment	Qualitative—in-depth interviews, participant observation, and focus groups	An enabling social environment plays a significant role in enabling participation in occupation(s). An enabling environment provides opportunity, choice, affirming individual's worth, support, enabling sense of belonging

(continued)

Author(s)	Year	Topic	Method	Conclusion
Sumsion & Smyth	2000	Barriers to client-centered practice and suggested strategies to address/resolve these barriers in enabling occupation	Survey—quantitative, non-experimental survey design, postal questionnaire	Different goals of clients and practitioners often viewed as the most common barrier to client centered practice. Most effective method to transform practice appears to be to provide occupational therapists with case examples of practicing in a client-centered, enabling manner

Christiansen, C., & Baum, C. M. (Eds.). (1991). *Occupational therapy: Overcoming human performance deficits*. Thorofare, NJ: SLACK Incorporated.

Christiansen, C., & Baum, C. M. (Eds.). (1997). *Occupational therapy: Enabling function and well-being* (2nd ed.). Thorofare, NJ: SLACK Incorporated.

Coburn, D. (1993). State authority, medical dominance, and trends in the regulation of the health professions: The Ontario case. *Sociology of Science and Medicine*, *37*, 129-138.

Cohen, C. I., D'Onofrio, A., Larkin, L., Berkholder, P., & Fishman, H. (1999). A comparison of consumer and provider preferences for research on homeless veterans. *Community Mental Health Journal*, *35*(3), 273-280.

Corring, D., & Cook, J. (1999). Client-centred care means that I am a valued human being. *Canadian Journal of Occupational Therapy*, *66*(2), 71-82.

Deegan, P. E. (1997). Recovery and empowerment for people with psychiatric disabilities. *Social Work in Health Care*, *25*(3), 11-24.

Department of National Health and Welfare & Canadian Association of Occupational Therapists. (1983). *Guidelines for the client-centred practice of occupational therapy H39-33/1983E*. Ottawa, ON: Department of National Health and Welfare.

Department of National Health and Welfare & Canadian Association of Occupational Therapists. (1986). *Intervention guidelines for the client-centred practice of occupational therapy H39-100/1986E*. Ottawa, ON: Department of National Health and Welfare.

Department of National Health and Welfare & Canadian Association of Occupational Therapists. (1987). *Toward outcome measures in occupational therapy H39-114/1987E*. Ottawa, ON: Department of National Health and Welfare.

Dewey, J. (1922). *Human nature and conduct*. New York, NY: Henry Holt.

do Rozario, L. (1994). Ritual, meaning and transcendence: The role of occupation in modern life. *Journal of Occupational Science*, *1*(3), 46-53.

Dunn, W., Brown, C., & McGuigan, A. (1994). The ecology of human performance: A framework for considering the effect of context. *American Journal of Occupational Therapy*, *48*(7), 595-607.

Dunst, C. J., Trivette, C., & Deal, A. (1998). *Enabling and empowering families: Principles and guidelines for practice*. Cambridge, MA: Brookline Books.

Dunst, C. J., Trivette, C., Davis, M., & Cornwell, J. (1988). Enabling and empowering families of children with health impairments. *Children's Health Care*, *17*, 71-81.

Dunst, C. J., & Trivette, C. M. (1989). An enablement and empowerment perspective of case management. *Topics in Early Childhood Special Education*, 8, 87-102.

Dunton, W. R. (1919). *Reconstruction therapy*. Philadelphia, PA: Saunders.

Egan, M., Dubouloz, C., von Zweck, C., & Vallerand, J. (1998). The client-centred evidence-based practice of occupational therapy. *Canadian Journal of Occupational Therapy*, *65*(3), 136-143.

Fearing, V. G., & Clark, J. (2000). *Individuals in context: A practical guide to client-centred practice*. Thorofare, NJ: SLACK Incorporated.

Frank, G. (1992). Opening feminist histories of occupational therapy. *American Journal of Occupational Therapy*, *46*, 989-999.

Gage, M., & Polatajko, H. (1995). Naming practice: The case for the term client-driven. *Canadian Journal of Occupational Therapy*, *62*, 115-118.

Grady, A. P. (1995). Building inclusive community: A challenge for occupational therapy. *American Journal of Occupational Therapy*, *49*, 300-310.

Hagedorn, R. (1997). *Foundations for practice in occupational therapy* (2nd ed.). London, England: Churchill Livingston.

Health Canada & Canadian Association of Occupational Therapists. (1993). *Occupational therapy guidelines for client-centred mental health practice*. Ottawa, ON: Canadian Association of Occupational Therapists.

Hong, C. S., Pearce, S., & Withers, R. A. (2000). Occupational therapy assessments: How client-centred can they be? *British Journal of Occupational Therapy, 63*(7), 316-318.

Hopkins, H. L. (1988). An historical perspective on occupational therapy. In H. Hopkins & H. Smith (Eds.), *Willard and Spackman's occupational therapy* (7th ed., pp. 16-37). Philadelphia, PA: J. B. Lippincott.

Kari, N., & Michels, P. (1991). The Lazarus project: The politics of empowerment. *American Journal of Occupational Therapy, 45*, 719-725.

Kidner, T. B. (1931). Occupational therapy: Its diagnosis, scope, and possibilities. *Archives of Occupational Therapy, 10*, 1-11.

Kielhofner, G. (1983). *Health through occupation: Theory and practice in occupational therapy*. Philadelphia, PA: F. A. Davis Company.

Kielhofner, G. (1995). *A model of human occupation: Theory and application* (2nd ed.). Baltimore, MD: Williams and Wilkins.

Kielhofner, G., & Burke, J. P. (1977). Occupational therapy after 60 years: An account of changing identity and knowledge. *American Journal of Occupational Therapy, 31*, 675-689.

Kinsella, E. A. (2001). Reflections on reflective practice. *Canadian Journal of Occupational Therapy, 68*(3), 195-198.

Klein, B. S. (1995). Reflections... An ally as well as a partner in practice. *Canadian Journal of Occupational Therapy, 62*, 283-285.

Kuyek, J. N. (1990). *Fighting for hope: Organizing to realize our dreams*. Montreal, PQ: Black Rose Books.

Lane, L. (2000). Client-centred practice: Is it compatible with early discharge hospital-at-home policies? *British Journal of Occupational Therapy, 63*(7), 310-315.

Law, M. (1991). Muriel Driver Memorial Lecture: The environment: A focus for occupational therapy. *Canadian Journal of Occupational Therapy, 58*, 171-180.

Law, M. (Ed.). (1998). *Client-centred occupational therapy*. Thorofare, NJ: SLACK Incorporated.

Law, M., Baum, C. M., & Baptiste, S. (Eds.). (2002). *Occupation-based practice: Fostering performance and participation*. Thorofare, NJ: SLACK Incorporated.

Law, M., Cooper, B. A., Strong, S., Stewart, D., Rigby, P., & Letts, L. (1996). The Person-Environment-Occupation Model: A transactive approach to occupational performance. *Canadian Journal of Occupational Therapy, 63*(1), 9-22.

Lefley, H. P. (1998). Families, culture, and mental illness: Constructing new realities. *Psychiatry, 61*(4), 335-355.

Letts, L., Fraser, B., Finlayson, M., & Walls, J. (1993). *For the health of it! Occupational therapy within a health promotion framework*. Toronto, ON: CAOT Publications ACE.

Low, J. F. (1992). The reconstruction aides. *American Journal of Occupational Therapy, 46*, 38-44.

Mader, C. (1998). Reverence for the ordinary. *Canadian Journal of Native Education, 22*(2), 171-187.

Mattingly, C. F., & Fleming, M. H. (1994). *Clinical reasoning: Forms of inquiry in a therapeutic practice*. Philadelphia, PA: F. A. Davis.

Maxwell, J. D., & Maxwell, M. P. (1983). Inner fraternity and outer sorority: Social structure and the professionalization of occupational therapy. In A. Wipper (Ed.), *The sociology of work: Papers in honour of Osward Hall*. Carleton Library series number 129. Ottawa, ON: Carleton University Press.

McCaugherty, D. (1991). The use of a teaching model to promote reflection and the experiential integration of theory and practice in first-year student nurses: An action research study. *Journal of Advanced Nursing, 16*, 534-543.

McColl, M. A. (1994). Holistic occupational therapy: Historical meaning and contemporary implications. *Canadian Journal of Occupational Therapy, 61*, 72-77.

Metz, T. (2000). Arbitrariness, justice, and respect. *Social Theory and Practice, 26*, 24-45.

Meyer, A. (1922). The philosophy of occupation therapy. *Archives of Occupational Therapy, 1*(1), 1-10.

Milhollan, F., & Forisha, B. (1972). *From Skinner to Rogers: Contrasting approaches to education*. Nebraska: Professional Educators Publications.

Mosher, L. R., & Burti, L. (1992). Relationships in rehabilitation: When technology fails. *Psychosocial Rehabilitation Journal, 15*, 11-17.

Oxford University Press. (2000). *Oxford advanced learner's dictionary*. Oxford, UK: Author.

Peloquin, S. M. (1993a). The depersonalization of patients: A profile gleaned from narratives. *American Journal of Occupational Therapy, 47*, 830-837.

Peloquin, S. M. (1993b). The patient-therapist relationship: Beliefs that shape care. *American Journal of Occupational Therapy, 47*, 935-942.

Pizzi, M. (1992). Women, HIV infection, and AIDS: Tapestries of life, death, and empowerment. *American Journal of Occupational Therapy, 46*, 1021-1027.

Polatajko, H. J. (1992). Muriel Driver Memorial Lecture: Naming and framing occupational therapy: A lecture dedicated to the life of Nancy B. *Canadian Journal of Occupational Therapy, 59*, 189-200.

Polatajko, H. J. (1994). Dreams, dilemmas, and decisions for occupational therapy practice in a new millennium: A Canadian perspective. *American Journal of Occupational Therapy, 48*, 590-594.

Pollock, N. (1993). Client-centered assessment. *American Journal of Occupational Therapy, 47*, 298-301.

Readman, T. (1992). Recruitment of men in occupational therapy: Past, present and future. *Canadian Journal of Occupational Therapy, 59*, 73-77.

Rebeiro, K. (2000). Client perspectives on occupational therapy practice: Are we truly client-centred? *Canadian Journal of Occupational Therapy*, *67*(1), 7-14.

Rebeiro, K. (2001). Enabling occupation: The importance of an affirming environment. *Canadian Journal of Occupational Therapy*, *68*(2), 80-89.

Redick, A. G., McClain, L., & Brown, C. (2000). Consumer empowerment through occupational therapy: The Americans with Disabilities Act Title III. *American Journal of Occupational Therapy*, *54*(2), 207-213.

Reed, K. L., & Sanderson, S. (1980). *Concepts in occupational therapy*. Baltimore, MD: Williams and Wilkins.

Reed, K. L., & Sanderson, S. N. (1999). *Concepts of occupational therapy* (4th ed.). Philadelphia, PA: Lippincott, Williams & Wilkins.

Rogers, C. R. (1939). *The clinical treatment of the problem child*. Boston, MA: Houghton Mifflin.

Rogers, C. R. (1953). *Client-centered therapy*. Boston, MA: Houghton Mifflin.

Rogers, C. R. (1961). *On becoming a person*. Boston, MA: Houghton Mifflin.

Rogers, C. R. (1965). *Client-centered therapy: Its current practice, implications and theory*. Boston, MA: Houghton Mifflin.

Rogers, C. (1969). *Freedom to learn: A view of what education might become*. Columbus, OH: C. E. Merrill Publishing Co.

Rogers, C. R. (1980). *A way of being*. Boston, MA: Houghton Mifflin.

Schon, D. (1987). *Educating the reflective practitioner: Toward a new design for teaching and learning in the professions*. San Francisco, CA: Jossey-Bass Publishers.

Schwartz, K. B. (1992). Occupational therapy and education: A shared vision. *American Journal of Occupational Therapy*, *46*, 12-18.

Sherwin, S. (1998). A relational approach to autonomy in health care. In S. Sherwin (Ed.), *The politics of women's health: Exploring agency & autonomy* (pp. 19-47). Philadelphia, PA: Temple University Press.

Staral, J. M. (2000). Building on mutual goals: The intersection of community practice and church-based organizing. *Journal of Community Practice*, *7*(3), 85-95.

Sumison, T. (Ed.). (1999). *Client-centred practice in occupational therapy: A guide to implementation*. London, UK: Churchill Livingston.

Sumison, T., & Smyth, G. (2000). Barriers to client-centredness and their resolution. *Canadian Journal of Occupational Therapy*, *67*(1), 15-21.

Townsend, E. (1996a). Institutional ethnography: A method for showing how the context shapes practice. *Occupational Therapy Journal of Research*, *16*(3), 179-199.

Townsend, E. (1996b). Enabling empowerment: Using simulations versus real occupations. *Canadian Journal of Occupational Therapy*, *63*, 113-128.

Townsend, E. (1998a). Client-centred occupational therapy: The Canadian experience. In M. Law (Ed.), *Client-centred occupational therapy* (pp. 47-65). Thorofare, NJ: SLACK Incorporated.

Townsend, E. (1998b). *Good intentions overruled: A critique of empowerment in the routine organization of mental health services*. Toronto, ON: University of Toronto Press.

Townsend, E. (1999). Enabling occupation in the 21st century: Making good intentions a reality. *Australian Occupational Therapy Journal*, *46*, 147-159.

Townsend, E. (2000). Occupational terminology interactive dialogue... Enabling occupation. *Journal of Occupational Science*, *7*(1), 42-43.

Townsend, E., & Wilcock, A. A. (2004a). Occupational justice. In C. H. Christiansen, (Ed.), *An introduction to occupation* (pp. 243-273). NJ: Prentice Hall Publishing Inc.

Townsend E., & Wilcock, A. A. (2004b). Occupational justice and client-centred practice: A dialogue in progress. *Canadian Journal of Occupational Therapy*, *71*, 75-87.

Watson, D. (1992). Documentation of paediatric assessments using the occupational therapy guidelines for client-centred practice. *Canadian Journal of Occupational Therapy*, *59*, 87-94.

Wilcock, A. A. (1998). *An occupational perspective of health*. Thorofare, NJ: SLACK Incorporated.

Wilcock, A., & Townsend, E. (2000). Occupational justice: Occupational terminology interactive dialogue. *Journal of Occupational Science*, *7*(2), 84-86.

Wilkins, S., Pollock, N., Rochon, S., & Law, M. (2001). Implementing client-centred practice: Why is it so difficult to do? *Canadian Journal of Occupational Therapy*, *68*(2), 70-79.

Wilson, V. (1999). Action learning: A "highbrow smash and grab" activity? *Career Development International*, *4*(1), 5-10.

Woodside, H. (1991). National perspective. The participation of mental health consumers in health care issues. *Canadian Journal of Occupational Therapy*, *58*, 3-5.

World Health Organization. (1986). Ottawa charter for health promotion. Retrieved February 18, 2000, from http://www.who.int/hpr/archive/ docs/ottawa.html.

Yerxa, E. J. (1994). Dreams, dilemmas, and decisions for occupational therapy practice in a new millennium: An American perspective. *American Journal of Occupational Therapy*, *48*, 586-589.

BIBLIOGRAPHY

Townsend, E., Birch, D., Langille, L., & Langley, J. (2000). Participatory research in a mental health clubhouse. *Occupational Therapy Journal of Research*, *20*, 18-44.

Chapter Twenty: Interventions in a Societal Context
Reflections and Learning Activities

Julie Bass-Haugen, PhD, OTR/L, FAOTA

Reflections

This chapter challenged us to explore our underlying values and beliefs about occupational therapy. Occupational therapy is often described as having both art and science as core attributes. Much of the focus of current occupational therapy literature is on the scientific basis for occupational therapy. The art of occupational therapy requires that we use self-reflection to understand how we feel and act as we enable others to achieve their goals through our client-centered, occupation-based practice.

One can look at client-centered care as a value. I can focus my interventions toward the needs, goals, and interest of the client. Using this approach, the concept of client-centered care is implicit. This chapter reminded us that people learn by doing, by participating in experiences that relate to their everyday occupations. In this way, client-centered care becomes the intervention with the therapist enabling the client—either an individual or group—to learn how to do what he or she needs and wants to do. This may occur through recovery of personal skills or by creating an inclusive, accessible environment.

Using a client-centered approach requires the practitioner to use complex professional reasoning to enable the individual to employ occupations as he or she explores practical approaches to everyday challenges. Such an approach also requires the practitioner to enlist the help of families, coworkers, teachers, and others who are drawn into the process to problem solve and find solutions that help clients realize their goals.

The enabling process often goes beyond individuals and groups. It may be targeted at policies, legislation, communities, agencies, or organizations. Such approaches are designed to eliminate barriers that limit the participation of people who have goals that can only be realized when there are supportive environments.

Four principles are central to enabling client-centered, occupation-based approaches. Participation in occupations encourages people to be active participants helping themselves. Generally, people don't want to be on the sideline in the "game of life." They want to have a chance to actually play the game. So, we must focus our enabling approaches on actual participation in occupations, not just 'talking' about occupations of interest to our clients. Collaboration with clients occurs when the clients' goals are driving the interventions. By collaboration, we mean the therapist-client relationship is intended to be a partnership regardless of the setting or model of service delivery. Holism in context is incorporated when clients are involved in self or organizational change. Holism requires attention to all dimensions of the person and the environment, not just the dimensions that seem inherent in the specific therapeutic approach. Empowerment and justice enable clients to be empowered and to experience hope. This in turn allows clients to have increased opportunity and quality of life.

These ideals and principles related to enabling and client-centered, occupation-focused approaches are important to retain throughout your professional life. You will no doubt encounter situations in which occupational therapy practice appears mechanical and limited by the restrictions in a particular setting. It is especially important during these times to continue your work toward the greater good of the profession and last, but not least, the people you serve. Enabling occupational performance and participation in life are the rewards that come from being an occupational therapy practitioner.

Journal Activities

1. Look up and write down a dictionary definition of enable. Highlight the component of the definition that is most related to the descriptions in Chapter Twenty.
2. Identify the most important new learning for you in this chapter.
3. Identify one question you have about Chapter Twenty.
4. Reflect on the experience of being enabled in your own life. Spend a few minutes alone or in a group jotting down a few thoughts about enabling. Think about three linked forces that enable you to live and learn with others: your personal qualities, your environment, and your occupations. Answer the questions in Table 20-1.

Technology/Internet Learning Activities

1. Use a discussion database to share specific journal activities.

Applied Learning Activities

Applied Learning Activity #1: Reflection on Enabling Others

Instructions:

- Complete the Reflection on Enabling Others in Table 20-2.
- Think about the things that you listed as enablers for these occupations. How would you classify these specific factors according to the Person and Environment categories in the PEOP Model?
- Think about the things that you listed as barriers for these occupations. How would you classify these specific factors according to the Person and Environment categories in the PEOP Model?
- Identify three specific goals that could promote improved performance of these occupations by the individual. For each goal, identify two to three strategies to build on the enablers and strategies to limit the influence of the barriers.

Applied Learning Activity #2: Reflection on Client-Centered, Occupation-Focused Enabling

Instructions:

- Complete the Reflection on Client-Centered, Occupation-Focused Enabling.
- Review Enabling Processes in Table 20-5.
- Think about yourself as an occupational therapy practitioner who uses client-centered, occupation focused enabling approaches with the individuals you serve.
  - ✧ What skills do you have that are important in enabling approaches?
  - ✧ What attitudes and beliefs do you have that are important in enabling approaches?
  - ✧ What skills would you like to develop to strengthen your ability to use enabling approaches?
  - ✧ What attitudes and beliefs would you like to develop/change to strengthen your ability to use enabling approaches?
- Identify three specific goals you have for yourself to improve your ability to use enabling approaches. For each goal, identify two to three strategies you could use to build on your strengths and address areas needing professional development.

Active Learning Activities

Group Activity #1: Enabling Paid Work With George

Preparation: Read Chapter Twenty
Time: 30 to 45 minutes
Instructions:

- Individually:
  - ✧ Read the case on George on pp. 507 and 508.
- In small groups:
  - ✧ Complete Enabling Audit #1: Enabling Paid Work With George on p. 508.

Discussion:

- Discuss the aspects of enabling that seemed easiest in this case.
- Discuss the aspects of enabling that seemed the most challenging.
- Discuss the enabling skills you would like to strengthen and identify possible strategies for doing this.

Group Activity #2: Enabling Community Change

Preparation: Read Chapter Twenty
Time: 30 to 45 minutes
Instructions:

- Individually:
  - ✧ Read the case on Sayed on pp. 509 and 510.
- In small groups:
  - ✧ Complete Enabling Audit #2: Sayed, the Occupational Therapist, Enabling Community Change on p. 509.

Discussion

- Discuss the aspects of enabling that seemed easiest in this case.
- Discuss the aspects of enabling that seemed the most challenging.
- Discuss the enabling skills you would like to strengthen and identify possible strategies for doing this.

Group Activity #3: Enabling Rehabilitation Following Stroke

Preparation: Read Chapter Twenty
Time: 30 to 45 minutes
Instructions:

- Individually:
  - ✧ Read the case on James on pp. 510 and 511.
- In small groups:
  - ✧ Complete Enabling Audit #3: James, the Occupational Therapist, Enabling Rehabilitation Following Stroke on p. 511.

Discussion:

- Discuss the aspects of enabling that seemed easiest in this case.
- Discuss the aspects of enabling that seemed the most challenging.
- Discuss the enabling skills you would like to strengthen, and identify possible strategies for doing this.

Chapter Twenty-One Objectives

The information in this chapter is intended to help the reader:

1. Understand that a profession is recognized and reimbursed for providing services to meet society's needs.
2. Recognize that most of the outcomes of concern to the profession today have not changed since occupational therapy was founded in 1917.
3. Discuss the difference in efficacy and effectiveness.
4. Relate occupational therapy outcomes to the World Health Organization's *International Classification of Function, Disability, and Health* (ICF).
5. Discuss the importance of role performance as an occupational therapy outcome.
6. Discuss the importance of identity and realization of self as an occupational therapy outcome.
7. Discuss life satisfaction as an occupational therapy outcome.
8. Discuss well-being and happiness as an occupational therapy outcome.
9. Discuss quality of life as an occupational therapy outcome.
10. Discuss meaning as an occupational therapy outcome.
11. Discuss participation as an occupational therapy outcome.
12. Describe why valid and reliable outcome measures are the therapist's tool in documenting the impact of occupational therapy intervention.

Key Words

identity: Participation and role performance are central to realization of self-hood and come largely through shaping the self through occupations (Christiansen, 1999).

life satisfaction: Being able to do what the person wants and needs to do. The central concepts are pursuing valued interests, meaningful experiences, and relationships consistent with one's life plan (Branholm, 1992; Lundmark, 1996; Neugarten, Havighurst, & Tobin, 1961).

meaning: Meaningful lives have an active life with opportunities for creative work, enjoyment with the experience of beauty, art and nature, and meaning. People are able to adapt when they perceive their world as comprehensible, manageable, and meaningful (Antonovsky, 1979; Frankl, 1984).

occupational role: Being able to carry out the occupations that are central to the person's role. Satisfaction with role performance (Kielhofner & Burke, 1980; Reilly, 1962).

participation: Extent to which individuals are engaged in a societal context (World Health Organization [WHO], 2001).

quality of life: Incorporates health, psychological state, level of independence, social relationships, and relationships with the environment (Group, 1994).

well-being (happiness): Having time, structure, and capacity to do what one wants to do. Physical and mental health and the person's perception of confidence and self-esteem (Christiansen, 1999; Wilcock, 1998).

> *Never doubt that a small group of thoughtful, committed citizens can change the world. Indeed, it is the only thing that ever has.*
> Margaret Mead

Chapter Twenty-One

Outcomes: The Results of Interventions in Occupational Therapy Practice

Carolyn M. Baum, PhD, OTR/L, FAOTA and Charles H. Christiansen, EdD, OTR, OT(C), FAOTA

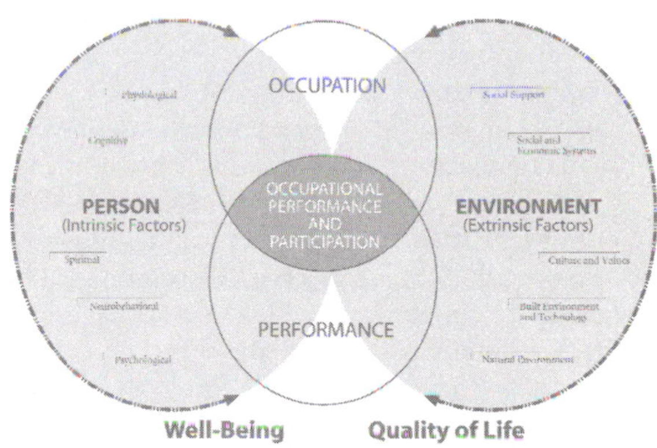

Setting the Stage

This chapter discusses the importance of using outcomes as the means to demonstrate that occupational therapy services meet society's needs. Role performance, identity, realization of self, life satisfaction, quality of life, well-being, happiness, meaning, and participation are the ideal outcomes of engagement in occupation. These outcome measures are increasingly important as we continue to gather evidence regarding the effectiveness and efficiency of our services.

Don't miss the companion Web site to *Occupational Therapy: Performance, Participation, and Well-Being, Third Edition.* Please visit us at http://www.cb3e.slackbooks.com.

Baum, C. M., & Christiansen, C. H. (2005). Outcomes: The results of interventions in occupational therapy practice. In C. H. Christiansen, C. M. Baum, and J. Bass-Haugen (Eds.), Occupational therapy: Performance, participation, and well-being *(3rd ed.). Thorofare, NJ: SLACK Incorporated.*

INTRODUCTION

For a profession to earn the respect of the people it serves, it must offer a service of demonstrable value. This means that the public must perceive that there is measurable benefit, result, or consequence for the services delivered. A profession must deliver what it says it will. Medicine has earned public support through, among other things, the provision of medical and surgical techniques that increase life expectancy, save lives, and reduce pain and suffering. These are outcomes, or results, that the public values and expects in exchange for its considerable support of organized medicine. Outcomes, then, are the deliverables or benefits that a profession brings to society.

All professions achieve their status by providing a service to society. Society will either accept or support that contribution with payment for services or will limit what professions can do by denying payment and the privileges to practice. In more recent times, accountability for results has increased. Regulatory bodies and financial authorities in the business and health sector and in local as well as national government are seeking to know the potential impact on interventions employed in health and social services. This interest has encouraged the use of outcomes focused on quality of life and other measures to assist in resource allocation and assessing the impact of policy decisions (Rogerson, 1995).

In this chapter, we explore the types of outcomes relevant to occupational therapy. We note that many of the outcomes of concern to the profession have not changed since occupational therapy was founded. The field remains dedicated to helping people achieve health, well-being, and a high quality of life. However, in directing their efforts toward these ultimate outcomes, therapy personnel may often set interim goals, which can also be viewed as outcomes.

Because of its broad scope of concerns about humans as occupational beings, occupational therapy personnel deliver services that range from helping children acquire the functional skills necessary for everyday living to helping older adults identify ways in which they can maintain their health and continue living in the community. With this range of concerns, the number of potential outcomes of interest is large. However, this broad scope does not reduce the importance of thinking carefully about how outcomes are identified, defined, measured, and demonstrated.

HOW DOES A PROFESSION DEMONSTRATE ITS OUTCOMES?

The words *efficacy* and *effectiveness* are often used as synonyms to describe the results of intervention demonstrated through research. Although they have slightly different meanings, they each refer to studies of outcome. Professions demonstrate the efficacy of their services through highly controlled clinical trials and the general effectiveness of their services through other types of outcome studies done under less controlled and more natural conditions. The idea in both instances is to objectively demonstrate whether or not an expected goal or result of intervention was achieved. Typically, the degree of confidence that one has in a given procedure or technique increases as the evidence accumulates in support of its effectiveness.

The public is interested in evidence that a procedure, treatment, or program of intervention provides the results or outcomes that were intended. The term *evidence-based practice* aptly describes the expectation that services delivered have been shown to result in expected outcomes (Law & Baum, 1998). The randomized clinical trial (RCT) is the "gold standard" for demonstrating efficacy. However, because of the difficulty and expense associated with conducting clinical trials, as well as ethical problems associated with denying potentially beneficial treatment to a control or comparison group, other types of evidence-related studies are often conducted. These effectiveness studies often have less stringent controls, and, as a result, the confidence that one may have in his or her findings is limited.

When several studies of this type, showing the same or similar results, have been completed, this adds to the level of confidence that one can have in the effectiveness of an intervention. The aggregate results of these types of studies (as well as RCTs) can be estimated using a technique called *meta-analysis*. A meta-analysis considers various characteristics of many studies by using statistical techniques to estimate the overall benefit of a particular type of intervention (Naylor, 1997).

PLACING OUTCOMES IN A HISTORICAL CONTEXT

As occupational therapy personnel consider the expected outcomes of their interventions, it is reassuring to find that many of the desired outcomes popular today in health care (such as participation, well-being, quality of life, life-satisfaction, and prevention) have been central to occupational therapy since its inception as an organized profession in the United States in 1917.

The earliest work of occupational therapists was focused primarily on individuals with mental illness (Bing, 1981). The interventions used in occupational therapy were designed to establish and reinforce personal habits and provide structure in the daily routines of individuals who were placed in institutions. The occupational therapists provided opportunities for experiences and practice in activities and tasks to build skills (this occurred at a time when drugs were not available to control behavior). Here, the expected outcomes were improvements in the client's daily habits and time use.

Eleanor Clarke Slagle, a distinguished practitioner of the period, emphasized the need for a balance between work and restorative activities. She also emphasized the need for graded activity and the use of the environment to support habits and occupations (Slagle, 1922). Other pioneers of the occupational therapy movement applied techniques to elicit natural interests and childhood occupations (such as care of self) to foster healthy development (Sellew, 1932; Whitter, 1923). The expected outcomes in these cases were well-being and the ability to care for one's self. The practical approach of using natural interests and opportunities for learning in these treatment programs was consistent with the emerging philosophy of pragmatism being advanced at the time by the American philosopher and educator John Dewey (Dewey, 1922).

The expectation that occupational therapy would lead to improved mental status and habits persisted well into the 1940s. For example, Dutton (1941) wrote of the importance of providing the patient with the activities to allow him or her to control attention and focus on productive thoughts. Stanley (1942) placed emphasis on establishing habits that would make the individual more aware of his or her environment and show interest in achievement. Here, the expected outcomes were improved attention and motivation.

Habits and mental function were not the only concerns of the occupational therapy workshops of the 1940s. With the emergence of physical therapy and physical medicine, there was a concurrent interest in how occupations could be used to improve a client's physical function. Licht and Reilly (1943) viewed occupational therapy as a treatment process to improve physical or functional performance. It should be noted that the outcomes for these clients during the early decades of occupational therapy were documented by observation of the patient's behavior. At the time, the availability of objective measures for these outcomes was limited.

Later, Ayres (1958) called attention to the importance of the treatment of physical disabilities through occupation. Purposeful function was used to achieve maximal rehabilitation. Ayres was convinced that because the human motor system evolved to permit purposeful motion, it was logical that purposeful activity would elicit the highest level of recovery of function for this system. Ayres was one of the first occupational therapists to engage in a program of research to demonstrate links between neuromotor components viewed as central to development and learning behaviors in children. This led to the emergence of sensory integration theory and a battery of tests that were used to identify deficits and measure function. Through her dedicated work, Ayres had identified maximum performance as a desired outcome of occupational therapy.

In 1968, Ainsley and colleagues (Ainsley et al., 1968) reported a program of occupational therapy services aimed at assisting older adults, people with mental retardation, criminals, and culturally deprived individuals with social adjustment. Their program focused on developing the skills to adjust to community life, and their desired outcome was community participation.

More recently, researchers at USC completed a study of occupational therapy with well elderly people living in the community. This study demonstrated that community-based services aimed at engaging clients in learning new occupations and lifestyle habits can improve health status and well-being. Table 21-1 highlights key statements that identify the importance of occupation. These can be directly translated into outcomes that practitioners can address today as they plan client-centered care for individuals, communities, and organizations.

Goals and Outcomes in Contemporary Occupational Therapy

The types of goals toward which occupational therapy personnel provide their expertise are as varied as the occupations of life. For a child, the goals may be to be able to engage in sports, to learn in a classroom, to be able to play with siblings, or to acquire the skills to be able to work when they are older. For an adult, the goals may be to return to work, to live safely in a community environment, to be able to care for a child, or to have the skills to support an important relationship. Older adults may want to be able to continue to work, to remain in their own homes, to be able to read to their grandchildren, or to go to a place of worship. Despite their variety, these goals have something in common. Each goal reflects an individual's desire to participate fully in society. Thus, it can be said that an important, perhaps universal outcome of occupational therapy services is to enable people to participate in society through engaging in the occupations that are meaningful and important to them.

An organization may want to reduce its absenteeism due to injury, help an employee return to work after an injury, or provide knowledge to employees on how to manage their aging parents. Communities may want to provide more services to enable older adults to remain in their own homes, design a new playground that will accommodate all children with and without disabilities, or plan new street signs that older adults will be able to use to navigate safely. Each of these goals can be support-

Table 21-1

Relationship of Historical Statements to Contemporary Outcomes

Historical Outcome	*Contemporary Outcome*
"Our conception of man is that of an organism that maintains and balances itself in the world of reality and actuality by being in active life and active use... It is the use that we make of ourselves that gives the ultimate stamp to our every organ" (Meyer, 1922, p. 640).	Health and participation
"A pleasure in achievement, a real pleasure in the use and activity of one's hands and muscles and a happy appreciation of time began to be used as incentives in the management of our patients" (Meyer, 1922, p. 640).	Satisfaction and achievement
Occupational therapy through the use of light manual occupations arouses interest and develops the initiative of men and women with handicapping or serious medical conditions (Hall, 1923).	Demonstration of initiative and participation
Occupational therapy uses objects to arouse interest, courage, and confidence to exercise mind and body in healthy activity to overcome disability and to re-establish capacity for industrial and social usefulness (American Occupational Therapy Association, 1923).	Health, work, and participation

Table 21-2

Descriptions of Occupations That Reflect Participation

- Occupation is the vehicle to acquire, maintain, or redevelop skills necessary to fulfill occupational roles and provides satisfaction to fulfill occupational roles and provide satisfaction (Fidler & Fidler, 1963).
- Occupation can contribute to a person's sense of well-being and state of health (Reed, 1999).
- Occupation can be used to help a person learn to organize his or her life and use resources to reduce the impact of disability (Reed, 1999).
- The lack of occupation leads to a breakdown in habits and physiological deterioration. This leads to loss of ability and competency to support daily life (Kielhofner, 1995).
- Individuals with cognitive loss who remain engaged in occupations retain higher levels of functional status and demonstrate fewer disturbing behaviors (Baum, 1995).
- Engagement in individually motivating and ongoing occupations supplies sustenance for survival and safety and enhanced health (Wilcock, 1993).
- Meaningful occupations provide individuals with exercise to maintain homeostasis, to keep body parts and neuronal physiology and mental capacities functioning at peak efficiency, and to enable maintenance and development of satisfying and stimulating social relationships (Wilcock, 1993).

ed by an occupational therapist using an occupational performance approach. In each case, the expected outcome is one of increased participation, brought about by increases in capacities or skills or the elimination of environmental barriers (Table 21-2).

Participation

Being able to go where you want to go and do what you want to do is central to personal freedom. Participation describes the extent to which a person is engaged in life situations in a societal context (WHO, 2001). The

International Classification of Function, Disability, and Health, known as ICF (2001), asks health professionals to measure participation across nine domains: 1) learning and applying knowledge, 2) general tasks and demands, 3) communication, 4) mobility, 5) self-care, 6) domestic life, 7) interpersonal interactions and relationships, 8) major life areas, and 9) community, social, and civic life.

While the concept of participation is not new to occupational therapists, the concept of participation as central to health care delivery has taken hold only in the past decade. In its report to the U.S. Congress, the National Medical Rehabilitation Research Center at the National Institutes of Health (National Center for Medical Rehabilitation Research [NCMRR], 1993) introduced the possibility that it is social limitation due to societal policy, attitudes, and actions, or lack of, that creates physical, social, or financial barriers to access health care, housing, and vocational/avocational opportunities (NCMRR, 1993).

In 1997, the Institute of Medicine developed the report *Enabling America: Assessing the Role of Rehabilitation Science and Engineering* (Brandt & Pope, 1997). This report introduced the Enabling-Disabling Process to describe the outcome of rehabilitation as both restoring the individual's function and employing environmental strategies to remove barriers that limit performance and participation. More recently, the WHO (2001) released the ICF. This model shifts the view of the indicators of health from one based on mortality rates of the populations to one focused on how people live with health conditions and how the individual can achieve a productive, fulfilling life. It introduces and defines the concept participation as an individual's involvement in life situations or occupations. Such reflect the individual's desire to participate fully in society, performing the occupations that are meaningful and important to them.

Participation enables other high-level outcomes, such as the creation of meaning, satisfactory role performance, life satisfaction, well-being (happiness), and the creation of meaning. Each of these outcomes is discussed briefly in the sections to follow.

Occupational Role Performance

Reilly (1962) first introduced the concept of occupational role to occupational therapy when she proposed a framework of occupational behavior. She emphasized that occupational therapy should help people achieve satisfaction in their occupational roles. This focus on occupational roles is related to the concept that, to be competent in daily life, the occupational therapist has to understand what daily activities are related to a patient's roles.

In the first description of the Model of Human Occupation, Kielhofner and Burke (1980) emphasized that social roles help organize daily life. Such roles are positions that individuals hold: worker, spouse, parent, friend, member, student, and scientist. Each social role carries obligations and expectations that influence actions and therefore help structure the daily lives of the people who occupy them. People with illness or injury whose role performance is compromised are clients in occupational therapy. Because performing their valued roles is important to them, satisfaction with role performance is often an important goal or outcome for occupational therapy intervention. Sadly, it is often overlooked, despite attention to it in the literature and the availability of role performance measures (Goodman, Sewell, Cooley, & Leavitt, 1993), some of which are specifically designed for use by occupational therapists (Good-Ellis & Spencer, 1985; Jackoway, Rogers, & Snow, 1987; Oakley, Kielhofner, Barris, & Richler, 1986).

Sue: A Case Study

Sue is a 49-year-old woman who loves her job as an administrative assistant to the president of a national church group. She plans to stay at her job until she retires because it is very satisfying to her and the work allows her to be involved with activities that are in balance with her values.

Sue is an independent woman who enjoys her roles as wife and mother. She and her husband share the activities that maintain their home and family. She loves to cook and entertains frequently. She organizes family events and plans social events with friends and family. She daily takes time for herself. Early morning walks are routine, as is reading the Bible, as it is important to her to keep a strong and growing relationship with the Lord.

Her leisure activities are with family and friends. She and her husband spend every Friday night during sports season at the local high school watching their youngest daughter cheer. This has been an activity for 10 consecutive years. She and her husband go to church and sing in the choir. Sue thrives on relationships and being with people she cares about and with people who care about her.

Sue might be your patient or client. What outcomes would be central to returning her to be able to fulfill her occupational roles? This description of Sue was abstracted from an assignment completed by first-year student

(continued)

Shauda Augsberger at Washington University in St. Louis, MO. The assignment required her to describe the occupational roles and occupations of an adult and then look at how the person's life would be altered if she was to have a severe crush injury to her dominate hand. Shauda identified many activities and roles that would be difficult. She ended her paper saying, "One does not think about the impact an accident would have on one's life until he or she goes through the person's day and realizes how many activities are dependent upon hand movement. Everything in Sue's life, her self-care, her activities in the home, her work, and her social activities with her family and friends would be interrupted. It will be my job as an OT to help people get back to what they need and want to do."

Identity and the Realization of Self

The areas of participation and role performance are critical elements in the creation and realization of self-hood. Existential philosophy proposes that throughout life, humans seek to answer questions about their existence: Who am I? What is the purpose of existence? Why am I here? What is the nature of reality? How shall I live my life? (Kaufmann, 1989). Christiansen (1999) and others (McAdams, 1992) have proposed that the realization of both meaning and identity come largely through self-construction or shaping the self through engagement in occupations. Both writers suggest that humans get their sense of self-hood from agency, or the reactions and changes they engender through participation in occupations that lead to creation, personal expression, and influencing others, particularly as these take place within an understandable life story.

Life Satisfaction

The concept of life satisfaction is very subjective because what is satisfying to one person is not necessarily satisfying to another. The concept reminds the occupational therapist of the importance of implementing a client-centered plan—helping the person do what he or she wants and needs to do. The concepts central to life satisfaction are pursuing valued interests, meaningful experiences, relationships, and a sense of comfort with one's life plan (Neugarten et al., 1961). Branholm and her colleagues (Branholm & Frolunde, 1998; Lundmark, 1996) have studied occupational roles and activity preferences as antecedents of life satisfaction. She describes satisfaction as based on the person's contentment in daily life. Branholm explains that the extent to which a person achieves his or her goals under different circumstances throughout life depends upon the person's abilities to adapt or to cope (Branholm, 1992). She identified eight life satisfaction domains that extend the concept of satisfaction to daily activities. The Life Satisfaction Checklist (Branholm, 1992) includes eight domains: 1) ability to manage self-care, 2) leisure situations, 3) vocational situation, 4) financial situation, 5) sexual life, 6) partnership relations, 7) family life, and 8) contacts with friends and acquaintances. Each of these domains is impacted by an injury or chronic condition, and each can be addressed as part of a client-centered plan to enable the client to do what he or she wants and needs to do.

Well-Being and Happiness

A concept closely related to life satisfaction is subjective well-being (SWB) or happiness. Much research has shown that SWB is explained by three factors: life satisfaction, negative affect or feelings, and positive affect or feelings (Diener et al., 1999). One of the foremost researchers in this area, Ed Diener of the University of Illinois, has developed a measure of happiness called the Satisfaction with Life Scale (SWLS). The SWLS was developed to assess satisfaction with people's lives as a whole and does not assess satisfaction with life domains such as health or finances, but allows subjects to integrate and weigh these domains in whatever way they choose. Research has consistently shown that economics and material goods do not predict happiness or SWB. Christiansen (1999) has studied the relationship between goal-directed occupations (called personal projects) and well-being. This research has shown that certain characteristics of a person's projects, such as their progress, structure, stressfulness, outcomes, importance, and time adequacy, help explain differences in well-being.

Another view holds that well-being includes the concepts of physical and mental health and includes the person's perception of confidence and self-esteem (Wilcock, 1993, 1998). Wilcock asserts that relationships, including friends, family, partnerships, neighbors, and strangers, as well as the availability of surroundings including home, school, place of worship, peace, and weather [and terrain] contribute to a person's perception of well-being.

Quality of Life

Well-being is also one of the concepts that contribute to an individual's perception of quality of life (QoL). The WHO defines QoL as an individual's perception of his or her position in life in the context of the culture and value

Table 21-3 WHO QoL Domains and Facets

Domain	*Facet*
Physical health	1 General health 2 Pain and discomfort 3 Energy and fatigue 4 Sexual activity 5 Sleep and rest
Psychological health	6 Positive affect 7 Sensory functions 8 Thinking, learning, memory, and concentration 9 Self-esteem 10 Body image and appearance 11 Negative affect
Level of independence	12 Mobility 13 Activities of daily living 14 Dependence on substances Medicinal substances Nonmedicinal substances 15 Communication capacity 16 Work capacity
Social relationships	17 Intimacy/loving relationships 18 Practical social support 19 Activities as provider/supporter
Environment	20 Physical safety and security 21 Home environment 22 Work satisfaction 23 Financial resources 24 Health and social care: accessibility and quality 25 Opportunities for acquiring new information and skills 26 Participation in and opportunities for recreation/leisure activities 27 Transport
Spiritual domain	28 Spirituality/religion/personal beliefs

systems in which he or she lives, and in relation to his or her goals, expectations, standards, and concerns. "It is a broad-ranging concept, incorporating in a complex way the person's physical health, psychological state, level of independence, social relationships, and his or her relationship to salient features of their environment" (Group, 1994, p. 43).

There are many measures of QoL described in the literature. Some focus on outcomes associated with specific disease states, and these instruments are often described as measuring health-related quality of life (HRQoL). The WHO has sponsored research on an international measure of quality of life called the WHO QoL (Group, 1998a). Efforts are being made to create an international scale that can be standardized across different populations and cultural groups (Group, 1998a, 1998b). The scale currently encompasses six domains and 28 facets, for which specific items have been developed. There are versions for younger and older adults being studied across 15 nations (Table 21-3).

The Creation of Meaning

Victor Frankl (1984), a psychologist who proposed the theory of logotherapy, suggested that all humans have a need to find meaning in existence and that this is an elementary driving force in who we become. Frankl observed that people can lead three types of meaningful lives: the active life, which affords the opportunity to realize values in creative work; the passive life of enjoyment, which allows the experience of beauty, art, and nature; and the life of moral excellence, which may impart meaning through suffering, as in the ascetic existence of some religious orders. It is easy to see the relationship between occupations and meeting the essential drive for meaning that Frankl described in his important psychological theory.

Another psychologist, Aaron Antonovsky, proposed a theory attempting to explain why some people adapt better to life's challenges and difficult circumstances than others. Antonovsky's salutogenic theory proposes that people are best able to adapt when they perceive that their world of existence is comprehensible, manageable, and meaningful (Antonovsky, 1979). Collectively, these three factors, which Antonovsky described as "the sense of coherence," are defined by what people do, how effectively they can do it, and what meanings they derive from their daily endeavors. The Sense of Coherence scale, which measures these factors, has consistently predicted well-being and other indicators of health in numerous studies (Antonovsky, 1993).

A related measure of personal meaning reported in the literature is the Life Regard Index (LRI) (Debats, 1998). This 28-item scale measures personal meaning from the standpoint of life structure (goals and purposes) and fulfillment. The scale has demonstrated impressive psychometric properties, and research has shown that it has evidence of conceptual validity (Debats, 1996). For example, it correlates significantly with measures of well-being, intimacy, commitment, happiness, and self-esteem (Debats & Wezeman, 1993). The scale has also been used as an outcome measure following psychological intervention, but there are no reports of its use following occupational therapy.

Another measure of personal meaning, the Personal Meaning Profile (PMP), has been reported by Wong (1998). This instrument hypothesizes the existence of eight domains that contribute to a meaningful life, including achievement, relationship, religion, self-transcendence (making a difference in the world), fulfillment, self-acceptance, intimacy, and fair treatment. The PMP, while still in its developmental stages, is designed for use in counseling and seems highly consistent with goal-setting and activity-related intervention strategies. The scale has satisfactory psychometric properties and has correlated with measures of physical and psychological well-being (Wong, 1989). No examples of its use as a measure of occupational therapy outcome have been reported in the literature.

Tristram Englehardt, a medical historian and philosopher, once observed the uniqueness of occupational therapy as a bridge between a patient's world of meaning and the scientific, technologically dominated world of medicine (Englehardt, 1977). He described therapists as "custodians of meaning" precisely because the field enables participation in the occupations of life through which people derive meaning. Clearly, life meaning is an important outcome of

Louise: A Case Study

Louise, age 66, married her high school sweetheart at 18 and worked to help him through college until they had their first of three children when she was 21. As her children grew older, she took evening classes at small colleges across the country as they moved frequently because of her husband's business. She eventually became a CPA, and at age 42 and with a concurrent move to southern California, she purchased her first of four tax business franchises. After a few years of business success, she sold 13 store locations and began her own private CPA firm at which she still works. Louise reports her most important occupations related to her involvement in the care and support of her children and 13 grandchildren. She expressed feelings of empowerment for her future because of the hard work, motivation, daily struggles, and success she has had.

Louise places a tremendous importance on her independence, the ability to enjoy the daily activities she chooses to engage in, and her involvement with her family and community relationships. She reports that she has found and cherished a great sense of quality and meaning in her life through the management of her everyday tasks and her business success. She also has planned for her retirement, having made good investments, and she now lives in the same neighborhood as her daughter. Her activities continue to be management of investments, cooking as a hobby, collecting artwork, reading for education and leisure, traveling to different parts of the world (including trips to Europe with her grandchildren), going out to dinner with family and friends, and serving as a volunteer with community organizations. Her family remains central. She visits those out of state frequently, attends the grandchildren's sports events, entertains family during the holidays, and enjoys her interactions and the intellectual stimulation of her children.

It is easy to see how Louise's everyday activities define her as a person. Should Louise need occupational therapy, it is essential that the therapist know about Louise and her activities as her recovery would be focused on these activities that bring meaning to her life.

therapy, and one that should continue to be studied and documented by practitioners and occupational scientists.

Defining Expectations for Evidence-Based Practice Outcomes

All health care professionals are expected to inform their clients about what results or outcomes they can expect from different intervention approaches and whether such approaches involve strategies to support recovery, remove barriers, educate consumers, or employ assistive technologies. This requires that the expected outcomes are made explicit to the client so that he or she can collaborate in the selection of approaches that are most likely to lead to the achievement of goals. Occupational therapy intervention should always be aimed at achieving improved occupational performance in occupations and tasks that the individual wants and needs to do.

When an occupational therapist interacts with clients, the clients have the right to know about the interventions that will be employed to help them meet their goals and the probability that the outcome will be achieved. This approach is becoming known as using an evidence-based approach to care. Evidence-based practice is about asking questions and "finding, appraising, and using contemporaneous research findings as the basis for clinical decisions" (Rosenberg & Donald, 1995, p. 1122).

Selecting Suitable Outcome Measures

In the earlier section on occupational therapy goals and outcomes, several outcome instruments were identified and described. However, the instruments listed were provided as examples. Any measure that can reliably and validly document change as a result of planned intervention can be a suitable measure of therapeutic outcome. Once occupational performance needs or issues have been identified, an appropriate assessment approach or instrument should be selected. Criteria for selection include theoretical consistency, clinical utility (which includes factors such as cost, time required for administration, training required for administration, and interpretation), and the reliability and validity of a measure. A reliable measure will yield consistent results over time and across therapists while also being sensitive to change in the performance of a client. A valid measure has face or content validity and yields findings that are intuitively sound, logical, and consistent with theory. Therapists are encouraged to consult test manuals and published reviews of measures to determine their suitability for use in measuring the attainment of specified client or program goals.

Summary

In this chapter, we have introduced the important concept of outcomes as a necessary and important way for occupational therapists to document the efficacy and effectiveness of their services, guide clinical decisions, and secure public trust and support. Many examples of occupational therapy outcomes were provided, ranging from improved sensorimotor and cognitive function to life satisfaction, well-being, and meaning. The ultimate goal of therapeutic effort, toward which targeted performance-oriented interventions contribute and through which grander outcomes are achieved, is participation.

Occupational therapists must target their interventions to help clients participate in daily life, enabling them to develop the skills or build the adaptive strategies to do what is necessary for them to carry out their occupation roles. By being able to carry out roles and do what they want and need to do, therapists contribute to the individual's sense of well-being, life satisfaction, and even life meaning.

There should be a bright future for a profession that uses its knowledge and skills to help people achieve their personal goals and improve the quality of their everyday lives. Educator and leader Mary Reilly wrote in 1962 that occupational therapy "readies an individual for action" (Reilly, 1962). Reilly also noted that occupational therapy would gain its professional credibility and acceptance only by offering the public services that were worthy of public support. Attention to the importance of documenting outcomes will enable occupational therapy to maintain its public acceptance and remain in its unique and important position of making a contribution to the health and quality of life of its clients, and collectively to society.

Danny: A Case Study

Let's look at the daily activities of Danny. Danny is a 9-year-old boy who has again moved to a new town with his mom and dad who move frequently because they are in the military. This interview was collected by Amanda McGee, a graduate student at Washington University, for an assignment in her Theory and Foundations class. "I was nervous to begin the interview because I really didn't know what a child his age would be capable of thinking. I assumed he would focus on the present, not even thinking that he would be able to comprehend the future. It didn't take long to discover the he liked his roles as a student, friend, family member, and game system player. He made it very clear to me that he would work when he was older stating, 'There is no other way to live.' Danny engages in a lot of daily activities. By himself, he takes out the trash and makes his bed. He also enjoys doing things with his parents like going to the store with his mom and to the barbershop with his dad. He also helps around the house with dishes and laundry. Danny does a lot of things by himself. He reads, draws, and enjoys creative writing. He is proud that he studies by himself and plays on his computer. He enjoys spectator sports, table games, and recreational shopping with others. He also likes to go to movies and watch movies on TV; he particularly likes action shows. His father is a musician and he likes to sing with him. Danny is an active child: he swims, runs, bicycles, plays tennis, and particularly likes to bowl. He is not comfortable with social activities. He does go to parties and family gatherings and enjoys visiting with friends and having friends to his home. Danny's five favorite activities are bowling, watching TV, playing his game system, bicycling, and playing on the computer. These and other activities define the occupations of a 9 year old. Danny's daily activities are done in his home, his school and community buildings, and in his neighborhood, none of which are difficult for him to navigate. Danny reported that he has made a new friend in his neighborhood and now he has somebody to do things with. What if Danny's friend had a mobility limitation or was homeless? Would the social, physical, and natural environment enable full participation of his or her activities? Certainly, the daily life of a child would be different if he or she could not access activities, play on a playground, enter a building, attend school, or engage in sports because of attitudinal, physical, or economic barriers that would limit participation. As the occupational therapist addresses the occupational performance of an individual, the community and organizational enablers and barriers must also be addressed in order to enable access to the activities necessary to support everyday life."

Evidence Worksheet

Author	*Year*	*Outcomes Achieved by Engagement in Occupation*	*Description of Terms*
World Health Organization	2001	Participation	Extent to which individuals are engaged in a societal context
Reilly Kielhofner & Burke	1962 1980	Occupational role	Being able to carry out the occupations that are central to the person's role Satisfaction with role performance
Christiansen	1999	Identity	Participation and role performance are central to realization of self-hood and come largely through shaping the self through occupations
Neugarten et al. Lundmark Branholm	1961 1996 1992	Life satisfaction	Being able to do what the person wants and needs to do The central concepts are pursuing valued interests, meaningful experiences, and relationships consistent with ones life plan
Christiansen Wilcock	1999 1998	Well-being (happiness)	Having time, structure, and capacity to do what one wants to do Physical and mental health and the person's perception of confidence and self-esteem

(continued)

Author	*Year*	*Outcomes Achieved by Engagement in Occupation*	*Description of Terms*
Group	1994	Quality of life	Incorporates health, psychological state, level of independence, social relationships, and relationships with the environment
Frankl Antonovsky	1984 1979	Meaning	Meaningful lives have an active life with opportunities for creative work, enjoyment with the experience of beauty, art and nature and meaning People are able to adapt when they perceive their world as comprehensible, manageable, and meaningful

REFERENCES

Ainsley, J., Barnes, S. S., Grove, E. A., Johnson, T, Koolman, C. A., & Stephens, F. (1968). On change. *American Journal of Occupational Therapy, 5*, 29-45.

American Occupational Therapy Association. (1923). *Principles of occupational therapy, Bulletin No. 4*. New York, NY: Author.

Antonovsky, A. (1979). *Health, stress, and coping: New perspectives on mental and physical well-being*. San Francisco, CA: Jossey-Bass.

Antonovsky, A. (1993). The structure and properties of the Sense of Coherence Scale. *Social Science & Medicine, 36*, 725-733.

Ayres, A. (1958). Basic concepts of clinical practice in physical disabilities. *American Journal of Occupational Therapy, 12*(6), 300-302, 311.

Baum, M. (1995). The contribution of occupation to function in persons with Alzheimer's disease. *Journal of Occupation Science: Australia, 2*(2), 59-67.

Bing, R. K. (1981). Occupational therapy revisited: A paraphrastic journey. *American Journal of Occupational Therapy, 35*, 499-518.

Brandt, E. N., & Pope, A. M. (1977). Executive summary. In E. N. Brandt & A. M. Pope (Eds.), *Enabling America: Assessing the role of rehabilitation science and engineering* (pp. 1-23). Washington DC: National Academy Press.

Branholm, I. F.-M., A. R. (1992). Occupational role preferences and life satisfaction. *Occupational Therapy Journal of Research, 12*(3), 159-171.

Branholm, I. F.-M., A. R., & Frolunde, A. (1998). Life satisfaction, sense of coherence and locus of control in occupational therapy students. *Scandinavian Journal of Occupational Therapy, 5*(1), 39-44.

Christiansen, C. H. (1999). Defining lives: Occupation as identity. An essay on competence, coherence and the creation of meaning. *American Journal of Occupational Therapy, 53*(6), 547-558.

Debats, D. (1996). Meaning in life: Clinical relevance and predictive power. *British Journal of Clinical Psychology, 35*, 503-516.

Debats, D. (1998). Measurement of personal meaning: The psychometric properties of the Life Regard Index. In P. F. PTP Wong (Ed.), *The human quest for meaning* (pp. 237-259). Mahwah, NJ: Lawrence Erlbaum.

Debats, D., & Wezeman, F. R. (1993). On the psychometric properties of the Life Regard Index: A measure of meaningful life. *Personality and Individual Differences, 14*, 337-345.

Dewey, J. (1922). *Human nature and conduct*. New York, NY: Henry Holt.

Diener, E., Suh, E. M., et al. (1999). Subjective well-being: Three decades of progress. *Psychological Bulletin, 125*(2), 276-302.

Dutton, W. R. (1941).The mechanisms of recovery by occupation. *Canadian Journal of Occupational Therapy, 8*, 42-46.

Englehardt, H. T. (1977). Defining occupational therapy: The meaning of therapy and the virtues of occupation. *American Journal of Occupational Therapy, 31*(10), 666-672.

Fidler, G. S., & Fidler, J. W. (1963). *Occupational therapy: A communication process in psychiatry*. New York, NY: MacMillan.

Frankl, V. (1984). *Man's search for meaning*. New York, NY: Washington Square Press.

Good-Ellis, M. F. S., & Spencer, J. H. (1985). Developing a role activity performance scale. *American Journal of Occupational Therapy, 41*(4), 232-241.

Goodman, S. H., Sewell, D. R., Cooley, E. L., & Leavitt, N. (1993). Assessing levels of adaptive functioning: The Role Functioning Scale. *Community Mental Health Journal, 29*(2), 119-131.

Group, T. W. (1994). The development of the World Health Organization Quality of Life Assessment Instrument (the WHOQoL). In *Quality of Life Assessment: International Perspectives*. Heidelberg: Springer-Verlag.

Group, T. W. (1998a). Development of the World Health Organization WHOQOL-BREF Quality of Life Assessment. *Psychological Medicine, 28*, 551-558.

Group, T. W. (1998b). The World Health Organization Quality of Life Assessment (WHOQOL): Development and general psychometric properties. *Social Science and Medicine, 46*, 1569-1585.

Hall, H. J. (1923). *OT: A new profession.* Concord, MA: Rumford Press.

Jackoway, I., Rogers, J., & Snow, T. (1987). Role change assessment. *Occupational Therapy Mental Health, 7*(1), 17-37.

Kaufmann, W. (1989). *Existentialism: From Dostoevsky to Sartre.* New York, NY: Penguin.

Kielhofner, G., & Burke, J. P. (1980). A model of human occupation. Part 1. Conceptual framework and content. *American Journal of Occupational Therapy, 34*, 572-581.

Kielhofner, G. W. (1995). *A model of human occupation: Theory and application.* Baltimore, MD: Williams & Wilkins.

Law, M., & Baum, C. (1998). Evidence-based occupational therapy. *Canadian Journal of Occupational Therapy, 65*(5), 131-135.

Licht, S., & Reilly, M. (1943). The correlation of physical and occupational therapy. *Occupational Therapy and Rehabilitation, 22*, 171-175.

Lundmark, P. B. I. (1996). Relationship between occupation and life satisfaction in people with multiple sclerosis. *Disability & Rehabilitation, 18*(9), 449-453.

McAdams, D. (1992). Unity and purpose in human lives: The emergence of identity as a life story. In R. A. Zuker (Ed.), *Personality structure in the life course* (pp. 323-376). New York, NY: Springer.

Meyer, A. (1922). The philosophy of occupational therapy. *American Journal of Occupational Therapy, 31*, 639-642.

Naylor, C. D. (1997). Meta-analysis and the meta-epidemiology of clinical research. *British Medical Journal, 315*, 617-619.

National Center for Medical Rehabilitation Research (NCMRR). (1993). Research Plan for the National Center for Medical Rehabilitation Research. (NIH Publication No. 93-3509). Washington DC: U.S. Government Printing Office.

Neugarten, B. L., Havighurst, R. J., & Tobin, S. S. (1961). The measurement of life satisfaction. *Journal of Gerontology, 16*(2), 134-143.

Oakley, F., Kielhofner, G., Barris, R., & Richler, R. K. (1986). The role checklist: Development and empirical assessment of reliability. *Occupational Therapy Journal of Research, 6*, 157-169.

Reed, K. S. S. N. (1999). *Concepts of occupational therapy.* Philadelphia, PA: Lippincott Williams & Wilkins.

Reilly, M. (1962). Occupational therapy can be one of the great ideas of 20th century medicine. *American Journal of Occupational Therapy, 16*, 300-308.

Rogerson, R. (1995). Environmental and health-related quality of life: Conceptual and methodological similarities. *Social Science and Medicine, 41*, 1373-1382.

Rosenberg, W., & Donald, A. (1995). Evidence-based medicine: An approach to clinical problem-solving. *British Medical Journal, 310*, 1122-1126.

Sellew, G. (1932). Occupational therapy for children. *Occupational Therapy and Rehabilitation, 11*, 379-381.

Slagle, E. C. (1922). Training aids for mental patients. *Archives of Occupational Therapy, 1*, 11-17.

Stanley, J. (1942). Habit training. *Occupational Therapy and Rehabilitation, 21*, 82-85.

Whitter, I. (1923). The modern hospital. *Occupational Therapy for Children, 21*, 330-334.

Wilcock, A. A. (1993). A theory of the human need for occupation. *Journal of Occupational Science: Australia, 1*(1), 17-24.

Wilcock, A. A. (1998). *An occupational perspective of health.* Thorofare, NJ: SLACK Incorporated.

Wong, T. (1998). Implicit theories of meaningful life and the development of the personal meaning profile. In P. F. P. T. P. Wong (Ed.), *The human quest for meaning* (pp. 111-140). Mahwah, NJ: Lawrence Erlbaum.

World Health Organization. (2001). Introduction to the ICIDH-2: The International Classification of Functioning and Disability. Retrieved June 23, 2004, from http://www.who.int/icidh/.

Chapter Twenty-One: Outcomes Reflections and Learning Activities

Julie Bass-Haugen, PhD, OTR/L, FAOTA

REFLECTIONS

You have come a long way on your journey to learn about occupational therapy from a framework of enabling participation and well-being. You now have a good foundation in both human occupation and occupational therapy.

This last chapter introduced various ways we can think about the outcomes of occupational therapy practice. It challenged us to look beyond the specific interventions we use and evaluate occupational therapy outcomes in terms of the real difference it makes in people's lives. The terms *participation*, *role performance*, *identity*, *realization of self*, *life satisfaction*, *well-being*, *happiness*, *quality of life*, and *meaning* provide us with a wonderful lens to examine the effect of occupational therapy services. All of these terms are trying to capture what we as humans mean by "the good life." The good life is what we want for ourselves and for the people we care about. We want to feel good about who we are, what we do, and how we fit in the larger society.

So, when an occupational therapy practitioner provides a service, how do we conceptualize the outcomes? What do we hope and envision the end result will be?

When occupational therapy interventions help children to be successful in the classroom, is the outcome the completion of class assignments during the school day? Or is the outcome the ability of the children to develop identities as motivated, bright, and capable?

When occupational therapy interventions help older adults organize their homes and their lives, is the outcome the ability to balance a checkbook? Or is the outcome the quality of life that is maintained by aging in place?

When occupational therapy interventions help workers prevent injuries, is the outcome the ability to do the job safely and effectively? Or is the outcome the ability to fully participate as a productive member of society?

When occupational therapy interventions help athletes who are disabled engage in a sport, is the outcome the ability to ski down a hill? Or is the outcome the sense of well-being and happiness that results from engaging in an occupation you really love?

Defining occupational therapy outcomes from the larger perspective helps us retain the energy and commitment that comes from knowing you really do make a difference in the world. Individuals and communities do benefit from your occupational perspective on life and your understanding of person and environment. As you provide occupational therapy services, remember that your work is important, as it enables occupational performance, participation, and well-being.

JOURNAL ACTIVITIES

1. Look up and write down a dictionary definition of outcomes. Highlight the component of the definition that is most related to the descriptions in Chapter Twenty-One.
2. Identify the most important new learning for you in this chapter.
3. Identify one question you have about Chapter Twenty-One.
4. Reflect on the types of services for which you would pay $50 an hour. $100 an hour? $200 an hour? How will you design your occupational therapy practice so it is perceived as valuable and essential by the recipients of your services? How will you design your occupational therapy practice so it is perceived as "worth every penny" by the recipients of your services? Think about these questions from the perspective of an individual client who has low income? A neighborhood organization who is trying to support elders in their homes? Other definitions of clients?

TECHNOLOGY/INTERNET LEARNING ACTIVITIES

1. Use a discussion database to share specific journal activities.
2. Use a good Internet search engine to find the Web site for the Canada Well-Being Measurement Act.
   - Enter the phrase "well-being Canada" in your search line.
   - Review the home page of the Web site.
   - What are the key points of this act?

- What are the limitations of using the GDP (Gross Domestic Product) to measure the health of a society?
- Are there other Web sites that address well-being and quality of life in public policy?

3. Use a good Internet search engine to find the Internet sites on outcomes of occupational therapy.
   - Enter the phrase "occupational therapy quality of life" in your search line.
   - Describe two to three Web sites on this topic.
   - Identify three to five occupational therapy resources on outcomes available on these Web sites.
   - Identify other words you could use to explore occupational therapy outcomes.
4. Use a good Internet search engine to find the Web site for the Canada Well-Being Measurement Act.
   - Enter the phrase "functional outcomes project" in your search line.
   - Describe two to three Internet sites on this topic.
   - How are functional outcomes related to occupational therapy outcomes as described in this chapter?
   - Identify three to five resources for learning more about outcomes related to occupational therapy.

Applied Learning Activities

Individual Learning Activity #1: Describing Outcomes for Case Studies

Instructions:

- Review the definitions of different occupational therapy outcomes provided in the chapter.
- Review the cases of Sue, Louise, and Danny provided in the chapter.
- Describe the current outcomes achieved by engagement in occupation for each case.
- Summarize the outcomes in the table.
- Summarize how you might feel as the person in each case.
- How might the outcomes of engagement in occupation change for each person if:
  - ✧ A family member with dementia moved in with the person?
  - ✧ The family had to declare bankruptcy and receive public assistance?
  - ✧ The person was in a terrible accident resulting in a traumatic brain injury or spinal cord injury?
  - ✧ The person was in an abusive relationship?
  - ✧ The family home was destroyed by fire?
- Identify the strategies that might be helpful in restoring the positive outcomes of engagement in occupation for each person.
- Identify other examples of things that would influence the outcomes of engagement in occupation (see chart on p. 537).

Outcomes achieved by Engagement in Occupation	*Sue*	*Louise*	*Danny*
Participation			
Occupational Role	Worker—loves her job Mother—attends daughter's events Homemaker—organizes, entertains, etc.		
Identity			
Life Satisfaction			Experiences—moving a lot, helping parents Interests—music, solitary activities, active activities Relationships—new friend, parents, etc.
Well-Being (Happiness)		Confidence—achieving work goals Structure—management of tasks Capacity—realizing educational goals, etc.	
Quality of Life			
Meaning			

Individual Learning Activity #2: Examining Life Satisfaction as an Outcome

Instructions:

- Review the section on life satisfaction in the chapter.
- Complete a self-assessment of your current status in each of the eight domains of life satisfaction (Branholm, 1992). Use a five-point rating scale with 5 being the absolute best and 1 being the absolute worst.
- Select two domains that you would like to work on to improve your life satisfaction. Write a personal goal for these two domains.

Domain	*Rating*	*Personal Goal*
Ability to manage self-care		
Leisure situations		
Vocational situation		
Financial situation		
Sexual life		
Partnership relations		
Family life		
Contacts with friend and acquaintances		

- Describe how you might use these domains in your occupational therapy practice.
- Critique the application of the domains for different periods of a person's life.

Individual Learning Activity #3: Examining Quality of Life as an Outcome

Instructions:

- Review the section on Quality of Life in the chapter.
- Complete a self-assessment of your current status in each of the WHO QoL domains and facets. Use a five-point rating scale with 5 being the absolute best and 1 being the absolute worst.
- Select two facets that you would like to work on to improve your life satisfaction. Write a personal goal for these two facets.

WHO QoL Domains and Facets

Domain	*Facet*	*Rating*	*Personal Goal*
Physical Health	1 General health		
	2 Pain and discomfort		
	3 Energy and fatigue		
	4 Sexual activity		
	5 Sleep and rest		
Psychological Health	6 Positive affect		
	7 Sensory functions		
	8 Thinking, learning, memory, and concentration		
	9 Self-esteem		
	10 Body image and appearance		
	11 Negative affect		
Level of Independence	12 Mobility		
	13 Activities of daily living		
	14 Dependence on substances		
	Medicinal substances		
	Nonmedicinal substances		
	15 Communication capacity		
	16 Work capacity		
Social Relationships	17 Intimacy/loving relationships		
	18 Practical social support		
	19 Activities as provider/supporter		
Environment	20 Physical safety and security		
	21 Home environment		
	22 Work satisfaction		
	23 Financial resources		
	24 Health and social care: accessibility and quality		
	25 Opportunities for acquiring new information and skills		
	26 Participation in and opportunities for recreation/leisure activities		
	27 Transport		
Spiritual Domain	28 Spirituality/religion/personal beliefs		

- Describe how you might use these domains in your occupational therapy practice.
- Critique the application of the domains for different periods of a person's life.

Active Learning Activities

Group Activity #1: Reflecting on Identity and Realization of Self

Preparation: Read Chapter Twenty-One, especially the section on identity and realization of self
Time: 45 minutes to 1 hour
Instructions:

- Individually:
  - ✧ Describe yourself by answering the following questions: Who am I? What is my purpose? Why am I here? How shall I live? Rather than writing an essay, answer the questions using short phrases or create an image to represent your answer to the question.
- In small groups:
  - ✧ Get in groups of three or four people.
  - ✧ Share your answers to the questions with other group members.

Discussion:

	Group Member #1 Name:	Group Member #2 Name:	Group Member #3 Name:	Group Member #4 Name:
Who am I?				
What is my purpose?				
Why am I here?				
How shall I live?				

- How does this activity support the idea that we are all unique in our view of self?
- How does this activity support the idea that there are similarities in people?

Group Activity #2: Reflecting on Identity and Realization of Self

Preparation: Read Chapter Twenty-One and reflect on your learning through this textbook
Time: 45 minutes to 1 hour
Instructions:

- Individually:
  - ✧ Answer the following questions:

    Identify three to five core beliefs and values you have about humans.

    Identify three to five core beliefs and values you have about human occupation.

    Identify three to five core beliefs or values you have about occupational therapy.

    Identify three to five core beliefs or values you have about outcomes of occupational therapy.
- In small groups:
  - ✧ Get in groups of three or four people.
  - ✧ Share your answers to the questions with other group members.

	Group Member #1 Name:	Group Member #2 Name:	Group Member #3 Name:	Group Member #4 Name:
Humans				
Human occupation				
Occupational therapy				
Outcomes of occupational therapy				

Discussion:

- How does this activity shape your personal philosophy of occupational therapy?
- What are your goals for learning more about human occupation and occupational therapy that are consistent with your beliefs and values?
- What are some learning activities you might use to continue building your knowledge and skill with regard to human occupation and occupational therapy?

Glossary

ability: Supports performance and engagement in activity and tasks, makes it possible to complete the tasks within time frame or to meet standards of performance.

action: Actions taken during a task may be a reflection of the individual's capabilities, skills, and experiences.

activity: Productive action required for development, maturation, and use of sensory, motor, social, psychological, and cognitive functions. Activity may be productive without yielding an object. It is also a valuable vehicle to acquire, maintain, or redevelop skills necessary to fulfill occupational roles and provide satisfaction.

activity analysis: Activity analysis is a process in which the practitioner determines the performance demands of the activity by determining the performance demands of the activity and breaking the activity down to components parts. This involves analyzing each task in terms of its contextual, temporal, psychological, social, cultural, and meaning dimensions.

activity limitations: Activity limitations occur because the activity is not adapted to accommodate a change in capability, and likewise, participation restrictions occur because the environment does not accommodate the loss of capability and limitations in activity.

activity synthesis: The process of modifying activities or the environment to better match the goals and the capabilities of the client with the environment in which performance is to occur.

affect: Emotions or feelings that are associated with evaluation of self.

affordance: Humans perceive possibilities based upon both the places and objects in the environment, and these influence meaning and action (Gibson, 1979).

agricultural age: The period of history when farming or crop production was the primary form of human work.

andragogy: The art and science of helping adults learn.

archetypal places: Propose the idea that space and furnishings should be designed to support the fundamental types of activities that people do in various built environments (Spivak, 1973).

arousal: The process through which environment influences our actions. Three groups of variables are associated with arousal. These include psychophysical characteristics such as noise or light, ecological events such as a storm or rough terrain, or situations (Berlyne, 1960).

attention: Ability to concentrate our perceptual experience on a selected portion of the available sensory information.

attentional focus: A term often used in motor tasks, relating to whether the focus of attention is internal (body alignment or movement) or external (environmental relationship or movement outcome).

attribution theory: Model of client education that focuses on the causal relationships a client attributes to events.

basic self-care (ADL): Personal activities such as eating, grooming, hygiene, and mobility that are necessary for maintenance of the self within the environment.

best practice assessment: The use of reliable and valid assessment strategies by occupational therapists to determine occupational performance issues from a client-centered perspective and to derive information to determine appropriate intervention.

biomedical rehabilitation: A team of rehabilitation professionals with recognized expertise, often headed by a physician, who collaborate to assess and diagnose functional problems of a patient, set goals and priorities, implement interventions to promote optimum functioning, assess progress, and discontinue services when an optimal level has been reached (Bakheit, 1995).

built environment: Physical environments can be built for accessibility, manageability, safety, aesthetics, comfort, and enjoyment. The suitability of the space to accommodate an individual's needs is central to physical or built environments. Built environments also include tools that support engagement in tasks and occupations. Tools that are usable within the person's capabilities are grouped under the category of assistive technology.

capitalism: An economic system based on a belief in private ownership of the means of production and distribution of goods and characterized by a free competitive market and profit as an incentive.

case study: A design from the qualitative paradigm consisting of a systematic description and analysis of a particular case or situation.

chromosomes: Microscopic structures inside the nucleus of the cells.

chronobiology: The study of the body's physiological clocks.

Civilian Conservation Corps: An agency created by the government during the Depression to create employment opportunities in the service of conservation projects to enhance and preserve the natural environment.

client-centered intervention plan: A plan that focuses on the individual's goals and has been constructed using a situational analysis that integrates evidence, the client's occupational history, and that what the client wants and needs to do to foster participation in family, work, and community life.

client-centered practice: Practice is focused on the needs expressed by the client; collaborative and partnership approaches used in enabling occupation with clients who may be individuals, groups, agencies, governments, corporations, or others; client-centered occupational therapists demonstrate respect for clients, involve clients in decision making, advocate with and for clients' needs, and otherwise recognize clients' experience and knowledge (Canadian Association of Occupational Therapists [CAOT], 2002).

client-centered rehabilitation: A therapeutic orientation whereby clients engage the assistance and support of a therapist to facilitate their problem solving and the achievement of their own goals. It is influenced by client-centered practice as a nondirective approach to therapy (Rogers, 1942).

clinical utility: The clinical usefulness of an assessment tool.

coaching: An enabling process to provide supportive comments, feedback, and input with the aim of enhancing physical or mental performance, insight, or growth in humans.

cognition: Mental processes that include thinking, perceiving, feeling, recognizing, remembering, problem solving, knowing, sensing, learning, judging, and metacognition.

cognitive rehabilitation: Systematic intervention, based on assessment, that may use the range of approaches from remedial to compensatory to address the variety of cognitive limitations experienced by a client.

collective agency: Operates through shared beliefs of efficacy, pooled understandings, group aspirations and incentive systems, and collective action (personal agency beliefs are not independent of, but rather formed through, a broad network of sociostructural influences) (Bandura, 2000).

community: A collective of people identified by common values and mutual concern for the development and well-being of their group or geographical area (Green & Kreuter, 1991, p. 504).

community-based practice: Provision of services in community settings where people live, play, and work.

community-based rehabilitation: A community development approach that uses the combined efforts of people with disabilities, families, and communities, and health, education, vocational, and social services for the purposes of rehabilitation, equalization of opportunities, and social integration of people with disabilities (International Labour Organization et al., 1994).

community capacity: "Combined assets that include a community's commitment, resources, and skills used to solve problems and strengthen the quality of life for its citizens" (2000 Joint Committee on Health Education and Promotion Terminology, 2001, p. 97).

community-centered interventions: Approach in which community members come together through partnerships and coalitions to identify common concerns and solve community problems.

community-level interventions: Population-based approaches that attempt to modify the sociocultural, political, economic, and environmental context of the community in order to achieve health goals.

community organization: "Process by which communities mobilize to identify common problems or goals, mobilize resources, and in other ways, develop and implement strategies for reaching the goals they have collectively set" (2000 Joint Committee on Health Education and Promotion Terminology, 2001, p. 97).

compensation/adaptation/modification: Interventions aimed at diminishing personal constraints or eliminating environmental barriers. **compensation:** Use of environmental supports to avert occupational performance problems associated with a personal performance constraint. **adaptation/modification:** Reducing environmental barriers by changing the existing environment or the features of the task in which the client will engage.

competence: The ability to interact effectively with the environment while maintaining individuality and growth. Achievement of skill equal to the demands of the environment.

competency: Occupational therapist needs to demonstrate the ability to understand the interaction among the person, occupation, and environment. Being able to influence occupational performance requires a thorough understanding of a person's capabilities, how identity is influenced by occupations, the way in which actions and tasks may be modified with technology, and how all the environmental influences create barriers and enablers for performance.

conspicuous consumption: Spending lavishly to impress others.

construct validity: The degree to which an assessment's findings fits with prior theoretical relationships among characteristics or individuals.

content validity: The comprehensiveness of an assessment tool; inclusion of all important aspects of the attribute that is being measured.

cultural environment: Culture refers to values, beliefs, customs, and behaviors that are transmitted from one generation to the next. Culture affects performance by prescribing norms for the use of time and space and influencing beliefs regarding the importance of activities, work, and play. It also influences choices in what people do, how they do it, and how important it is to them (Altman & Chelmers, 1984; Hall, 1973).

culture: Provides people with a set of values, assumptive beliefs, and implicit inferences about how the world operates that enable them to find meaning in and make sense of the events in their lives. "Culture provides the cognitive tools through which we understand and regulate behavior" (Cantor & Zirkel, 1990, p. 140).

declarative knowledge: Knowledge of information or facts that can be named and recited.

descriptive study: The collection and measurement of data to describe the characteristics of a variable of interest.

design: The particular approach used by a researcher to answer a question.

development: The process of growth and maturation occurring across the lifespan.

disability: The cause of disability has shifted from being viewed as a pathology that could be medically managed to one of an interaction between the characteristics of the individual and his or her impairments and the characteristics of the environment (Brandt & Pope, 1997).

disabling process: A misfit between a person's abilities and the environment in which they perform their daily activities.

educating: An enabling process to facilitate learning in others using a variety of methods in various sites and times. While educators may facilitate learning, learning may or may not actually occur.

ego-involved activity: Activity in which a person's self-esteem depends on attaining a specific level of performance (Ryan, 1982).

employment: Choosing a course of action with the context of a personal narrative.

enabler: An environmental feature or attribute that supports a person's ability to perform their daily activities.

enabling occupation: Enabling people to choose, organize, and perform those occupations they find useful and meaningful in their environment (CAOT, 2002).

encouraging: An enabling process of promoting hope through verbal support, compassion, practical help, advocacy, or the provision of resources to others.

environment: The external social and physical conditions or factors that have the potential to influence an individual.

environmental attributes: Aspects of the environment that can influence an individual's occupational performance in either a negative or positive way.

environmental press: Places influence behavior by creating demand or expectations for behavior (Barris, Kielhofner, Levine, & Neville, 1985; Lawton, 1980; Murray, Barrett, & Hamburger, 1938); demands placed on an individual by the environment.

epidemiology: Study of the distribution, frequencies, and determinants of disease, injury, and disability in human populations and the application of this study to the control of health in populations (Last, 2001; MacMahon & Trichopoulos, 1996).

errorless learning: A teaching technique in which individuals are not allowed to make errors during the acquisition of a skill.

ethnography: An approach to studying groups that involves gathering subjective information through interaction, observation, and direct participation with subjects.

evidence: The basis for your decisions; the knowledge on which to base your treatment.

evidence-based practice: Evidence based clinical practice (EBCP) is an approach to health care practice in which the clinician is aware of the evidence that bears on [his or] her clinical practice, and the strength of that evidence.

experimental study: A research design involving the random assignment of subjects to at least one group that receives an experimental intervention and one group, serving as a control, that does not, with the intention of comparing the results of the two groups to determine differences.

explicit learning: Knowledge of information or facts that can be identified, like declarative knowledge.

facilitating: An enabling process that involves people as active participants in collaborative decision making and action toward identified goals.

function: Reflects an individual's performance of activities, tasks, and roles during daily occupations (Baum & Edwards, 1995).

functional limitations: Restrictions or lack of ability to perform an action or activity in the manner or within the range considered normal that results from impairment or failure of an individual to return to the preexisting level or function. This is synonymous with occupational therapists' description of performance components.

generalization: Performing a variation of a task in a new environment.

genes: Individual units of hereditary material.

genetics: Subject concerned with variation and heredity in all living organisms.

genotype (i.e., DNA): The genetic constitution of an individual (Jewell & Abate, 2001).

grounded theory: A qualitative design involving multiple stages of data collection, where the researcher collects, codes, and analyzes observational and interview data until the data, being collected, become redundant and relevant categories and relationships are discovered.

guiding: An enabling process to offer directional clues to those who are seeking assistance in finding their way in thinking out an issue, deciding what to do, or developing an action plan. Those seeking assistance may or may not choose to follow the guidance of the enabler.

habit: A recurring, largely automatic pattern of time use within the context of daily occupations.

habits: Influence behavior in a semiautomatic way without need for conscious, deliberate action.

health: From an occupational perspective, health is a balance of physical, mental, and social well-being attained through socially valued and individually meaningful occupation, enhancement of capacities and opportunity to strive for individual potential, community cohesion and opportunity, and social integration, support, and justice, all within and as part of a sustainable ecology, beyond the absence of illness, but not necessarily beyond disability (Wilcock, 1998).

health belief model: Client education model based on the client's perception of susceptibility to the consequences of a disease or set of behaviors.

health promotion: Any planned combination of educational, political, regulatory, environmental, and organizational supports for actions and conditions of living conducive to the health of individuals, groups, or communities (Green & Kreuter, 1991).

health protection: "Any planned intervention or services designed to provide individuals and communities with resistance to health threats, often by modifying policy or the environment to decrease potentially harmful interactions" (2000 Joint Committee on Health Education and Promotion Terminology, 2001, p. 101).

health services: Interventions typically provided by organizations staffed with health care and medical professionals to improve access to quality health services by organizing and distributing resources more effectively.

human agency: People are naturally motivated to explore their world and demonstrate mastery within it. To do this, the person must effectively use the resources (personal, social, and material) available in his or her environment (Baum & Christiansen, 2005).

identity: Participation and role performance are central to realization of self-hood and come largely through shaping the self through occupations (Christiansen, 1999).

impairment: The loss and/or abnormality of mental, emotional, physiological, or anatomical structure or function; this term includes all losses or abnormalities, not just those attributable to the initial pathophysiology, and also includes pain as a limiting experience.

implicit learning: Procedural knowledge, such as routines and habits, as well as automatic behaviors and motor skills, such as force generation and the development of skilled movement.

incidence: Refers to the number of new cases of disease, injury, or disability within a specified time frame and measures how quickly a disease is spreading.

independent living: An approach based on self-help and peer support, research and service development, and referral and advocacy aimed to ensure people with disabilities access to resources and full participation in society, including housing, health care, transportation, employment, education, and mobility (Canadian Association of Independent Living Centres, 1989; Cole, 1979; DeJong, 1979; DeLoach, Wilkins, & Walker, 1983).

Industrial Revolution: The social and economic changes in Great Britain, Europe, and the United States that began in the second half of the 18th century and involved widespread adoption of industrial methods of production.

instrumental activities of daily living (IADL): Include telephone, food preparation, housekeeping, laundry, shopping, money management, use of transportation, and medication management as important occupations necessary for living independently in the community (Lawton, 1971).

inter-rater reliability: Consistency of measurement between assessors.

intervention: The skilled process of effecting change in the client's occupational performance (American Occupational Therapy Association, 2002).

intra-rater reliability: Consistency of measurement within one assessor.

intrinsic motivation: That aspect of motivation that is based in innate, organismic needs for competence and self-determination, even in the face of obstacles offered by the social environment (Deci & Ryan, 1985).

learning: The enduring ability of an individual to comprehend and/or competently respond to changes in information from the environment and/or from within the self. As one learns about the environment, alterations occur in the definition of the self and possible behaviors; as one learns about the self, alterations occur in the definition of the environment and possible behaviors.

leisure: That category of occupations for which freedom of choice and enjoyment seem to be the primary motives.

life satisfaction: Being able to do what the person wants and needs to do. The central concepts are pursuing valued interests, meaningful experiences, and relationships consistent with one's life plan (Branholm, 1992; Lundmark, 1996; Neugarten, Havighurst, & Tobin, 1961).

life-world: The subjective experiences of an individual within the context of his or her daily activities and relationships.

lifestyle: A distinctive pattern of living that is both observable and recognizable, and over which an individual has choice; defined by habits, routines, and occupational preferences to address personal needs and the demands of the environment (Elliott, 1993).

linear theories of development: View the developmental process as comprised of sequential stages, such as connecting the links in a chain.

listening: An enabling process that requires full attention to another person to hear his or her words, watch his or her body language, consider the meaning behind his or her words and actions, and be aware of what is being communicated but not stated in words.

locus of control: A psychological term referring to one's orientation to the world of events. Persons with an internal locus of control believe they can influence the outcome of events. Those with an external locus of control, conversely, believe that the outcome of events is largely a matter of fate or chance (i.e., that they cannot have influence over the outcome of events).

making the best fit: Matching the capabilities of the person/population with the environment and/or task that is the most enabling.

meaning: Meaningful lives have an active life with opportunities for creative work, enjoyment with the experience of beauty, art and nature, and meaning. People are able to adapt when they perceive their world as comprehensible, manageable, and meaningful (Antonovsky, 1979; Frankl, 1984).

mediate, enable, advocate: Roles that health professionals need to play to build healthy public policy, create supportive environments, strengthen community action, develop personal skills, and reorient health services.

medical genetics: The science of human biological variation as it relates to health and disease.

medieval period: The period in European history between antiquity and the Italian Renaissance, often considered to be between the end of the Roman Empire in the 5th century and the early 15th century.

mental well-being: A feeling of contentment associated with emotional, intellectual, and spiritual satisfaction enabling effective interaction with others and peace with self.

method: Processes through which data are collected and measured in a study.

motivation: Drive toward action.

motivational processes: Mediate the formation of decision; create the impulse or intention to act (Kuhl, 1985, 1986).

narrative: The personal story or account of an experience over time that provides a framework for understanding events.

natural environment: The natural environment includes geographical features such as terrain, hours of sunlight, climate, and air quality. The natural environment can be a significant factor in determining whether or not an individual's physical limitations are disabling (Brandt & Pope, 1997).

nature: Primitive state of existence, untouched and uninfluenced by civilization (Jewell & Abate, 2001).

nature versus nurture: An age old controversy about human development that questions the relative influences of genetics and environment in determining what people are like.

neurobehavioral factors: The sensory (olfactory, gustatory, visual, auditory, somatosensory, proprioceptive, and vestibular) and motor systems (somatic, cerebellum, basal ganglia network, and thalamic integration) that underlie all neuromotor performance (Baum & Christiansen, 2005).

neuroscience: Study of the nervous system structure, function, and development.

nurture: The sum of environmental influences acting upon an organism (Jewell & Abate, 2001).

obligatory activities: Refer to required activities, including self-care, employment, and sleep (Csikszentmihalyi & Larson, 1984).

occupation: Engagement in activities, tasks, and roles for the purpose of productive pursuit, maintaining one's self in the environment, and for purposes of relaxation, entertainment, creativity, and celebration; activities in which people are engaged to support their roles.

occupational balance: A regular mix of physical, mental, social, spiritual, and rest occupations that provide an overall feeling of well-being.

occupational choices: "Deliberate commitments to enter into an occupational role, acquire a new habit, or undertake a personal project" (Kielhofner, 1992, p. 192).

occupational delay: Atypical schedule of occupational development generally associated with developmental disabilities or at-risk populations.

occupational deprivation: Lack of occupational opportunities due to certain personal or environmental characteristics.

occupational disparities: Inequalities in occupational patterns due to different choices/values or unequal opportunities.

occupational disruption: A temporary condition of being restricted from participation in necessary or meaningful occupations.

occupational history: The individual's current roles, responsibilities, future roles, lifestyle issues, routines, and necessary and chosen occupations.

occupational imbalance: Patterns of occupations that do not meet unique needs, interests, and commitments (Wilcock, 1998).

occupational interruption: A change in occupational engagement or performance due to changes in personal or environmental factors.

occupational justice: The just and equitable distribution of power, resources, and opportunity so that all people are able to meet the needs of their occupational natures without compromising the common good.

occupational performance: Occupational performance is central to the development of occupational therapy models. It operates as a means of connecting the individual to roles and to the sociocultural environment (Reed & Sanderson, 1999).

occupational performance assessment: Evaluation of the performance and satisfaction of a person participating in everyday occupations.

occupational performance or function: "The point when the person, the environment, and the person's occupation intersect to support the tasks, activities, and roles that define that person as an individual" (Baum & Law, 1997, p. 281).

occupational perseverance: Perceived progress toward meeting an important or valued goal (Carlson, 1995, p. 145).

occupational profile: The term adopted by the American Occupational Therapy Association to reflect the occupational history.

occupational role: Being able to carry out the occupations that are central to the person's role. Satisfaction with role performance (Kielhofner & Burke, 1980; Reilly, 1962).

occupationologist: The person who studies occupation.

occupations: Goal-directed pursuits that typically extend over time, have meaning to the performer, and involve multiple tasks (Christiansen & Baum, 1997).

participation: Extent to which individuals are engaged in a societal context (World Health Organization [WHO], 2001); involves active engagement in daily life, in families, and in community.

performance: Performance is supported by a complex interaction of biological, psychological and social phenomena that requires a satisfactory match between person, task and situational characteristics (Engel, 1977; Meyer, 1922; Mosey, 1974; Reilly, 1962); ability to complete a task after practice or cueing, may or may not indicate that learning has occurred.

Person-Environment-Occupation-Performance Model: A model of occupational therapy practice that considers the individual, the situations or environments in which they find themselves, and their engagement in daily occupations with the objective of providing multiple options for client-centered intervention.

phenomenology: The study of events that happen as they are perceived.

phenotype: Emerges through the process of development and exposure to a variety of experiences; is a set of observable characteristics of an individual or group as determined by its genotype and environment (Jewell & Abate, 2001).

physical well-being: A feeling of bodily health and wellness.

physiological factors: Endurance, flexibility, movement, and strength are necessary requirements for occupations requiring moderate or sustained effort. People who are physically active are healthier and live longer than those who are sedentary (Minor, 1997).

physiology: Physical health and fitness factors that include endurance, flexibility, movement, and strength.

plasticity: Capable of being molded or shaped.

play: The primary occupation of childhood; also a term often used interchangeably with leisure to describe the nonwork activities of adults.

population at risk: Groups of individuals who are vulnerable to a disease or condition (McKenzie, Pinger, & Kotecki, 1999).

possible selves: "Cognitive manifestations of enduring goals, aspirations, motives, fears, and threats" (Markus & Nurius, 1986).

postindustrial age: The period following industrialism where service-oriented work rather than production of goods created most employment opportunity.

prevalence: Total number of cases of disease, injury, or disability that exist in a community at one point in time (Pickett & Hanlon, 1990).

prevent: Supporting occupational performance by anticipating problems and taking actions to avert problems that will impact occupational performance.

procedural knowledge: Knowledge about how to do something; the sequences, habits, and routines used to perform operations.

process memory: Reproducing or recalling what has been learned.

productivity: "Activities and tasks which are done to enable the person to provide support to the self, family and society through the production of goods and services" (CAOT, 1995, p. 141).

promote: Supporting occupational performance by focusing on enhancing well-being and quality of life.

prompting: An enabling process of reminding others through supportive comments, written notes, organizational clues, or the use of time-sensitive technology, such as clocks or computer prompts. Prompting could be to remind a person to perform in a particular way to avoid pain; to increase effectiveness; or to refine the efficiency, power, or quality of performance. Prompting could also be to encourage a person or organization to follow through on intentions or plans.

proxy agency: The efforts of intermediaries can contribute to a person's sense of self-efficacy (Bandura, 2000).

psychological: Personality traits, motivational influences, and internal processes used by an individuals to influence what they do and how events are interpreted to contribute to a sense of self.

psychology: Study of the behavior of individuals and their mental processes.

Puritan ethic: A belief in strict moral or religious principles with emphasis on the value of work and diminished respect for pleasurable activity.

purposeful activity: Actions that are goal directed.

pyramidal theories of development: View the developmental process as the formation of levels of function and capacity that support the later development of more sophisticated and elaborate behaviors and capacities.

qualitative paradigm: A tradition in research that emphasizes the collection of descriptive data.

quality of life: Incorporates health, psychological state, level of independence, social relationships, and relationships with the environment (Group, 1994).

quantitative paradigm: A tradition in research that emphasizes the collection, measurement, and objective analysis of observable phenomena.

reflecting: An enabling process of thinking to become more aware of one's self, of others, or of the surroundings for the purpose of contemplation or action.

remediation/restoration/establishment: Interventions aimed at enhancing personal performance capabilities and/or diminishing constraints. **remediation:** Correct the problem; **restoration:** Recover a skill that was lost; **establishment:** Attain a new skill.

resolve: Supporting occupational performance by identifying performance problems and taking action to correct them.

risk factors: Those lifestyle behaviors or environmental conditions that, on the basis of scientific evidence or theory, are thought to influence susceptibility to a specific health problem (Turnock, 2001).

ritual: A prescribed occupation that is intentional in nature and that typically holds special significance and meaning for those performing them.

roles: Positions in society having expected responsibilities and privileges (Christiansen & Baum, 1997).

role scripts: "Appreciative tendencies that allow one to comprehend social situations and expectations and to construct behavior that enacts a given role" (Kielhofner, 1992, p. 193).

routine: Habitual, repeatable, and predictable ways of acting.

routines: Provide an orderly structure for daily living that extends over time and pertains to a particular set of activities within a defined situation (Bond & Feathers, 1988).

routinization: A psychological disposition to rely on routines for everyday function.

scaffolding: A teaching technique in which a complex cognitive task is taught by breaking it down into a hierarchy of skills and building from the most basic to the complex.

self-concept: The way in which individuals perceive themselves.

self-determination theory: Theory of motivation by Edward Deci and Richard Ryan in which drives for competence, autonomy, and relatedness influence development and well-being.

self-efficacy: An estimate by an individual as to his or her ability to manage a situation; the likelihood of something occurring.

self-esteem: The relative value in which the individual holds the attributes that contribute to self-concept.

self-identity: The composite, unique view of self that a person works at shaping to establish acceptance in the social community.

self-maintenance: Occupations pursued to enable participation in the social world, related to personal care and existence in the community.

self-monitoring: A metacognitive skill that involves a self-assessment of behavior (e.g., the self-assessment of the effectiveness of problem-solving strategies or self-assessment of the safeness and correctness of performance).

situational analysis: A process that involves the collection of information and the analysis of factors intrinsic and extrinsic to the individual, the organization or the population to determine the occupational performance issues that will impact the ability to reach client-centered goals. The Situational Analysis will identify strengths, weaknesses, opportunities, and goals and will help the practitioner choose the appropriate evidenced-base intervention to help the client achieve his or her goals.

sleep: Obligatory and necessary for self-maintenance. Current theories suggest that sleep provides important restorative functions by repairing tissue, allowing for the consolidation of memory traces and information, and conserving energy (Horne, 1988; Meddis, 1983; Webb, 1983).

social cognitive theory: Analyzing behavior in terms of the person's characteristics, the behavior in question, and the intended context.

social ecology: Study of the effects of the physical and social environments on people.

social environment: Social support is an experienced rather than an observed phenomenon and is essential to maintain health. There are three types of social support that enable people to do what they need and want to do, These include practical support, informational support, and emotional support (Dunkel-Schetter & Bennett, 1990; McColl, 1997; Orth-Gomer, Rosengren, & Wilhelmsen, 1993; Pierce, Saroson, & Sarason, 1990; Thoits, 1997).

social support: The social relatedness and interactions with others that are perceived by the individual as supplying emotional, physical, and social resources.

social well-being: A feeling of contentment and freedom in interpersonal relationships enabling the development of ideas and action deemed of benefit to society. Also applicable to communities and societies at large.

societal environment: The standing of an individual within the group shapes behavior and attitudes toward self. Social rejection and isolation can have devastating psychological consequences. Societal policies govern the availability of resources that controls access to services and work (Christiansen, Baum, & Bass-Haugen, 2005).

societal limitations: When societal policy, attitudes, and actions (or lack of actions) create a physical, social, or financial barrier to access health care, housing, or vocational/avocational opportunities.

SOC theory: Theory by Baltes that views development as a process of responding to environmental demands in a way that optimizes gains and minimizes losses.

sociocultural: Involving both social and cultural factors.

specificity of learning: The condition of learning exactly what is taught, including environmental variables.

spiritual dimension: An individual's beliefs and practices that reflect significant connections with self, with others, with nature, and with a higher power or source of ultimate meaning.

spirituality: Everyday places, occupations, and interactions are filled with meaning that is interpreted by the person based on his or her goals, values, and experiences. Spirituality is socially and culturally influence but become internal to the individual through personal interpretation. As meanings contribute to personal understanding about self and one's place in the world they are described as spiritual. People develop a self-identity and serve a sense of fulfillment as they master and accomplish goals that have personal meaning (Christiansen, 1997).

stages of life: The idea that chronological development from birth to death is marked by distinct age periods with common developmental life tasks and concerns associated with the stage.

stakeholders: Those who are affected by an outcome or have an interest in an outcome in the occupational therapists terms this would be family, teachers, policy makers, elected officials, managers, etc.

structural memory: Memory store; short, long, sensory.

system of national accounts: An approach used to identify and account for the activities that contribute to the economy of a country.

tasks: Combinations of actions sharing a common purpose recognized by the performer (Christiansen & Baum, 1997).

task-involved activity: Activity characterized by engagement because a task is interesting, challenging, or has other inherent qualities (Ryan, 1982).

taxonomy: A method for organizing objects or events in nature.

temporal: Occupations across the lifespan in the context of time.

test-retest reliability: Consistency of measurement over time.

theory of reasoned action: Theory of client education that highlights the client's net attitude toward the proposed behavioral change.

threats to community health: Environmental, social, organizational, and political factors that interfere with the physical and mental health of individuals and families in a community.

time use diary: A structured approach for gathering information on how people use time.

top-down client-centered strategy: An occupational performance approach requires the practitioner to determine what the client perceives to be issues that are causing difficulty in occupations that support productivity, work, personal care, home maintenance, sleep, and recreation of leisure (Trombly, 1995; Mathiowetz & Bass-Haugen, 1994; Fisher, 1998).

transfer of learning: Performing a previously learned task in a new environment.

transtheoretical theory: Model of client education that frames the client's readiness for change into successive steps.

volitional processes: Control intentions and impulses so that an action is carried out; mediate the enactment of decisions to act and protect them (Kuhl, 1985, 1986).

volitional structure: "A stable pattern of dispositions and self-knowledge generated from and sustained by experience" (Kielhofner, Borell, Helfrich, & Nygard, 1995, p. 41).

volitional subsystem: "A system of dispositions and self-knowledge that predisposes and enables people to anticipate, choose, experience, and interpret occupational behavior" (Kielhofner, 1995, p. 30).

well-being: An individual perception of a state of happiness, physical and mental health, peace, confidence, and self-esteem that for many is associated with occupations, relationships, and environments.

well-being (happiness): Having time, structure, and capacity to do what one wants to do. Physical and mental health and the person's perception of confidence and self-esteem (Christiansen, 1999; Wilcock, 1998).

work: An activity required for subsistence.

work ethic: A belief in the moral value of hard work.

Work Progress Administration: An agency created during the Depression to provide work through commissioned projects in the arts and humanities.

References

2000 Joint Committee on Health Education and Promotion Terminology. (2001). Report of the 2000 joint committee on health education and promotion terminology. *American Journal of Health Education, 32*(2), 90-103.

Altman, I., & Chelmers, M. M. (1984). *Culture and environment.* New York: Cambridge University Press.

American Occupational Therapy Association. (2002). *Occupational therapy practice framework: Domain and process draft XVII.* Bethesda, MD: Author.

Antonovsky, A. (1979). *Health, stress, and coping: New perspectives on mental and physical well-being.* San Francisco, CA: Jossey-Bass.

Bakheit, A. M. O. (1995). Delivery of rehabilitation services: An integrated hospital-community approach. *Clinical Rehabilitation, 9,* 142-149.

Bandura, A. (2000). Social cognitive theory: An agentic perspective. *Annual Review of Psychology*. *52*, 1-26.

Barris, R., Kielhofner, G., Levine, R. E., & Neville, A. M. (1985). Occupation as interaction with the environment. In G. Kielhofner (Ed.), *A model of human occupation: Theory and application* (pp. 42-62). Baltimore: Williams & Wilkins.

Baum, C. M., & Christiansen, C. H. (2005). Person-environment-occupation-performance: A model for planning interventions for individuals, organizations, and populations. In C. H. Christiansen, C. M. Baum, & J. Bass-Haugen (Eds.), *Occupational therapy: Performance, participation, and well-being* (3rd ed.). Thorofare, NJ: SLACK Incorporated.

Baum, C. M., & Edwards, D. (1995). Position paper: Occupational performance: Occupational therapy's definition of function. *American Journal of Occupational Therapy*, *49*(10), 1019-1020.

Baum, C. M., & Law, M. (1997). Occupational therapy practice: Focusing on occupational performance. *American Journal of Occupational Therapy*, *51*, 277-288.

Berlyne, D. E. (1960). *Conflict, arousal and curiosity*. New York, NY: McGraw-Hill.

Bond, M. J., & Feathers, M. T. (1988). Some correlates of structure and purpose in the use of time. *Journal of Personality and Social Psychology*, *55*(2), 321-329.

Brandt, E. N. Jr., & Pope, A. M. (1997). *Enabling America. Assessing the role of rehabilitation science and engineers*. Washington, DC: National Academy Press.

Branholm, I. F.-M. (1992). Occupational role preferences and life satisfaction. *Occupational Therapy Journal of Research*, *12*(3), 159-171.

Canadian Association of Independent Living Centres. (1989). *Independent living promotion kit*. Ottawa, Canada: Author.

Canadian Association of Occupational Therapists. (1995). *Guidelines for client-centred practice of occupational therapy*. Toronto: Author.

Canadian Association of Occupational Therapists. (2002). *Enabling occupation: A Canadian occupational therapy perspective*. Ottawa, Ontario: Author.

Cantor, N., & Zirkel S. C. (1990). Personality cognition and purposive behavior. In L. A. Pervin (Ed.), *Handbook of personality: Theory and research*. New York, NY: The Guilford Press.

Carlson, M. (1995). The self perpetuation of occupations. In R. Z. F. Clark (Ed.), *Occupational Science: The emerging discipline* (pp. 143-158). Philadelphia: F. A. Davis.

Christiansen, C. H. (1997). Acknowledging a spiritual dimension in occupational therapy practice. *American Journal of Occupational Therapy*, *51*, 169-172.

Christiansen, C. H. (1999). Defining lives: Occupation as identity. An essay on competence, coherence and the creation of meaning. *American Journal of Occupational Therapy*, *53*(6), 547-558.

Christiansen, C., & Baum, C. M. (Eds.) (1997). *Occupational therapy: Enabling function and well-being* (2nd ed.). Thorofare, NJ: SLACK Incorporated.

Christiansen, C. H., Baum, C. M., & Bass-Haugen, J. (Eds.). (2005). *Occupational therapy: Performance, participation, and well-being* (3rd ed.). Thorofare, NJ: SLACK Incorporated.

Cole, J. A. (1979). What's new about independent living? *Archives of Physical Medicine and Rehabilitation*, *60*, 458-461.

Csikszentmihalyi, M., & Larson, R. (1984). *Being adolescent: Conflict and growth in the teenage years*. New York: Basic Books.

Deci, E. L., & Ryan, R. M. (1985). *Intrinsic motivation and self determination in human behavior*. New York, NY: Plenum.

DeJong, G. (1979). Independent living: From social movement to analytic paradigm. *Archives of Physical Medicine and Rehabilitation*, *60*, 435-446.

DeLoach, C. P., Wilkins, R. D., & Walker, G. W. (1983). *Independent living: Philosophy, process and services*. Baltimore, MD: University Park Press.

Dunkel-Schetter, C., & Bennett, T. L. (1990). Differentiating the cognitive and behavioral aspects of social support. In B. R. Sarason, I. G. Sarason, & G. R. Pierce (Eds.), *Social support: An interactional view* (pp 267-296). New York, NY: John Wiley & Sons, Inc.

Elliott, D. S. (1993). *Health enhancing and health compromising lifestyles*. New York: Oxford University Press.

Engel, G. (1977). The need for a new medical model: A challenge for biomedicine. *Science*, *196*, 129-136.

Fisher, A. G. (1998). Uniting practice and theory in an occupational framework: 1998 Eleanor Clarke Slagle Lecture. *American Journal of Occupational Therapy*, *52*, 509-521.

Frankl, V. (1984). *Man's search for meaning*. New York, NY: Washington Square Press.

Gage, M., & Polatajko, H. (1994). Enhancing occupational performance through an understanding of perceived self-efficacy. *American Journal of Occupational Therapy*, *48*(5), 452-462.

Gibson, J. J. (1979). *The ecological approach to visual perception*. Boston, MA: Houghton Mifflin Company.

Green, L. W., & Kreuter, M. W. (1991). *Health promotion planning: An educational and environmental approach* (2nd ed.). Mountainview, CA: Mayfield.

Group, T. W. (1994). The development of the World Health Organization Quality of Life Assessment Instrument (the WHOQoL). In *Quality of Life Assessment: International Perspectives*. Heidelberg: Springer-Verlag.

Hall, E. T. (1973). *The silent language*. Garden City, NJ: Anchor Books.

Horne, J. A. (1988). *Why we sleep. The functions of sleep in humans and other mammals*. Oxford: Oxford University Press.

International Labour Organization, United Nations Educational, Scientific and Cultural Organization, World Health Organization. (1994). *Community-based rehabilitation for and with people with disabilities*. Geneva, Switzerland: WHO.

Jewell, E. J., & Abate, F. (Eds.). (2001). *New Oxford American dictionary*. New York: Oxford University Press.

Kielhofner, G. (1992). *Conceptual foundations of occupational therapy* (2nd ed.). Philadelphia, PA: F. A. Davis.

Kielhofner, G. (1995). Internal organization of the human system for occupation. In G. Kielhofner (Ed.), *A model of human occupation: Theory and application* (2nd ed.). Baltimore, MD: Williams and Wilkins.

Kielhofner, G., Borell, L., Helfrich, C., & Nygard, L. (1995). Volitional subsystem. In G. Kielhofner (Ed.), *A model of human occupation: Theory and application* (2nd ed.). Baltimore, MD: Williams and Wilkins.

Kielhofner, G., & Burke, J. P. (1980). A model of human occupation. Part 1. Conceptual framework and content. *American Journal of Occupational Therapy, 34*, 572-581.

Kuhl, J. (1985). From cognition to behavior: Perspectives for future research on action control. In J. Kuhl & J. Beckmann (Eds.), *Action control: From cognition to behavior* (pp. 267-275). New York, NY: Springer-Verlag.

Kuhl, J. (1986). Motivational and information processing: A new look at decision making, dynamic change and action control. In R. M. Sorrentino & E. T. Higgins (Eds.), *Handbook of motivation and cognition* (pp. 404-434). New York, NY: Guilford Press.

Last, J. M. (Ed.). (2001). *A dictionary of epidemiology* (4th ed.). New York, NY: Oxford University Press.

Lawton, M. P. (1971). The functional assessment of elderly people. *Journal of the American Geriatric Society, 19*(6), 465-481.

Lawton, M. P. (1980). *Environment and aging*. Monterey, CA: Brooks-Cole.

Lundmark, P. B. I. (1996). Relationship between occupation and life satisfaction in people with multiple sclerosis. *Disability & Rehabilitation, 18*(9), 449-453.

MacMahon, B., & Trichopoulos, D. (1996). *Epidemiology principles and methods*. Boston, MA: Little, Brown.

Markus, H., & Nurius, P. (1986). Possible selves. *American Psychologist, 41*, 954-969.

Mathiowetz, V., & Bass-Haugen, J. B. (1994). Motor behavior research: Implications for therapeutic approaches to central nervous system dysfunction. *American Journal of Occupational Therapy, 48*(8), 733-745.

McColl, M. A. (1997). Social support and occupational therapy. In C. Christiansen & C. Baum (Eds.), *Occupational therapy: Enabling function and well-being* (2nd ed.). Thorofare, NJ: SLACK Incorporated.

McKenzie, J., Pinger, R., & Kotecki, J. (1999). *An introduction to community health* (3rd ed.). Boston, MA: Jones and Bartlett.

Meddis, R. (1983). *The evolution of sleep. Theories in modern sleep research. Sleep mechanisms and functions in humans and animals-an evolutionary perspective*. Wokingham, England: Van Nostrand-Reinhold; 57-106.

Meyer, A. (1922). The philosophy of occupation therapy. *Archives of Occupational Therapy, 1*(1), 1-10.

Minor, M. A. (1997). Promoting health and physical fitness. In C. Christiansen & C. Baum (Eds.), *Occupational therapy: Enabling function and well being* (2nd ed.). Thorofare, NJ: SLACK Incorporated.

Mosey, A. C. (1974). An alternative: The biopsychosocial model. *American Journal of Occupational Therapy, 28*(3), 137-140.

Murray, H. A., Barrett, W. G., & Hamburger, E. (1938). *Explorations in personality*. New York, NY: Oxford University Press.

Neugarten, B. L., Havighurst, R. J., & Tobin, S. S. (1961). The measurement of life satisfaction. *Journal of Gerontology, 16*(2), 134-143.

Orth-Gomer, K., Rosengren, A., & Wilhelmsen, L. (1993). Lack of social support and incidence of coronary heart disease in middle-aged Swedish men. *Psychosomatic Medicine, 55*(1), 37-43.

Pickett, G., & Hanlon, J. J. (1990). *Public health: Administration and practice*. Bethesda, MD: American Occupational Therapy Association.

Pierce, G. R., Sarason, I. G., & Sarason, B. R. (1990). General and relationship-based perceptions of social support: Are two constructs better than one? *Journal of Personality and Social Psychology, 612*(6), 1028-1039.

Reed KL & Sanderson S (1999) Concepts of occupational therapy. 4th ed. Williams and Wilkins.

Reilly, M. (1962). Occupational therapy can be one of the great ideas of 20th century medicine. *American Journal of Occupational Therapy, 16*, 300-308.

Rogers, C. (1942). *Counselling and psychotherapy: Newer concepts in practice*. Boston, MA: Houghton-Mifflin Co.

Ryan, R. M. (1982). Control and information in the intrapersonal sphere: An extension of cognitive evaluation theory. *Journal of Personality and Social Psychology, 43*, 450-461.

Spivak, M. (1973). Archetypal place. *The Architectural Forum, 140*, 44-49.

Thoits, P. A. (1997). Stress, coping, and social support process: Where are we? What next? *Journal of Health and Social Behavior*, Spec No., 53-79.

Trombly, C. A. (1995). Occupation: Purposefulness and meaningfulness and therapeutic mechanisms. *American Journal of Occupational Therapy*, 49, 960-972.

Turnock, B. J. (2001). *Public health: what it is and how it works*. Gaithersburg, MD: Aspen Publishers, Inc.

Webb, W. B. (1983). Theories in modern sleep research. Sleep mechanisms and functions in humans and animals-an evolutionary perspective. A. Mayes. Wokingham, England, Van Nostrand-Reinhold: 1-17.

Wilcock, A. A. (1998). *An occupational perspective of health*. Thorofare, NJ: SLACK Incorporated.

World Health Organization. (2001). Introduction to the ICIDH-2: The International Classification of Functioning and Disability. Retrieved June 23, 2004, from http://www.who.int/icidh/.

Appendix A

Comparing the Languages of: * the ICF, * the PEOP Model, * the AOTA *Practice Framework*

Charles H. Christiansen, EdD, OTR, OT(C), FAOTA; Carolyn M. Baum, PhD, OTR/L, FAOTA; and Julie Bass-Haugen, PhD, OTR/L, FAOTA

Christiansen, C. H., Baum, C. M., & Bass-Haugen, J. (2005). Comparing the languages of: the ICF, the PEOP Model, and the AOTA practice framework. *In C. H. Christiansen, C. M. Baum, and J. Bass-Haugen (Eds.),* Occupational therapy: Performance, participation, and well-being *(3rd ed.). Thorofare, NJ: SLACK Incorporated.*

Key Concepts	*ICF*	*PEOP Model*	*AOTA Practice Framework*
Occupational Performance (OP)	--------------	OP is the doing of occupations resulting from the complex interactions between the person and the environments in which he or she carries out actions, tasks and roles (occupations) that are important and meaningful	OP is the ability to carry our activities of daily life... the accomplishment of the selected activity or occupation resulting from the dynamic transaction among the client, the context, and the activity (Adapted from Law et al., 1996)
Occupation	----------------	Occupations are what we do. They provide the basis for feelings about ourselves. They engage us in the world around us, and in so doing, enable us to survive and maintain ourselves. They develop our abilities and skills, allow us to pursue our interests, relate with other people, and express our values	Activities of every day life, named, organized, and given value and meaning by individuals and a culture. Is everything people do to occupy themselves, including looking after themselves, enjoying life, and contributing to the social and economic fabric of their communities
Role	* See Participation	Positions in society with expected responsibilities and privileges	A set of behaviors that have some socially agreed upon function and for which there is an accepted code of norms (Christiansen & Baum, 1997)
Task	* See Activity	Sets of activities determined as purposeful by the person	
Action	--------------	A basic unit consisting of behaviors directed toward the performance of a task	--------------

(continued)

Key Concepts	*ICF*	*PEOP Model*	*AOTA Practice Framework*
Activity	The execution of a task or action by an individual Activities and Participation— Chapter 1. Learning and Applying Knowledge Chapter 2. General Tasks and Demands Chapter 3. Communication Chapter 4. Mobility Chapter 5. Self-Care Chapter 6. Domestic Life Chapter 7. Interpersonal Interactions and Relationships Chapter 8. Major Life Areas Chapter 9. Community, Social, and Civic Life	A productive action required for development, maturation, and use of sensory, motor, psychological, and cognitive function. A valuable vehicle to acquire, maintain, or redevelop skills	A class of human actions that are goal directed
Participation	Involvement in a life situation Activities and Participation— Chapter 1. Learning and Applying Knowledge Chapter 2. General Tasks and Demands Chapter 3. Communication Chapter 4. Mobility Chapter 5. Self-Care Chapter 6. Domestic Life Chapter 7. Interpersonal Interactions and Relationships Chapter 8. Major Life Areas Chapter 9. Community, Social, and Civic Life	Participation involves active engagement in daily life, in families, in work, and in communities. Participation may be denied because physical, attitudinal, social, or societal barriers limit an individual's ability to engage in the occupations that are necessary and meaningful	Involvement in a life situation
Person	An individual as defined by different domains including what a person does do or can do. Creates a profile of an individual, functioning, and health in various domains	An individual's characteristics, including physiological, cognitive, psychological, neurobehavioral, and spiritual that can either support capacities or limit the person's engagement in occupations	A client

(continued)

Key Concepts	*ICF*	*PEOP Model*	*AOTA Practice Framework*
Psychological	Body Function— Chapter 1. Mental Functions Activities and Participation— Chapter 3. Communication Chapter 7. Interpersonal Interactions and Relationships	Personality traits, motivational influences, and internal processes used by an individual to influence what they do, how these events are interpreted, and how they contribute to a sense of self	* See ICF, also Process Skills Communication/ Interaction Skills
Cognitive	Body Function— Chapter 1. Mental Functions Activities and Participation— Chapter 1. Learning and Applying Knowledge Chapter 2. General Tasks and Demands Chapter 3. Communication	Mechanisms of language comprehension and production, pattern recognition, task organization, reasoning, attention, and memory (Duchek, 1991)	*See ICF, also Process Skills Communication/ Interaction Skills
Spirituality	* See Activity and Participation— Chapter 9. Community, Social, and Civic Life	Meanings that contribute to a greater sense of personal understanding about the self and one's place in the world	* See Environment—Spiritual
Neurobehavioral	* See Body Functions— Chapter 2. Sensory Functions and Pain Chapter 7. Neuromusculoskeletal and Movement-Related Functions * See Body Structures— Chapter 1. Structure of the Nervous System Chapter 2. Eye, Ear, and Related Structures Chapter 7. Structures Related to Movement Activities and Participation— Chapter 4. Mobility	Sensory and motor factors that support performance. Includes ability to control movement, modulate sensory input, coordinate and integrate sensory information, compensate for sensorimotor deficits, and modify neural structures through behavior	*See ICF, also Motor Skills.

(continued)

Key Concepts	*ICF*	*PEOP Model*	*AOTA Practice Framework*
Physiological	* See Body Functions— Chapter 4. Functions of the Cardiovascular, Hematological, Immunological, and Respiratory Systems Chapter 7. Neuromusculoskeletal and Movement-Related Functions * See Body Structures— Chapter 4. Structures of the Cardiovascular, Hematological, Immunological, and Respiratory Systems Activities and Participation— Chapter 4. Mobility	Physical health and fitness factors. Includes abilities such as endurance, flexibility, movement, and strength	*See ICF, also Motor Skills.
Personal Factors	Particular background of an individual's life and living. Comprised of features of the individual that are not a part of a health condition or health status. Factors include gender, race, age, other health conditions, fitness, lifestyle, habits, upbringing, coping styles, social background, education, profession, past and current experience, behavioral patterns, character style, psychological assets, or any other characteristic which may play a role in disability at any level	Factors include gender, race, age, background, education, profession, and any other factor that indicates genetics or choice that influences the person's occupational performance	Features of the individual that are not part of a health condition or health status
Body Functions	Physiological functions of body systems (including psychological functions). Includes functions of mental, sensory and pain, voice and speech, cardiovascular, hematological, immunological and respiratory, digestive, metabolic, endocrine, genitourinary, reproductive, neuromusculoskeletal, movement-related, skin, and related structures	*See Person Intrinsic Factors	* See ICF

(continued)

Key Concepts	*ICF*	*PEOP Model*	*AOTA Practice Framework*
Body Structures	Anatomical parts of the body such as organs, limbs and their components. Includes structures of nervous system, eye, ear and related structures, voice and speech, cardiovascular, immunological, respiratory, digestive, metabolic, endocrine, genitourinary, reproductive, movement, skin, and related structures	* See Person Intrinsic Factors	* See ICF
Environment	Physical, social, and attitudinal environment in which people live and conduct their lives	Extrinsic factors that have the potential to enable or create barriers for the occupational performance of individuals, including social support mechanisms, social policies and attitudes, cultural norms and values, built environment/geography	* See Context
Context	Represents the complete background of an individual's life and living. Includes two components: environmental factors and personal factors, which may have an impact on the individual with a health condition and that individual's health and health-related states	* See Environment	Interrelated conditions within and surrounding the client that influence performance. Includes cultural, physical, social, person, spiritual, temporal, and virtual
Social Support Mechanisms	Environmental Factors—Chapter 3. Support and Relationships Activities and Participation— Chapter 9. Community, Social, and Civic Life	Practical, informational, and emotional supports that are central to the idea of community and supportive of occupational performance	Availability and expectations of significant individuals... and larger social groups that are influential in establishing norms, role expectations, and social routines

(continued)

Key Concepts	*ICF*	*PEOP Model*	*AOTA Practice Framework*
Social Policies and Attitudes	Environmental Factors— Chapter 4. Attitudes Chapter 5. Services, Systems, and Policies Activities and Participation— Chapter 8. Major Life Areas Chapter 9. Community, Social, and Civic Life	Laws, policies, or attitudes that enable or create barriers and support or limit individual's full participation in society. These may include economic or social conditions that alter people's behaviors	
Cultural Norms and Values	Environmental Factors— Chapter 4. Attitudes	Values, beliefs, customs, and behaviors that are passed on from one generation to the next	Customs, beliefs, activity patterns, behavior standards, and expectations accepted by the society of which the individual is a member Includes political aspects... and opportunities for education, employment, and economic support
Built Environment/ Geography	Animate and inanimate elements of the natural or physical environment and components of that environment that have been modified by people, as well as characteristics of human populations within that environment	Physical properties and geographical features, including physical modifications, adaptive equipment, terrain, weather, and light conditions	* See Physical
Physical	* See Built Environment/ Geography	* See Built Environment/ Geography	Nonhuman aspects of contexts
Spiritual	* See Activity and Participation— Chapter 9. Community, Social, and Civic Life	Social and cultural influences that have become internal to the individual, providing personal meaning	The fundamental orientation of a person's life; that which inspires and motivates that individual
Temporal	----	Occupation across the lifespan	Location of occupational performance in time (Neistadt & Crepeau, 1998)
Virtual	----	----	Environment in which communication occurs by means of airways or computers and an absence of physical contact

References

American Occupational Therapy Association. (2002). The occupational therapy practice framework. Bethesda, MD: The American Occupational Therapy Association.

Christiansen, C., & Baum, C. M. (Eds.) (1997). *Occupational therapy: Enabling function and well-being* (2nd ed.). Thorofare, NJ: SLACK Incorporated.

Duchek, J. (1991). Cognitive dimensions of performance. In C. Christiansen & C. Baum (Eds.), *Occupational therapy: Overcoming performance deficits* (pp. 284-303). Thorofare, NJ: SLACK Incorporated.

Law, M., Cooper, B., Strong, S., Stewart, S., Rigby, P., & Letts, L. (1996). The person-environment-occupational model: A transactive approach to occupational performance. *Canadian Journal of Occupational Therapy, 63*, 9-23.

Neistadt & E. B. Crepeau (Eds.), *Willard and Spackman's occupational therapy* (9th ed., pp. 13-21). Philadelphia, PA: Lippincott.

World Health Organization. (2001). *International Classification of Functioning, Disability and Health (ICF)*. Geneva, Switzerland: World Health Organization.

* This material is adapted from the models listed in the table.

Appendix B

An Annotated History of the Concepts Used in Occupational Therapy

Kathlyn L. Reed, PhD, OTR, MLIS, AHIP

Introduction

As occupational therapy moves into its second century, reflection and analysis of what has gone before is one strategy for looking into the future. Occupational therapy was organized around ideas and applications that served the context of clients and practitioners at the time they were developed. Changes in ideas and applications occur as the context for practice has changed. Some of the original ideas and some of the changes may be useful in the future. The question is which ideas and how can they be evaluated? One approach is to examine the concepts.

Why Concepts Are Important

In scientific theories, ideas are called concepts and occasionally constructs (Kerlinger, 1986, p. 26). Concepts are words or phrases used to label similarities between phenomena (Mosey, 1981, p. 32). Concepts are used to organize and synthesize thinking processes. Kim (1983) suggests concepts serve six functions, which are summarized in Table B-1. The most important functions are the naming and framing of ideas and the definitions or descriptions that explain the parameters of the concept.

A distinction should be made between concept and term. A term is "a word or group of words designating something;" in other words a name or label (Barnes & Noble, 1995, p. 1958). A term becomes a concept when characteristics, particulars, or elements are added to form an idea or notion. Sometimes a writer is using a word as a term and other times the writer is trying to convey a concept. Thus, in this chapter the word *term* appears when it is unclear to the author whether a concept is really intended or when both term and concept may be implied.

Organizing Concepts

The organization of concepts clarifies communication of thought by encouraging the sharing of ideas that may facilitate elaboration and refinement (Rodgers & Knafl, 2000). Thus, concepts shape a profession's point of focus. Every profession needs to examine, clarify, and establish the boundaries of what constitutes its field of study and domain of concern. For occupational therapy, occupation is the field of study and occupational therapy is the application of that study. Concepts can also clarify the difference between the state of being (end result or product) and the state of action or becoming (process). Occupation may be described as a product (task or role), but occupational therapy is primarily concerned with the process of performing (doing) occupation(s). In addition, concepts can describe the thing pictured (entity) or a family of resemblances. In other words, a concept can apply to a single occupation such as getting dressed or to a group of occupations such as activities of daily living.

Furthermore, concepts are a key element in constructing and understanding models and theories. Concepts act as the construction units or scaffolding of a model or theory. To know and articulate the concepts is to understand in principle what the model or theory is about. For example, if a person understands the concepts of volition, habituation, and mind-brain-body performance, that person has a grasp of the important ideas expressed in the Model of Human Performance (Kielhofner, 1985). In addition, in a practice (applied) discipline, concepts become the basic units for the development and application of assessment instruments.

Reed, K. L. (2005). An annotated history of the concepts used in occupational therapy. In C. H. Christiansen, C. M. Baum, and J. Bass-Haugen (Eds.), Occupational therapy: Performance, participation, and well-being *(3rd ed.). Thorofare, NJ: SLACK Incorporated.*

Table B-1

Functions of Concepts

- Facilitate the process of thinking about ideas by permitting the naming, labeling, and framing of things, events, events, and realities
- Are best explained as definitions or descriptions
- Can express symbolic constructs of real world phenomena (e.g., spirituality expresses an idea that has no specific physical structure and may represent several cognitive meanings)
- May refer to a single, unique case or entity or to a class of phenomena (e.g., a person can speak about what is a purposeful activity to one individual or speak about purposeful activity as it relates to all media used in occupational therapy)
- Can reference concrete or abstract phenomena using the same criteria (e.g., the same rules can be applied to discussing a concrete concept such as eating as to an abstract concept such as wellness)
- May be developed and used at either the specific or general level (e.g, the concept of competence may be discussed as it used in one model or as it is applied to all models)

Thus, to understand how a client's volition subsystem is functioning, a therapist might want to obtain information by assessing the person's sense of personal causation, values, and interests. As a result of that knowledge, plus information obtained from the other two subsystems, the occupational therapy practitioner has the data on which to base the selection of media, methods, and approaches designed to help a client gain or regain the skills and occupations needed for better living. Therefore, concepts not only help build and understand a model, they also contribute to the assessment and intervention strategies associated with a practice model.

Finally, Chinn & Kramer (1995) suggest that concepts can be viewed in a range from relatively empiric or concrete to relatively abstract. Within the range, concepts can be organized into three types: those which are directly observable and measurable such as height and weight, those which are indirectly observed and measured such as physical fitness and perceptual skills, and those which are inferred from multiple direct and indirect observations such as self-efficacy and well-being. Figure B-1 shows how some concepts used in occupational therapy might be viewed.

Models developed using empiric concepts are fairly easy to understand and apply in practice. An example may be the biomechanical model, which is based in the principles of physics and kinesiology. However, models developed using more abstract concepts may be more difficult to understand and to apply in practice situations. Examples include models such as occupational behavior (Reilly, 1966), occupational adaptation (Schkade and Schultz, 1992), and the Model of Human Occupation (Kielhofner & Burke, 1980). Likewise, research studies based on empiric concepts are fairly easy to perform, and the results are understandable to most students and practitioners. On the other hand, research based on relatively abstract concepts is more challenging to conduct and results may not be easily understood.

In summary, concepts are useful tools within the profession of occupational therapy. Better understanding and use of concepts can clarify how occupation should be studied and what occupational therapy does as an applied discipline. Finally, concepts facilitate communication among occupational therapy personnel with clients and their families and to other professionals.

Where Concepts Begin

Concepts derive from and are part of the language. Two language systems are recognized. One is the commonly used language of daily communication. The other is the language used mostly within a particular trade or profession, often called professional jargon. Dictionaries may address both but usually begin with the common language and then note the specialized definitions used in that trade or profession.

Concepts developed within a specialized group are used to convey ideas needed to express the work of that group. In trade groups, the concepts often refer to particular equipment or materials used by that the group. For example, to most people, a nail is a nail. However, to a carpenter, a nail may be a common nail, a finishing nail, a brad nail, a roofing nail, a screw nail, a cut nail, or a boat nail. Each was designed for a particular purpose. Carpenters find the distinctions useful because they get better results by using the nail designed for the project at hand. Professions also have developed specialized concepts to convey ideas useful to them. Occupational therapy has developed a number of concepts and has also borrowed many concepts from both the common language and from other professions. The source of the concepts may be lost or forgotten over the years. For example, the activities of daily living concept was not developed by occupational therapists but came to the profession through physical medicine and rehabilitation, special education for orthopedically handicapped children, and physical therapy. This knowledge explains why there are many different definitions of activities of daily living and why the emphasis varies from one profession to another. Activities of daily living in occupational therapy are usually described in terms of tasks such as eating or dressing. Activities of daily living in physical therapy is more often described in terms of mobility such as rolling

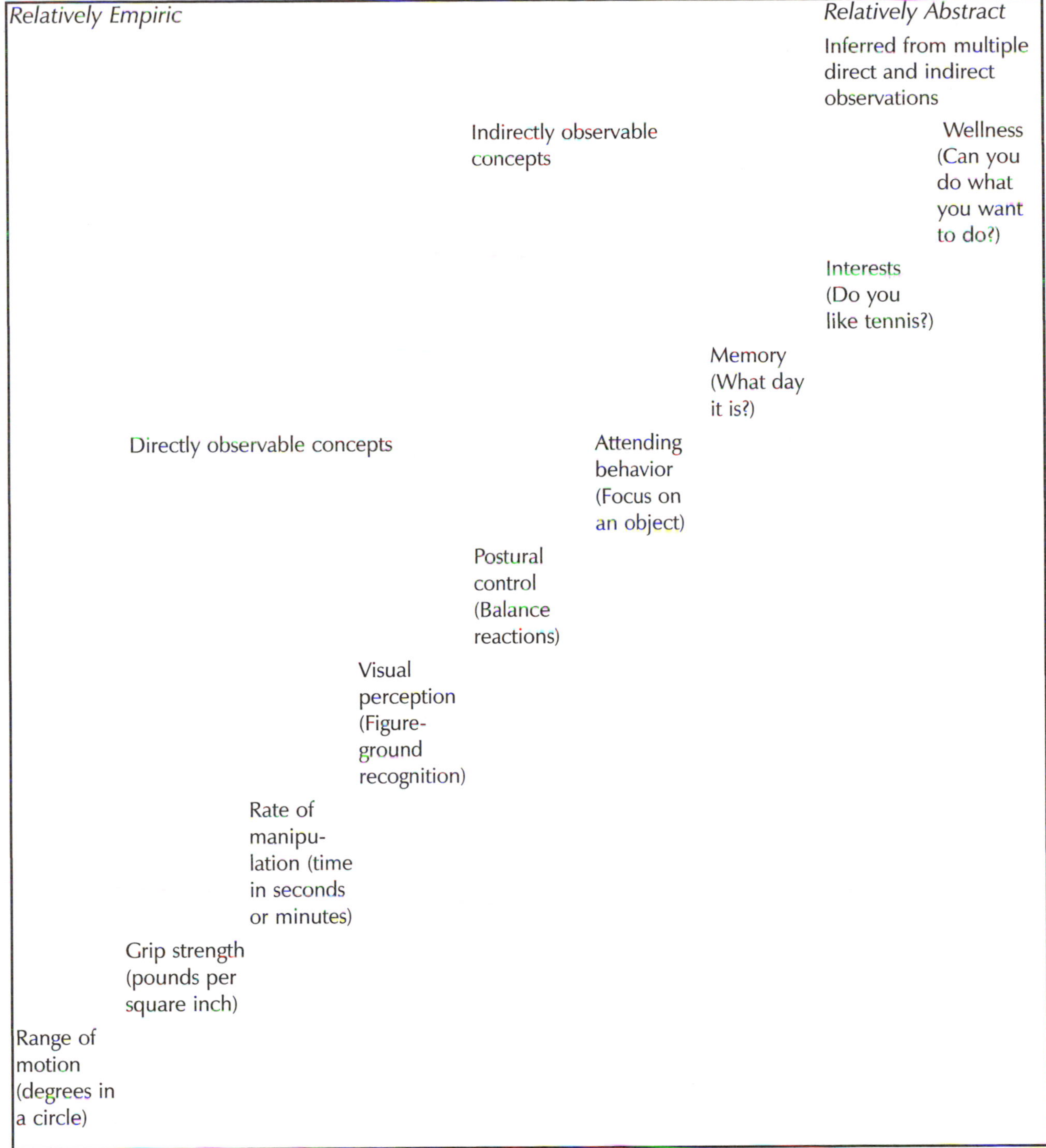

Figure B-1. Example of empiric-abstract continuum. (Adapted from Chinn, P. L., & Kramer, M. K. (1995). *Theory and nursing: A systematic approach* (4th ed., p. 59). St. Louis, MO: Mosby.)

Table B-2

Significant Time Periods in the Development of Occupational Therapy

Period	*Time Period*	*Major Influences and Contributions*
Preformative	1800 to 1899	Major influences: moral treatment and the arts and crafts movement. Major contribution: initial ideas that lead to the development and application of occupational therapy to clients in mental health institutions
Formative	1900 to 1929	Major influences: philosophy of pragmatism and publications of early leaders and scholars. Major contribution: many of the basic terms and concepts used today were developed during this period
Mechanistic	1930 to 1965	Major influences: push by physicians to adopt the scientific (quantitative) method. Major contribution: many of the formative concepts were forgotten and few new concepts were developed
Modern	1966 to present	Major influences: Return to ideas expressed in the publications of the formative period and acceptance of qualitative methods. Major contribution: development of useful models of practice and expansion of the ideas about occupation and its contribution to performance of tasks and roles in everyday life

over in bed or walking. Neither profession, however, owns the concept since it was developed from ideas synthesized from several different disciplines.

Another major influence on the development of concepts is philosophy. Models based on mechanistic philosophy, in which the person is viewed as passive, have one set of concepts and definitions for these concepts, while models based on organismic or vitalistic philosophy have another. Occupational therapy was organized primarily around the concepts from organismic or vitalistic philosophy in which the individual is viewed as an active agent. However, during the middle part of the 20th century, the profession was strongly urged to adopt mechanistic philosophy as an organizing base. In the latter half of the 20th century, the profession began to resist the pressure to use mechanistic philosophy and to return to the original philosophic ideas. As a result, four periods of time can be used to roughly describe the development of concepts in the profession of occupational therapy. These are the preformative period, the formative period, the mechanistic period, and the modern period. These time periods, major influences, and major contributions are detailed in Table B-2.

What Concepts Are Needed?

While concepts are useful, too many concepts may clutter the information channels and confuse the intended audience. On the other hand, an insufficient number of concepts may lead to inadequate communication, causing gaps in understanding and possibly failures in application. Obviously, the right number of concepts is important, although the exact number may be difficult to determine. One way of determining how many concepts of what kind are needed or useful is to develop a working model of concept usage. The author has suggested that useful models in occupational therapy need to contain concepts in three areas: outcome, doing, and tools (Reed & Sanderson, 1999). Outcome concepts address the question, "What are the goals, purposes or results of occupational therapy?" and explain why occupational therapy personnel should be allowed to intervene in a person's life and what change might result. Doing concepts address the question, "What beliefs and assumptions underlie our views of humans as occupational beings?" and explain how occupational therapy "works" as an applied profession to facilitate the change process. Tool concepts address the question, "Given those beliefs and assumptions, what concepts support where and how occupational therapy personnel choose to achieve their goals and purposes with individual or groups of clients?" Tool concepts explain the instruments of change or therapeutic interventions, what strategies are used, and why the strategies are viewed as useful. Tools include media, modalities, methods, techniques, approaches, and contexts or environments.

Outcomes

Outcomes may be examined by looking at statements made by various authors or by analyzing concepts in detail that purport to be outcome concepts. Some samples of statements from early leaders suggest a variety of outcomes were advanced. Examples of statements and the outcomes advanced are summarized in Table B-3.

The problem of discordance regarding outcome is also evident in the analysis of concepts related to outcome in occupational

Table B-3 Examples of Outcome Statements in the Early Literature of Occupational Therapy

- The "aim of all curative work is to salvage the patient from a state of disability and unproductiveness and make him once more a useful unit of society" (Burnette, 1918, p. 20). The outcomes focused on decreasing the effects of disability and increasing productiveness.
- "A distinct advantage processed by the work-shop type of therapy consists in the fact that the patient here is a member of a social group and turns out a tangible product of economic value; he is thus brought to full realization of his social fitness and economic usefulness..." (Baldwin, 1919, p. 7). Thus, socialization and economic usefulness were the desired outcomes.
- "It (occupational therapy) attempts through the introduction of light manual occupations to rouse the interest and develop the initiative of men and women who are permanently handicapped, or who are convalescing from serious illness or injury" (Hall, 1923, p. 1). The outcomes focused on initiative and motivation to engage in occupation.
- "The objects sought are to arouse interest, courage, and confidence to exercise mind and body in healthy activity; to overcome disability; and to re-establish capacity for industrial and social usefulness" (American Occupational Therapy Association, 1923, p. 1). The outcomes focus on health, work, and citizenship.
- "The handicrafts are used... for the purpose of developing physical and mental effectiveness..." (Hall, 1923, p. 1). Thus, fitness is stressed as an outcome.
- "The present concept of therapy is that a person disabled by disease or injury... at the earliest possible moment shall be given active occupation that is graded, as rapidly as his strength permits, to normal levels of activity" (Willard & Spackman, 1947, p. vii). The outcome is normal activity.

therapy literature. A total of 19 concepts related to outcome statements were identified in occupational therapy literature. They include, in alphabetical order, achievement, adaptation, autonomy, balance (of mind and occupation), competence, coping, function, health, independence, mastery, normal or normalcy, occupational performance, person-activity-environment fit, quality of life, reconditioning, satisfaction, self-efficacy, well-being, and wellness. Of these 19 concepts, five seem to be discussed most often in current thinking: adaptation, competence, independence, occupational performance, and balance of occupation. Each of the first four is closely associated with another concept: adaptation/coping, competence/mastery, independence/autonomy, and occupational performance/function. These four pairs will be discussed. Balance of occupation is discussed by itself. The remaining concepts are summarized in Table B-4.

Adaptation/Coping

Adaptation has been a concept since the beginning of the profession. Meyer (1922) said, "No branch of medicine has learned as clearly as psychiatry that after all many of these formidable diseases are largely problems of adaptation..." (p. 1). Meyer was referring to the idea that mental health problems were, in his opinion, more related to problems in adaptation or adjustment to the contextual situations than to pathology of the brain, constitutional weakness, or poor upbringing. His use of the term *adaptation* appears to be consistent with one of four definitions proposed by Corsini (1999), which states the adaptation is "changes of attitudes toward external stimulations resulting in better adjustment to these situations" (p. 17). In the occupational therapy literature, the attitudinal description of adaptation seems to appear most often. King (1978) states that "individual adaptation refers to adjustments made by the individual that primarily enhance personal rather than species survival, and secondarily contribute to actualization of personal potential" (p. 431). Schkade & Schultz (1992) define adaptation as "a change in the functional state of the person as a result of movement toward relative mastery over occupational challenges" (p. 831). The term *movement* refers to a cognitive change, not a physical motion. Ryan (1993) says that adaptation is "satisfactory adjustment of individuals within their environment over time" (p. 357). Christiansen and Baum (1997) define adaptation as "a change a person makes in his or her response approach when that person encounters an occupational challenge. This change is implemented when the individual's customary response approaches are found inadequate for producing some degree of mastery over the challenge" (p. 591). This definition appears to be a restatement of the Schkade and Schultz definition (1992). Gillen and Burkhardt (1998) seem to describe the same type of adaptation, which is "coping with the changing characteristics of a task, the environment, or the method of carrying out a task so that an activity can be completed" (p. 536). Stein & Roose (2000) also follow the attitude approach by defining adaptation as "the adjustment of a person to his or her environment as a reaction to a stressor or environmental demand" (p. 2).

A second set of definitions appear to emphasize both internal factors such as changes in attitude and external factors in the environment, which may affect or contribute to adaptation.

Table B-4

Other Outcomes

Achievement

- Achievement is mentioned in Meyer's article: "to get the pleasure and pride of achievement... is the basic remedy for the blasé tedium that characterizes the indifference or the hopeless depression" (Meyer, 1922, p. 7).
- Achievement means "getting some work or things done" (Meyer, 1951).
- Achievement is "competition with a standard of excellence" (McClelland, 1953 as stated in Reilly, 1974, p. 147).
- Parham and Fazio (1997a) provide two definitions of achievement: "1) performance that is linked to public expectancies or standards of excellence, and 2) something accomplished, especially by ability or special effort; connotes final accomplishment of something noteworthy; an attainment" (p. 248).
- In both Reilly's Model of Occupational Behavior and Kielhofner's Model of Human Occupation, achievement is the third or highest level of occupational functioning.

Health

- First definition located in 1976, although the concept is mentioned in the formative period.
- Health "is an individual state of biological, social, and emotional well-being whereby an individual is capable and able to perform those tasks or activities which are important or necessary to him to promote and maintain a sense of well-being. The individual state of health is influenced by forces such as heredity, behavior, physical environment, and the economic and social system in which he lives" (AOTA, 1976a, p. 262).
- Other definitions of health have suggested that integrity of body, mind, spirit, and emotions create a condition of well-being or wholeness that permits the individual to function adequately or optimally in his or her environment in a balanced variety of roles and patterns of occupation, allows the person to contribute to the social and economic fabric of a community over the lifespan, is conducive to independent choice, opportunity, enjoyment of life, optimal function, life satisfaction and is available even in the presence of illness, disease, or disability (Christiansen & Baum, 1997, p. 597; Creek, 1997, p. 529; Johnson, 1986, p vii; Spencer, 1989, p. 92; Townsend, 1997, p. 181).
- Smith (1986), a nurse, has suggested that there are four models included in the concept of health:
    - ✧ Clinical model, which views health as the absence of disease
    - ✧ Role performance model, which considers health the state of optimum capacity of an individual for the effective performance of the roles and tasks for which one has been socialized
    - ✧ Adaptive model, which considers the environment as a central factor
    - ✧ Eudaemonistic model, which defines health as well-being and self-realization
- Occupational therapy has models of practice that address all four models of health.

Normal

- Term appears in formative period but is not defined.
- "Our occupation is considered not chiefly diversional but remedial, reconstructive, curative, convalescent, normalizing" (Brush as quoted in Upham, 1918a, p. 41).
- "The aim of the worker should be to restore the patient to a condition of normal manhood" (Burnette, 1918, p. 11).
- "A person... shall be given active occupation that is graded, as rapidly as his strength permits, to normal levels of activity" (Willard & Spackman, 1947, p. vii).
- Normalization is the process of "making available to people with disabilities patterns and conditions of everyday life that are as close as possible to the norms and patterns of the mainstream of society" (Trombly, 1995a, p. 352).

(continued)

Table B-4

Prevention

- Prevention became a concept in the occupational therapy literature in the late 1960s. West (1969), Wiemer (1972), and Finn (1972) discuss prevention as an aspect of community health and suggest several roles occupational therapy personnel could fill.
- The Uniform Reporting System describes prevention as referring "to skill and performance in minimizing debilitation. It may include programs for persons where predisposition to disability exists, as well as for those who have already incurred a disability" (AOTA, 1979a, p. 905). Examples provided include energy conservation, joint protection and body mechanics, positioning, and coordination of daily living activities.
- Prevention involves "efforts that limit progression of disease at any point along the course" (Christiansen and Baum, 1997, p. 601). Note 18-year gap.
- Neistadt and Crepeau (1998) define the word prevent that "involves therapeutic interventions designed to prevent the occurrence or evolution of barriers to performance—may address person context, or task variables" (p. 872).
- Prevention involves "minimizing the possibility of disease, dysfunction, or disability" (Punwar & Peloquin, 2000, p. 283).
- Stein and Roose (2000) define the three levels as follows: primary prevention involves "prevention of the initial onset of a disease, for example, the prevention of polio with a vaccination" (p. 237). Secondary prevention is "prevention of the recurrent of a disease, for example, preventing a second stroke in an individual" (p. 273). Tertiary prevention is "prevention of secondary problems that can result from a disability, such as prevent decubiti in individuals with spinal cord injury" (p. 311).
- Reed and Sanderson (1980) include prevention as a service function. They state that the goal of a prevention program has been attained "when that person is able to avoid developmental regression, and biogenic, psychogenic or sociogenic disorders to the extent that current knowledge and technology will permit. In other words, the client has been provided with the knowledge and skills to avoid certain health problems" (p. 790).

Quality of Life

- Concept first appears in the modern period in 1985.
- Is a concept defined by an individual's perceptions of overall life satisfaction and happiness with his or her living circumstances, including physical status and needs, abilities and capacities, psychological well-being, social interactions, and economic conditions? Involves choosing and participating in occupations that foster hope, generate motivation, offer meaning and satisfaction, create a driving vision of life, promote health, and enable empowerment; includes factors such as being with one's family, being in one's home, ability to travel independently, food choices, expressing one self through music and art, socialization with friends, and working at an interesting job and which can be maintained by finding meaning in life, expanding horizons, renewing old interests, and learning new talents and skills (Christiansen & Baum, 1997, p. 602; Kielhofner, 1985, p. 507; Mann, Edwards, & Baum, 1986, p. 784; Punwar & Pelloquin, 2000, p. 284; Stein & Roose, 2000, p. 245; Townsend, 1997, p. 182).
- Eisenberg (1995) suggests that there are three meanings for the term quality of life in the field of rehabilitation:
    - ✧ Aspects of daily life that collectively are construed as positive and render a feeling that life is worth living
    - ✧ Aspects of a person's ability to perform ordinary activities of daily living
    - ✧ Ability to realize life plans (p. 202)

  The first is based on affect, the second on performance, and the third on cognition.
- Quality of life is a complex concept that requires clarification to be useful as an outcome measure because the term has both subjective and objective components that must be addressed in determining whether a person has a quality of life that is acceptable, good, or better.

(continued)

Table B-4

Satisfaction and Life Satisfaction

- Hall (1905) describes satisfaction as "the one great end to be obtained is self-forgetfulness and a pride and satisfaction in work and in life" (p. 32). Meyer (1922) uses satisfaction several times in his article (p. 8).
- Dunton (1928) suggests that "stimulating heart action, respiration and blood circulation... yield some of the joy and satisfaction that wisely selected wholesome occupation provides in normal life" (p. 4).
- Hopkins and Smith (1983) state simply that life satisfaction is a "subjective sense of well-being" (p. 923).
- McGuire (1983) describes a model of life satisfaction in which "satisfaction depends on the degree of congruence between an individual's perceived resources and his or her expectations for participation in valued activities" (p. 167). Four assumptions are proposed:
    - ✧ A person's individual activity resources either enhance or constrain his or her ability to act
    - ✧ Activity expectations vary with each individual and particular social situation
    - ✧ Activity expectation may prescribe relative activity levels
    - ✧ A person's individual expectations may vary from the social norms of a particular situation

Self-Efficacy

- The concept of self-efficacy or efficacy expectation was originated in 1977 by Bandura, a psychologist, and was originally defined as "the conviction that one can successfully execute the behavior required to produce the outcome" (p. 193). In 1986, Bandura further defined perceived self-efficacy as "people's judgements of their capabilities to organize and execute course of action required to attain designated types of performances" (p. 391). He continues by stating that judgment or perception of what a person can do is more critical than the skills or skill level per se. In 1988, he changed it to read "concerned with beliefs in one's capabilities to mobilize the motivation, cognitive resources and courses of action needed to meet given situational demands" (Bandura, Cioffi, Taylor, & Brouillard, 1988, p. 479).
- Self-efficacy appears in occupational therapy literature in 1992.
- Crist & Stoffel (1992) refer to Bandura's (1977) four sources of judgments about one's self-efficacy that affect performance: emotional arousal, verbal and social persuasion, vicarious experience, and performance accomplishment (p. 436).
- Gage & Polatajko (1994) suggest there are three parameters of perceived self-efficacy: magnitude, strength, and generality.
- Self-efficacy is the feeling or perception that a person has about his- or herself to be successful in using a particular coping strategy or problem-solving approach and the person's belief or self-confidence in his or her performance capabilities with respect to the effectiveness or power to produce effects or intended results on a specific functional task or occupation. The feeling or belief is assumed to be an important determinant of actual performance and predicts the likelihood that one will attempt a given behavior and continue working at it, despite possible difficulties, in new situations (Cara & MacRae, 1998, p. 688; Christiansen & Baum, 1997, p. 433; Gage, Noh, Polatajko, & Kaspar, 1994, p. 783; Hagedorn, 2000, p. 311; Jacobs, 1999, p. 132; Stein & Roose, 2000, p. 284).
- The definition appears to be congruent with Bandura's original definitions, which is important because when concepts enter the occupational therapy literature, changes in the limitations on meaning or descriptors may occur that are different from the original source or usage.

Well-Being

- Well-being became a concept in the occupational therapy literature in the 1980s.
- Johnson (1986) defines well-being as "a state that transcends the limitations of body, space, time, and circumstances and in which one is at peace with one's self and with others" (p. vii).
- Christian and Baum (1997) state that well-being is "a subjective sense of overall contentment, thought to be defined by affective state and life satisfaction" (p. 606).

(continued)

Table B-4

- Wilcock (1998) suggests the concept of well-being should be explored from three individual aspects: physical, mental, and social and two contexts: community and ecology. In other words, well-being is an interactive process between the individual and the surrounding in which the person lives.
- The ICIDH-2 prefinal draft (World Health Organization, 2000) includes the following definition of well-being: "Well-being is a general term encompassing the total universe of human life domains including physical, mental and social aspects, that make up what can be called a 'good life'. Health domains are a subset of domains that make up the total universe of human life" (p. 163).
- The concept of well-being does not appear to be well developed in the occupational therapy literature although Wilcock (1998) has provided some direction.

Wellness

- According to Johnson (1986), the concept of wellness began in the 1960s.
- Earliest reference in the occupational therapy literature is Reed and Sanderson (1980) in which wellness is described as "an optimal or ideal condition toward which to strive" (p. 92).
- In 1985, Johnson described wellness "as a context for living" (p. 129). In 1986, White defined wellness as "a lifestyle for well-being that a person chooses, regardless of the presence or absence of disabling conditions, to reach optimum potential" (p. 745).
- Reed and Sanderson (1992) suggest there are three uses of the term *wellness*:
  - Wellness as the polar opposite of illness
  - Wellness as a graduated scale with illness
  - Wellness as a separate or nearly separate dimension from illness (p. 48)
- None of the three has been developed adequately in occupational therapy to be used as a consistent indicator of outcome. In addition, wellness is often associated with health promotion
- Sources outside the field may be helpful in clarifying the concept. *Taber's Cyclopedic Medical Dictionary* (Thomas, 1997) defines wellness as "the condition of being in good health, includes the appreciation and enjoyment of health. Wellness is more than a lack of disease symptoms; it is a state of mental and physical balance and fitness" (p. 2110).
- Dunn (1977), one of the early advocates of wellness, defined wellness as an "integrated method of functioning which is oriented toward maximizing the potential of which the individual is capable; it requires that the individual maintain a continuum of balance of purpose and direction within the environment where he/she is functioning" (p. 4).
- Corsini (1999) says that wellness is "the emphasis in health and medical counseling toward healthy lifestyles, preventive measures, and self-treatment" (p. 1068).
- Wellness is another example of a concept that appears in the occupational therapy literature without adequate development and refinement to make it useful as an outcome criterion for occupational therapy services at this time.

Webster's New Universal Unabridged Dictionary (Barnes & Noble, 1995) includes two definitions that may apply here: "the state of being adapted, adjustment" and "a form or structure modified to fit a changed environment" (p. 22). Note that the focus has changed from person to object. In this use of the term *adaptation*, an object is changed or altered in some manner to make it more suitable for use by a person. The person is not the only focus of change. Parham and Fazio (1997a) include both emphases in their definition of adaptation. The first is "a change or response to stress of any kind; may be normal, self-protective, and developmental" and the second is "a change in routine, materials, or equipment that enables a person with a disability to function independently or to participate more fully in an activity" (p. 248). Neistadt and Crepeau (1998) also follow the idea of changes generated external to the individual in their definition of adaptation: "Making the task simpler or less physically demanding to promote independent function" before proceeding to the second part: "changing in response to new demands or expectations (p. 866). The first part of the definition appears to be directed at the therapist, while the second part appears directed at the client. Unsworth (1999) says that adaptation involves "promoting quality of occupational performance by modifying the method used to accomplish a task, modifying the task itself, or changing the environment" (p. 473). Finally,

Hagedorn (2000) describes both internal and external adaptation in one definition by suggesting that adaptation is:

> Any change in the occupational habits or organization of person which is made in order to meet environmental demands and restore fit or an alteration made by a therapist or client to an object or environment in order to provide therapy or to improve the client's ability to perform. (p. 307)

The foregoing discussion of definitions is one way to examine concepts to determine how the term is being applied in the profession. As the review of dictionary definitions illustrate, occupational therapy uses one of four major definitions of the term *adaptation* and, in addition, has expanded the use of the term to include changes made in the environment to facilitate individual adaptation. Selective and expanded use of a term as a concept in a field is not unusual. Many other fields do the same thing. Selective use becomes a problem when the field does not know which dictionary definition is being applied. Without clarification, the number of dictionary definitions may appear overwhelming and become confusing. Occupational therapy in particular is prone to confusion over the various dictionary definitions because so many of the terms and concepts used in the field are words commonly found in a standard dictionary with multiple definitions attached. Examples include work, play, and balance, which are discussed later in the chapter.

Another use of dictionaries is to compare the origin of the term with the concept used in the field. The origin of the term *adaptation* is the verb *adapt*. The verb came from the Latin word "adaptive" possibly from the French word *adapter*, which means to fit or adjust. Both meanings appear consistent with the usage in occupational therapy. Occupational therapy practice is designed to assist the person to fit with the environment and to adjust to the environment. At the same time, the second usage of adaptation may also be applied. Occupational therapy practice is designed to initiate external changes that may better fit or adjust the environment to the person.

A third method of examining concepts is to compare the concept with a similar concept to determine if both are useful because they have different purposes or if both serve the same purpose and are redundant. Coping is an example of such a concept. The terms *adaptation* and *coping* have been linked together (Coelho, Hamburg, & Adams, 1974). Lazarus (1984), a psychologist, says that "coping has been widely and long regarded as having a central role in adaptation, yet it has defied universal agreement on definition..." (p. 294). White (1974), also a psychologist, suggests that adaptation is the master concept with three superordinate terms: *coping*, *mastery*, and *defense*. Coping is viewed as a special type of adaptation that occurs "under relatively difficult conditions" (p. 49). *Taber's Cyclopedic Medical Dictionary* (Thomas, 1997) defines coping skills as "the characteristics or behavior patterns of a person that enhance adaptation. Coping skills include a stable value or religious belief system, problem solving, social skills, health-energy, and commitment to a social network" (p. 411).

Coping does not have as long a history with occupational therapy as does adaptation. The first definition was located in 1973 in a grant report on roles and functions. The definition of coping behavior "includes abilities and limitations in ability to sublimate drives, find sources of need gratification, tolerate frustration and anxiety, experience gratification and control impulses" (AOTA, 1973, p. 42). Coping does not appear in the terms listed in the first *Uniform Terminology*, but does in the second in which the definition for coping skills is "identify and manage stress and related reactors" (McGourty, Foto, Marvin, Smith, & Smith, 1989, p. 815). Kielhofner (1985) describes coping as "the active psychosocial process through which persistent efforts are made to overcome and solve the problems and dilemmas of the person or those imposed by the environment" (p. 502). Zeitlin, Williamson, and Szczepanski (1988) define coping as " a general term for the process of using learned adaptive behaviors to manage one's world. Coping is the process of making adaptation to meet personal needs and to respond to the demands of the environment" (pp. 1-2). Gage (1992) describes coping as the process though which the individual manages to deal with the demands of stressful situations that tax or exceed the person's resources and the emotions generated by those situations in the person-environment relationship. Williamson (1997) describes coping as "(a)n adaptation to environmental stress that is based on conscious or unconscious choice and that enhances control over behavior or gives psychological comfort" (p. 439). Punwar and Peloquin (2000) state the coping skills are "those abilities that enable an individual to identify and manage stress and related reactions" (p. 278). Stein & Roose (2000) define coping skills as "an individual's ability to self-regulate stress and master the environment" (p. 80).

Three themes can be identified from the previous definitions: drive-reinforcement learning theory leading to stress reduction, ego psychology and gratification, and cognitive appraisal processes and adaptation. These themes correspond to three identified by Lazarus (1984). Apparently, occupational therapy personnel have accepted all three interpretations of coping over the years, but the later definitions favor the third interpretation: cognitive appraisal processes and adaptation. Coping then is viewed as a process that affects adaptation outcome. In therapy, interventions to improve coping skills and behaviors should contribute to the outcome of adaptation. Although it is unclear if occupational therapy scholars and practitioners accept the idea that coping is a subset of adaptation, that would be the author's recommendation.

Competency/Mastery

The concept of competency and competence discussed in this section refers to client outcomes. Therefore, the issue of professional competence or the ability of occupational therapy personnel to perform the job or role of therapy is not discussed.

The term *competency* related to clients first appears in occupational therapy literature in an article by Reilly (1966). She is discussing the specifications for a psychiatric occupational therapy program and states that "the fourth specification, therefore, speaks for the building of a milieu which acknowledges competency..." (p. 63). The term is not defined. The term *incompetence* appears in an article by Taylor (1930, p. 54). Again, the term in not defined. The first definition of competency appears in 1975 as the "ability to perform at a predetermined level" (AOTA, 1976b, p. 262).

The term *competence* is defined in 1971 by Robert White, a psychologist, who originated the concept in 1959. He states that competence is "sufficient or adequate behavior to meet the demands of the situation or task" (1971, p. 273). Competence is also called *effectance motivation*. Hopkins & Smith (1977) define competence as the "quality of adequacy or possession of required skill, knowledge, or capacity" (p. 730). Rogers (1982) describes competence as:

> A transactional concept that involves effectiveness in interacting with the environment. It (competence) arises from an urge to learn about the environment by testing our actions upon it. Competence implies adaptability in organizing skills into integrated courses of action to serve innumerable purposes. Competence is an overall strategy of adaptation consisting of thinking, deciding, doing, and evaluating. (p. 709)

Note the suggestion that competence may be viewed as a subtype of adaptation. Competence is defined by Allen (1985) as "an inference we make about the prerequisite ability required to do the task procedure" and "an estimate of the level of thought required to do a step in the task" (p. 73). Kielhofner (1985) states that competence is "the quality of being able or having the capacity to respond effectively to the demands of one or a range of situations" (p. 502). Competence, according to Mocellin (1988), "refers to the ability required to carry out a task; to the quality of being functionally adequate or having sufficient skill for a particular; and to a potential which is realized at the moment of performance" (p. 5). Competence has also been defined as "the ability to answer all the requirements of an environment" (Polatajko, 1992, p. 196) or "achievement of skill equal to the demands of the environment (Christiansen & Baum, 1997, p. 593). Creek (1997) adds the idea of life role to her definition, which is "the ability to perform skills to a level that allows satisfactory performance of life roles" (p. 529). Parham and Fazio (1997a) return to the theme that competence is "the state of being adequate to meet the demands of a task or situation" (p. 249). Finally, Hagedorn (2000) defines competence as "skill and adequately successful completion of a piece of performance, task, or activity" (p. 308), while Punwar and Peloquin (2000) state that competence is "the individual's adequacy or capacity in a given task" (p. 278).

The basic term *competence* or *competency* has been modified by occupational therapists to the terms *competency behavior* and *occupational competence*. Therefore, these definitions need to be considered as well. Parham and Fazio (1997b) define competency behavior as "play that involves practice or repetition of fragments of activity sequences in pursuit of mastery of skills" (p. 249). They further explain that competency behavior is:

> Reilly's second hierarchical stage of play behavior, in which the play is driven by effectance motivation and practice tasks repeatedly in pursuit of competence and mastery of skills. In this stage, play builds on trust in the environment and generates self confidence. (p. 249)

Occupational competence, by definition, "is determined by the interaction of the individual and environment. (It) is the product of the dynamic interaction between the environment and the individual, each changing in response to the other" (Polatajko, 1992, pp. 196-197). The definition was slightly rephrased as "occupational competence is the product of the dynamic interaction of the three dimensions of the individual, the environment, and occupation" (Martini, Polatajko, & Wilcock, 1995, p. 16). A third rephrasing reads as "Occupational competence is adequacy or sufficiency in an occupational skill, meeting all requirements of an environment" (Law, Polatajko, Baptiste, & Townsend, 1997, p. 40). Occupational competence seems to imply the ability to cope adequately with the three "duties of care," to self, neighbor and state, while occupational dysfunction implies a breakdown in one or more of these areas (Hagedorn, 1995, p. 53).

The terms *competence* and *competency* are based on the word *competent*, which is from *competence*, meaning to meet or agree. *Webster's New Universal Unabridged Dictionary* (Barnes & Noble, 1995) defines competent as having suitable or sufficient skill, knowledge, experience, etc. for some purpose, properly qualified; adequate but not exceptional. Synonyms include fit, capable, proficient, and able (p. 417). *Taber's Cyclopedic Medical Dictionary* (Thomas, 1997) defines competence as "performance in a manner that satisfies the demands of a situation; interaction effectively with the environment" (p. 424). All of these descriptors and synonyms seem to fit the meaning applied in occupational therapy to the terms *competence*, *competency*, and *occupational competence*. Additional descriptors used by occupational therapy writers include perform, capacity, effectiveness, adaptation, adaptability, achievement, and cope. Also, the dictionary definitions do not address the object of the competence such as dealing with the environment or performing life roles

The other concept in this pair is mastery. Wantanabe (1968) defined mastery as the "ability and skill in recognizing and comprehending the options that society offers and make choices appropriately using one's human and nonhuman environment to meet one's own needs and abilities" (p. 440). Hopkins and Smith (1978) define mastery as "command or grasp of a subject" (p. 734). Llorens (1976) uses the term *mastery* but does not define it. Phrases include "mastery of the developmental tasks and adaptive skills according to the age" and "developmental mastery for successful adaptation" (p. 1). In 1991, Llorens states that "accomplishment of tasks is prefaced on the ability to achieve mastery of skills" and describes "levels of mastery for successful adaptation" (pp. 46-47). Level 1 is called "occupational performance enablers," which includes the subskills of sensory perception, sensory integration, motor coordination, psychosocial and psychodynamic responses, sociocultural development, and social language responses. Level 2 is called "activities and task of occupational performance" and includes the skill areas of self-care/self-maintenance, play/leisure, work/education, and rest/relaxation. Level 3 is called "occupational roles" and includes worker, student, volunteer, homemaker, parent, child, sibling, peer, and best friend or chum. Likewise, Fidler and Fidler (1978) describe mastery but do not define the term. They say "the meaning and worth of one's doing or mastery is appreciably determined by the views and values of significant others" (p. 307). Christiansen and Baum (1991) define mastery as "the achievement of skill to a criterion level of success" (p. 854). Schkade and Schultz (1992) use the term *relative mastery*, which is defined as:

> The extent to which the person experiences the occupational response as efficient (use of time and energy), effective (production of the desired result), and satisfying to self and society, that is, it is pleasing not only

> to the self but also to relevant others as agents of the occupational environment. (p. 835)

Ryan (1993) defines mastery as "the desire to explore, understand, and to some extent, control oneself and an environment" (p. 362). Muñoz and Kielhofner (1995) also use the term *mastery* but do not define it. They state that the achievement level "represents the fullest mastery over one's self and the environment" (p. 346). Parham and Fazio (1997a) define mastery as "the state of being competent" or of "having adequate skills to exert some degree of control over one's environment and situation" (p. 250). In *Webster's New Universal Unabridged Dictionary* (Barnes & Noble, 1995), mastery is defined as command or grasp as of a subject; superiority or victory; expert skill or knowledge; power of command or control (p. 1184). Of these four definitions, the first and third seem to best fit the intent of occupational therapy writers. A working definition might be mastery is the knowledge, grasp, or understanding of a subject; or command of, control of, or ability to perform a skill. The meanings related to superiority, victory, expertness, or power do not seem to apply to usual intent of occupational therapy writers.

When comparing the two terms *competence* (competency) and *mastery*, they appear to be similar in ideas of having knowledge and skill for a purpose. Where they differ is the mastery includes descriptors that imply a high degree, superiority, or expertness that descriptors of competence do not seem to imply. Therefore, while both terms can be applied with meaning to occupational therapy ideas, competence provides a more consistent meaning. Mastery has more descriptors that could be misinterpreted to mean that more of or higher levels of knowledge and skill are needed than is actually intended by the author's or practitioner's use of the word.

Independence/Autonomy

The term *independence* came into the occupational therapy literature much earlier that the term *autonomy*. Independence has been used since 1905 when Hall stated that "to encourage a feeling of independence it has been decided that when a patient can turn out work of value, this product may be sold..." (1905, p. 31). Upham (1918b) states that "the sooner he sees tangible evidence of his returning ability... the sooner he will believe independence possible" (p. 36). Independence in these two references refers to economic independence (i.e., earning one's own paycheck). By the 1950s and '60s, the definition of independence began to be related to self-care, activities of daily living, and self-care devices. Zimmerman (1957) illustrates and discusses several self-help devices designed to increase independence. Hightower (1966) continues the theme stating, "In achieving independence, training in the use of the residual ability is always necessary and training in the use of self-help devices or specialized equipment is often indicated" (p. 449). By the 1970s, the focus of independence has turned to independent living for the elderly in their own homes and communities as evidenced by the articles written by Hasselkus and Kiernat (1973) and Warren (1974). Warren's statement (1974) seems typical: "While most older people prefer to live independently as long as they can manage for themselves, coping becomes increasingly strenuous with advanced age" (p. 439). In the first edition of the *Uniform Terminology* adopted in 1979, the three themes of economy, self-care, and living in community are integrated into one definition which reads, "Independent living/daily living skills refer to the skill and performance of physical and psychological/emotional self-care; work, and play/leisure activities to a level of independence appropriate to age life-space, and disability" (AOTA, 1979b, p. 900). Rogers (1982) expands the concept of independence by stating, "Functional independence is not just a core concept of occupational therapy theory, it is the goal of the occupational therapy process" and that "independence connotes self-reliance, self-determination, self-directedness, and a perspective of personal control" (p. 709). Christiansen and Baum (1991) define independence as "having adequate resources to accomplish everyday tasks" (p. 853), while Hagedorn (1995) states that independence means "able to do what is required to remain healthy, without needing someone else to help" (p. 53). In 1997, Christiansen and Baum also use the phrase *functional independence* and define it to mean "the ability to successfully perform the day-to-day activities expected of the person (depending on culture, age, and gender)" (p. 596). Jacobs (1999) defines independence as the "lack of requirement or reliance on another; adequate resources to accomplish everyday tasks" (p. 69).

A specialty dictionary on rehabilitation has several definitions of independence or independent and provide a variety of descriptors. Cammack and Eisenberg (1995) define independence as "the ability to perform a task without physical or cognitive assistance or supervision in a reasonable amount of time" (p. 70). They continue by stating, "This term is used in the rehabilitation taxonomy to reflect the highest level of functioning. It may be used to refer to independence with all activities of daily living (or) with one specific activity..." (p. 70). Davis (1996) seems to agree with this description when she states that to encourage independence, the patient should begin with simple ADL tasks (p. 445). Rock (1996) also supports the "independence is activities of daily living view" when he says, "The person is encouraged to analyze and perform the activities of personal hygiene and grooming, dressing, feeding, home management, communication, avocation and vocation as independently as possible" (p. 584). The concept of independence is further reinforced by its use in definitions of levels of function. As an example, Trombly (1995a) suggests a goal be stated as, "the patient will demonstrate independent sitting balance and truck flexion and extension required for independently putting on and removing shoes and stocking" (p. 33).

Webster's New Universal Unabridged Dictionary (Barnes & Noble, 1995) lists 23 definitions for the word *independent* (p. 970). Of those, the following seem to most closely fit the idea expressed above: "an independent person or thing," "not replying on another or others for aid or support," "possessing a competency," "expressive of a spirit of independence; self-confident; unconstrained," "not influenced or controlled by others in matters of opinion, conduct, etc; thinking or acting for oneself," and "not subject to another's authority or jurisdiction; autonomous; free." Under the term *independence*, the definitions are "freedom from the control, influence, support, aid, or the yoke of others" and "a competency," which is considered to be an archaic use of the term. Themes appear to be free; freedom; autonomous; competency; not influenced or controlled by others; and not dependent, contingent, or relying on others.

The earliest use of the term *autonomy* appears in Moorhead (1969) who speaks about occupational role history and the critical variables to occupational function. The first listed variables are autonomy and independence and are described as including "realistic perception of one's own assets and liabilities; ability to make stable decisions and implement them effectively; and (c)ompetence in management of time, space, and personal needs" (p. 330). Hopkins and Smith (1978) define autonomy as the "quality of being self-governing and self-determining" (p. 729). In addition to the definition, Erikson's eight stages of development are listed. The second stage is called autonomy versus shame. Erikson's concept of autonomy is discussed in Pratt and Allen (1985) as follows: "Erikson specified the relationship of autonomy to the child's increasing control over his body. This permits independent movement into the outer world" (p. 25). This description marks the change in definitions from being able to perform to being able to take control as well as perform.

Reed & Sanderson (1983) define autonomy as "the ability to act or perform according to one's own volition or direction" (p. 237). In 1997, Christiansen and Baum defined autonomy as "reflected in the ability to make choices and have control over the environment" (p. 592). In 1995, Hagedorn defines autonomy as "capable of exercising choices and control over one's personal life" (p. 53). Cara and MacRae (1998) provide a more comprehensive definition by stating that autonomy means:

> ...self-determination and independence. The process of becoming autonomous is characterized by a gradual reduction in dependency and steady movement toward ever-greater independence. The process of and timing for becoming autonomous are largely determined by the cultural context of the family. (p. 666)

Jacobs (1999) provides a succinct definition to autonomy as the "state of independence and self-control" (p. 13).

The dictionary definitions include "a state of independence and self-determination either in a society or an individual, a basic tendency and desire to be free to control the self" (Corsini, 1999, p. 4). Reber (1995) defines autonomy simply as independence but gives a slightly more explained definition of the term *autonomous* as "controlled from within, internally directed, self-regulatory" (p. 75). *Webster's New Universal Unabridged Dictionary* (Barnes & Noble, 1995) states "independence or freedom, as of the will or one's action; the condition of being autonomous; self-government, or the right of self-government; independence; a golf-governing community" (p. 141). In addition, the term *autonomous* includes a definition used in biology that states "existing and functioning as an independent organism" (p. 141). The word *autonomy* comes from the Greek words *autos*, meaning self, and *nomos*, meaning law, self-law, or law of the self. The term can be applied to either an individual or a governmental unit. The major themes are independence, independent, self-determination, self-regulatory, self-control, volition, and will.

The terms *autonomy* and *independent* have many similar meanings. They also convey a similar view of life: a person should be as independent of others as possible for as long (in age) as possible. Brown and Gillespie (1992) have reminded occupational therapy personnel that "the concept of independence has permeated the cultural understanding of mental and physical health" (p. 1001). As Jackson (1996) has stated, "The spirit of independence is a tenacious American value that permeates many social institutions in this country..." (p. 351). Kielhofner (1997) encourages occupational therapy personnel not to impose values derived from their own professional perspectives onto the client. He summarizes the view of Hocking and Whiteford's (1995) article on values, saying, "the traditional occupational therapy values of independence and self-determination may conflict with cultural values of clients that emphasize interdependence" (p. 87). Not all clients want to be independent of others or living independent lives. Some clients value interdependence or prefer to be taken care of by family members. Whiteford and Wilcock (2000) suggest that occupational therapy personnel not view the concept of independence as a given in occupational therapy practice but rather attempt to explore what independence may mean for the client.

In summary, several authors have made the point that independence as a predetermined outcome for occupational therapy practice should be discontinued. The same suggestion should also apply to autonomy. Independence is not a universal value even in the United States and adherence to it as an outcome creates a division between occupational therapy services and the people the profession purports to serve. Another option might be to include the concept of interdependence with independence. One drawback of the dual approach is that more explanation is needed. Perhaps, American occupational therapy practitioners should begin to expand the values of occupational therapy to address the multicultural nature of the United States, and the world, in the 21st century.

Occupational Performance/Function

Both the concepts of function and performance have appeared in occupational therapy since the formative period. In addition, both have been used in ways that are overlapping and confusing. The overlapping has been acknowledged in the position papers entitled "Occupational Performance" (Baum & Edwards, 1995) and "Fundamental Concepts of Occupational Therapy" (Hinojosa & Kramer, 1997). Both references include statements that function and performance are seen as interchangeable or equivalent terms, in other words, synonyms. Furthermore, function and performance are used both as outcome and doing. Hinojosa and Kramer (1997) acknowledge this duality of use in the statement "function is part of the process, rather than an outcome alone" (p. 865). The duality occurs because occupational therapy personnel view "the process (of doing) as being as important as the product" (p. 865). To further add to the confusion when the terms *functional activities* or *occupational activities* are added, the use of function and performance become tools used in occupational therapy intervention. In other words, the following statement could be considered acceptable within occupational therapy: Through occupational therapy services, a person should be able to function (outcome) by functioning (doing) while engaged in functional occupation (tool). While the sentence may make sense to occupational therapy personnel, it probably makes no sense to those outside the profession. Nevertheless, this section will address primarily the outcome aspect but some overlapping is inevitable.

The concept of function as used in occupational therapy seems to be consistent with the idea of functionalism as expressed in functional psychology. Central figures in the founding of functionalism at the end of the 19th century were William James and John Dewey (Wolman, 1989). In functionalism, "the process of adjustment of the organism to the environment is central, as is a purposivistic interpretation of the process in which stimuli and responses are a chain of deeds and not separate entities" (Wolman, 1989, p. 141). Functionalism is the "philosophical doctrine of W. James which considers mental phenomena is their dynamic unity as a system of functions (geared to adapting the organism to its environment) for the satisfaction of needs that are biological in origin" (Eysenick, Arnold, & Meili, 1982, p. 395). Functionalism is a "theory claiming that the best, or only, way of defining something is in terms of what is does or the role it plays in the ongoing course of events" (Bothamley, 1993, p. 217).

Functional psychology is the doctrine that conscious processes or states such as those of willing (volition), thinking, emoting, perceiving, and sensating are activities or operations of an organism in physical interrelationship with a physical environment and cannot be given hypostatized, substantive existence. These activities facilitate the organism's control, survival, adaptation, engagement or withdrawal, recognition, direction, etc. (Angeles, 1981, p. 107). Functional psychology considers the mental process of sense perception, emotion, volition, and thought as functions of the biological organism in the adaptation to and control of its environment. Functionalism arose as a protest against structural psychology for which the task of psychology is the analysis and description of consciousness. The functional theory of mind is characteristic of the pragmatism and instrumentalism of Pierce, James, Mead, and Dewey (Runes 1962, p. 114). Many of the words used in these definitions and descriptions are familiar to occupational therapy personnel. Since none were written by occupational therapists, there appears to be an agreement of thought between the concept of functionalism and the use of function as a concept in occupational therapy.

The word *function* appears in occupational therapy literature from the formative period. Meyer (1922) speaks of the "laws of function" as expansions of the laws of physics and chemistry (p. 9). Definitions, however, do not appear until 1981. Mosey (1981) states that "function is the ability to engage comfortably at an age-appropriate level in performance components and the areas of occupational performance within the context of one's cultural, social, and nonhuman environment" (p. 82). Baum and Edwards (1995) state that practitioners focus "their efforts on function by using interventions to improve the occupational performance of persons who lack the ability to perform an action or activity considered necessary for their everyday lives" (p. 1019). Turner, Foster, and Johnson (1996) define function as "an action performed to fulfill an allocated task" (p. 873). According to Christiansen and Baum (1997), "function as used by an occupational therapist, describes a behavior related to the performance of a task" (p. 596). Creek (1997) states that function is the "possession of the skills necessary for successful participation in the range of roles expected of the individual" (p. 529). Hinojosa and Kramer (1997) state that the term *function* "(is) viewed as the ability to perform activities required in one's occupations" (p. 866). Punwar and Peloquin (2000) define function as "a person's ability to perform those tasks necessary in his or her daily life" (p. 280). Stein & Roose (2000) chose to define functional rather than function. Functional is "the degree of a client's independence in the performance areas of work/productivity and leisure" (p. 108).

In addition, to the concept of function as a single noun, occupational therapy personnel use function as an adjective to modify several other nouns. A few examples are presented. Functional ability is "the skill to perform activities in a normal or accepted manner" (Reed & Sanderson, 1992, p. 339). Functional assessment is the "observation of motor performance and behavior to determine if a person can adequately perform the required tasks of a particular role or setting" (Christiansen & Baum, 1991, p. 852). Functional group is a "group that includes the group leader's capitalizing on the use of group structure and therapeutic use of self to enhance the group process and individual function" (Unsworth, 1999, p. 477). Functional independence is the "ability to successfully perform the day-to-day activities expected of the person" (Christiansen & Baum, 1997, p. 596). Functional limitations are the "restrictions or lack of ability to perform an action or activity in the manner or within the range considered normal that results from impairment or failure of an individual to return to the preexisting level or function" (Christiansen & Baum, 1997, p. 596). Functional mobility is "the ability to move from one position or place to another" (Punwar & Peloquin, 2000, p. 280). Functional performance is defined as "having the ability to perform competently the roles, relationships and occupations required in the course of daily life" (Hagedorn, 2000, p. 209). Functional position is a "position that allows a person to complete necessary functional activities, even if that position is fixed so that movement is limited to that single position" (Stein & Roose, 2000, p. 108). Functional skills are those "that if not performed by the person in part or in full must be completed or performed by another" (Christiansen, 2000, p. 402). Functional training is "a remedial intervention system that uses cognitive or behavioral strategies to train and compensate for disabilities in the day-to-day activities expected of the person" (Christiansen, 2000, p. 402).

Other combinations incorporating function include executive functions, which are "a group of capacities and mental processes that occur within the brain" (Unsworth, 1999, p. 477) and occupational functioning, which Gillen and Burkhardt (1998) define as "the ability to perform the tasks that have a role in their natural context" (p. 540).

Occupational therapy personnel need to be aware that the concept of function is also used in rehabilitation. For example, Coulter (1950) describes functional therapy as "prescribed activities planned to assist in the restoration of articular and muscular function..." (p. 452). Bennett (1950) defines functional training as:

> The specific use of physical, occupational and recreational therapy to assist the patient to "pass" the test items, representing the common obstacles encountered in daily living in a normal environment. Functional training is the attempt to teach a physically handicapped individual to safely and practically perform the basic physical activities that will be required of him when he returns home. (p. 351)

Pattee (1951) describes functional occupational therapy as "for patients needing remedial exercise for the restoration of function of muscles or joints and for coordination... (p. 83). Kamenetz (1983) defines functional training or therapy as "therapeutic motions or exercises in the form of purposeful activities, such as balancing, walking, eating, dressing, in which a combination of motions is practiced rather than isolated motions of individual muscle groups or body parts" (p. 132). In addition, functional capacity was originally evaluated on a functional evaluation form (Bennett, 1950), which today would be renamed functional assessment or activities of daily living form. In Kamenetz (1983), functional assessment includes activities of daily living but adds locomotion and communication.

Clearly, the profession of occupational therapy has incorporated the concept of function into the professional terminology. In the process, however, the concept has been overused to the point that clarity of communication is lost. Function has become a buzzword and a stand-in for more precise descriptors. Among the problems are the need to sort out the professional functions (role or purpose) of occupational therapy from the client functions. In addition, as already cited, the use of function as an outcome (person can function, or person is functional), as doing (person is functioning or performing), or as a tool (use of a functional occupation such as ADL, work, and play in intervention) is difficult to follow at best and probably adds to the difficulty in communicating with other professions. Furthermore, function is used to refer to intervention based on remedial or restorative techniques in which the parts are fixed in the hopes that the whole will work to do whatever the person chooses to do, as well as intervention based on adaptation and coping in which the focus is on what occupations the client needs to do and how such occupations can be done effectively and efficiently. Finally, there is a problem of clarifying the use of the concept of function within the profession without creating additional communication gaps with other groups who also use the term. For example, the revised International Classification of Functioning, Disability and Health defines functioning as "an umbrella term for body functions, body structures, activities and participation. It denotes the positive aspects of the interaction between an individual (with a health condition) and that individual's contextual factors (environmental and personal factors)" (WHO, 2000, p. 164). Such a broad use of the concept of function is even greater than used in occupational therapy since discussion of function and structures within body is usually not the primary focus of discussion by occupational therapy personnel but rather function in relation to activities and participation. Another example is mathematics in which the concept of function refers to a variable quantity that is expressed in relation to another quantity. Perhaps, the concept of function should be replaced with other concepts. Baum and Edwards (1995) suggested as much by titling their position paper *Occupational Performance: Occupational Therapy's Definition of Function*, thus substituting occupational performance for function. A discussion of occupational performance follows after a discussion of performance as a single term.

The concept of performance has also appeared in the occupational therapy literature since the formative years. Meyer (1922) used the term *performance* nine times. A typical comment is, "We all know how fancy and abstract thought can go far afield... while *performance* is its own judge and regular and therefore the most dependable and influential part of life" (p. 5, italics in original article). Performance is discussed as reality while thinking is sometime subject to "flights of fancy." Therefore, performance is more desirable in the real world. There are few definitions of performance found in the current occupational therapy literature. Fidler and Fidler (1978) describe performance "as the ability, throughout the life cycle, to care for and maintain the self in a more independent manner, satisfy one's personal needs for intrinsic gratification, and contribute to the needs and welfare of others" (p. 310). This appears to be an outcome statement. Allen (1985) states that "performance is the task behavior we see the patient do" (p. 73). Allen's definition relates more to doing, which brings up the same problem as noted with the word *function*. Performance may be used as an outcome or to describe a process. When used as an adjective, performance may also be used to describe a tool. Therefore, each use of the term *performance* must be analyzed for intent and meaning. Jackson and Banks (1997) suggest that performance is "routine task behavior" (p. 460). Law et al. (1996) define performance as "the actual execution or carrying out of an occupation" (p. 40). Both of the previous definitions also pertain to doing. Performance has also been used in combination with other words such as *performance areas*, *performance components*, and *performance contexts*. In the *Uniform Terminology III* (Dunn, 1994), performance areas are defined as the "activities that the occupational therapy practitioner emphasizes when determining functional abilities" (p. 1047). They include activities of daily living, work and productive activities, and play or leisure. Performance areas are tools. Performance components "are the elements of performance that practitioners assess and, when needed, in which they intervene for improved performance" (Dunn, 1994, p. 1047). They include sensorimotor, cognitive, psychosocial, and psychological aspects. Performance components become part of the doing process. Performance contexts are "situations or factors that influence an individual's engagement in desired and/or required performance areas" (Dunn, 1994, p. 1047). Performance contexts consist of temporal aspects and environmental aspects. As such, they are examples of tools.

There seems to be an assumption that everyone knows what performance means because it's a common English word. However, when a word becomes a concept in a profession, that word needs to be defined for clarity and appropriate application within the profession. The term *performance*, like *function*, is being used to communicate multiple meanings, which may confuse rather than clarify the communication.

Although the term *performance* appears in Meyer's article (1922), the term *occupational performance* does not appear in the occupational therapy literature until 1973 in a grant report in which occupational performance is described as:

> ...the individual's ability to accomplish the tasks required by his role and related to his developmental stage. Roles include those of a pre-schooler, student, homemaker, employee, and retired worker. Occupational performance includes self-care, work and play/leisure time performance. Occupational performance requires learning and practice experiences with the role and developmental stage-specific tasks, and the utilization of all performance components. Deficits in task learning experiences, performance

> components, and/or life space, any result in limitations in occupational performance. (AOTA, 1973, p. 41)

This definition describes both the outcome (accomplish the tasks required of the role) and describes the doing process (requires learning and practice). The following year, occupational performance is defined as:

> The ability to accomplish the tasks related to a development stage; it includes the ability to develop and sustain a life style that is equally balanced among goal-directed activities—toward self-care, independence, contributions to others and gratification of personal needs. (Johnson, 1974, p. 232)

Johnson's definition primarily addresses outcome. In 1978, occupational performance is defined as "the performance of self-care, work, and play/leisure activities, the activities of daily living. The performance of these activities requires self-care, work, and play/leisure skills" (AOTA, 1978, p. 74). Nelson (1988) defines occupational performance as "the doing, the action, the active behavior, or the active responses exhibited within the context of an occupational perform" (p. 634). Clearly, Nelson is describing a doing process. Christiansen and Baum (1997) describe occupational performance as the "accomplishment of tasks related to self-care/self-maintenance, work/education, play/leisure, and rest/relaxation; the unique term used by occupational therapy to express function as it reflects the individual's dynamic experience of engaging in daily occupations within the environment" (p. 600). This is an outcome definition. Creek (1997) defines occupational performance as "the actions of the individual elicited and guided by the occupational form" (p. 529). This is a doing process definition. Hagedorn (1997) describes occupational performance as "human behavior having three areas: self-care, productivity and leisure which are based on the interaction of the individual's mental, physical, sociocultural and spiritual performance components" (p. 145). This definition suggests criteria for an outcome statement. Jackson and Banks (1997) define occupational performance as "task accomplishment in everyday living with a desirable role" (p. 460). Their definition is more consistent with the concept of tool. Townsend (1997) states that occupational performance is the "ability to choose, organize and satisfactorily perform meaningful occupations that are culturally defined and age appropriate for looking after oneself, enjoying life, and contributing to the social and economic fabric of one's community" (p. 181). Again, criteria for an outcome statement are described. Gillen and Burkhardt (1998) explain that occupational performance is the ability to accomplish the tasks required by a certain role (p. 540). This definition suggests the doing application of the concept. Punwar and Peloquin (2000) define occupational performance as "an individual's total pattern of activities, i.e., self-care, work, leisure, and organization of time" (p. 282). Yet another description of possible criteria for outcome.

A trend of usage may be appearing. Performance appears to be used more frequently in occupational therapy literature to describe a doing process in which perform and performing may appear. Occupational performance appears to be defined more in relation to a desired outcome. An important note should be addressed here. *Perform*, *performing*, and *performance* are common English words. The profession of occupational therapy can only clarify their use within the profession. The concept of occupational performance is more unique to the profession and thus, the profession can more easily direct its use. The same can be said for the concepts of performance areas, performance components, and performance contexts. These concepts developed primarily within the profession and their usage can be controlled by the profession. However, there may be some help from the new International Classification of Functioning, Disability and Health document. In the prefinal draft (WHO, 2000), performance is defined as "a construct that describes, as a qualifier, what individuals do in their current environment, and in this way, brings in the aspect of a person's involvement in life situations" (p. 166).

Balance of Occupation

Balance as related to occupation has been a concept in the occupational therapy literature from the formative years. Meyer (1922) says "...and finally the big four—work and play and rest and sleep, which our organism must be able to balance even under difficulty. The only way to attain balance in all this is *actual doing, actual practice*, a program of wholesome living as the *basis* of wholesome feeling and thinking and fancy and interests" (p. 6, italics in original text). The concept of balance was familiar to anyone who read the literature of the day. For example, Dewey (1990) originally wrote in 1900 that "the fundamental point in the psychology of an occupation is that it maintain a balance between the intellectual and the practical phases of experience" (p. 133). Reilly (1966) reestablished balance as an important concept in occupational therapy. She states that "the concept of balanced daily living" should become "highly valued by us and that skills pertaining to planning and implementing daily living schedules" should be acquired (Reilly, 1966, p. 64). Later she says that the rehabilitation milieu should be structured so it "presses for the exercising of life skills in a balanced pattern of daily living," which takes into account individual interests and abilities and is tailored to age, sex and occupational role (Reilly, 1966, p. 64). The term *balance* is not defined in Reilly's article. However, in an article based on master's thesis from the University of Southern California where Reilly was a professor, Marino-Schorn (1985-1986) elected to operationally define balance as "equality in amount" (p. 51). Mosey (1981) also seems to interpret the temporal aspect of balance to mean equal amounts. She states that "temporal adaptation refers to one's ability to satisfy these needs (work, play, and rest) in a relatively equal manner" (p. 78).

A review of the literature from the formative period does not address the concept of balance as time budgeting in terms of equal time or amounts. Hall (1910) speaks of dividing the "twenty-four hours into changeable periods of work, rest and recreation," but he did not say the time units should be equal (p. 13). In his intervention programs, however, he used 15 minute intervals as a time unit that could be interchanged equally between work, rest, or recreational tasks. Meyer (1922) also did not say the time periods should be equal. He was referring to naturally occurring rhythms such as night and day or sleep and waking hours that the person must balance. The terms *equal* or *divided equally* do not appear.

Mocellin (1995) returns to the theme of equal time, speaking of "activity balance" and reports that in Australia the 8-hour working day was established in the skilled trades in the 1850s when the idea of 8 hours of work, 8 hours of play, and 8 hours of sleep was established (p. 505). While this temporal meaning of balance may be useful in Australia, the meaning is not universal nor should it limit the concept of balance to the three divisions. Meyer, after all, said there were four: work, play, rest, and sleep. Therefore, in Meyer's scheme, the 24-hour day would be divided by four equal periods of 6 hours, not three periods of eight.

Perhaps, mention should also be made that dividing occupation into categories, except for Meyer, is also recent. Christiansen (1994) has reviewed several categorization systems in his article on classification. The division into three groups is the most common and may have been an unintended consequence of the term *occupational performance* as it was first defined in 1973, which states that "occupational performance includes self care, work, and play/leisure time performance" (AOTA, 1973, p. 41). Thereafter, the documents from the AOTA have used three groups of occupations, although the names of groups have changed over the years.

Llorens (1984) suggests another interpretation for the concept of balance. She says that "balance in the individual environment supports functional performance in activities of daily living, and independent living skills, in work and play, and learning and leisure" (p. 30). She does not suggest that balance means equal but does not provide her own definition. Spencer (1989) further elaborates this second view of balance in her definition. She defines balance as "a state of equilibrium or stability of opposing forces, harmony in the relationship of component parts, the proportion of which may or may not be equal" (Spencer, 1989, p. 90). In other words, balance is viewed as related to resolving opposing or competitive forces, not to equal amounts of time.

Christiansen and Baum (1997) do not define balance as a single word but rather define the phrase *balance of occupations* as "a belief, not substantiated by research, that a general configuration of daily occupation can contribute to health and well-being" (p. 592). Kielhofner (1985) speaks of role balance as "integration of an optimal number of appropriate roles into one's life" (p. 508). Wilcock (1998) may have had a similar idea in mind when she defines occupational balance as "a balance of engagement in occupation that leads to well-being. For example, the balance may be among physical, mental, and social occupations; between chosen and obligatory occupations; between strenuous and restful occupations; or between doing and being" (p. 257). This definition suggests there are several choices or options available to a person in achieving a balanced state. One choice or option is not automatically viewed as better than another but is left to the individual to determine. The choice may be between several types of occupation, which may be organized in a variety of temporal frameworks. The issues of choice and diversity are further supported by her definition of occupational imbalance as "a lack of balance or disproportion of occupation resulting in decreased well-being" (Wilcock, 1998, p. 257).

Christiansen (1996) has suggested the profession actually incorporates three different ideas within the concept of balance. One is the time budget approach based on the assumption that daily activities can be classified according to intrinsic characteristics and that equivalent time spent among these categories will result in improved well-being. Examples can be found in the assessment instruments called *activity configurations*. The second approach, chronobiology, suggests that well-being results when internal clocks and external behaviors (and occupations) are synchronized. The idea of natural rhythms and living in harmony with nature were popular during the founding of occupational therapy. Meyer (1922) speaks to both. The third approach, called *complementarity*, is described as "an individual's unique array of goal-oriented and time-extended endeavors or personal projects" (Christiansen, 1996, p. 447). Such an approach suggests a person may use more than one method for classifying and balancing personal occupations.

Tracking changes in the definitions and meanings of concepts provides a means of documenting changing views in the profession. The new meanings may expand or reduce the intentions of the original authors. Whether such changes are positive or negative must then be evaluated using current criteria. For example, one use of the term *balance* has not been discussed at all. That usage involves balance as "the ability to maintain a functional posture through motor actions that distribute weight evenly around the body's center of gravity" (Jacobs, 1999, p. 15). The concept of balance as it relates to equilibrium, posture, and muscle tone is not viewed as an outcome statement. Thus, it was not discussed even though the same word is used. Multiple use of the same term is common in occupational therapy literature.

Summary of Outcome Concepts

The choice of outcome criteria in occupational therapy includes a wide variety of concepts. The variety suggests several issues and possibilities that can be summarized as follows:

- There are many factors affecting outcome, both positive and negative, which may internal to the person or external in the environment. Table B-5 is a simple classification of the factors.
- There are many potential outcomes of occupational therapy services and all should be recognized as legitimate within certain service delivery systems.
- The variety of outcomes should be organized into a logical sequence such as easy to difficult, or short- term versus long-term goals.
- The variety of models of practice in occupational therapy leads to different outcomes and thus, variety is inevitable.
- Occupational therapy is based on a complex discipline of study, and different outcomes are a natural reflection of the complexity.
- Occupational therapy personnel have tried to "fit" occupational therapy practice into a number of delivery systems developed outside the field, and the outcomes for occupational therapy services reflect occupational therapy's role in those systems.
- Some outcomes may be viewed as goals to be obtained while other outcomes are stages that may occur in the process of reaching a given state. Table B-6 provides a possible organization.
- Some concepts related to outcome may be unclear and need further development and refinement to be useful as objectives and goals for establishing outcome criteria.

Table B-5

Simple Classification of Factors Affecting Outcome

	Person	*Environment*
Positive Factors	Strengths Capacities Skills Abilities Knowledge Learning potential Experience Motivation Interests Aspirations Goals Objectives Mastery Competence Achievement Attitudes (may also be negative) Accomplishments Sense of self-efficacy Sense of self-control	Therapists Enablers (may also be negative) Facilitators Consultants Social support Helpers Problem solvers Advocates Occupation (may also be negative) Activities (may also be negative) Tasks (may also be negative) Solutions Adapted equipment Assistive technology Universal design Modified/adapted environment
Negative Factors	Limitations Weaknesses Problems Needs (may also be positive) Disease Disorder Dysfunction Lack of motivation Lack of interest Lack of control Lack of confidence Lack of skill Lack of knowledge Lack of information Lack of goals Immaturity Stresses	Barriers Constraints Demands Disease-causing agents Lack of services Lack of access to services Gaps in services Delays in services Stressors Blockages Too much "red tape" Lack of or inadequate reimbursement

- More study is needed to determine what the outcome or outcomes of occupational therapy services actually are.

Any one or combination of these explanations is plausible at this time. Nevertheless, there continues to be a need for clearly articulated outcomes to occupational therapy services that can facilitate communication and interaction with consumers, other health care and education providers, and reimbursement sources.

Doing

Doing has always been a central concept in occupational therapy. However, the meaning of doing, the rationale for doing, and the organization of the doing process have been explained in many ways over the years. The verb "to do" has numerous meanings, all of which can become part of doing. Examples include act, accomplish, achieve, approve, arrange, cause,

Table B-6

Changes in Rationale for Intervention Using Occupational Therapy

Intervention Rationale	*Time Period*	*Primary Goal of "Doing" Occupational Therapy*
Moral behavior (Barton, 1987; Bockoven, 1971)	1800 to 1899	Provide consistent role model for performing daily routines. (Helped shape development of occupational therapy when it was formally recognized as a discipline)
Habit and time organization (Hall, 1905, 1910; Meyer, 1951; Slagle, 1922)	1900 to 1939 Mental Health 1966 to Present All practice areas	Re-establish/reinforce personal habits and structure the daily routine into specific units of clock time. (Mental illness is viewed as the result of "habit disorder and faulty living" and thus, habits must be corrected/reinstated and organized into a daily living routine called *habit training*)
Pragmatism (Dewey, 1902; James, 1890; Tracy, 1910)	1900 to 1939 Mental Health 1966 to Present All practice areas	Provide opportunity for experience and practice in real occupation(s). (Experience and practice shape the interpretation of ideas, the meaning of concepts, and the understanding of reality)
Curative work (Baldwin, 1919; Mock, 1918)	1918 to 1946 Physical Disabilities	Provide functional re-education and functional restoration to persons with orthopedic conditions. (Restore person to usefulness, overcome deformities, or teach new functions through use of specific voluntary movements involved in occupations)
Thought substitution (Dunton, 1915, p. 27; Farrar, 1906)	1915 to Present Mental Health	Focus attention on desired (reality-based) actions. (Will prevent the person from focusing on an undesired [hallucination, depressive thought, non-reality] thinking because brain can only focus on one thought at a time)
Emotional release and gratification (AOTA, 1958; Azima & Azima, 1959; Fidler & Fidler, 1958)	1940 to 1965 Mental Health	Provide constructive outlets in a controlled setting to meet and satisfy emotional needs. (The id, ego, and superego and/or psychosexual stages of development must be satisfied to permit the person to function normally in everyday life)
Kinetic and metric occupational therapy (Licht, 1947; Spackman, 1947)	1947 to Present Physical Disabilities	Restore or improve muscle strength, joint mobilization, and coordination. Improve work tolerance (now called the biomechanical model)
Functional training (Deaver & Brown 1945, now called rehabilitation model)	1945 to Present Physical Disabilities	Teach persons with long-term disability how to perform the physical demands of daily life using adapted or compensatory techniques and altered equipment as needed. (Persons who cannot have "normal" function restored should be taught alternate methods of performing the functional tasks of daily living)

(continued)

Table B-6

Intervention Rationale	Time Period	Primary Goal of "Doing" Occupational Therapy
Skill and role building (Muñoz & Kielhofner, 1995; Reilly, 1966; Robertson, 1998)	1966 to Present All practice areas	Gain or regain the skills that support task, role, and occupational performance in daily life. (Occupational performance requires competence in performing skills, and tasks necessary to carry out each occupational role, as expected by the situation/context in which the person lives and to the level of satisfaction, purpose, and meaning desired by the individual)
Environmental interaction (Dunning, 1972; Howe & Briggs, 1982)	1972 to Present All practice areas	Changing the context or ecological system can facilitate or hinder an occupational performance as much as changing the individual's functional skills. (The external environment should be viewed as having potential to adapt to the individual's needs and to change to promote the individual's participation)

change, clean, complete, conduct, condone, create, effect, execute, exert, explore, finish, fit, form, give, make, manage, move, pay, perform, prepare, proceed, render, serve, study, translate, travel, traverse, and work (Barnes & Noble, 1995, p. 576). The mere lack of specificity creates its own problem in explaining the role of doing in occupational therapy.

The meaning of "to do" is sometimes compared to the meaning of the verb "to occupy." Meanings provided for the word *occupy* include to take up, to fill up, to engage, to employ, to hold, to take, to control, to be a resident of, or to be a tenant of. Synonyms include use, busy, capture, and seize (Barnes & Noble, 1995, p. 1340). In essence, the meanings of the two words do not overlap. The verb "to occupy" is not a synonym for the concept of doing but rather relates to the rationale or purpose for selecting an occupation "to do" but not the process of actually doing or performing that occupation.

The rationale, explanation, or justification for "doing" in occupational therapy has been explained in several ways. Nine major rationales have been discussed in the literature, beginning with the formative ideas of occupational therapy, which can be traced to the concept of moral treatment (Bockoven, 1971). The rationales can be labeled moral (role modeling) behavior, habit and time organization, practice and experience, mechanotherapy, thought substitution, emotional release and gratification, functional training, skill and role building, and environmental interaction. Each rationale, an approximate time period, and corresponding goal(s) in occupational therapy practice has been summarized in Table B-6. Some of the rationales remain in practice today while others have been discarded, reorganized, or of limited used. Because of the influence of moral treatment on the early development of occupational therapy, some pertinent thoughts about moral behavior and treatment have been summarized in Table B-7.

Values and Beliefs About Doing

The rationales described in Table B-6 provide some explanations of why doing is viewed as important process, but do not explain why a given individual engages in doing. Polatajko (1992) and Mayer (2000) suggest there are several values or beliefs about occupation from an individual's perspective. Six of the values and beliefs can be related to doing: 1) doing occupation is a basic human need, 2) doing occupation is an essential component of life, 3) doing occupation organizes behavior, 4) doing occupation gives meaning to life, 5) doing occupation improves an individual's quality of life, and 6) doing occupation enables a healthy lifestyle. These values and beliefs provide some of the rationale for why humans do occupations based on current models of practice. The same values and beliefs support the use of occupation as a therapeutic tool that is discussed in the next section.

The values and beliefs regarding doing require special consideration because of the literature written about them. *Uniform Terminology III* (Dunn, 1994) defines values as "identifying ideas or beliefs that are important to self and others" (p. 1054). Jacobs (1999) added that values are "operational beliefs that one accepts as one's own and determines behavior" (p. 154). Punwar and Peloquin (2000) define values as "those ideas or beliefs that are intrinsically important to an individual" (p. 285). According to *Webster's New Universal Unabridged Dictionary* (Barnes & Noble, 1995), a belief involves "confidence in the truth or existence of something not immediately susceptible to rigorous proof" (p. 190). Eleven concepts were identified. Of these, the following are discussed: effectiveness, efficiency, indirect and direct focus of attention, learning by doing, meaning or meaningfulness, occupational behavior, purposeful doing and purposeful activity, and sociocultural relevant doing. The other three—busy work, moral rules, and practical doing—are summarized in Table B-8.

Effectiveness

The value of the concept of effectiveness is beginning to receive serious attention in the occupational therapy literature. Schkade and Schultz (1992) discuss effectiveness as one measure of evaluating the concept of relative mastery. They state that

Table B-7

The Influence of Moral Treatment on Occupational Therapy

- The formative ideas of occupational therapy can be traced to the concept of moral treatment (Bockoven, 1971).
- Moral treatment was used to treat moral insanity of the moral senses in the 18th and 19th centuries.
- The rationale was based on the belief that "the brain could be damaged by 'moral' agencies such as emotional stress, overwork, religious fanaticism, and self-abuse" (Barton, 1987, p. 58).
- "Any stressor of a psychological nature was referred to as a 'moral' cause of damage to the brain" (Barton, 1987, p. 58).
- There were several moral sense theories but basically they proposed that there was a special moral sense that either enabled a person to perceive special moral qualities of virtue and vice or would arouse feelings of approval or disapproval of the ordinary human actions (Bothamley, 1993).
- The philosophy of moral treatment was based on the belief that a mentally deranged person would recover moral reason in the company of persons of sound mind and kindly nature who helped the individual with the regimen of daily life (Bockoven, 1971).
- Caregivers (staff) lived with the clients in small units or houses and were with the clients at all times to provide role models and maintain the daily routine.
- Essential attitudes of the caregivers were respect for human beings as individual persons, respect for the rights of individuals under the law, and respect for the need of every individual to be engaged in creative and recreational activity with others (Bockoven, 1971).
- The ideas and ideals of moral philosophy and treatment set the stage for occupational therapy personnel to view clients from a humanitarian (kind care), humanistic (person is source of action and change), and holistic (person is an indivisible whole) perspective.
- Moral treatment broke down for three major reasons:
    - ✧ A rapid increase in the number of clients admitted to the psychiatric hospitals overwhelmed staff
    - ✧ Ethnic prejudice against new and different immigrant populations who had different cultures, attitudes, and beliefs
    - ✧ A shift in medical view from regarding mental illness as a moral-emotional problem to belief in cellular damage in the brain, which was incurable (Bockoven, 1971)

"relative mastery is the extent to which the person experiences the occupational response as... effective (production of the desired result)" (p. 835). Jacobs (1999) defines effectiveness as the "degree to which the desired result is produced" (p. 47). Hagedorn (2000) suggests that "the effective level is the level of occupation at which productive, meaningful activities are performed in order to enable the individual to achieve an adaptive fit with the individual's environment, which enhances and maintains survival, health and well-being" (p. 308).

Webster's New Universal Unabridged Dictionary (Barnes & Noble, 1995) defines effective as "adequate to accomplish a purpose; producing the intended or expected result" (p. 622). Synonyms include capable or competent, and closely related concepts are effectual, efficacious, and efficiency. The concept of effective doing or doing that is effective is probably part of the subculture or "underground practice" of occupational therapy. The idea is so ingrained it has only recently surfaced for careful analysis. The knowledge of occupational therapy practice could be further enhanced by studying what constitutes "effective doing" and how occupational therapy personnel can promote in the client "doing which is effective?"

Efficiency

Like effectiveness, the concept of efficiency is an old idea but has only recently received serious attention in the occupational therapy literature. Hall (1905) states that "it is hoped that the treatment of work will... substitute a simple but positive efficiency which will reorganize the life of the individual on better lines" (p. 32). Schkade and Schultz (1992) use efficiency in relation to relative mastery: "Relative mastery is the extend to which the person experiences the occupational response as efficient (use of time and energy)" (p. 835). *Webster's New Universal Unabridged Dictionary* (Barnes & Noble, 1995) defines efficient as "performing or functioning in the best possible manner with the least waste of time and effort" and "having and using requisite knowledge, skills, and industry" (p. 622). Synonyms include competent, capable, and reliable. These descriptions seem to relate to the treatment methods of work simplification, motion economy, and energy conservation. Thus, efficiency appears to

Table B-8

Other Concepts Concerned With Doing

Busy Work

- Dewey (1900) may have set the tone for occupational therapy regarding busy work in his statement first published in *The School and Society*: "By occupation is not meant any kind of 'busy work' or exercises that may be given to a child in order to keep him out of mischief or idleness when seated at his desk. By occupation I mean a mode of activity on the part of the child when reproduces, or runs parallel to, some form of work carried on in social life" (p. 132).
- Idleness was viewed as a major causative factor in the loss of health.
- The issue of what constitutes valued work (business) and what is simply keeping a person "out of mischief or idleness" has been a issue in occupational therapy for many years.
- Woodside (1976) may summarize the current view by stating, "Do not simply keep clients busy. Maintain a relationship which rests on feedback, dialogue, pacing and guidance" (p. 13).
- The concept of real work or business is elusive. For example:
    - ✧ Must real work be performed or can it be discussed and planned at one time to be performed later?
    - ✧ Must persons who are acutely deconditioned perform real work or can selected tasks, single actions, or simulated work be used until the person has regained some endurance and cognitive skills are functioning?

Moral Rules

- Moral rules of right conduct is probably the oldest value related to doing from the preformative years of occupational therapy. The use or moral or following the rules of right conduct was the basis for moral treatment.
- *The Concise Oxford Dictionary* (Thompson, 1995) defines moral as concerned with goodness or badness of human character or behavior or with the distinction between right and wrong. It continues by stating the moral is concerned with accepted rules and standards of human behavior.
- These ideas are not often expressed as the rationale for asking or guiding clients into doing certain tasks but the moral implication is often apparent. Teaching dressing skills does require motor and cognitive skills but putting on clothes is also a required moral act in society when a person enters a social setting especially in the community.
- More often, occupational therapy personnel write about the cultural customs that are closely related but not necessarily the same. Moral behavior may have legal consequences whereas customs may have social sanctions that do not include legal consequences.
- Moral rules and the result, moral behavior, are another example of a concept without definition in current occupational therapy literature. Several occupational therapy textbooks talk about moral treatment as a historical treatment approach but do not discuss the embedded concept of moral rules as they apply to choices of intervention strategies today.
- The only concept that comes close to this topic is Reilly's (1974) interest in Piaget's discussion of rule-bound behavior in her chapter "Defining a Cobweb."

Practical Doing

- The concept of practical doing or doing what is practical dates to the formative years. Upham (1918b) states:

    > An occupation may be said to be practical which in some way trains or prepares the patient for his future vocation or employment. An occupation which is merely time-wasting and which contributes no improved knowledge or skill or awakened interest and which possess no special therapeutic advantages may be said to be trivial and useless. That occupation is most practical which best restores the patient's mental and physical vigor. After this first consideration that occupation is most useful which is most closely related to his economic future. (p. 36)

(continued)

Table B-8

- Practicality is a cornerstone to the pragmatic philosophy. *Webster's New Universal Unabridged Dictionary* (Barnes & Noble, 1995) defines pragmatism as "a philosophical movement or system having various forms, but generally stressing practical consequences as constituting the essential criterion in determining meaning, truth, or value" (p. 1518).
- *The Concise Oxford Dictionary* (Thompson, 1995) makes a similar statement. Pragmatism is "a philosophy that evaluates assertions solely by their practical consequences and bearing on human interests" (p. 1073).
- Current occupational therapy literature does not seem to reflect the idea of doing what is practical. Instead, the current term seems to be doing what is meaningful or purposeful.
- Is the concept of practical doing a subconcept within the ideas of meaningfulness or purposefulness or is it an overlooked concept that should be reinstated in current models of practice?

be a type or quality of doing valued in occupational therapy practice. Additional clarification may enhance the understanding of how efficiency or efficient doing can benefit clients in their daily lives. On the other hand, some rituals or ceremonies are probably not efficient in terms of time, effort, knowledge, or skills. In what situations is nonefficiency acceptable or even desirable in human occupation?

Indirect and Direct Focus of Attention

Doing can be focused indirectly or directly on the person's problems and was the subject of an ongoing debate in the formative years of the profession. Upham (1918b) summarized the debate as follows:

> ...the concrete value of occupation is its power to turn the patient's attention away from his disability... into healthy channels of interest and effort. This is especially necessary for patients inclined to self-analysis and morbid introspection. There is... (a)... group of occupational therapists who believe the patient's disability should be uppermost in his mind. They related the occupation so closely to his disability that he is keenly conscious that occupation is a fundamental part of his cure. He is taught to be faithful in that occupation as he would be in taking a drug... (p. 18).

Which side of the debate a practitioner took frequently depended on whether mental or physical disabilities were being addressed. In mental disability, the approach to health and living often includes redirecting attention away from the symptoms and behaviors that lead to dysfunctional living. In place of the dysfunctional behavior, attempts are made to attract the person's attention to more healthy and useful behaviors. Therefore, the person was asked to do occupations that redirected attention from immediate problems. In contract, in physical disabilities, frequently the focus of attention was directed to the dysfunction so that weakened muscles can be strengthened, range of motion can be increased, and endurance improved, for example. Specific occupations directed at the dysfunction were assumed necessary for the objectives to be obtained.

Both approaches are valued today. In many cases, occupations are selected that directly address the nature of the person's problems. On the other hand, a person in pain may need occupations that focus awareness away from the particular location of that pain toward some other situation or object, which can command attention. As attention is refocused, awareness and response to pain may decrease. Perhaps the real issue is to understand when to select occupations that will most benefit the client at a particular point in the therapeutic process. More study is needed to clarify whether to focus doing and attention indirectly or directly on the identified client problems.

Learning by Doing

Learning by doing is a basic principle of the pragmatic philosophy. Although learning is a central part of the doing process, the value of learning was discussed only in the term *learning academic subjects* in the early literature. In 1977, Hopkins and Smith defined learning as the "relatively permanent change in behavior or in the capacity for behavior resulting from either experience or practice" (p. 734). Both experience and practice require doing an occupation. Christiansen and Baum (1991) state that learning is:

> The enduring ability of an individual to comprehend and/or competently respond to changes in information from the environment and/or from within the self. As one learns about the environment, alterations occur in the definition of the self and possible behaviors; as one learn about the self, alterations occur in the definition of the environment and possible behaviors. (p. 855)

The focus of this definition is the contribution of learning through doing on the development of the self. Mosey (1994) states that learning is:

> A process wherein there is a change in an individual's behavior in a given situation brought about by repeated experience in that situation, providing that the behavior cannot be explained on the basis of native response tendencies, maturation, or temporary states of the organism such as fatigue or drugs. (p. 26)

In other words, learning through doing changes a person's behavior. Learning is a permanent change in behavior as a result of experience and practice according to Schmidt (1988) as stated in Poole (1995, p. 265).

Learning may also be modified by an adjective. For example, Pedretti and Umphred (1996) use another definition of Schmidt's (1991) for motor learning, which is "a set of processes associated with practice or experience leading to relatively permanent changes in the capability for responding" (p. 65). Kielhofner

(1985) defines formal learning as "the transmission of cultural norms in situations where right and wrong ways of doing something are so taken for granted that explanations are not given" (p. 504). He also defines informal learning as " the transmission of cultural norms through imitation of role models, trial and error, and other intuitive processes that tend to be difficult to describe or pin down" (p. 504). Kielhofner's definitions could have been included in the section on socially and culturally relative doing, which is discussed later.

The importance of the relationship of learning to doing is apparent. Therefore, the lack of attention to learning as a doing process in occupational therapy textbooks is surprising. Perhaps, the obvious is easy to overlook. Of special concern should be the types of learning approaches and which is useful for what disability, especially where cognitive disabilities are involved.

Meaning or Meaningfulness

The concepts of meaning or meaningfulness and their opposites, meaningless or meaninglessness, do not appear as issues in the early literature on occupational therapy. The first definitions appear in 1985. Kielhofner speaks of the meaningfulness of activities as "an individual's disposition to find importance, security, worthiness and purpose in particular occupations" (Kielhofner, 1985, p. 505). Nelson (1988) says that "meaning or meaningfulness is the term to be used in labeling the individual's interpretation of the occupational form" and that "meaningfulness refers both to the perceptual sense it makes to the individual as well as to the cognitive associations elicited in the individual" (p. 635). In 1994, he defines meaning as "the entire interpretive process in which an individual engages when encountering an occupational form" (p. 21). Christiansen and Baum (1997) explain:

> Meanings reflect our overall interpretations of life events. Most of our intentions and actions are filled with meaning. This meaning comes from the nature of a situation and how we interpret its significance based on our current goals, values and past experiences. There are individual meanings and collective or shared meanings" (p.53)

They define the word *meaning* as "the personal significance of an event as interpreted by an individual" (Christiansen & Baum, 1997, p. 599). Meaninglessness is lack of belief in the value, usefulness, or importance of daily occupations or lives (Christiansen & Baum, 1997, p. 599). Hagedorn (2000) suggests there is a problem with therapeutic meaningful doing because it is often simulated doing and performed in a protected and artificial environment.

As stated above the concept of meaningful occupation or meaningfulness came into the occupational therapy literature in the modern period. The early literature contains the concept of interest and focuses on productivity and social usefulness. The term appears to be closely related to the concept of purpose. In *Webster's New Universal Unabridged Dictionary* (Barnes & Noble, 1995), the words *meaning* and *meaningful* both list the word *purpose* as a synonym. Perhaps the intent of using the term *meaningful* or *meaningfulness* is an attempt to expand the idea of practical or purposeful doing.

Occupational Behavior

Behavior as a means of doing has been accepted in the occupational therapy literature for many years. The term *occupational behavior*, however, was introduced by Reilly in 1966 when she stated that "society programs its members for occupational behavior through sequential experience in play, family living, school and recreation" and that "occupational behavior is developmentally acquired and is capable of being divided into various substrates for corrective purposes" (p. 64). In 1969, Reilly provides a definition of the concept, stating that occupational behavior is the "entire developmental continuum of work and play" (p. 302). Matsutsuyu (1969) expanded Reilly's idea of occupational behavior by suggesting the "adult occupational behavior reflects an attempt to assimilate oneself into some identified group that meets one's own need for productivity, belonging, and life structuring activities" (p. 292). In 1973, occupational behavior was defined as "the person's use of time, energy, and attention to rest, play, and work" (Johnson, 1973, pp. 160-161). A more comprehensive definition was provided by Woodside, a student of Reilly's, in 1976, "Occupational behavior is that aspect of growth and development represented by the developmental continuum of play and work as they support competency, achievement, and occupational role" (p. 11).

Additional definitions have expanded the concept of occupational behavior. In 1977, occupational behavior was defined as "organization and action based on skills, knowledge, and attitudes to make functioning possible in life roles" (Hopkins & Smith, 1997, p. 735). In 1997, Christiansen and Baum state that occupational behavior is "the set of responses which allow the individual to maintain role competence" (p. 433). In the same year, Law et al. state occupational behavior "is that aspect or class of human action that encompasses mental and physical doing" (1997a, p. 40). Finally, Creek (1997) says that occupational behavior is the "active engagement in occupation" (p. 529). Jacobs (1999) states that occupational behavior is a "set of responses which allow the individual to maintain role competence" (p. 97). Punwar and Peloquin (2000) define occupational behavior as "those behaviors or activities that an individual engages in to fulfill his or her occupational roles" (p. 282).

This is a good example of how terms evolve in a profession beyond the original parameters. Reilly does not include phrases such as skills, knowledge, and attitudes; make functioning possible; maintain role competence; encompasses mental and physical doing; or active engagement in occupation. She did, however, stress that occupational behavior was a developmental continuum involving work and play. Woodside (1976) added "support competency, achievement, and occupational role," which may be assumed to be acceptable to Reilly. Concepts that take on a life of their own, may stray considerably from the original meaning. Redefinition is not necessarily undesirable but failure to acknowledge that new definitions have been written does create a discontinuity of thought about the concept and confusion in the minds of the readers.

Purposeful Doing and Purposeful Activity

Purposeful doing has been widely used as a concept in occupational therapy literature. The most common phrase is purposeful activity. The phrase may have been adopted from the literature of the early 20th century. Dewey (1916) uses the phrase in talking about work: "Like play, it (work) signifies purposeful activity and differs not in that activity is subordinated to an external result, but in the fact that a longer course of activity is occasioned by the idea of a result" (p. 204). Burnette (1918) states, "This improved state is our chance to turn the awakened activities towards more purposeful and dignified occupation" (p. 11). Upham (1919) states, "In all countries purposeful exercise has been found the expedient way to cure weakened muscles and stiffened joints" (p. 211). (*Note*: Purposeful exercise is related to active doing as opposed to passive.) Perhaps the best explanation for purposeful activity comes from Bowman (1922) when she explains that "... the fundamental principle of occupational therapy is a psychological principle: the substitution of a coordinated, purposeful activity, mental or physical, for scattered activities or the idleness which comes with weakened body or mind" (p. 172).

Mosey (1981) provides a current definition, stating, "Purposeful activities are doing processes directed toward a planned or hypothesized end result. They provide an opportunity for investigating, trying out and gaining evidence of one's capacities for experiencing, responding managing, creating and controlling" (p. 62). Hinojosa, Sabari, and Pedretti (1993) state that "an activity is purposeful if the individual is an active, voluntary participant and if the activity is directed toward a goal that the individual considers meaningful... Purposeful activity is goal-directed behaviors or tasks that comprise occupations" (p. 1081). Christiansen and Baum (1997) provide a short-hand definition, stating that purposeful activities are "actions which are goal directed" (p. 602). Punwar and Peloquin (2000) define purposeful activity as "meaningful occupation; an occupation with a goal" (p. 283).

The idea of purpose and doing in occupational therapy probably began with the philosophy of pragmatism as the statement by Dewey (1916) suggests. However, there were psychologists whose primary interest was purposive psychology. Of these, William M. McDougall (1923) and Edward C. Tolman (1932) are best known. Peters (1953) summarizes the assumptions of purposive psychology as 1) all behavior is purposive and that 2) there are certain innate goal-seeking tendencies (p. 669). The development of purposive psychology parallels the early years of occupational therapy. Basically, purposive psychology is "the doctrine that behavior is distinguished from purely mechanical change or from physiological activity... (English & English, 1958, p. 432). Purposiveness has a history of controversy according to English & English (1958):

> Some theorists regard purposiveness as an inadmissable concept in science because it cannot be directly observed. Others use purposiveness as the defining characteristic of human behavior. A third group distinguish between purposive behavior, in which persistent striving is clearly evident, and nonpurposive behavior in which striving, if present, is not so evident. (p. 432)

If occupational therapy model builders and theorists are using purpose as one type of behavior in which an aim, end, plan, result, or goal is established to be attained by the person, the study of pragmatic philosophy should be the focus for clarification of the concept. If, on the other hand, occupational therapy model builders view purpose as purposiveness, in which all behavior is viewed as having a purpose, then the works of McDougall and Tolman should be studied further. The statement of *The Philosophic Base of Occupational Therapy* (AOTA, 1979b) appears to using purposeful activity as the primary or central means of facilitating adaptation. If this interpretation is correct, occupational therapy is using purposive psychology as an important source of philosophical base.

However, a third use of the concept of purpose relates to the values or beliefs a society or culture has about various types of doing. Certain "doings" are usually more valued than others. Purpose in doing can be related to the project or product and to the use of the time needed to do it. Making a buggy or horsewhip may be important to a society that uses buggies and horses for transportation. Thus, making buggy whips becomes a "good" use of time. A society that relies on fossil fuels or nuclear power may find little use for buggy whips and consider the making of a whip a waste of time. As is evident, therefore, use of the concept of purpose or purposiveness is not simple or straight forward. Occupational therapy model builders and theorists need to clarify the concept of purpose as a means of explaining human behavior within and without the profession.

Sociocultural Relevant Doing

The issue of socially and culturally relevant doing began to surface in the 1970s. Klavins (1972) was one of the first to point out the work and play had different values and beliefs in different cultures and subcultures. For example, culture determines what sort of play experiences are encouraged or permitted. What constitutes a good job in one society may be considered unacceptable in other.

Uniform Terminology III (Dunn, 1994) defines social as "availability and expectations of significant individuals, such as spouse, friends, and caregivers. Also includes larger social groups which are influential in establishing norms, role expectations, and social routines" (p. 1054). The same document defines cultural in this way:

> Customs, beliefs, activity patterns, behavior standards, and expectations accepted by the society of which the individual is a member. Includes political aspects, such as laws that affect access to resources and affirm personal rights. Also includes opportunities for education, employment and economic support. (p. 1054)

Kielhofner (1985) defines culture as "the beliefs and perception, values and norms, and customs and behaviors that are shared by a group or society and passed from one generation to the next through both formal and informal education" (p. 503). Christiansen and Baum (1991) state that culture is "patterns of behavior learned through the socialization process, including anything acquired by humans as members of society: knowledge, values, beliefs, laws, morals, customs, speech patterns, economic production patterns, etc." (p. 850). Cara and MacRae (1998) state that culture is "a conscious and unconscious internal process of identification with overt manifestations of traditions, beliefs and values, often involving the use of objects, which guide human beings in organizing their lives" (p. 667).

Ryan (1992) defines cultural shift as "movement in response to societal forces that results in a dynamic change" (p. 359). Clark, Ennevor, and Richardson (1996) define cultural place as "the place in which development occurs, the ecology and locally adapted environment which includes meanings, beliefs, values and conventional practice learned and shared by members of a community" (p. 390).

The relationship of doing and sociocultural issues has always been recognized to some degree as a significant issue in occupational therapy evaluation and intervention strategies. However, the full impact is beginning to be understood as multiculturalism becomes a larger factor in the delivery of occupational therapy services. Doing is a multifaceted concept that will require additional study to understand and use as a therapeutic process.

Related Concepts

There are several concepts that are related to doing. These concepts organize doing into sequences, patterns, or chains of doing which are done with regular frequency or are memorized and written down to be done in a certain way. The concepts have a common theme of being familiar or known to the person performing them. These related concepts include habit, interests, motivation and intrinsic motivation, role, routine, and volition. Flow, learning style, and ritual are mentioned in Table B-9.

Habit

The concept of habit has been discussed in the occupational therapy literature since the early years. Hall (1905) talks about the potential of systematic work for a patient to "...change his occupation and habits of life" (p. 30). Upham (1918a) states that the instructors in occupational therapy should be able "...to develop in them (war invalids) regular habits of work, habits which are self-disciplinary and will render the mean valuable members of civil communities" (p. 18). Slagle continues the dialogue about habits by saying, "Occupation used remedially serves to overcome some habits, to modify others and construct new ones, to the end that habit reaction will be favorable to the restoration and maintenance of health" (1922, p. 14). Meyer summarizes the view of habits common to the formative years of occupational therapy by stating:

> Habits are the essential fabric of the reactive resources of the organism. The doing of things forms the basic structure of the mental life, and habit formation is a process that applies to every item of human. Habits of action and bringing things to completion are the basic conative resources of the organism. Disorganization of habits is the deterioration of the learned but fundamental ways of meeting life. (1951, p. 201)

Habit continued to be an important concept into the 1930s as evidenced by Pollack (1938) who said that "habit, as is well known, is responsible for practically all the daily activities of an individual, comprising as they do the habits of dressing, eating, drinking, speech, thought, play or work" (p. 292). Pollack, a physician, knew how to get the attention of his occupational therapy audience. He said all the right words.

The current view of habits is expressed by Kielhofner (1985) as "images guiding the routine and typical ways in which a person performs" (p. 504). In 1995, Kielhofner added habits are defined as "latent tendencies acquired from previous repetitions, mainly operating at a preconscious level and influencing a wide range of behavioral patterns that correspond to familiar habitats" (p. 65). Trombly (1995a) defines habits as "chains of subroutines that are so well learned that the person does not have to pay attention to do them under ordinary circumstances" (p. 19). Parham and Fazio (1997b) state that habits are "skills that are performed so routinely that they have become automatic" and they "allow for efficiency in daily occupations" (p. 250). Neistadt and Crepeau (1998) explain that a habit is "automatic behavior that is integrated into more complex patterns that enable people to function on a day-to-day basis; skills that are habituated are typically performed easily and with little effort" (p. 869). A summary of key assumptions in these definitions are that habit formation is useful; that habits are learned and can be changed or modified through new learning; that habits can facilitate the attainment of a positive health status; that habits can organize a person's life, can simplify life and reduce energy demand; that habits can disorganize a person's life; that habits have an automatic and repetitive quality; that habits are mental or cognitive operations but may function with little conscious attention, that habits affect a range of behaviors and that habits are most likely to occur in familiar contexts..

Dunn (2000) has taken the concept of habit one step further and suggested that there is a continuum of habit beginning with habit impoverishment, followed by habit utility and habit domination. Habit impoverishment occurs when "habits are not established and cannot support daily life" (p. 8S). Examples given are ADHD and depression. Habit utility occurs when "habits support performance in daily life and contribute to life satisfaction" and there is the "ability to follow rhythms of daily life" (p. 8S). Habit domination is a situation in which "habits are so inherent that they interfere with daily life" (p. 8S). Examples given are autism, addiction, and obsessive-compulsive disorder. Kielhofner (1985) may have had a similar idea in mind when he defined degree of organization in habits as "the degree to which one has a typical use of time which supports competent performance in a variety of environments and roles and provides a balance of activity" (p. 503) and rigidity/flexibility of habits as "the degree to which a person is able to change routines of behavior to accommodate periodic contingencies" (p. 508). Yet another aspect of habit is added by Kielhofner (1985) when he defines the social appropriateness of habits as "the degree to which one's typical behaviors are those expected and valued by the environments in which one performs" (p. 508).

The word *habit* derives from the Latin verb *habere*, meaning "to have" and ordinally referred to external appearance, manner or bearing such that one would recognize a person or class of persons. Reading (1994), a psychologist, says there are two key elements. First, the behavior is evoked by a group of conditions, which in turn are dependent on an intrinsic "set," disposition, or readiness to response to those conditions. Second, a habit is "always acquired, representing the end-product of a process of learning" (p. 478). Reading also points out that the concept of habit has been used to refer to a frequently repeated act such as

Table B-9

Other Concepts Related to the Doing Process

Flow

- Flow is a concept developed and defined by Csikszentmihalyi over several years of work which culminated in books published in 1975, 1988, and 1990. According to Csikszentmihalyi, he began studying optimal experience leading to the use of the concept of flow with his doctoral dissertation in 1965 at the University of Chicago.
- Flow began appearing in occupational therapy literature in the 1990s. Jacobs (1994) describes flow as "a positive feeling that occurs when there is a balance between perceived challenges and one's skills, and may include enjoyment, intense or total involvement, deep concentration or the loss of one's sense of time" (p. 989).
- Christiansen and Baum (1997) define flow as a "term describing the subjective quality of an experience" (p. 596).
- Neistadt and Crepeau (1998) expand the explanation as a "state of deep concentration in which consciousness is well ordered; elements present are a feeling of control, loss of self-consciousness, transformation of time, and concentration on the task at hand" (p. 868).
- Wilcock (1998) defines flow as "a state of consciousness when people are so involved in an activity that nothing else seems to matter; of optimal experience, transcendence, and enjoyment when individuals are challenged but engaged within the scope of their abilities" (p. 255).
- Rebeiro and Polgar (1999) suggest that "flow may be useful in understanding those aspects of the occupation, environment and person that contribute to a 'just right' challenge, and to enabling occupational performance through enjoyable, structured and purposeful activity" (p. 14).
- Flow appears to have a relationship to the doing process as developed within occupational therapy:
    - ✧ Additional studies should clarify at what point flow can be identified along a continuum of doing. Such identification might be a marker toward a desired outcome such as adaptation, health, or wellness.
    - ✧ Another aspect to be explored is the role of attention or concentration that must be available or attained for the flow experience to occur. For example, is it possible for a person with a short attention span to attain flow?
    - ✧ Finally, can occupational therapy personnel assess the qualities or characteristics needed for a person to experience flow?

Learning Style

- The concept of learning styles or modes in relation to clients has received little attention in the occupational therapy literature.
- Turner, Foster, and Johnson (1996) is the only major text to mention learning style as an issue. However, the focus is on the practitioner's knowledge of styles of learning and not on the effect of the style on the doing process.
- Trombly (1995b) does devote a chapter to learning but only generally addresses the effect of the learning style on client's doing in the occupational therapy setting.
- Of potential value to practitioners would be whether instruction should be focused more on visual input versus auditory input for some clients.
- Much of the current instruction appears to be auditory with visual demonstration used only when auditory does not get the desired response. Persons with visual preference learning styles may be at a disadvantage in doing what the practitioner requests. Could the disadvantage slow the progress of intervention and achievement of goals and outcomes?
- How much learning time is wasted giving instruction in the learning style less effective for a particular client? In these days of limited client contact time, using the preferred learning style might increase therapy efficiency and effectiveness.

(continued)

Table B-9

Ritual

- The concept of ritual does not appear in the literature with any frequency until 1987.
- Low (1987) writes about ritual time "as the texture of experience, with patterns overlapping, interwoven, leading in all directions through all dimensions, like movement in dance" (p. 19).
- The first definition of rituals located is by do Rozario (1994) who defines them as "mythological activities and symbolic expression" (p. 48).
- Christiansen and Baum (1997) suggest that rituals are "patterns of behavior that have strong elements of symbolism attached to them" (p. 603).
- Crepeau (1994) states that "ritual is distinguished from day-to-day routine by its connection to the symbols, beliefs, and values of the social group" (p. 6). She continues by stating that "ritualization structures social life and imbues it with meaning... Rituals have two major characteristics: repetition and dramatic presentation. Rituals involve repetition of occasion, content, or form. Occasion such as weddings, funerals, holiday celebrations, family dinners, and work-related meetings. Content refers to the particular words or actions of a ritual. Form refers to the sequence of actions" (p. 9).
- *Webster's New Universal Unabridged Dictionary* (Barnes & Noble, 1995) includes twelve definitions for the term *ritual*. Among these are four dealing with religious and worship services, two concern books containing rites, one is from psychiatry, and two pertain to a ritual or rite. Other definitions have a broader application such as a prescribed or established rite, ceremony, proceeding, or service; any practice or pattern of behavior regularly performed in a set manner; and a prescribed code of behavior regulating social conduct (p. 1661).
- Corsini (2002) provides three definitions for ritual: 1) An elaborate formal process usually art of a celebration; 2) a ceremonial procedure, repeated in the same way over a long period of time, usually conducted during religious and fraternal services, the military and other settings; and 3) an established formal ceremony, often used to mark an important occasion, for example, baptism, bar mitzvah, burials, citizenship-granting, indoctrination, and marriage (p. 848).
- At this point, the concept of ritual has not been widely used in the profession. There may be some resistance from practitioners in mental health and psychiatry because of the close relationship between ritual behavior and obsessive compulsive behavior as a problem. The consideration of ritual behavior as energy conservation and stress reduction has not appeared in occupational therapy literature to date. There may be some value in exploring the concept further.

getting dressed or to modes of thinking leading to a particular attitude or value. Reference may be made to one instance of doing as a habit or to a broad range of doings over an extended period of time. Habit may be viewed as one type of learning that humans use to organize their lives or be viewed as the only mechanism used to develop verbal, manual, and emotional acts. Thus, habit may be used in a variety of ways. Occupational therapy personnel must be sure to keep the meaning of the concept clearly in mind when using the term *habit*.

Interests

Interest is another term that appeared in the early literature of occupational therapy. The major supporter of the concept of interest was Dr. Dunton. In 1918, he says that "...any form of work to be curative must be able to create some interest for the patient" (p. 318). In 1928, he defines interest as follows: "By interest is meant the state of consciousness in which the attention is attracted to a task, companies by a more or less pleasurable emotional state" (p. 6). The pragmatist philosopher William James is probably one source of influence. In his famous text (1890), he states, "Only those items which I notice shape may mind—without selective interest, experience is an utter chaos. Interest alone gives accent and emphasis, light and shade, background and foreground—intelligible perspective, in a word" (p. 402). Matsutsuyu (1969) suggests that "interests are described as feelings, drives or reactions which are interest states and related to attitudes, values and other motivation indices such as attention, direction and sentiments" (p. 324). In her study, she suggested that there are six assumptions about interests:

1. Interests are family influenced.
2. Interests evoke affective response.
3. Interests are choice states.
4. Interests can be manifest in effective action.
5. Interest can sustain action.
6. Interests reflect self-perception.

Borys (1974) suggests that interests are "developmentally permanent, learned and related to achievement" (p. 36). She summarizes the major issues and influences in interest theories as developmental learning, motivational learning, choice, and personality development and self-concept. Ryan (1993) states that interests are "activity that the individual finds pleasurable...and... are those that maintain one's attention" (p. 361). *Uniform Terminology III* (Dunn, Foto, et al., 1994) defines interests as "identifying mental or physical activities that create pleasure and maintain attention" (p. 1054). Kielhofner (1997) defines interests as "dispositions to find pleasure and satisfaction in occupations, and the self-knowledge of our enjoyment of occupations; encompasses attraction and preference " (p. 207). Punwar and Peloquin (2000) state that interests are "those mental or physical activities that create pleasure and maintain attention" (p. 281). Stein & Roose (2000) provide an extensive definition:

> Psychological components that include an individual's choice in engaging in activities such as sports, reading, music, films, theater, arts and crafts, cuisine, and table games. The motivation to engage in activities depends upon the opportunities available to the individual, ability to do the activity, and the pleasure related to the activity. (p. 131)

The concept of interest is established in the occupational therapy literature and basic elements of the concept have been identified. However, the concept has not won wide acceptance in occupational therapy practice except in the area of leisure due to the popularity of the Interest Check List (Matsutsuyu, 1969). Occupational therapy theorists and practitioners should consider giving the concept of interest more attention. The concept of interest would seem to be highly related to the concept of meaning and meaningfulness. Both seem to address such ideas as likes and dislikes, preferences, and willingness to engage in a particular occupation. What are the similarities and differences between meaning and interest? Do interests express meaningfulness? Kielhofner (1985) has suggested as much when he defines discrimination of interests as "the degree to which one differentiates a liking or expectation of enjoyment in certain occupations" (p. 503).

Motivation and Intrinsic Motivation

The concept of motivation, especially intrinsic motivation or effectance motivation, appears in 1969. Florey (1969) says that there is general agreement that the "motivational construct refers to a mediating system, process, or mechanisms that attempts to account for the purposive aspects of behavior" (p. 319). She suggests that "intrinsic motivation builds toward self-reward in independent action that underlies competent behavior" (p. 320). In 1977, Hopkins and Smith defined intrinsic motivation as the "will to act based on personal internal standards incentives, desires, and needs" (p. 734). Sharrott and Cooper-Fraps (1986) defined intrinsic motivation as "a biologically inherent or innate urge to explore and master the environment," which is characterized by the desire to be a causative agent resulting in behavior that is self-satisfying. Creek (1997) defines intrinsic motivation as "an innate drive to use one's capacity for action" (p. 529). In the same year, Parham and Fazio (1997a) state that intrinsic motivation is "a prompt to action that comes from within the individual and is not prompted by outside influence" and a "drive to action that is rewarded by the doing of the activity itself rather than some external reward. Intrinsic motivation is widely accepted as an essential ingredient of play" (p. 250). Jacobs (1999) states that intrinsic motivation is a "concept in human development that proposes that people develop in response to an inherent need for exploration and activity" (p. 72). Punwar and Peloquin (2000) suggest that intrinsic motivation is "motivation that comes from within the individual; self-motivation" (p. 281). Stein & Roose (2000) define intrinsic motivation as "the internal motivation to achieve or perform an activity without external rewards. For example, an artist will continue painting without expecting any reward or praise. Individuals with intrinsic motivation have an internal locus of control" (p. 132).

Deci (1975), a psychologist, defines intrinsic motivations as "behaviors which a person engages in to feel competent and self-determining" (p. 61). He continues by saying that the primary effects of intrinsic motivation are on the tissues of the central nervous system, not on non-nervous system tissues. He states there are two types of intrinsic motivation. One occurs where there is no stimulation and the person seeks it out. A person who does not get stimulation will not feel competent and self-determining. The other kind of intrinsic motivation occurs when a person attempts to conquer challenges or reduce incongruity that reduces dissonance. In conquering the challenges, the person feels competent and self-determining. An individual seeks out pleasurable stimulation and deals with any overstimulation effectively. Therefore, the individual is able to engage in seeking and conquering challenges that are optimal for that person. Reber (1995) defines intrinsic motivation as "any behavior that is dependent on factors that are internal in origin" (p. 387) and is derived from feelings of satisfaction and fulfillment. Corsini (1999) defines intrinsic motivation with two definitions. The first is "behavior done for its own sake rather than for some kind of reward or payoff, for example, fishing for the pleasure of doing so versus fishing to make a living" and "the intellectual satisfaction derived form the understanding of a meaningful solution: engaging in an activity for its own sake" (p. 505).

Although the term *intrinsic motivation* is fairly new in the occupational therapy literature, the concept itself is probably very old. For example, Dunton (1925) discusses the use of upholstery as a therapeutic medium. He says "There are numerous small problems constantly arising which must be solved... Their solutions may demonstrate a variety of mental mechanisms. It is believed that this has much to with creating enjoyment in the task, but there also seems to be a marked satisfaction when the work has been completed" (p. 221). When a client is willing to continue a task with many steps and shows enjoyment in dealing with "small problems," one interpretation might be that intrinsic motivation is occurring. There are probably many more examples.

Doble (1988) has suggested there are four determinants of intrinsic motivation that influence the amount and use of the concept within an individual. The determinants are identified as the orientation of the person to the task environment, meaningfulness of the activity to the person, provision of opportunities for personal control, and generation of feelings of competence. Consideration of the four determinants suggests a variety of possible responses on the part of the person that affect the doing process.

Intrinsic motivation is thus an example of a term being created outside the field but brought into the field to explain a phenomenon that had existed for some time. The term and concept increase the clarity of communication about the phenomenon.

Role and Occupational Role

The concept of role entered the occupational therapy literature as an important concept in 1966 when Reilly talked about occupational role but did not define it. Moorhead (1969), a student of Reilly's, states that the role concept:

> ...has been constructed as a frame of reference for conceptualizing man's interaction with his human and task-oriented environment. Social roles are viewed as institutionally prescribed and proper ways for an individual to participate in society and thus satisfy his needs and wants. (p. 329)

She continues her discussion by stating that occupational role is one of three types of roles used in sociology. The other two are family roles and personal-sexual roles. Occupational role can be identified by social position and by the tasks performed. Matsutsuyu (1969), another student of Reilly's, adds that the concept occupational role includes "housewife, student, retiree, and preschooler as well as worker" (p. 292). Moorhead (1969) also suggests that people identify each other by the occupational roles they perform and that the roles become incorporated into a personal identification system.

Writers in occupational therapy do not consistently distinguish the concept of role from occupational role. The reader should probably assume that role and occupational role are synonyms when reading occupational therapy literature unless the writer defines the terms or concepts differently. Several examples appear in Table B-10. They can be summarized as follows: A role is a set of socially agreed upon exceptions, functions, or obligations that involve patterns, scripts, or codes of behavior, routines, habits, and occupation that a person assumes and which become part of that person's social identity.

Creek (1997) states that an occupational role is "the main social position held by an individual and the tasks performed in that position, for example, student, worker or volunteer" (p. 529). Parham and Fazio (1997a) define occupational role as "the expected pattern of behavior associated with occupancy of a distinctive position in society and that contributes to society in an economic sense. Examples of occupational roles include player, preschooler, student, worker, homemaker, retiree" (p. 251). No other definitions of occupational role were identified in occupational therapy literature. However, Stein & Roose (2000) define role performance:

> A social component that includes the individual's position in a family, job, culture, nation, or religion. The role functions include husband/wife, occupational title, political leader, spiritual, counselor, parent/homemaker, and professional soldier. These role functions are gained through education and social and family expectations. Throughout one's life, role functions are assumed and changed. (p. 265)

In summary, there are two separate but overlapping concepts here. One concerns roles in general and their relationship to human doing. The other concerns the specific occupational roles that humans do to fulfill the productivity aspects of social participation and responsibility. Reilly apparently felt that a specific concept of occupational role was the most appropriate concern for occupational therapy (Moorhead, 1969). Kielhofner (1997), on the other hand, has used the general concept of role in the Model of Human Occupation. He speaks of people seeing themselves as "spouses, parents, workers, or students" and that their identity is shaped by those roles (p. 393). At this time it appears the field has not established whether one or the other concepts related to role is most useful to occupational therapy.

Routine

The concept of routine in relation to clients is discussed by Allen (1985) and was used as the basis for the development of the Routine Task Inventory. However, the concept is not defined. The focus is on routine task behavior that "is observed during the process of completing a routine task" (Allen, 1985, p. 11). Hagedorn (1995) defines routine as "an automated and habitual chain of task with a fixed sequence" (p. 301). Christiansen and Baum (1997) state that routines (plural) are "occupations with established sequences, such as the related sequence of tasks that characterizes personal care (bathing, dressing, grooming) at that start of the day" (p. 603). Christiansen (2000) defines routines as "behaviors that are repeated over time and organized into patterns and habits" (p. 404).

The Concise Oxford Dictionary (Thompson, 1995) defines routine as a regular course or procedure or a set sequence in a performance (p. 1202). *Webster's New Universal Unabridged Dictionary* (Barnes & Noble, 1995) lists three different definitions: 1) a customary or regular course of procedures; 2) commonplace tasks, chores, or duties as must be done regularly or at specified intervals; typical or everyday activity; and 3) regular, unvarying, habitual, unimaginative or rote procedure (p. 1676). Synonyms given are habitual, ordinary, and typical. Reber (1995) suggests that some rituals become routines whenever the symbolic elements of the behaviors are lost. He states that there is a connotation "that somehow a routine is a more mundane, stereotyped behavior pattern that a ritual" (p. 676). Corsini (1999) defines routine as "a set of coordinated behaviors usually conducted without conscious intention, such as always putting shoes first on the left rather than on the right foot" (p. 865). Habit is given as a synonym.

Use of the concept of routine will need to be clarified as to how it is different from habit. New concepts are most useful if they solve a problem created by an older concept or fill a void. If routine refers to tasks while habit refers to behavior, then the concept of routine may become useful in the occupational therapy literature. Another problem is to differentiate routine tasks from activities of daily living. What doing behavior is involved in performing routine tasks that is not found in performing activities of daily living? Without such clarification, the concept of routine becomes yet another term students and practitioners

Table B-10 Definitions of Role

- Ryan (1993) states that roles are "functions of the individual in society that may be assumed or acquired (homemaker, student, caregiver, etc)" (p. 364).
- Creek (1997) states that role is "the set of expectations placed on an individual in a particular social context that become part of his identity and influence his behavior. Each person plays a large number of roles, such as worker, parent, friend" (p. 530).
- Hagedorn (1997) defines role as "a social or occupational identity which directs the individual's social, cultural and occupational behavior and relationships" (p. 145).
- Kielhofner (1997) defines an internalized role "as a broad awareness of a particular social identify and related obligations that together provide a framework for appreciating relevant situations and constructing appropriate behavior" (p. 193).
- Jackson and Banks (1997) suggest that roles are a "set of expectations governing the behavior of persons holding a particular position in society" (p. 460).
- Parham and Fazio (1997a) state that a role is "the expected pattern of behavior associated with occupancy of a distinctive position in society" (p. 252).
- Townsend (1997) defines role as "a culturally defined pattern of occupation that reflects particular routines and habits; stereotypical role expectations may enhance or limit persons' potential occupational performance" (p. 182).
- Neistadt and Crepeau (1998) state that "roles give people scripts to behave in ways consistent with their social roles, such as student, worker, or parent" (p. 872).
- Jacobs (1999) states that a role is a "set of behaviors that have some socially agreed-upon functions and for which there is an accepted code of norms" (p. 127).
- Punwar and Peloquin (2000) define role as "those functions that one assumes or acquires in society, i.e., the roles of worker, parent, student, etc. (p 284).

must learn and deal with in practice. Duplication of terms and concept is not useful or desirable. Concepts must be clearly separate from each other in terms of meaning and purpose.

Volition

The concept of volition appears in the early occupational therapy literature. Upham (1919) says that "in healthy minds, volition precedes action, and disordered minds may be normalized if volition can be born, and action and decision made clear and enforced. Volition may be helped by the selection of the right occupation..." (p. 211). The concept seems to have come from J. Madison Taylor, a physician, who wrote at the beginning of the 20th century. It was reintroduced by Kielhofner in the 1980s. He uses the concept as a volition subsystem that is "an interrelated set of energizing and symbolic components which together determine conscious choices for occupational behavior" (Kielhofner, 1985, p. 509). In 1997, Kielhofner defines the term volition as "a system of dispositions and self-knowledge that predisposes and enables a person to anticipate, choose, experience, and interpret occupational behavior" (p. 208). Creek (1997) defines volition as "the ability to choose between alternative actions; exercise of the will or the inner condition of the organism that initiates or directs its behavior toward a goal" (p. 530). Unsworth (1999) states that volition is "the capacity to determine what one needs and wants to do and the capacity to conceptualize a future realization of one's needs and wants. Volition requires the capacity to formulate a goal or an intention and then to initiate task performance" (p. 484).

Reber (1995) defines volition as "conscious, voluntary selection of particular action or choice from many potential actions or choices" (p. 848). *The Concise Oxford Dictionary* (Thompson, 1995) states "the exercise of the will" or "the power of willing" (p. 1570). *Webster's New Universal Unabridged Dictionary* (Barnes & Noble, 1995) gives three definitions: 1) the act of willing, choosing, or resolving; 2) a choice or decision made by the will, and 3) the power of willing" (p. 2130).

Volition as a concept has received limited attention in recent years. Except for the Model of Human Occupation, the concept of volition has not been considered a major concept by model builders and theorists today. Whether subsequent model builders will confirm the usefulness of the concept remains to be seen.

Personal Characteristics

Recently, additional concepts related to doing have begun to appear. These concepts can be grouped as personal characteristics of the doer. The specific concepts are ability, action, capacity, and skill. Because the concepts are new to models of occupational therapy, their utility and usefulness is difficult to establish at this time.

Ability and Abilities

Ability is defined by Trombly (1995a) as referring to a "general trait that an individual brings with him when he begins to learn a new task" (p. 19). Christiansen and Baum (1997) provide a similar definition by suggesting the ability refers to "general traits which are a product of genetic make-up and learning much of which occurs during childhood and adolescence" (p. 56). Both of the definitions are based on the work of Fleishman (1975), a human factors scientist and researcher. *Webster's New Universal Unabridged Dictionary* (Barnes & Noble, 1995) defines abilities as "talents, special skills or aptitudes" (p. 4). The singular form, ability, is defined as 1) power or capacity to do or act physically, mentally, legally, morally, financially, etc. and 2) competence in an activity or occupation because of one's skill, training, or other qualification (Barnes & Noble, 1995, p. 4). The difference may be significant. The plural form, abilities, seems to imply inborn or genetic characteristics that are refined through learning. The singular form makes no reference to inborn or genetic characteristics, only to well learned behaviors. Corsini (1999) also suggests well learned behaviors in his definitions, which is "1) the physical, mental or legal competence to function; and 2) A present skill, such as being able to spell a certain word, perform arithmetic, ride a bicycle, or recite a poem" (p. 2).

One important problem to solve is the relation of ability to skill and capacity. Although there is a trend toward considering ability as more associated with inborn or genetic characteristics and skill with learning, the trend is not universally accepted. The difference between ability and capacity is less defined. Both are being used to convey inborn, genetically endowed, or innate characteristics. Once again, clarity in use of concept is important to the communication of ideas.

Action and Actions

Christiansen and Baum (1997) define actions as "any observable behavior that is recognizable, can be described as an 'action', the basic building block of occupation" (p. 56).

Unsworth (1999) defines purposive action as the "capacities for productivity and self-regulation (including the capacity to structure an effective and fluent course of action by initiating, maintaining, switching, and stopping complex action sequences in an orderly manner) to realize a goal" (pp. 481-482). *Webster's New Universal Unabridged Dictionary* (Barnes & Noble, 1995) defines action as "1) the process or state of acting or of being active; 2) something done or performed; and 3) an act that one consciously wills and that many be characterized by physical or mental activity," whereas actions is defined as "habitual or usual acts or conduct" (p. 20). On the other hand, *Taber's Cyclopedic Medical Dictionary* (Thomas, 1997) lists fifteen definitions for the word *action*, all of which have to do with physiological or drug actions.

The problem of using the terms *action* or *actions* will be similar to that of function or functions. Usage must be clearly directed toward the organism or person as a whole, not a specific part or internal organ. The action(s) results in a behavior(s) the individual makes.

Capacity and Capacities

Christiansen and Baum (1997) define capacity as "the immediate potential of the individual to perform tasks which support occupational performance" (p. 592). Jackson and Banks (1997) suggest that capacity "is the ability to perform a task" (p. 460). Wilcock (1998) says that capacity means "the innate and perhaps undeveloped potential, aptitude, ability, talent, trait, or power with which each individual is endowed" (p. 42). Jacobs (1999) states that capacity is "one's best, includes present abilities as well as potential to develop new abilities" (p. 21). Unsworth (1999) describes capacity as "possessing normal psychological, physiological, or anatomical structure or function" (p. 474).

Of the nine definitions in *Webster's New Universal Unabridged Dictionary* (Barnes & Noble, 1995), only one comes close to the meanings expressed in the definitions by occupational therapy authors. The fourth definition is "actual or potential ability to perform, yield, or withstand" (p. 308). Corsini (1999) states that capacity "refers to potential ability" (p. 2). The World Health Organization (2000) states that capacity is a "construct that indicates... the highest probable level of functioning that a person may reach... Capacity is measured in a uniform or standard environment and, thus, reflects the environmentally adjusted ability of the individual" (p. 166). The most consistent word used to describe capacity in the foregoing definitions is potential. Generally, the meaning seems to pertain to function or perform. As stated under the discussion of ability, the problem is to decide if capacity or ability are basically the same concept or if both are needed to convey ideas about personal characteristics.

Skill or Skills

The word *skill* has become a popular concept in modern occupational therapy literature. Kielhofner (1985) defines skills as "the abilities that a person has for the performance of various forms of purposeful behavior" (p. 508). Hagedorn (1992) describes skill as "a specific ability or integrated set of abilities such as motor, sensory, cognitive or perceptual, learnt and practiced to a standard required for the effective performance of a task or subtask" (p. 92). In 1995 she rephrased the description, saying skill is "the ability to put skill components together in smoothly integrated and sequenced, competent, performance" (p. 301). Trombly (1995a) defines skill as "an individual's ability to achieve goals under a wide variety of conditions with a degree of consistency and economy" (p. 19). Turner, Foster, and Johnson (1996) state skill is "a performance component which evolves with practice" (p. 873). Christiansen and Baum (1997) write that skill "pertains to the level of proficiency in a specific task" (p. 57). Parham and Fazio (1997a) state that skills are:

> ...consolidations of rule-based subroutines of behavior that produce goal-directed behavior; for example, the subroutines of grasping the handle of a pitcher, pouring and holding a glass are combined in the skill of pouring a drink. Skills, when practiced repeatedly until automatic, become habits. (p. 253)

Webster's New Universal Unabridged Dictionary (Barnes & Noble, 1995, p. 1791) provides five current meanings for the term *skill*; however, only three are relevant:

1. The ability, coming from one's knowledge, practice, aptitude, etc. to do something well.
2. Competent excellence in performance, experience, dexterity.
3. A craft, trade, or job requiring manual dexterity or special training in which a person has competence and experience.

Corsini (1999) defines skill as "an acquired high-order ability to perform complex motor acts smoothly and precisely" (p. 906). However, he also adds that the term "sometimes includes knowledge or keen cognition" in some definitions outside psychology (p. 906).

The practice of defining one term by using another is of limited assistance in clarifying the use of the term. Many of the definitions of skill begin by using the term *ability*. If both concepts are to be used, they must have separate meaning and be used for different purposes. As stated in the discussion on ability, there appears to be a trend in usage that may be useful.

Summary of Doing Concepts

Doing has both an internally and externally directed process. Internally, the person must be able to initiate some action through the sensorimotor or cognitive system and must have some direction toward interest, meaning, and purpose from the cognitive system. Externally, the context, especially the sociocultural environment, moderates and influences the doing process. In the past, occupational therapy literature has contained many articles concerning the internal processes but more recently attention has also focused on the external process. Examples of external factors that affect the occupational therapy process are listed in Table B-11.

There are many concepts associated with the doing process. As occupational therapy practitioners have experienced, doing is not a simple concept because any single act of doing has many factors contributing to the action. As occupational therapy continues to develop its own philosophy and rationale for practice, understanding the doing process becomes more important to the explanation of why occupational therapy is useful in developing, maintaining, and restoring health and well-being. Since the concepts selected for communicating the process of doing require exploration, some of the concepts related to doing will be given special attention in the following discussions.

Tools

Tools are the instruments of change used during the intervention stage. Common descriptors have included media, modalities, methods, techniques, and approaches. At issue are the things, strategies, and "stuff" occupational therapy personnel use when working with clients. The particular tool is not so important as the process of selection as Upham (1918a) stated:

> The success of occupational therapy does not lie in any particular craft or trade, but rather in the skill with which it is selected for a particular disability of the patient and the technique of allowing the patient's reaction, temperament, and fatigue to form the basic teaching (p. 51)

Although the exact tool may not be important, the use of tools as a group is very important because they are actual means of initiating the doing process. The discussion of tools begins with a naming problem and continues with discussions of assumptions about purposes and classification systems.

Occupation and Activity

Two terms have been used frequently to describe the major tool used in occupational therapy: *occupation* and *activity*. Both concepts are defined from various sources and discussed.

The definitions presented in Table B-12 are those located in the past 10 years. They are presented in reverse chronological order to permit the reader to see the building process that has occurred. Also, each definition has been analyzed to determine whether it addresses the outcome, doing, or tools aspect of occupational therapy most directly. The analysis is stated as a word at the end of each definition.

Because these definitions were all written by authors in the profession, two conclusions are evident. First, more than one idea is being conveyed in the use of the term *occupation*. Because these definitions were all written by authors in the profession, a second conclusion is evident. Occupational therapy personnel use the term *occupation* to convey the essential reality of the profession—occupation is both process and product. As Trombly (1995b) has said, occupation is both means and ends. Occupation is both the means by which occupational therapy is delivered and the result of having engaged in or received occupational therapy services. In other words, clients engage in occupation in the present to learn or relearn how to engage in occupation in the future. There is both a present and future time-reference. Clients supposedly do in the present the occupations they will need to do in the future. The process takes time and energy and is composed of actions, tasks, and roles with labels such as washing clothes (action) to provide clean clothing (task) as one part of the homemaker role. The product is influenced by factors such as health or disability status, sociocultural customs, economic means, geography, political situation, religious rituals, and personal preferences. All of the factors that affect the use of the term *occupation* as used in occupational therapy should appear in the description of the term as used by occupational therapy personnel.

The second conclusion is that the term *occupation* is not often used to describe the tools used in occupational therapy. The definitions either define occupation in terms of outcome or occupation in terms of doing, some do both, only one mentions the use of occupation as a therapeutic tool. None define occupation in terms of being a therapeutic tool. However, occupation in occupational therapy is used primarily as a therapeutic tool. Clarification is clearly in order. The profession must come to some agreement about the central term and concept in the field. A solution may be to use therapeutic occupations, at least in clinical situations.

Based on a word analysis of the definitions above, 10 assumptions are proposed that should be considered in a comprehensive definition of occupation as it is used in occupational therapy today. These are listed in Table B-13.

Another term seen frequently in occupational therapy literature is *activity*. The term *activity* has been with the profession

Table B-11 Factors That Can Influence the Nature of Doing

Physical Factors (Location)	*Temporal Factors (Time)*	*Sociocultural Factors*
Place: home or institution	Age/life span	Gender
Built or natural environment	Time of day	Race
Terrain	Sequence: 1st, 2nd, 3rd	Ethnicity
Climate	Season of the year	Socioeconomic status
Temperature	Speed and accuracy	Role: parent/child
Altitude	Taking turns	Role: supervisor/worker
Weather	Waiting in line	Role: staff/patient
Location (indoors or outdoors)	Being on time	Crowds
Location (clinic or ward)	Following directions	Consumer
Location: community	Stage/course of illness	Customer
Light and color	Expectation for recovery	Citizenship
Sound or noise	Start/stop a movement	Laws/rules and regulations
Odors/smells	Start/stop an activity	Values, beliefs, and attitudes
Safety or fire hazard	Repetitive motion	Economics
Indoor climate control	Amount of time needed to perform a task	Politics
Furniture	Number of steps to finish	Customs, mores, and social norms
Room arrangement	Short-term memory	Personal habits and preferences
Supplies/materials available	Long-term memory	Country of origin/birth
Equipment available		
Steps/stairs/ramps		
Doors		
Windows		
Tastes/texture		
Tactile sensations		
Gravity		
Humidity		
Soil		
Water		
Chemicals		
Architecture		
Technology		

Table B-12

Definitions of Occupation

- Occupation is a form of human endeavor that provides longitudinal organization of time and effort in a person's life (Hagedorn, 2000, p. 309). ***Doing***
- Human occupation is the total range of productive, purposeful, and meaningful occupations in which people participate. The area of human life with which occupational therapists are concerned (Hagedorn, 2000, p. 309). ***Outcome***
- Occupation is the active or "doing" process when one is engaged in goal-directed activity (Punwar & Peloquin, 2000, p. 282). ***Doing***
- Occupation is the culturally and personally meaningful and purposeful activities that humans engage in during their everyday lives. These occupations include the major functions of life such as work, leisure, play, self-care, rest, sleep, and social interactions (Stein & Roose, 2000, p. 201). ***Doing***
- Occupation is the ordinary tasks of human existence in which people create their self-image and identify and organize their lives (Cara & MacRae, 1998, p. 669). ***Outcome***
- Occupation is the engagement in daily life activities that are meaningful and purposeful, including self-care, instrumental, vocation, educational, play and leisure, and rest and relaxation activities of daily living (Gillen & Burkhardt, 1998, p. 540). ***Doing***
- Occupation is the daily activities typical for a culture that form a pattern of activity (Neistadt & Crepeau, 1998, p. 870). ***Outcome***
- Occupation is all the "doing" that has intrinsic or extrinsic meaning (Wilcock, 1998, p. 257). ***Doing***
- Occupation is the engagement in activities, tasks, and roles for the purpose of productive pursuit; maintaining one's self in the environment; and for purposes of relaxation, entertainment, creativity, and celebration; activities in which people are engaged to support their roles (Christiansen & Baum, 1997, p. 600). ***Outcome***
- Occupations are the ordinary and familiar things that people do every day (Christiansen & Baum, 1997, p. 600). ***Doing***
- Occupation defines and organizes a sphere of action over a period of time and is perceived by the individual as part of his or her social identify (Creek, 1997, p. 529). ***Outcome***
- Occupations are groups of activities and tasks of everyday life, named, organized, and given value and meaning by individuals and a culture; occupation is everything people do to occupy themselves, including looking after themselves (self-care), enjoying life (leisure), and contributing to the social and economic fabric of their communities (productivity); the domain of concern and the therapeutic medium of occupational therapy (Townsend, 1997, p. 181). ***Doing/Outcome***
- Occupations are defined as "chunks" of activity within the stream of human behavior that are names in the lexicon of the culture (Zemke & Clark, 1996, p. 48). ***Doing***
- Occupation is appropriate to use when the person's abilities, motivations, and goals come together to enable role performance (Trombly, 1995a, p. 237). ***Tool***
- Human occupation is "doing culturally meaningful work, play or daily living tasks in the stream of time and in the contexts of one's physical and social world" (Kielhofner, 1995, p. 3). ***Doing***
- Occupation is the relationship between an occupation form and an occupational performance. Occupational form is the objective set of circumstances, external to the person, that elicits, guides, or structures the person's occupational performance. Occupational performance is the voluntary doing of the person in the context of the occupational form (Nelson, 1994, pp. 10-11). ***Doing***
- Occupation is defined as groups of self-directed, functional tasks and activities in which a person engages over the lifespan (Law et al., 1996, p. 16). ***Doing***
- That which defines and organizes a sphere of action over a period of time and is perceived by the individual as part of his personal and social identity (Turner, Foster, & Johnson, 1996, p. 873). ***Outcome***

(continued)

Table B-12

- Activity or task that engages a person's resources of time and energy, especially self-maintenance, productivity, and leisure (Reed & Sanderson, 1992, p. 345). ***Doing***
- Chunks of culturally and personally meaningful activity in which humans engage that can be named in the lexicon of the culture (Clark et al., 1996, p. 301). ***Doing***
- Occupation is used as a general term that refers to engagement in activities, tasks, and roles for the purpose of meeting the requirement of living (Christiansen & Baum, 1991). ***Doing/Outcome***

Table B-13

Assumptions About Occupation(s) Based on Definitions

- Occupation(s) can be named and defined.
- Occupation is composed of activities, tasks, and roles.
- Occupation has an organizing, organizational, or sequencing effect on people.
- Occupation occurs in a physical dimension of time (temporal) and space (spatial).
- Occupation occurs in a social and cultural dimension, environment, or context.
- Occupation involves a doing process that includes effort and/or energy.
- Occupation may be done or performed for a variety of reasons, interests, meanings, purposes, values, or beliefs.
- Occupation can meet a variety of personal or individual goals or outcomes such as self image, self-identify, or self-efficacy.
- Occupation can met a variety of sociocultural goals or outcomes such as economic, political, and institution.
- Occupation can be subdivided into a number of categories for convenience, clarification, or classification.

since the formative years. Perhaps the best known use of the term is in Patterson's (1922) definition of occupational therapy which is "any activity, mental or physical, definitely prescribed and guided for the distinct purpose of contributing to, and hastening recovery from, disease or injury" (p. 21). Thus, the earliest use of the term *activity* is as a synonym for occupation. Some definitions appearing in the last 10 years are listed in Table B-14. However, several definitions suggest that activity is a behavior unit of a task, an action, or an event that is separate from occupation. Other definitions suggest that activity is a subpart or subtask of occupational performance.

Once again, the failure of the profession to arrive at a standard usage of the term and concept of activity increases the difficulty of communicating effectively within and without the field. Is activity a synonym for occupation or is activity a subpart of occupation? When reading about activity in the occupational therapy literature, how will the reader know what meaning is intended?

Therapeutic Occupation or Occupation as Therapy

Why is occupation therapeutic? What are the therapeutic characteristics of occupation? What is therapeutic about occupation? Why and what is therapeutic about occupation has most often been addressed in terms of the therapeutic value of work. The broader topic of occupation is less often addressed. One example is Prout (1931) who says:

> When we think of life in terms of the opportunity for doing things and for being occupied we don't have to apologize for being committed to the proposition of the real value of various forms of occupation as therapeutic measures. In a sense the human mind is never in its waking moments without occupation. (p. 235)

Prout continues, saying, "Occupational therapeutics in order to be therapeutic at all must of necessity be in line to satisfy the instinctive drive that has to do with self-expression or personal accomplishment, or the aesthetic and the altruistic..." (1931, p. 237). Nearly 70 years later, Punwar and Peloquin (2000) define therapeutic occupation as "any purposeful activity used to prevent physical or mental dysfunction to restore or improve function to a normal level" (p. 282). In 1986, the AOTA did not define therapeutic occupation but did describe therapeutic activities in occupational therapy as including "self-care, work, home management, child care, educational, play/leisure, and cultural activities that have been selected and adapted to meet specific occupational therapy goals" (p. 355). Creek (1997) does not define therapeutic occupation either but does define therapeutic medium as "any activity which is used to develop competence in skills that the individual can use to sustain a satisfactory range of life roles" (p. 530). Likewise, Parham and Fazio (1997a) do not define therapeutic occupation but instead define therapeutic use of objects, materials, and activities as:

> ...the therapists' strategic presentation of tangible things in the environment to facilitate treatment goals

Table B-14

Definitions of the Concept of Activity

- Activity is a series of linked episodes of task performance that take place on a specific occasion during a finite period for a particular reason. An activity is composed of an integrated sequence of chained tasks. A completed activity results in a change in the previous state of objective reality or subjective experience (Hagedorn, 2000, p. 307).
- Activity is productive action required for development, maturation, and use of sensory, motor, social psychological, and cognitive functions. Activity may be productive without yielding an object. It is also a valuable vehicle to acquire, maintain, or redevelop skills necessary to fulfill occupational roles and provide satisfaction (Christiansen & Baum, 1997, p. 591).
- An activity is performed by an individual for a specific purpose on a particular occasion (Creek, 1997, p. 529).
- Activity is an integrated sequence of tasks that takes place on a specific occasion, during a finite period, for a particular purpose (Hagedorn, 1997, p. 142).
- Activity is considered to be the basic unit of a task. It is designed as a singular pursuit in which a person engages as part of his or her daily occupational experience (Law et al., 1996, p. 16).
- Activities are the basic units of occupational performance and consist of specific behaviors directed toward the completion of a task, whereas tasks are a set of activities that share some purpose (Watson, 1997, p. 32).
- Activity is being active in mind and/or body. Doing something, usually for a particular purpose (Turner, Foster, & Johnson, 1996, p. 873).
- Activities are smaller units of behavior that comprise tasks (Trombly, 1995b, p. 19).
- Activity is a specific action, function, or sphere of action that involves learning or doing by direct experience (Reed & Sanderson, 1992).

> via the child's active engagement in organized play; including reducing the number of objects in the environment and carefully selecting when and how to present materials that are motivating to the child. (p. 254)

If occupations are therapeutic, the profession needs to come to a consensus regarding the use of concept to express the idea. Examination of assumptions may provide some insight. Yerxa (1996) says that occupation can be used therapeutically because of eight factors. Reed and Sanderson (1992) also suggest a different set of eight factors. These have been combined in Table B-15. Although the lists are slightly different, some common themes appear. Occupation can facilitate attainment of adaptation, master, competence, autonomy, efficacy, and sense of control. These ideas are supported by the concepts discussed under outcomes. Other ideas about the therapeutic use of occupation include expression of interests, discovery of resource potential, fulfillment of social roles, reduction of impact of disability, organization of life tasks, meet individual needs and social demands, orient person to reality, and create of levels of achievement. In summary, occupation is a versatile tool but versatility needs to be channeled into effective and efficient strategies to achieve the best therapeutic results.

Considering that the use of occupation therapeutically or therapeutic occupation is the essential medium of occupational therapy, it is surprising that more definitions and descriptions were not found. Once again the profession may be assuming the obvious simplicity of the term without giving thought to complexity of the concept in application.

Types of Occupation

Just as the uses of occupation vary, so do the types of occupation. Definitions were located for specific types of occupation such as activities of daily living, self-maintenance, instrumental activities of daily living, self-care, work, leisure, play, and task or tasks.

Activities of Daily Living

The term *activities of daily living* first appears in the occupational therapy literature in 1954. Holdeman (1954) states that "the function, or activities of daily living (ADL), test is a guide in evaluating his (the client's) process..." (p. 262). Activities of daily living, however, is not the original name for what is now called ADL. The original name for the assessment of daily living skills was the "achievement record" (Sheldon, 1935). An example of an achievement record appears in Livingstone (1950). A second name was "physical demands of daily life" (Deaver & Brown, 1945). Deaver, a physician, and Brown, a physical therapist, developed a scale with three headings: location, self-care activities, and hand activities. An assessment protocol based on Deaver and Brown appears in MacLean's (1949) article on the management of polio. Smith (1945) credits Deaver with initiating the program of training in daily life tasks. Smith says that

Table B-15

Assumptions About the Therapeutic Use of Occupation

- Occupation can enable the person to express his or her unique pattern of interests possessed by each individual.
- Occupation involves the engagement of the whole person in the performance of occupational activities or tasks.
- Occupation can contribute to a person's sense of well-being and state of health.
- Occupation can enable a person to meet individual needs and societal demands.
- Occupation can facilitate the attainment of adaptive behavior, mastery, autonomy, efficacy, control, or sense of competence within the environment because the person is able to produce an effect.
- Occupation can be used to attain, maintain, or regain skills necessary to fulfill social roles.
- Occupation can be used to prevent or slow the loss of skills.
- Occupation can be used to help a person learn to organize his or her life and use resources to reduce the impact of disability.
- Occupation can facilitate normal development throughout the lifespan.
- Occupation can be graded to accommodate different learning abilities.
- Occupation can be used to enhance skills in a variety of performance components, areas, or contexts.
- Occupation can be used to increase the level of performance and level of responsibility assumed by a person.

Based on Reed, K. L., & Sanderson, S. R. (1992). *Concepts of occupational therapy* (3rd ed., pp. 43-44). Baltimore: Williams & Wilkins and Yerxa, E.J. (1996), The social and psychological experience of having a disability. In L.W. Pedretti (Ed), *Occupational therapy: Practice skills for physical dysfunction* (4th ed. pp. 265-266). St Louis: Mosby.

Deaver became concerned with the number of clients who in spite of many months of treatment "could not perform the ordinary routine tasks required in daily life although they were capable of being taught to do so" (Deaver & Brown, 1945, p. I). Between the years 1945 and 1949, the name changed from "physical activities of daily life" to "functional activities" to "activities of daily living" (Buchwald, 1949, p. 491). Since then the phrase activities of daily living has been defined in numerous ways in the occupational therapy literature. Examples of definitions are provided in Table B-16. While some definitions are primarily lists of tasks a person might perform, others attempt to relate activities of daily living to meeting the demands of everyday life that a person must perform to participate in social life, work roles, and live independently.

Self-Maintenance

Self-maintenance has also been used to describe similar groups of tasks. Reed and Sanderson (1992) define self-maintenance occupations as "those activities or tasks that are done routinely to maintain the person's health and well-being in the environment, i.e., dressing, feeding" (p. 352). Christiansen (2000) also suggests that self-maintenance can be used as a synonym for activities of daily living. He defines self-maintenance as "the ability to handle tasks ranging from basic personal care, including dressing, eating, grooming, toileting, and getting around (mobility), to doing laundry, using the telephone, shopping, banking, and managing medications" (p. 404).

One central problem to the concept of activities of daily living or self-maintenance is the lack of agreement as to what constitutes an individual item as belonging to the group. There is no uniform list of terms or concepts in the literature on activities of daily living or self-maintenance. Each article and each assessment instrument provides a different list, making comparison difficult, if not impossible. Another problem is that the concept of activities of daily living done not belong safely to occupational therapy. Physiatrists, physical therapists, and nurses also use the concept. Any attempt to develop a consistent definition and list of activities would have to be a joint effort.

Instrumental Activities of Daily Living

Instrumental activities of daily living (IADL) became a phrase in 1971 when Lawton published an assessment of tasks not usually included in the standard activities of daily living assessment. According to Pedretti and Umphred (1996), IADL involve "more advanced problem-solving skills, social skills, and complex environment interaction such as home management and community living skills, health management, and safety preparedness" (p. 463). Jackson and Banks (1997) define IADL as "higher-order activities that support independence, including housekeeping duties, shopping, budgeting, and money management" (p. 460). Unsworth (1999) states that IADL are "domestic and community activities of daily living, such as cleaning, shopping, and driving" (p. 478). Piersol and Ehrlich (2000) state that IADL are "activities other than basic activities of daily liv-

Table B-16

Definitions of Activities of Daily Living

- AOTA (1978) defined activities of daily living as "the components of everyday activity including self-care, work and play/leisure activities (p. 73).
- Mosey (1986) says that activities of daily living are "all those activities that one must engage in or accomplish in order to participate with comfort in other facets of life. These activities may be subdivided into self-care, communication and travel... and... responsibilities of being a homemaker or home manager" (p. 8).
- Reed and Sanderson (1992) defined activities of daily living as "the tasks that a person must be able to perform in order to care for the self independently, including self-care, communication and travel" (p. 330).
- Ryan's (1993) definition is "area of occupational performance that refers to grooming, oral hygiene, dressing, feeding and eating, medication routine, socialization, functional communication, functional mobility and sexual expression activities" (p. 357).
- Trombly (1995a) says that activities of daily living "include those tasks that a person regularly does to prepare for, or as an adjunct to, participating in his or her social and work roles" (p. 289).
- Pedretti and Umphred (1996) state that "ADL require basic skills and include task of mobility, self-care, communication, management of environmental hardware and devices, and sexual expression" (p. 463).
- Christiansen and Baum (1997) define activities of daily living as "typical life tasks required for self-care and self-maintenance, such as grooming, bathing, eating, cleaning the house and doing laundry" (p. 591).
- Gillen and Burkhardt (1998) state that activities of daily living are "the activities usually performed in the course of a normal day, such as eating, toileting, dressing, washing, and grooming" (p. 536).
- Neistadt and Crepeau (1998) suggest activities of daily living are "self-maintenance tasks considered necessary for meeting the demands of daily living including such activities as bathing, dressing, grooming, oral hygiene, eating, taking medication and communication" (p. 866).
- Christiansen (2000) says that activities of daily living are "activities or tasks that a person does every day to maintain personal independence" (p. 399).
- Finally, Stein and Roose (2000) define activities of daily living as "tasks that are essential for self-care, including dressing, grooming, feeding, mobility/transferring, bathing, and toileting" (p. 1).

ing (ADL) that relate to the ability to manage independently at home, e.g., laundry, shopping and money management" (p. 200). Stein and Roose (2000) define IADL as "tasks that involve participation of a client with the physical and/or social environment, including home management, money management, communication, safety, community living skills, work and leisure activities" (p. 130).

As evidenced by the five definitions, this concept also contains a variety of items that cover a wide range of roles and tasks from doing laundry to safety preparedness. The most consistent items are shopping and money management. Clearly, if the concept of IADL is to be useful, criteria for what elements are to be included must be established. Again, however, occupational therapy must work with others because the term came from psychology and is used in other health care professions, especially nursing.

Self-Care

In some definitions of activities of daily living, the term *self-care* is viewed as a subcategory. In other categories, self-care is viewed as a separate entity. The definitions that follow show some of the diversity of description regarding the concept of self-care. The AOTA (1978) defined self-care skills as "skills such as dressing, feeding, hygiene/grooming, mobility, and object manipulation" (p. 75). Letts, Fraser, Finlayson, and Walls (1993) define self-care as "the decisions and actions individuals take in the interest of their own health and for the health of family members, e.g. eating a balanced diet, choosing to exercise regularly, pre-natal care" (p. 8). Trombly (1995b) suggests self-care involves "activities or tasks done routinely to maintain the client's health and well-being, considering the environment and social factors" (p. 352). Jacobs (1999) says that self-care is the "personal activities an individual performs to prepare for and maintain a daily routine" (p. 131). Christiansen (2000) uses the term *self-care occupations*, which are defined as "those basic personal care activities such as eating, grooming, dressing, mobility, and personal hygiene" (p. 404). Finally, Stein and Roose state that self-care includes "activities that are completed daily to maintain good hygiene and good appearance, meet basic needs such as eating and voiding, and move from one necessary area (such as the kitchen) to another (the bathroom)" (2000, p. 273).

Is there an advantage to using self-care over activities of daily living or vice versa? There appears to be no real consensus either way. Of interest may be definitions used in the MEDLINE database in which self-care is the individual's ability to perform the tasks for him- or herself whereas activities of daily living require the help or supervision of another person to perform. Which idea is being conveyed in the occupational therapy literature?

Work

The term *work* has also had a variety of definitions, descriptions, and interpretations. The definitions in Table B-17 provide examples of the diversity. These definitions illustrate the concern over what constitutes work. Is it paid activity only or are there other legitimate forms of work? The consensus in occupational therapy seems to be that there are several categories of work or productive activity and that the work occurs in a variety of settings. A summary of ideas expressed in the definitions is that work involves participating in socially purposeful, meaningful, and productive activities that include services or commodities to maintain or advance society and individuals with labels such as remunerative employment, subsistence, home management, care of others, education, avocation, or vocation and which is characterized as having a predetermined manner or standard of performance.

Leisure

The term *leisure* comes from the Latin verb *licere*, which means "to be permitted." Leisure is not as widely defined as work. However, the diversity of opinion as to what constitutes leisure is evident in the seven definitions in Table B-18.

Themes include a temporal relationship to other occupations (done in free time or nonwork time), control of choice (freedom to chose, not obligatory), related to health and well-being (promote health, enjoyment, quality of life), may be considered an adult form of play, and variety of activities from which to chose. The lack of consensus on what constitutes leisure may be one factor in the lack of development of leisure in many practice settings.

Play

The concept of play became popular in the models of occupational therapy due to Reilly's (1966) interest. Thereafter, most discussions of occupational therapy media include play. Nine definitions are presented in Table B-19. Based on these definitions, play is also a complex term that has only received serious study in occupational therapy in the modern period. The role of play in child development and the relation of play to adult work skills have been discussed but consensus has not been achieved. A summary of ideas is that play is characterized by pleasure, fun, experimentation, exploration, self-expression, competition, and make believe; that play does not have a utilitarian goal but does contribute to learning or rehearsing a wide range of skills that can be applied to productive occupations and permits self-expression; that play involves intrinsic motivation, choice, and voluntary participation that may be spontaneous or organized and is process rather than product or goal oriented; that play does have rules that govern the conduct of the specific play activity; and that play may result in entertainment, amusement, diversion, passing time, and/or relaxation.

Task or Tasks

Task has been discussed under tools because most, but not all, definitions imply that task or tasks are performances required or expected of the individual and not based on the individual's unique being. Eleven definitions appear in Table B-20. The relation of task to activity or occupation is being explored but has not achieved consensus. For example, is a task a unit of activity or is a task composed of units of activity?

Successful Application of Tools

Tools can be conceptualized based on their success as therapeutic agents. Turner and MacCaul (1996) suggest there are eight factors that determine the success of a tool for use within occupational therapy practice. These are flexibility, adaptability, relevance, therapeutic richness, usability, defensible and justifiable, robust and replaceable, and finally appropriateness and acceptability. These characteristics are presented in Table B-21.

Factors Influencing the Choice of Tools

Tools can also be conceptualized based on the factors that influence their choice in application for occupational therapy intervention. Reed (1986) suggested there are eight factors that include the choice or abandonment of tools by occupational therapy practitioners. These are cultural, social, economic, political, technological, theoretical, historical, and research influences. These factors are listed in Table B-22.

While occupation may be the major tool used in occupational therapy, the application of occupation must be translated by occupational therapy personnel into a therapeutic form. Thus, the person must be considered a tool as well. The technique or approach of the person becomes part of the tool as it is delivered to the client.

Therapeutic use of self has been discussed formally in the occupational therapy literature since 1958 (Frank, 1958). Parham and Fazio (1997a) describe therapeutic use of self as:

> The therapist's conscious or unconscious utilization of personal traits and interactions as a tool to facilitate treatment goals; may include strategies such as initiating an activity, providing emotional support and assistance, giving positive feedback and encouragement, exhibiting a playful attitude, and giving assurance of safety. (p. 254)

Punwar and Peloquin (2000) summarize the concept by defining use of self as "a therapist's planned use of his or her personality and perceptions as part of the therapeutic process" (p. 285).

Therapeutic use of self includes the concept of therapeutic rapport, which Tickle-Degnen (1995) defines as "the qualities of patient and therapist experience and behavior doing interaction with one another that affect patient performance and involvement in therapy" (p. 278). The qualities of experience include concentration on the interaction between therapist and client, communication that is clear and shared by both, and enjoyment and satisfaction with the interaction. The qualities of verbal and nonverbal behavior include attentiveness to each other, interpersonal responsiveness to each other, and positive feelings toward each other. The beneficial effects for the patient or client include enhanced performance and best follow through with therapeutic activities.

Table B-17

Definitions of Work

- Work refers to skill and performance in participating in socially purposeful and productive activities. These activities may take place in the home, employment setting, school, or community (AOTA, 1979a).
- Work is any formal activity that prepares one for or involves earning a living, being a student or remunerative employment (Mosey, 1986, p. 71).
- Work includes activities or tasks in the areas of home management, care of others, education, vocation, and avocation (McGourty et al., 1989).
- Work involves serious mental and/or physical effort directed toward purposeful production of something, a known objective or outcome, self-imposed or other imposed utilitarian activity to be performed in a predetermined manner and standard of performance (Spencer, 1989, p. 92).
- Work includes skill in socially productive activities, which include gainful employment, homemaking, child care-parenting, and work preparation activities (Ryan, 1993, p. 366).
- Refers to activities (both paid and unpaid) that provide services or commodities to others (e.g., ideas, knowledge, help, information-sharing, utilitarian or artistic objects, and protection (Kielhofner, 1995, p. 3).
- Work involves activities or tasks done to provide support to the self, family, and society (Trombly, 1995b, p. 352).
- Work is any activity, physical or mental, undertaken to achieve a desired outcome (Turner et al., 1996, p. 873).
- Work is a category of occupation in which an individual engages for the primary purpose of subsistence (Christiansen & Baum, 1997, p. 606).
- Work is any productive activity, whether paid or unpaid, that contributes to the maintenance or advancement of society as well as the individual. The work in which an individual spends most time usually becomes both an occupation and a major social role (Creek, 1997, p. 530).
- Work and productive activities are activities that enable people to contribute to society; to support themselves and others dependent on them through work-related activities; and to manage day-to-day activities such as shopping and cleaning (Neistadt & Crepeau, 1998, p. 873).
- Work includes paid or unpaid activity that contributes to subsistence, produces a serve or product, and is culturally meaningful to the worker (Stein & Roose, 2000, p. 327).

Table B-18

Definitions of Leisure

- Leisure is time when one is free from family and other social responsibilities, activities of daily living, and work (Mosey, 1986, p. 85).
- Leisure includes those activities or tasks done for the enjoyment and renewal that the activity or task brings to the person, which may contribute to the promotion of health and well-being (i.e., bowling, collecting antiques) (Reed & Sanderson, 1992, p. 343).
- Leisure is nonwork or free time spent in adult play activities that have an influence on the quality of life (Ryan, 1993, p. 361).
- Leisure includes activities or tasks that are not obligatory and that are done for enjoyment (Trombly, 1995a, p. 44) or components of life free from work and self-care activities (Trombly, 1995b, p. 352).
- Leisure is that category of occupations for which freedom of choice and enjoyment seem to be the primary motives (Christiansen & Baum, 1997, p. 598).
- Leisure includes activities driven by internal motivation, implies freedom of choice, is not usually done within time constraints (Neistadt & Crepeau, 1998, p. 870).

(continued)

Table B-18

- Leisure is a major occupation and performance area that relates to the individual's use of free time. It is related to intrinsic motivation, quality of life, personal freedom, life satisfaction, relaxation, health, lifestyle, amusement, self-actualization, and pleasure. Leisure occupations include a wide range of activities such as gardening, sports, hobbies, social clubs, music, and traveling that are related to the specific interests of an individual. Cultural, psychological, social, developmental, family, and educational factors may influence leisure choices (Stein & Roose, 2000, p. 142).

Table B-19

Definitions of Play

- Play is activity voluntarily engaged in for pleasure (Hopkins & Smith, 1983, p. 925).
- Play is spontaneous behavior initiated for pleasure, fun, or experimentation; a motive or activity characterized by freedom to explore, unrestricted by a utilitarian goal or expected result (Spencer, 1989, p. 92).
- Play includes activities carried on as part of one's leisure occupation that develop skills in and permit self-expression, competition, exploration, and make believe. Most play has rules that govern the conduct of the specific play activity. Skills learned in play may be applied to work and productive occupations (Reed & Sanderson, 1992, p. 347).
- Play is an intrinsic activity that involves enjoyment and leads to fun; spontaneous, voluntary, and engaged in by choice (Ryan, 1993, p. 363).
- Play includes a variety of occupations that constitute a pleasurable way of passing time and are also the medium through which a wide range of skills can be learned and rehearsed (Creek, 1997, p. 529).
- Play is a category of occupation characterized by choice, expression, and development (Christiansen & Baum, 1997, p. 601).
- Play is an attitude or mode of experience that involves intrinsic motivation; emphasis on process rather than product and internal rather than external control; and an "as-if" or pretend element; takes place in a safe, unthreatening environment with social sanctions. Also any spontaneous or organized activity that provides enjoyment, entertainment, amusement, or diversion (Parham & Fazio, 1997a, p. 252).
- Play involves choosing, performing, and engaging in an intrinsically motivated activity (attitude or process) that is experienced as pleasurable (Jacobs, 1999, p. 112).
- Play and leisure activities are intrinsically motivating activities that provide pleasure, relaxation, and expression of creativity (Neistadt & Crepeau, 1998, p. 871).

Table B-20

Definitions of Task

- Tasks are the sequence of actions engaged in to salsify either societal requirements or internal motivations to explore and be competent (Kielhofner, 1985, p. 509).
- Task is a stage in or component of an activity (Hagedorn, 1992, p. 92).
- Tasks are objective set of behaviors necessary to accomplish a goal (Dunn, Brown, & McGuigan, 1994, p. 599).
- A task is a self-contained stage in an activity. Tasks chain to form an activity (Hagedorn, 1995, p. 301).
- Tasks are composed of activities that are smaller units of behavior (Trombly, 1995b, p. 17).
- Task is defined as a set of purposeful activities in which a person engages (Law et al., 1996, p. 16).
- A task is the constituent parts of an activity (Turner et al., 1996, p. 873).
- Tasks are viewed as combinations of action sharing some purpose recognized by the task performer (Christiansen & Baum, 1997, p. 56).
- Tasks are work assigned to, selected by, or required of a person related to a skill. A collection of activities related to accomplishment of a goal (Jackson & Banks, 1997, p. 460).

(continued)

Table B-20

- Tasks are a set of activities that share some purpose (Watson, 1997, p. 32).
- Tasks involve the work assigned to, selected by, or required of a person related to development of occupational performance skills; collection of activities related to accomplishment of a specific goal (Jacobs, 1999, p. 146).

Table B-21

Characteristics of Good Tools for Practice in Occupational Therapy

- Tools should be flexible so that they can be used in variety of ways for long and short periods of time, and to offer a side variety of therapeutic components.
- Tools should be adaptable so they can be used within and without its normal domain of expected use. Tools should be relevant to the therapeutic needs and cultural, age, and gender requirements of the people who use them.
- Tools should be rich in therapeutic components, so that the occupation offers sufficient therapeutic value as opposed to nontherapeutic elements.
- Tools should be used by a variety of therapy staff and not dependent on the skills of one or two people with specialized training.
- Tools should be therapeutically and professionally justifiable and defended within the scope of occupational therapy practice.
- Tools should be useable within existing resources, including staff, time, environment, and cost.
- Tools should be robust and replaceable and conform to health and safety regulations.
- Tools should be aesthetically pleasing; culturally, gender, and age appropriate; and acceptable to the clients who will use them.

Table B-22

Effectiveness vs. Noneffectiveness in Relation to Doing

- Schkade and Schultz (1992) discuss effectiveness in relation to relative mastery stating that "relative mastery is the extent to which the person experiences the occupational response as... effective (production of the desired result)" (p. 835).
- Jacobs (1999) defines effectiveness as the "degree to which the desired result is produced" (p. 47).
- Hagedorn (2000) suggests that "the effective level is the level of occupation at which productive, meaningful activities are performed in order to enable the individual to achieve an adaptive fit with the individual's environment, which enhances and maintains survival, health and well-being" (p. 308).
- *Webster's New Universal Unabridged Dictionary* (Barnes & Noble, 1995) defines effective as "adequate to accomplish a purpose; producing the intended or expected result" (p. 622). Synonyms include capable or competent, and closely related concepts are effectual, efficacious, and efficiency.
- The idea of effective doing or doing that is effective is probably part of the subculture or underground practice of occupational therapy. The idea is so ingrained it rarely surfaces for careful analysis.
- Could the knowledge of occupational therapy be enhanced by a careful study of what constitutes "effective doing" and how occupational therapy personnel can promote in client "doing which is effective"?

Pierce (1997) talks about therapist design skill, which Parham and Fazio (1997a) define as "the ability of the occupational therapist to create activities that are tailored to meet the unique needs and goals of each child" (p. 254). Hagedorn (2000) defines a therapeutic relationship as "the relationship which develops between client and therapist during the process of therapy, through which the client is empowered and enabled to achieve specified goals" (p. 312).

The use of the therapist (OT or OTA) as a tool has been most often discussed in the mental health literature. However, the concept is valid in all areas of practice. Models of practice have frequently viewed the therapist as a neutral tool or agent who automatically carries all the intervention strategy as designed by the model. Clients and consumers might choose to disagree, as might some therapists.

Therapist-Client Relationship Tools

More recent models have focused directly on the therapist-client relationship as a significant tool in its own right. Two examples are provided: empowerment and enablement.

Empowerment is a very new concept in the occupational therapy literature. The term appears in Bowman and Marzouk (1992) but is not defined. Townsend (1996) described empowerment "as a process of change towards sharing rather than controlling power" (p. 115). The following year empowerment is defined as "personal and social process that transform visible and invisible relationships so that power is shared more equally" (Townsend, 1997, p. 180). *Webster's New Universal Dictionary* (Barnes & Noble, 1995) states that to empower is to give power or authority to or to enable or permit. The concept of empowerment has been examined by nursing using concept analysis. Rodwell (1996) concludes that the nursing profession must develop a philosophy of valuing and empowering its members in order for nursing to take charge of its practice and empower its clients. The same could be said for occupational therapy.

Polatajko (1992) describes enablement as incorporating the concepts of skill, ability, and competence where skill is a developed proficiency or dexterity in some art, craft, or the like; ability is the power to do something whether physical or mental; and competence is adequacy, sufficiency, answering all requirements of an environment (p. 196). Brintnell (1993) defines enablement as "an education process which occurs within the client-occupational therapist relationship. Enablement helps people to learn about themselves and their situation, and about their ability to make decisions which fulfill their sense of purpose in life" (p. 80). Letts et al. (1993) state that to enable means "providing people and communities with information and support to identify and address health issues, so that they can achieve their fullest potential" (p. 9). *Webster's New Universal Unabridged Dictionary* (Barnes & Noble, 1995) states that the verb *enable* means "to give power, means, competence, or ability to authorize; or to make possible or easy." Synonyms are empower, qualify, allow, permit (p. 639). Townsend (1997) defines enabling, stating that the term "refers to the processes of facilitating, guiding, coaching, educating, prompting, listening, reflecting, encouraging, or otherwise collaborating with people so that individuals, groups, agencies, or organizations have the means and opportunity to be involved in solving their own problems" (p. 180).

Enablement and empowerment appear to have similar characteristics. Which is the better concept, if either, is unclear at the present time. There is one cautionary note about the use of enablement. In the United States, the term *enable* also has a negative connotation in the language of addiction where an enabler is a person who performs tasks that the addicted person is responsible for performing, thus allowing the addicted person to continue being addicted without suffering the consequences of irresponsibility. In mental health especially, the negative connotation may outweigh the positive meaning implied by the definitions of enable in the occupational therapy literature.

Context as a Tool

Although context, environment, and ecology have always been considered as a part of the therapy situation, their roles as tools in and of themselves has been recognized more recently. *Uniform Terminology III* (Dunn et al., 1994) includes, for the first time, a separate section on contextual issues. Some definitions of context and environment are provided as examples in the terminology list.

The concept of context is a recent addition to the occupational therapy literature. Ryan (1993) states that context "refers to the social, physical and psychological milieu of the situation" (p. 358). Gillen and Burkhardt (1997) define context as the "circumstances associated with a particular environment or setting" (p. 537). Parham and Fazio (1997a) suggest that context is "the situation in which an event occurs; includes physical, symbolic, social cultural, and historical dimensions" (p. 249). Neistadt and Crepeau (1998) divide context into two aspects: temporal and environmental: "temporal aspects [include] chronological, culture, developmental, life cycle, [and] disability status; environmental aspects [include] physical, social, [and] cultural" (p. 868). This description is based on the *Uniform Terminology III* (Dunn et al., 1994).

Unsworth does not define context but does define two concepts based on context. Contextual congruence is " a simple environment that requires minimal processing demands... A congruent environment is designed to match the task with the goal" (p. 476). Contextual interference is described as "potential destructors that are normally found in an environment. An environment with contextual interference is complex, requires higher processing demands, and is usually designed to make a goal more difficult to achieve in order to strengthen a learning pattern" (p. 476).

Although environmental issues such as the arrangement and organization of space have been discussed in the occupational therapy literature for many years, the formal interest in environment seems to have started with Dunning's article (1972). Dunning (1972, p. 292) summarized five environmental issues:

1. The function and meaning of space.
2. The satisfaction of need through spatial organization.
3. The effect of the environment on social interaction and role performance.
4. Environmental influences as these shape psychological processes of learning, perception, cognition, and emotion.

5. The importance of environmental design and urban planning on human behavior and the quality of life.

Thereafter, definitions of environment began to appear. These are presented in Table B-23. A summary of the ideas are the environment is a composite of all external forces, influences, surroundings such as physical factors or conditions (geography, building, objects) and social factors or conditions (people, events, culture, social norms and expectation) which have the potential to influence or affect the development and maintenance of an individual. Hagedorn (1995) makes an additional distinction between external environment, which is "the physical and psychosocial environment; the world and universe" (p. 298) and the internal environment, which is "the abstract area in which the individual experiences his inner personal existence and actions" (p. 299). Gillen and Burkhardt (1997) also define environment as including both "the external and internal surroundings that influence a person's development (including the person's own psyche)" (p. 538).

AOTA defined environmental adaptations and structuring environment in 1978. Environmental adaptations are defined as "structural or positional changes designed to facilitate independent living and/or increase safety in the home, work or treatment settings: i.e., the installation of ramps, bar; change in furniture heights; adjustment of traffic patterns" (p. 74). Structuring environment is defined as "the organization of the client's time, activities, and/or physical environment in order to enhance performance" (AOTA, 1978, p. 75). Hagedorn (1997) also defines environmental adaptation, environmental analysis, and environmental demand. Environmental adaptation includes "changing the physical or social features of an environment to enhance performance, promote or restrict a behavior, or provide therapy" (p. 144). Environmental analysis is the "observation of features in the physical or social environment and interpretation of their significance or patient performance or therapy" (p. 144). Environmental demand is "the combined effect of elements in the environment to produce expectations for certain human actions and reactions" (p. 144). She also defines environmental demand as "the challenges presented by an environment which press the individual to respond by appropriate occupational performance" (Hagedorn, 2000, p. 308). Parham and Fazio (1997a) define environmental negotiation as "those transactions required to succeed in moving through, over, or around obstacles in the physical surroundings; involves the organization of space, time and social interactions." They define environmental control system as "any structure, design, instrument, contrivance or device that enables a person with a disability to effect changes in the surroundings in which daily routines take place and thereby gain more functional independence" (p. 249).

There are relatively few definitions of ecology in the current occupational therapy literature. The first appears in Howe and Briggs (1982) who define ecology as "the study of the relationship between organisms and their environments" (p. 322). Dunn, Brown, et al. (1994) state that ecology "is concerned with the interrelationships of organisms and their environments" (p. 595). Wilcock (1998) defines ecology as "the scientific study of organisms in their natural environment, including the relationships of different species with each other and the environment" (p. 254).

Ecological sustainability is defined as "to uphold and support the ecology and ecosystems by practices which maintain, and continue to maintain, the natural environment and relationships of different species" (Wilcock, 1998, p. 254). Ecological systems analysis is described as "a model that presents behavior as the result of interaction between an individual with an inherent biopsycholosocial makeup and a given environmental system (Neistadt & Crepeau, 1998, p. 868). Ecology of human performance is described as "a framework for considering the transaction among persons, tasks, and the contexts (i.e., temporal, cultural, social, and physical environments) for daily life (Christiansen & Baum, 1997, p. 595) and as "a framework that emphasizes that the ecology, or the interaction between a person and the context, affects human behavior and task performance" (Neistadt & Crepeau, 1998, p. 868).

Clearly, the interest in occupational therapy for considering contextual issues is expanding. As occupational therapy practice moves further away from controlled environments such as a hospital or clinic, the need to understand the context becomes more important because the therapist enters the client or consumer's world in which the rules are not determined by the therapist. Concepts of practice must describe these tools as well as more tradition tools. Table B-24 lists models that use environment or ecology as a major concept and briefly states the application.

Summary of Concepts About Tools

Occupational therapy practice does not lack for tools or concepts related to tools. The important issue is to organize the tools and their concepts into a better classification system. Such a system must be easy for occupational therapy personnel to comprehend and articulate to others. The field has incorporated many new tools since the formative period when arts and crafts were the primary tools of choice. However, the inclusion of new tools has not been accompanied by a narrative or graphic organization of those tools. Thus, practitioners lack a succinct means of describing the tools to others within the profession and to persons outside the field. Outsiders in particular may see a bewildering array of media, modalities, and methods that seem to lack a cohesive logic or framework.

Toward Better Concepts

This section discusses some of issues concerning the organization and refinement of concepts that can improve their usefulness in occupational therapy practice and communication of occupational therapy as an applied discipline to improve health and well-being of people.

Organizing Concepts

Clearly, one major problem in occupational therapy is the number of terms and concepts and the lack of organization. This chapter has been written using one system of organization: outcome, doing, and tools. While the organization is acceptable for the purpose of the chapter, such an organization is not necessar-

Table B-23 Definitions of Environment

- Hopkins and Smith (1977) define environment as "a composite of all external forces and influences affecting the development and maintenance of an individual" (p. 731).
- Kielhofner (1985) defines environment as "the objects, persons and events with which a system interacts" (p. 503).
- Christiansen and Baum (1997) define environment as "the external social and physical conditions or factors which have the potential to influence an individual" (p. 595).
- Creek (1997) defines environment as "the human and nonhuman surroundings of the individual, including objects, people, events, cultural influences, social norms and expectations" (p. 529).
- Neistadt and Crepeau (1998) describe environment as including "physical (geography, buildings, objects) and social (people, culture, surroundings)" (p. 868).

Table B-24 Development of the Concept of Environmental Context/Ecology in Occupational Conceptual Models for Occupational Therapy

Model	*Author*	*Year*	*Summary of How Environment is Used and Author(s) Within the Model*
Environmental Occupational Therapy	Dunning	1972	There is a total environment of which man is one component but for purpose of analysis it can be divided. Dunning used space, person, and task
Personal Adaptation Through Occupation Model	Reed & Sanderson	1980, 1983, 1992	Environment is divided into three parts: physical or inorganic, psychobiological (organic), and societal/cultural (superorganic). These environments are viewed as interacting forces that shape the performance of an individual's occupation
Ecological Systems Model	Howe & Briggs	1982	Environment is viewed as composed of nested environmental layers that are embedded within each other beginning with the first layer, which is the immediate setting; the second is social networks; the third is the ideological system
Model of Human Occupation	Kielhofner	1985, 1995	Environment includes the objects, persons, and events with which a system interacts. Environment affords or presses occupational behavior

(continued)

Table B-24

Model	*Author*	*Year*	*Summary of How Environment is Used and Author(s) Within the Model*
Person-Environment-Occupation-Performance Model	Christiansen & Baum	1991, 1997,	Environment enables or acts as a barrier to occupational performance. Types of environment include social support mechanisms, social policies and attitudes, cultural norms and values, and built environment/geography
Enablement Model Occupational Competence Model	Polatajko	1992	Environmental dimensions include physical, social, and cultural. Occupational competence is the product of the dynamic interaction between the environmental demand and individual ability
Model for the Practice of Occupational Therapy	Stewart	1992	Environment includes human and physical. Occupational therapy process involves interaction between client, therapist, environment, and activities
Occupational Adaptation Model	Schkade & Schultz	1992	Occupational environments are those that call for an occupational response and include the contexts in which occupations occurs (self-maintenance, work, and play and leisure
Ecology of Human Performance Model	Dunn, Brown, et al.	1994	Environmental cues and features are used by a person to support performance of tasks
Competent Occupational Performance in the Environment Model	Hagedorn	1995, 2000	Environmental demand is defined as the challenges presented by an environment that press the individual to respond by appropriate occupational performance
Contemporary Task-Oriented Approach Model	Bass-Haugen & Mathiowetz	1995	Environmental and performance context (physical, socioeconomic, and cultural) as well as personal characteristics are important factors in determining occupational and role performance
Person-Environment-Occupation Model	Law et al.	1996	Environment is defined as those contexts and situations that occur outside the individual and elicit responses from the person and include social, political, economic, institutional, and cultural considerations

(continued)

Table B-24

Model	Author	Year	Summary of How Environment is Used and Author(s) Within the Model
Canadian Model of Occupational Performance	Canadian Association of Occupational Therapists	1997	Environment includes physical, institutional, cultural, and social factors and form the outer ring of the conceptual model. The middle ring is called occupa tion while the inner triangle is labeled person

ily best for all concepts. Two approaches may be useful. One is to take small sections of the concepts and create an organization structure for them first.

Next, the small sections are combined into a large framework. While such an approach may lead to misfitting concepts and require reassembly of some sections, working initially on smaller units of concepts may make each section a more manageable task. An example might be to classify all media, modalities or methods used in occupational therapy practice. Table B-25 provides a starting point. The other approach is to start with an overall scheme and work from the top down until all concepts are included. The final product of either approach is a taxonomy or classification system that organizes the concepts of the profession into a chart that can be viewed by all. The chart must be a working or dynamic document because the knowledge and application within the field changes over time. Nevertheless, the outline provides a starting point for analyzing what the profession includes, its domain of concern, and allows analysis of the status of current concepts. Table B-26 is an example of taking one section of concepts, occupation, and attempting to create an organizing classification.

The concept of occupation continues to challenge the field in terms of classifying its elements or attributes. Since occupation is a major concept, organizing it is a good starting point.

Concept Organization Using Existing Models

Another approach is organizing concepts is by examining the various models of occupational therapy using a overall scheme. Since the chapter used outcome, doing and tools, one approach to organization of models could be to examine which focus on outcome, which stress doing, and which are concerned most with occupation as a therapeutic tool. A simple organization scheme is presented in Table B-27.

A second potential organizational scheme is to use the new International Classification of Functioning, Disability and Health published by the World Health Organization (2000). The major concepts employed are health domains, health-related domains, functioning, disability, context, body functions and structures, activities and participation, and the environment in which health and functioning occur. Thus, the major focus of the model is on functioning and contextual factors within the health domain. Table B-28 is an example of how the classification system might look.

Although organizational approaches are useful, consideration should also be given to their limitations. The ICIDH-2 model clearly states that it

> ...does not cover circumstances that are not health-related, such as those brought about by socio economic factors. For example, because of their race, gender, religion or other socio-economic characteristics people may be restricted in their execution of a task in their current environment, but these are not health-related restrictions of participation as classified in ICIDH-2. (p. 10)

In other words, where occupation therapy practitioners are primarily concerned with health status, the new ICIDH-2 model is useful. Where others factors such as socioeconomic issues impact the delivery of occupational therapy services, the ICIDH-2 model would be of limited value and would need to be abandoned or combined with another model that addresses outcome in a broader context than health alone.

A third possible approach is to explore a practice model developed within the profession to clarify major ideas such as outcome, doing, and tools. Occupational adaptation (Schkade & Schultz, 1992) might serve as a starting point for outcomes. The major outcome concepts suggested in the model are adaptation, competency, relative mastery, and competency. "Adaptation is a change in functional state of the person as a result of movement toward relative mastery over occupational challenges. Occupational adaptation... is a state of competency in occupational functioning toward which human beings aspire" (Schkade & Schultz, 1992, p. 831). Competency is not defined. Relative mastery is defined as "the extent to which the person experiences the occupational response of efficient (use of time and energy), effective (production of the desired result), and satisfying to self and society (Schkade & Schultz, 1992, p. 835). While the definitions may suggest that adaptation competency and mastery are different outcomes, they may actually be difference stages of outcome. Competency and relative mastery may be stages in the final outcome of adaptation. Rogers (1992) suggested as much when she stated that competency was an overall strategy of adaptation.

Nelson's article (1994) might be used to begin examining the statements on doing. He states that "occupation involves the doing of something. The 'doing' is the occupational performance, and the 'something' to be done is the occupational form" (p. 11). Nelson has tried to articulate how occupation interacts with the person through doing. The interactive process involves

Table B-25 Classification of Media, Modalities, and Methods

Media and Modalities		*Methods, Approaches and Techniques*		
Media or Agent Types	**Modalities Agent Groups**	**Teaching Methods**	**Therapeutic Approaches**	**Specialize Techniques**
A. Inanimate	1. ADL tasks	1. Demonstration and performance	1. Normal developmental sequencing	1. One-handed techniques
1. Creative arts	2. IADL tasks	2. Exploration and discovery	2. Normal activity sequencing	2. Work simplification techniques
2. Manual Skills	3. Productive occupations	3. Explanation and	3. Task analysis	3. Energy conservation techniques
3. Games and sports	4. Leisure/play occupations	4. Problem solving and decision making	4. Graded activities	4. Prosthetic/orthotic training
4. Education and learning	5. Homemaking tasks	5. Audiovisual aids	5. Adapted activity	5. Joint protection
5. Toys	6. Functional tasks	6. Role playing and stimulation	6. Consulting	6. Adapted techniques
B. Animate		7. Practice and repetition	7. Normal	7. Adapted equipment and devices
1. Self		8. Behavioral management	8. Adapted environment	8. Adapted therapy equip-
2. Dyad		9. Cuing	9. One client/one therapist	9. Work tolerance
3. Group		10. Learning strategies	10. Activity group	10. Modified learning sequences
4. Animals			11. Time budgeting/ management	11. Sensory integration and modulation
5. Plants and nature			12. Progressive resistive exercise	12. Making splints
			13. Relaxation	13. Home modification
			14. Reality orientation	14. Activity configuration
			15. Normal environment analysis	15. Architectural barriers
			16. Adapted environment analysis	16. Sensorimotor
				17. Driver's training

Adapted from Bueker, K. (2000). *Classifications of media and modalities.* Denton, TX: Master's professional project (unpublished).

Table B-26

Possible Taxonomy of Occupations

Person Centered Doing (Process)	*Environment Centered Result (Product)*	*Type*
Personal occupational roles	Social roles Self-care/maintenance ADL, IADL Productivity or work Leisure and play Life stage	Organizational
Occupational performance (occupation performed)	Occupational form	Organizational
Routine Habits Patterns Sequence Series	Goods and services	Effective
Action Interaction Reaction	Activity (chained tasks) Tasks	Effective
Performance unit	Stages/segments Steps	Developmental
Skills Components Sensorimotor Cognitive Psychosocial		Developmental
Abilities		Personal characteristics
Capacities		Personal characteristics

Definitions

abilities: Talents, special skills, aptitudes (Barnes & Noble, 1995, p. 4).

ability: Power or capacity to do or act physically, mentally; legally, morally, financially; competence in an activity or occupation because of one's skill, training, or other qualification (Barnes & Noble, 1995, p. 4).

actions: A repertoire of movements and emotional and cognitive responses (Hagedorn, 2000, p. 26). Actions are intentional and goal-directed (Hagedorn, p. 30). Habitual or usual acts; conduct (Barnes & Noble, 1995).

activity: A sequence of linked episodes (chained tasks) of task performance that takes place on a specific occasion during a finite period for a particular reason (Hagedorn, 2000, p. 27). Extended chunks of related performance that take place during a finite period for a particular purpose. The outcome or product of an activity is a change in the previous state of objective reality or subjective experience (Hagedorn, 2000, p. 26).

capabilities: Qualities, abilities, features that can be used or developed, potential (Barnes & Noble, 1995, p 308).

cognitive-perceptual components: Those involved in learning and the application of knowledge or processing of information from the environment (Hagedorn, 2000, p. 32).

occupation: Organized form of human endeavor that has a name and associated role title (Hagedorn, 2000, p. 27). Names units of daily activity that provide longitudinal organization of time and effort in a person's life and provide that person with an occupational role (Hagedorn, 2000, p. 26).

performance unit: The smallest piece of performance that can be separately identified within a task stage (Hagedorn, 2000, p. 26).

psychosocial components: Those required for communication with and response to others. Awareness of self and of self in relation to others (Hagedorn, 2000, p. 32).

(continued)

Table B-26

routines: Habitual and fixed sequences of activities (Hagedorn, 2000, p. 26).

sensorimotor components: Those required for the execution of movement and the reception of input from the environment (Hagedorn, 2000, p 32).

skill: Coming from one's knowledge, practice, aptitude, etc., to do something well; competent excellence in performance; expertness; dexterity (Barnes & Nobel, 1995, p. 1791).

skill components: Potentials for performance in the areas of action, interaction, and reaction. Skills components are divisible into areas or domains: sensorimotor, cognitive, psychosocial (Hagedorn, 2000, p. 26).

social roles: Designation of relationships, responsibilities, or status within a culture or group that directs the individual's engagement in certain occupations, activities, or tasks related to the role over extended periods of time (Hagedorn, 2000, p. 26). The behavior expected of a person occupying a given status or social position. Roles are governed by certain norms or expectations, but are also by some extend interpreted by the individuals playing them (O'Donnel, 1992, p. 27).

tasks: Each task is a self-contained part of an activity. A task is composed of a sequence of stages, often in a predetermined order, each of which contributes to task completion (Hagedorn, 2000, p 26). A task is a "piece of doing," a self-contained stage in an activity (Hagedorn, 2000, p. 29).

Adapted from Hagedorn, R. (2000). Glossary. In Hagedorn, R. *Tools for practice in occupational therapy: A structured approach to core skills and processes*. Edinburgh: Churchill Livingstone.

Table B-27

Examples of Outcome, Doing, and Tool Models

Outcome Models	*Doing Models*	*Tool Models*
Individual adaptation (King, 1978)	Doing and becoming (Fidler & Fidler, 1978)	Communication process (Fidler & Fidler, 1963)
Model of human occupation (Kielhofner & Burke, 1980)	Sensory integration (Ayres, 1968)	Activity therapy (Mosey, 1973)
Person-environment-occupation performance (Christiansen & Baum, 1991)	Cognitive disorders (Allen, 1985)	Activities model (Cynkin, 1979)
Occupational adaptation (Schkade & Schultz, 1992)	Playfulness (Bundy, 1997)	Group work (Howe & Schwartzberg, 1995)

Table B-28

Outline of a Classification System Based on ICIDH-2

Functioning and Disability				*Contextual Factors*		*Parts*
Body functions and structures		Activities and participation		Environmental factors	Personal factors	Components
Body function	Body structure	Capacity	Performance	Facilitator/ barrier	Personal characteristics	Construct/ qualifiers
Items	Items	Items	Items	Items	Items	Domains

Adapted from World Health Organization (2000). *International classification of functioning, disability and health*. Geneva, Switzerland: Author.

doing or performing, which connects the occupational form, the external element, with the occupational performance, the internal element. "Occupational performance is the voluntary doing of the person in the context of the occupational form" (Nelson, 1994, p. 11).

The tools of occupational therapy can be viewed from a number of perspectives. One is to look at models that examine the tools from a macro or top-down approach and those that view the tools from a micro or bottom up approach. Top-down approaches emphasize a macrolevel function level of analysis and is based on concepts while bottom-up approaches emphasize a microlevel functional level of analysis and is based on data (Christiansen & Baum, 1997).

The Occupational Behavior model presented by Reilly (1966) is an example of the macro approach. Her primary concept involved work-play as the major occupational behavior of the individual. Work-play is viewed as developing over a lifetime through the process of exploration, competence, and achievement. Intervention is thus designed to address the person's use of exploratory behavior to learn about the task, practice to facilitate competence, and competition to promote achievement.

Another macro model is the Model of Human Occupation. Kielhofner (1995) defines human occupation as "doing culturally meaningful work, play or daily living tasks in the stream of time and in the contexts of one's physical and social world" (p. 3). Thus, the Model of Human Occupation focuses on occupational behavior to increase understanding of how people engage in occupational functioning and occupational dysfunction and on how to support change to reorganize occupational behavior when dysfunction occurs. The model is concerned with the motivation for occupation, the patterning of occupational behavior into routines and lifestyles, and the nature of skilled performance.

On the other hand, the micro approach addresses only one aspect of occupation as a tool. An example is Allen's Cognitive Disabilities model. Basically, "a cognitive disability restricts the cognitive ability to do a voluntary motor action" (Allen, 1985, p. 31). Cognition occurs at more than one level of brain action or activity. Allen has suggested there are six levels useful to consider in occupational therapy intervention (Allen, 1985). By selecting tasks that can be performed at a specific level of cognition, occupational therapy personnel attempt to increase or maintain the performance of cognitive skills. Another example of a bottom up approach is the model of sensory integration, which focuses on the integration of sensory information to achieve an adaptive response.

In addition, top down and bottom up models tend to emphasize different views of the same concept. For example, environment or content is usually viewed as an essential or central concept by top down models because the performance of occupation occurs in some situation that is defined by the context of the environment. Occupation is supported (enabled) or constrained by the environmental situation, which is as much external to the individual as internal. Bottom-up models tend to focus on the internal functioning of the individual. While the external environment may be acknowledged (but often is not) attention is concentrated on the individual's ability and capacity to perform in any external environment without regard to which environmental situation may actually occur. One of the problems of bottom up approaches has been the tendency to use any occupation in any environment to elicit function. For example, stacking cones or square blocks does illustrate the person's functional capacity to grasp and release the objects and place them in a relation (stacked) that requires coordination. What is ignored or overlooked in the bottom up models is that occupation performed in an environment context usually has purpose, direction, and meaning to the person performing the occupation. When a person stacks towels for example, the focus is not on grasp, release, and coordination but on creating an organized pile of towels which can be placed in the storage area or closet. Thus, bottom up models tend to facilitate therapy oriented outcomes based on ability or capacity while top down approaches facilitate client oriented outcomes based on actual occupational performance observed in the environment or context.

The Person-Environment-Occupation-Performance (PEOP) model can be used to illustrate the differences in emphasis between the top down and bottom up models in actual practice. The PEOP model starts with a top down approach. The focus is the performance of personal activities in relation to roles and tasks established in the external environment. Therefore, assessment of the client should start with a history of the person's previous activities, perceptions about those activities and the occupational roles and tasks the person performs which are based on those activities. In other words, what activities, roles and tasks the person did in the past and which activities, roles and tasks the person wants or needs to do in the present and future. Intervention is then based on enabling the person to perform those activities, roles and tasks which are of most importance to the person. If personal limitations or constraints are present those are addressed but as the same time environment barriers are reduced or eliminated wherever or whenever possible. The outcome to be achieved is better occupational performance of the person in his/her environment.

If the PEOP model were a bottom up approach, the focus would be on determining the capabilities or constrains present in the psychological, cognitive, spiritual, neurobehavioral and physiological body structures and functions. Intervention would address the limitations or weaknesses found in those body structures and functions. Examples might include increasing attention span or muscle strength. The outcome would be body structures and functions that work better or are stronger. The individual could then use the improved function to do whatever the person wants or needs to do or the environmental situation permits that individual to do. Note that the tasks or roles the person is performing in the environment were not addressed directly. Body structures and functions could have been increased or improved that the person does not value or that the roles and tasks do not require.

Increasing models are being developed and utilized so that both the top down and bottom up approaches are being incorporated. Starting from a top down perspective does not prohibit a bottom up perspective from occurring. However, starting from the top down helps identify which personal constraints or environmental barriers are contributing directly to the loss of performance in activities, roles, and tasks the person actually wants or needs to perform. Intervention addresses the problems that the person identifies as important rather than fixing a problem the person may not need to have fixed or even see as important.

In summary, there are a variety of ways to analyze the concepts of occupational therapy to explore and develop organizational and classification systems that provide an integrated framework of concepts used within the field. Different viewpoints or focuses, however, tend to produce different results. The process (means) and the product (end or outcome) are important.

Summary of Techniques Used in This Chapter to Study Concepts

Several techniques have been used to study the concepts in this chapter. All of these techniques can be used to better organize and refine concepts in occupational therapy. Some have been discussed as they appeared in the text but a review list may be useful. The specific techniques have included the following:

- Use in context as the term or concept appeared in the original text of an article written by a prominent writer in the occupational therapy literature
- Definitions of terms and concepts as they appear in glossaries of textbooks of occupational therapy including multiple meanings of the same term
- Definitions appearing in standard dictionaries of the English language, especially unabridged dictionaries that list multiple meanings of the same term
- Definitions appearing in specialized dictionaries such as psychology and rehabilitation
- Origin of a term as stated in a dictionary
- Comparison of terms and concepts using synonyms and antonyms
- Comparison of concepts using word/phrase themes from published articles or books
- Explanation of concepts has developed from philosophy and different philosophical views of the world
- Explanation of the use of concepts from another discipline especially whether the concept is used as described in the originating discipline or if the concept has been changed in the occupational therapy literature
- Comparison of definitions of a term or concept over a time period by examining definitions from dictionaries published several years apart
- Comparison of usage of a term or concept over a time period by examining use from articles or books published several years apart
- Examination of the assumptions stated in the development of a concept or associated with an existing conceptual model
- Examination of how concepts have appeared and been organized in various models of practice in occupational therapy

A technique not used in this chapter, but used in the nursing literature (Rodgers & Knafl, 2000; Walker & Avant, 1995) is the case method in which the term or concept is developed in a short case study that is designed to convey the current usage in context so that other usages can be compared and contrasted against the case. The case method approach is useful for examining one concept but would have been too lengthy to use in this chapter.

SUMMARY

Members of the occupational therapy profession need to better understand and utilize the concepts within the field. Many of the concepts used in occupational therapy models, theories, and position papers originated outside the field of occupational therapy. Some concepts have been adopted without modification; other concepts have been modified to suit the intent of occupational therapy writers, leaders, and practitioners. If occupational therapy as a profession is to articulate and communicate with other professions, occupational therapy writers and leaders must identify and understand the source of the concept or concepts being discussed and indicate what, if any, modifications have been made to the formative ideas about that concept from the original discipline's literature. Doing one's professional "homework" is part of the scholarly advancement of knowledge and professional literature. To date, the homework has generally not been done. Occupational therapy writers, leaders, and practitioners cannot or do not identify the source of many important concepts, do not explain how the concept developed without and within the profession, and what position that concept holds in current models of practice. Without such explanation within the profession, communication to other professionals will continue to be unclear and fuzzy. There must be an attempt to document and trace the source of major concepts used within the field and to place those concepts in relationship to each other in a taxonomy. In other words, if you do not know from whence you came, how can you be sure of where you are going? The profession needs to get its terminology and concepts into a format that can be followed.

Furthermore, the concepts of occupational therapy must be better integrated with each other. Hierarchies and taxonomies are examples of classification systems but models and theories can perform a similar purpose of structuring and organizing the concepts into logical groups and sequences. Currently, the number of concepts and the lack of organization are barriers to effective student earning and to sharing ideas within the profession. Terms and concepts translate into learning definitions and understanding where and when to apply the information. Occupational therapy does encompass a wide range of ideas so the number of terms and concepts is likely to be large. However, no one knows how many terms of concepts there really are because no one has ever really listed or organized them.

Finally, the nursing literature can a useful source of ideas because the application of nursing in the practice arena is also broad and covers many similar concerns for health, well-being, and prevention. Also, the basic philosophy is congruent with occupational therapy since the discipline of occupational therapy has many roots in the field of nursing. Using ideas from another profession is nothing new to occupational therapy. Borrowing and adapting is also a useful way to avoid "reinventing the wheel" when time and effort could be better spent building a better wheelbarrow.

REFERENCES

Allen, C. A. (1985). *Occupational therapy for psychiatric diseases: Measurement and management of cognitive disabilities*. Boston: Little, Brown and Company.

American Occupational Therapy Association. (1923). *Principles of occupational therapy, Bulletin No. 4*. New York: Author.

American Occupational Therapy Association. (1958). *Objectives and functions of occupational therapy*. Dubuque, IA: William C. Brown Book Co.

American Occupational Therapy Association. (1973). *The roles and functions of occupational therapy personnel*. (Grant Contract No. N01-AH-24172). Rockville, MD: Author.

American Occupational Therapy Association. (1976a). Glossary: Essentials for an approved program for the occupational therapy assistant. *American Journal of Occupational Therapy, 30*, 261-263.

American Occupational Therapy Association. (1976b). Essentials of an approved education program for the Occupational Therapy Assistant. *American Journal of Occupational Therapy, 30*(4), 245-263.

American Occupational Therapy Association (1978). Glossary of terms used in the occupational therapy standards of practice. In *Manual on Administration* (pp. 73-75). Dubuque, IA: Kendall/Hunt Publishing Co.

American Occupational Therapy Association. (1979a). Uniform terminology for reporting occupational therapy services (899-907). In H. L. Hopkins & H. D. Smith (Eds.), *Willard and Spackman's occupational therapy* (6th ed.). Philadelphia: J. B. Lippincott.

American Occupational Therapy Association. (1979b). The philosophical base of occupational therapy. *American Journal of Occupational Therapy, 33*, 785.

American Occupational Therapy Association. (1986). Definitions: Entry-level role delineation for OTRs and COTAs. In *Reference manual of the official documents of the American Occupational Therapy Association, Inc* (VII.11-VII.15). Rockville, MD: The Association.

Angeles, P. W. (1981). *Dictionary of philosophy*. New York: Barnes & Noble.

Ayres, A. J. (1968). Sensory integrative processes and neuropsychological learning disabilities. In J. Hellmuth (Ed.), *Learning disorders* (Vol. 3., pp. 41-58). Seattle: Special Child Publications.

Azima, H., & Azima, F. (1959). Outline of a dynamic theory of occupational therapy. *American Journal of Occupational Therapy, 13*(5), 215-221.

Baldwin, B. T. (1919). *Occupational therapy applied to restoration of function of disabled joints* (Walter Reed Monograph). Washington, DC: Walter Reed General Hospital.

Bandura, A. (1977). Self-efficacy: Toward a unifying theory of behavioral change. *Psychological Review, 84*, 191-215.

Bandura A. (1986). *Social foundations of thought*. Englewood Cliffs, NJ: Prentice Hall.

Bandura, A., Cioffi, D., Taylor, C. B., & Brouillard, M. E. (1988). Perceived self-efficacy in coping with cognitive stressors and opiate activation. *Journal of Personality and Social Psychology, 55*, 479-488.

Barnes & Noble. (1995). *Webster's new universal unabridged dictionary*. New York: Barnes & Noble Books.

Barton, W. E. (1987). *The history and influence of the American Psychiatric Association*. Washington, DC: The Association.

Baum, C., & Edwards, D. (1995). Occupational performance: Occupational therapy's definition of function. *American Journal of Occupational Therapy, 49*(10), 1019-1020.

Bennett, R. L. (1950). Rehabilitation in poliomyelitis. In H.H. Kessler (Ed.), *The principles and practice of rehabilitation* (pp. 324-360). Philadelphia: Lea & Febiger.

Bockoven, J. S. (1971). Occupational therapy—A historical perspective, legacy of moral treatment—1800's to 1910. *American Journal of Occupational Therapy, 25*(5), 223-225.

Borys, S.S. (1974). Implications of interest theory for occupational therapy. *American Journal of Occupational Therapy, 28*(1), 35-38.

Bothamley, J. (1993). *Dictionary of theories*. London: Gale Research International Ltd.

Bowman, E. (1922). Psychology of occupational therapy. *Archives of Occupational Therapy, 1*(3), 171-178.

Bowman, O. J., & Marzouk, D. K. (1992). Using the Americans with Disabilities Act of 1990 to empower university students with disabilities. *American Journal of Occupational Therapy, 46*(5), 450-456.

Brintnell, E. S. (1993). *Occupational therapy guidelines for client-centred mental health practice*. Ottawa: Canadian Association of Occupational Therapists.

Brown, K., & Gillespie, D. (1992). Recovering relationships: A feminist analysis of recovery models. *American Journal of Occupational Therapy, 46*(11), 1001-1005.

Buchwald, E. (1949). Functional training. *Physical Therapy Review, 29*(11), 491-496.

Bundy, A. C. (1997). Play and playfulness: What to look for. In: L.D. Parham & L. Fazio (Eds.), *Play in occupational therapy for children* (pp. 52-66). St. Louis: Mosby.

Burnette, N. (1918). *Invalid occupation in war hospitals* (Manual No. 1). Ontario, Canada: Department of Soldiers Civil Re-establishment, Invalid Soldiers' Commission, Vocational Branch.

Cammack, S., & Eisenberg, M. G. (Eds.). (1995). *Key words in physical rehabilitation: A guide to contemporary usage*. New York: Springer Publishing Co.

Cara, E., & MacRae, A. (1998). Glossary. In E. Care & A. MacRae (Eds.), *Psychosocial occupational therapy: A clinical practice*. New York: Delmar Publishers.

Chinn, P. L., & Kramer, M. K. (1995) *Theory and nursing: Integrated knowledge development* (4th ed.). St. Louis, MO: Mosby.

Christiansen, C. (1994). Classification and study in occupation: A review and discussion of taxonomies. *Journal of Occupational Science: Australia, 1*(3), 3-21.

Christiansen, C. (1996). Three perspectives on balance in occupation. In R. Zemke & F. Clark (Eds.), *Occupational science: The evolving discipline* (pp. 431-451). Philadelphia: F. A. Davis.

Christiansen, C. (Ed.). (2000). *Ways of living* (2nd ed.). Bethesda: American Occupational Therapy Association.

Christiansen, C., & Baum, C. (1991). Glossary. In C. Christiansen & C. Baum. (Eds.), *Occupational therapy: Overcoming human performance deficits* (pp. 847-860). Thorofare, NJ: SLACK Incorporated.

Christiansen, C., & Baum, C. (1997). Glossary. In C. Christiansen & C. Baum (Eds.), *Occupational therapy: Enabling function and well-being* (2nd ed., pp. 591-606) Thorofare, NJ: SLACK Incorporated.

Clark, F., Ennevor, B. L. & Richardson, P. L. (1996). A grounded theory of techniques for occupational storytelling and occupational story making. In F. Clark & R Zemke (Eds.), *Occupational science: The evolving discipline* (pp. 373-392). Philadelphia, PA: F. A. Davis.

Coelho, G. V., Hamburg, D. A., & Adams, J. E. (Eds.). (1974). *Coping and adaptation*. New York: Basic Books.

Corsini, R. J. (1999). *The dictionary of psychology*. Philadelphia: Brunner/Mazel.

Corsini, R. (2002) *The dictionary of psychology*. New York: Brunner-Routledge (paperback edition)

Coulter, J. S. (1950). Occupational therapy in a private general hospital. In American Medical Association (Ed.), *Handbook of physical medicine and rehabilitation* (pp. 452-483). Philadelphia: Blakiston Co.

Crepeau, E. B. (1994). Rituals. In C. B. Royeen (Ed.), *The practice of the future: Putting occupation back into therapy. AOTA self-study series #6* (pp. 1-32). Bethesda, MD: American Occupational Therapy Association.

Creek, J. (1997). Glossaries—Occupational therapy terms. In J. Creek (Ed.), *Occupational therapy and mental health* (2nd ed., pp. 529-530). New York: Churchill Livingstone.

Crist, P. A. H., & Stoffel, V. C. (1992). The Americans with Disabilities Act of 1990 and employees with mental impairments: Personal efficacy and the environment. *American Journal of Occupational Therapy, 46*(5), 434-443.

Cynkin, S. (1979). *Occupational therapy: Toward health through activities*. Boston: Little, Brown and Co.

Davis, J.Z. (1996). Neurodevelopmental treatment of adult hemiplegia: The Bobath approach. In L. W. Pedretti (Ed.), *Occupational therapy: Practice skills for physical dysfunction* (4th ed., pp. 435-461). St. Louis, MO: Mosby-Year Book.

Deaver, G. G., & Brown, M. E. (1945). *Physical demands of daily life: An objective scale for rating the orthopedically exceptional*. (Studies in rehabilitation I). New York: Institute for Crippled and Disabled.

Deci, E. L. (1975). *Intrinsic motivation*. New York: Plenum Press.

Dewey, J. (1900). *The school and society: Being three lectures*. Chicago: University of Chicago Press

Dewey, J. (1902). *The child and the curriculum*. Chicago: University of Chicago Press.

Dewey, J. (1916). *Democracy and education: An introduction to the philosophy of education*. New York: Macmillian Company.

Dewey, J. (1990). *The school and society and the child and the curriculum*. Chicago: University of Chicago Press.

Doble, S. (1988). Intrinsic motivation and clinical practice: The key to understanding the unmotivated client. *Canadian Journal of Occupational Therapy, 55*(2), 75-81.

do Rozario, L. (1994). Ritual, meaning and transcendence: The role of occupation in modern life. *Journal of Occupational Science: Australia. 1*(3), 46-53.

Dunn, H. L. (1977). *High level wellness*. Thorofare, NJ: SLACK Incorporated.

Dunn, W. (1994). Uniform terminology for occupational therapy—Third edition. *American Journal of Occupational Therapy, 48*, 1047-1054.

Dunn, W., Brown, C., & McGuigan, A. (1994). The ecology of human performance: A framework for considering the effect of context. *American Journal of Occupational Therapy 48*(7), 595-607.

Dunn, W., Foto, M., Hinojosa, J., Schell, B., Thomson, L. K., & Hertfelder, S. D. (1994). Uniform terminology—Third edition. *American Journal of Occupational Therapy, 48*(11), 1047-1054.

Dunn, W. W. (2000). Habit: What's the brain got to do with it? *Occupational Therapy Journal of Research, 20*(Suppl.), 6S-20S.

Dunning, H. (1972). Environmental occupational therapy. *American Journal of Occupational Therapy, 26*(6), 292-298.

Dunton, W. R. (1915). *Occupation therapy*. Philadelphia: W. B. Saunders.

Dunton, W. R. (1918). The principles of occupational therapy. *Public Health Nurse, 18*, 316-321.

Dunton, W. R. (1925). Economic studies of crafts: 1. Upholstery. *Occupational Therapy and Rehabilitation, 4*(2), 219-222.

Dunton, W. R. (1928). *Prescribing occupational therapy*. Springfield, IL: Charles C Thomas.

Eisenberg, M. G. (1995). *Dictionary of rehabilitation*. New York: Springer Publishing Co.

English, H. B., & English, A. C. (1958). *A comprehensive dictionary of psychological and psychoanalytical terms: A guide to usage*. New York: David McKay Company, Inc.

Eysenick, H. J., Arnold, W., & Meili, R. (1982). *Encyclopedia of psychology*. New York: Continuum Publishing Co.

Farrar, C. B. (1906). The making of psychiatric records. *American Journal of Insanity, LXII*, 479-485.

Fidler, G. S., & Fidler, J. W. (1958). *Introduction to psychiatric occupational therapy*. New York: Macmillian Co.

Fidler, G. S., & Fidler, J. W. (1963). *Occupational therapy: A communication process in psychiatry*. New York: Macmillan

Fidler, G. S., & Fidler, J. W. (1978). Doing and becoming: Purposeful action and self-actualization. *American Journal of Occupational Therapy, 32*(5), 305-310.

Finn, G. L. (1972). The occupational therapist in prevention programs. *American Journal of Occupational Therapy, 26*(2), 59-66.

Fleishman, E. A. (1975). Toward a taxonomy of human performance. *American Psychologist, 30*(12), 1127-1149.

Florey, L. (1969). Intrinsic motivation: The dynamics of occupational therapy theory. *American Journal of Occupational Therapy, 23*(4), 319-322.

Frank, J. D. (1958). The therapeutic use of self. *American Journal of Occupational Therapy, 12*(4), 215-225.

Gage, M. (1992). The appraisal model of coping: An assessment and intervention model for occupational therapy. *American Journal of Occupational Therapy, 46*(4), 353-362.

Gage, M., Noh, S., Polatajko, H. J., & Kaspar, V. (1994). Measuring perceived self-efficacy in occupational therapy. *American Journal of Occupational Therapy, 48*(9), 783-790.

Gage, M., & Polatajko, H. J. (1994). Enhancing occupational performance through an understanding of perceived self-efficacy. *American Journal of Occupational Therapy, 48*(5), 452-461.

Gillen, G., & Burkhardt, A. (1998). Glossary. In G. Gillen & A. Burkhardt (Eds.), *Stroke rehabilitation: A function-based approach* (pp. 536-541). St. Louis, MO: Mosby-Year Book.

Hagedorn, R. (1992). *Occupational therapy: Foundations for practice: Models, frames of reference and core skills.* Edinburgh: Churchill Livingstone.

Hagedorn, R. (1995). Glossary. In R. Hagedorn (Ed.), *Occupational therapy: Perspectives and processes* (pp. 297-302). Edinburgh: Churchill Livingstone.

Hagedorn, R. (1997). Glossary. In R. Hagedorn (Ed.), *Foundations for practice in occupational therapy* (2nd ed., 141-147). New York: Churchill Livingstone.

Hagedorn, R. (2000). Glossary. In R. Hagedorn (Ed.), *Tools for practice in occupational therapy: A structured approach to core skills and processes* (pp. 307-312). Edinburgh: Churchill Livingstone.

Hall, H. J. (1905). The systematic use of work as a remedy in neurasthenia and allied conditions. *Boston Medical and Surgical Journal, CLII*(2), 29-32.

Hall, H. J. (1910). The work-cure. *Boston Medical and Surgical Journal, LIV*(1), 13-15.

Hall, H. J. (1923). *OT: A new profession.* Concord, MA: Rumford Press.

Hasselkus, B. R., & Kiernat, J. M. (1973). Independent living for the elderly. *American Journal of Occupational Therapy, 27*(4), 181-190.

Hightower, M. D. (1966). Independence through activities of daily living. *Delaware Medical Journal, 38*(8), 449-455.

Hinojosa, J., & Kramer, P. (1997). Fundamental concepts of occupational therapy: Occupation, purposeful activity, and function. *American Journal of Occupational Therapy, 51*(10), 864-866.

Hinojosa, J., Sabari, J., & Pedretti, L. (1993). Position paper: Purposeful activities. *American Journal of Occupational Therapy, 47*(12), 1081-1082.

Hocking, C., & Whiteford, G. (1995). Multiculturalism in occupational therapy: A time for reflection on core values. *Australian Occupational Therapy Journal, 42*(4), 172-175.

Holdeman, E. E. (1954). Occupational therapy for patients with anterior poliomyelitis. In H. S. Willard & C. S. Spackman, (Eds.), *Principles of occupational therapy* (pp. 256-273). Philadelphia: J. B. Lippincott.

Hopkins, H. L., & Smith, H. D. (1977). Glossary. In H. L. Hopkins & H. D. Smith (Eds.), *Willard and Spackman's occupational therapy* (5th ed., pp. 727-740). Philadelphia: J. B. Lippincott.

Hopkins, H. L., & Smith H. D. (Eds.). (1978). *Willard and Spackman's occupational therapy* (5th ed.). Philadelphia: J. B. Lippincott

Hopkins, H. L., & Smith, H. L. (1983). Glossary. In H. L. Hopkins & H. L. Smith (Eds.), *Willard and Spackman's occupational therapy* (pp. 915-930) Philadelphia: J. B. Lippincott.

Howe, M. C., & Briggs, A. K. (1982). Ecological systems models for occupational therapy. *American Journal of Occupational Therapy, 36*, 322-327.

Howe, M. C., & Schwartzberg, S. L. (1995) *A functional approach to group work in occupational therapy* (2nd ed). Philadelphia: J. B Lippincott.

Jackson, J. (1996). Living a meaningful existence in old age. In R. Zemke & F. Clarke (Eds.), *Occupational science the evolving discipline* (pp. 339-362). Philadelphia: F. A. Davis.

Jackson, S. J., & Banks, R. M. (1997). Home management—Glossary. In J. Van Deusen & D. Brunt (Eds.), *Assessment in occupational therapy and physical therapy* (pp. 459-460). Philadelphia: W. B. Saunders.

Jacobs, K. (1994). Flow and the occupational therapy practitioner. *American Journal of Occupational Therapy, 48*(10), 989-996.

Jacobs, K. (1999). *Quick reference dictionary for occupational therapy* (2nd ed.) Thorofare, NJ: SLACK Incorporated.

James, W. (1890). *The principles of psychology.* New York: Henry Holt & Co.

Johnson, J. (1973). Task force on target populations: Part 1. *American Journal of Occupational Therapy, 28*(3), 158-163.

Johnson, J.A. (1974). Task force on target populations: Association report II. *American Journal of Occupational Therapy, 28*, 231-236.

Johnson, J. A. (1985). Wellness: Its myths, realities, and potential for occupational therapy. *Occupational Therapy in Health Care, 2*(2), 117-138.

Johnson, J. A. (1986). *New dimensions in wellness: A context for living.* Thorofare, NJ: SLACK Incorporated.

Kamenetz, H. L. (1983). *Dictionary of rehabilitation medicine.* New York: Springer Publishing Co.

Kerlinger, F. N. (1986). *Foundations of behavioral research* (3rd ed.). San Diego: Academic Press.

Kielhofner, G. (1985). Glossary. In G. Kielhofner (Ed.), *A model of human occupation: Theory and application* (pp. 501-509). Baltimore: Williams & Wilkins.

Kielhofner, G. (1995). *A model of human occupation: Therapy and application* (2nd ed.). Baltimore: Williams & Wilkins.

Kielhofner, G. (1997). *Conceptual foundations of occupational therapy* (2nd ed.). Philadelphia: F. A. Davis.

Kielhofner, G., & Burke, J. (1980). A model of human occupation, part one. Conceptual framework and content. *American Journal of Occupational Therapy, 34*, 572-581.

Kim, H. S. (1983). *The nature of theoretical thinking in nursing*. Norwalk, CT: Appleton-Century-Crofts.

King, L. J. (1978). Toward a science of adaptive responses. *American Journal of Occupational Therapy, 32*(7), 429-437.

Klavins, R. (1972).Work-play behaviors: Cultural influences. *American Journal of Occupational Therapy, 26*(4), 176-179.

Law, M., Cooper, B., Strong, S., Steward, D., Rigby, P., & Letts, L. (1996). The person-environment-occupation model: A transactive approach to occupational performance. *Canadian Journal of Occupational Therapy, 63*(1), 9-23.

Law, M., Cooper, B., Strong, S., Steward, D., Rigby, P., Letts, L. (1997). Theoretical contexts for the practice of occupational therapy. In C. Christiansen & C. Baum (Eds.), *Occupational therapy: Enabling function and well-being* (2nd ed., pp. 73-102) Thorofare, NJ: SLACK Incorporated.

Law, M., Polatajko, H., Baptiste, S., & Townsend, E. (1997). Core concepts of occupational therapy. In E. Townsend (Ed.), *Enabling occupation: An occupational therapy perspective* (pp. 29-56). Ottawa: Canadian Association of Occupational Therapists.

Lawton, M. P. (1971). The functional assessment of elderly people. *Journal of the American Geriatric Society, 19*(6), 465-481.

Lazarus, R.S. (1984). Coping. In R. J. Corsini (Ed.), *Encyclopedia of psychology* (Vol. 1., 294-296). New York : John Wiley & Sons.

Letts, L., Fraser, B., Finlayson, M., & Walls, J. (1993). *For the health of it!: Occupational therapy within a health promotion framework*. Ottawa: Canadian Association of Occupational Therapists.

Licht, S. (1947). Kinetic analysis of crafts and occupations. *Occupational Therapy and Rehabilitation 26*, 75-78.

Livingston, D.M. (1950), Achievement recording for the cerebral palsied. *American Journal of Occupational Therapy, 4*, 66-67, 74.

Llorens, L. A. (1976). *Application of a developmental theory for health and rehabilitation*. Rockville, MD: American Occupational Therapy Association.

Llorens, L. A. (1984). Changing balance: Environment and individual. *American Journal of Occupational Therapy, 38*(1), 29-34.

Llorens, L. A. (1991). Performance tasks and roles throughout the life span (45-66). In C. Christiansen & C. Baum (Eds.), *Occupational therapy: Overcoming human performance deficits*. Thorofare, NJ: SLACK Incorporated.

Low, J. F. (1987). Time perception and rehabilitation of the elderly. *Physical and Occupational Therapy in Geriatrics, 5*(4), 17-30.

MacLean, F. M. (1949). Occupational therapy in the management of poliomyelitis. *American Journal of Occupational Therapy, 3*(1), 20-27.

Mann, M., Edwards, D., & Baum, C. M. (1986). OASIS: A new concept for promoting the quality of life for older adults. *American Journal of Occupational Therapy, 40*(110), 784-786.

Marino-Schorn, J. A. (1985-1986). Morale, work and leisure in retirement. *Physical & Occupational Therapy in Geriatrics, 4*(2), 49-59.

Martini, R., Polatajko, H. J., & Wilcock, A. (1995). ICIDH-PR: A potential model for occupational therapy. *Occupational Therapy International, 2*(1), 1-21.

Matsutsuyu, J. S. (1969). The Interest Check List. *American Journal of Occupational Therapy, 34*(4), 323-328.

Mayer, C. A. (2000). The Casson Memorial Lecture 2000: Reflect on the past to shape the future. *British Journal of Occupational Therapy, 63*(8), 358-366.

McDougall, W. (1923). Purposive or mechanical psychology. *Psychological Review, 30*, 273-289.

McGuire, G. H. (1983). An exploratory study of the relationship of valued activities to the life satisfaction of elderly persons. *Occupational Therapy Journal of Research, 3*(3), 164-172.

McGourty, K., Foto, M., Marvin, J. K., Smith, N. M., & Smith, R. O. (1989). Uniform Terminology for occupational therapy—Second edition. *American Journal of Occupational Therapy, 43*(12), 808-815

Meyer, A. (1922). The philosophy of occupation therapy. *Archives of Occupational Therapy, 1*(1), 1-10.

Meyer, A. (1951) Remarks on habit disorganization in the essential deteriorations, and the relation of deterioration to the psychasthenic, neurasthenic, hysterical and other constitutions. In E. Winters (Ed.), *The collected papers of Adolf Meyer: Vol. II Psychiatry*. Baltimore: Johns Hopkins Press.

Mocellin, G. (1988). A perspective on the principles and practice of occupational therapy. *British Journal of Occupational Therapy, 51*(1), 4-7.

Mocellin, G. (1995). Occupational therapy: A critical overview, Part 1. *British Journal of Occupational Therapy, 58*(12), 502-506.

Mock, H. E. (1918). Curative work. *Carry On, 1*(9), 12-15.

Moorhead, L. (1969). The occupational history. *American Journal of Occupational Therapy, 23*(4), 329-334.

Mosey, A. C. (1973). *Activities therapy*. New York: Raven Press.

Mosey, A. C. (1981). *Occupational therapy: Configuration of a profession*. New York: Raven Press.

Mosey, A. C. (1986). *Psychosocial components of occupational therapy*. New York Raven Press.

Mosey, A. C. (1994). Working taxonomies. In C. B. Royeen (Ed.), *Introduction to cognitive rehabilitation. AOTA self-study series* (Vol. 1., pp. 23-34). Bethesda, MD: American Occupational Therapy Association.

Muñoz, J. P., & Kielhofner, G. (1995). Program development (343-370). In G. Kielhofner (Ed.), *A model of human occupation: Theory and application* (2nd ed.). Baltimore: Williams & Wilkins.

Neistadt, M. E., & Crepeau, E. B. (1998). Glossary. In M. E. Neistadt & E. B. Crepeau (Eds.), *Willard & Spackman's occupational therapy* (9th ed., pp. 866-873). Philadelphia: Lippincott.

Nelson, D. L. (1988). Occupation: Form and performance. *American Journal of Occupational Therapy, 42*(10), 633-641.

Nelson, D. L. (1994). Occupational form, occupation performance, and therapeutic occupation. In C. B. Royeen (Ed.), *The practice of the future: Putting occupation back into therapy. #2* (pp. 10-48). Rockville, MD: American Occupational Therapy Association.

Parham, L. D., & Fazio, L. S. (1997a). Glossary. In. L. D. Parham & L. S. Fazio (Eds.), *Play in occupational therapy for children* (pp. 248-254). St. Louis, MO: Mosby-Year Book.

Parham, L. D., & Fazio, L. S. (1997b). *Play in occupational therapy for children*. St. Louis: Mosby

Pattee, G. (1951). Occupational therapy for the medical patient. In F. H. Krusen (Ed.), *Physical medicine and rehabilitation for the clinician* (pp. 83-94). Philadelphia: W. B. Saunders Co.

Patterson, H. A. (1922). The trend of occupational therapy for the tuberculous. *Archives of Occupational Therapy, 1*(1), 19-24.

Pedretti, L. W., & Umphred, D. A. (1996). Motor leaning and teaching activities in occupational therapy. In L. W. Pedretti (Ed.), *Occupational therapy: Practice skills for physical dysfunction* (4th ed., pp. 65-75). St. Louis, MO: Mosby-Year Book.

Peters, R. S. (1953). *Brett's history of psychology*. London: Macmillian Company.

Pierce, D. (1997). The power of object play fir infants and toddlers at risk for developmental delays. In L. D. Parham & L. S. Fazio, (Eds.). *Play in occupational therapy for children* (pp. 86-111). St. Louis, MO: Mosby-Year Book.

Piersol, C. V., & Ehrlich, P. L. (2000). Glossary. In C. V. Piersol & P. L. Ehrlich (Eds.), *Home health practice: A guide for the occupational therapist* (pp. 99-202). Bisbee, AZ: Imaginart.

Polatajko, H. J. (1992). Naming and framing occupational therapy: A lecture dedicated to the life of Nancy B. *Canadian Journal of Occupational Therapy, 59*(4), 189-200.

Pollack, B. (1938). Aims and ideals of occupational therapy in state hospitals. *Occupational Therapy and Rehabilitation*, 11, 291-300.

Poole, J. L. (1995). Learning. In C.A. Trombly (Ed.), *Occupational therapy for physical dysfunction* (4th ed., pp. 265-276). Baltimore: Williams & Wilkins.

Pratt, P. N., & Allen, A. S. (1985). *Occupational therapy for children* (2nd ed.). St. Louis: Mosby

Prout, T. P. (1931). The instinctive basis for occupational therapeutics. *Occupational Therapy and Rehabilitation*, 10(4), 235-240.

Punwar, A. J., & Peloquin, S. M (2000). Glossary. In A. J. Punwar & S. M. Peloquin (Eds.), *Occupational therapy: Principles and practice* (3rd ed., pp. 277-286). Philadelphia: Lippincott Williams & Wilkins.

Reading, P. (1994). Habit. In V. S. Ramachandran (Ed.), *Encyclopedia of human behavior* (Vol. 2., pp. 477-489). San Diego: Academic Press.

Rebeiro, K. L., & Polgar, J. M. (1999). Enabling occupational performance: Optimal experiences in therapy. *Canadian Journal of Occupational Therapy*, 66(1), 14-22.

Reber, A. S. (1995). *Dictionary of psychology* (2nd ed.). London: Penguin Books.

Reed, K. L. (1986). Tools of practice: Heritage or baggage. *American Journal of Occupational Therapy*, 40(9), 597-505.

Reed, K. L., & Sanderson, S. R. (1980). *Concepts of occupational therapy*. Baltimore: Williams & Wilkins.

Reed, K. L., & Sanderson, S. R. (1983). Glossary. In K. L. Reed & S. R. Sanderson (Eds.), *Concepts of occupational therapy* (2nd ed., pp. 329-357). Baltimore: Williams & Wilkins.

Reed, K. L., & Sanderson, S. R. (1992). *Concepts of occupational therapy* (3rd ed.). Baltimore: Williams & Wilkins.

Reed, K. L., & Sanderson, S. N. (1999). *Concepts of occupational therapy* (4th ed.). Philadelphia: Lippincott Williams & Wilkins.

Reilly, M. (1966). A psychiatric occupational therapy program as a teaching model. *American Journal of Occupational Therapy, 20*(2), 61-67.

Reilly, M. (1969). The educational process. *American Journal of Occupational Therapy, 23*(4),299-307.

Reilly, M. (1974). *Play as exploratory learning*. Beverly Hills, CA: Sage Publications.

Robertson, S. C. (1998). Treatment for psychosocial components: Intervention for mental health. In M. E. Neistadt & E. B. Crepeau. (Eds). *Willard and Spackman's occupational therapy* (9th ed., pp. 450-454). Philadelphia: Lippincott.

Rock, L. M. (1996). Upper extremity amputations and prosthetics: Section 1: Amputations and body-powered prostheses. In L. W. Pedretti (Ed.), *Occupational therapy: Practice skills for physical dysfunction* (4th ed., pp. 576-585). St. Louis, MO: Mosby-Year Book.

Rodgers, B. L., & Knafl, K. A. (2000). *Concept development in nursing: Foundations, techniques, and applications* (2nd ed.). Philadelphia: W. B. Saunders Co.

Rodwell, C. M. (1996). An analysis of the concept of empowerment. *Journal of Advanced Nursing, 23*, 305-313.

Rogers, J. C. (1982). The spirit of independence: The evolution of a philosophy. *American Journal of Occupational Therapy*, 36(11), 709-715.

Ryan, S. E. (1992). *The certified occupational therapy assistant: Principles, concepts and techniques* (2nd ed.). Thorofare, NJ: SLACK Incorporated.

Ryan, S. E. (1993). Glossary. In S. Ryan (Ed.), *Practice issues in occupational therapy: Intraprofessional team building*. Thorofare, NJ: SLACK Incorporated.

Runes, D. D. (1962). *Dictionary of philosophy*. Totowa, NJ: Littlefield, Adams & Co.

Schkade, J. K., & Schultz, S. (1992). Occupational adaptation: Toward a holistic approach for contemporary practice, Part 1. *American Journal of Occupational Therapy*, 46(9), 829-837.

Schmidt, R. A. (1988). *Motor control and learning: A behavioral emphasis*. Champaign, IL: Human Kinetics Publishers.

Schmidt, R. A. (1991). Motor learning principles for physical therapy. In *Contemporary management of motor control problems: Proceedings of the II step conference*. Alexandria, VA: American Physical Therapy Foundation.

Sharrott, G. W., & Cooper-Fraps, C. (1986). Theories of motivation in occupational therapy: An overview. *American Journal of Occupational Therapy*, *40*(4), 249-257.

Sheldon, M. P. (1935). Physical achievement record for use with crippled children. *Journal of Health and Physical Education*, 6(5), 30-31, 60.

Slagle, E. C. (1922). Training aides for mental patients. *Archives of Occupational Therapy, 1*(1), 11-17.

Smith, J. N. Jr. (1945). Preface. In: Deaver, G.G., & Brown, M.E. (1945). Physical demands of daily life: An objective scale for rating the orthopedically exceptional. (Studies in rehabilitation, No. 1). New York: Institute for the Crippled and Disabled

Smith, J.A. (1986). The idea of health: Doing foundational inquiry. In P. L. Munhall & C. J. Oiler (Eds.), *Nursing research: A qualitative perspective* (pp. 251-262). Norwalk, CT: Appleton-Century-Crofts.

Spackman, C. S. (1947). Occupational therapy for patients with physical injuries. In H. S. Willard & C. S. Spackman (Eds.), *Principles of occupational therapy* (pp. 175-273). Philadelphia: J.P. Lippincott.

Spencer, E. A. (1989). Toward a balance of work and play: Promotion of health and wellness. *Occupational Therapy in Health Care*, *5*(4), 87-99.

Stein, F., & Roose, B. (2000). *Pocket guide to treatment in occupational therapy*. San Diego, CA: Singular Publishing Co.

Taylor, M. (1930). Rehabilitation of the disabled through occupational therapy. *Hospital Social Service*, *23*, 54-56.

Thomas, C. L. (Ed.). (1997). *Taber's cyclopedic medical dictionary* (18th ed.). Philadelphia: F. A. Davis

Thompson, E. (Ed.). *The concise oxford dictionary* (9th ed.). Oxford: Clarendon Press.

Tickel-Degnen, L. (1995). Therapeutic rapport. In C. A. Trombly (Ed.), *Occupational therapy for physical dysfunction* (4th ed., pp. 277-285). Baltimore: Williams & Wilkins.

Tolman, E. C. (1932). *Purposive behavior in animals and men*. New York: Century.

Townsend, E. (1996). Enabling empowerment: Using simulation versus real occupations. *Canadian Journal of Occupational Therapy*, *63*(2), 114-128.

Townsend, E. (1997). Key terms. In E. Townsend (Ed.), *Enabling occupations: An occupational therapy perspective* (pp. 179-182). Ottawa, Ontario: Canadian Association of Occupational Therapists.

Tracy, S. E. (1910). *Studies in invalid occupations*. Boston: Whitcomb & Barrows

Trombly, C. A. (1995a). Planning, guiding, and documenting therapy. In C. A. Trombly (Ed.), *Occupational therapy for physical dysfunction* (4th ed., pp. 29-40). Baltimore: Williams & Wilkins.

Trombly, C.A. (1995b) Occupation: Purposefulness and meaningfulness as therapeutic mechanisms: 1995 Eleanor Clarke Slagle Lecture. *American Journal of Occupational Therapy*, 49, 960-972.

Turner, A., Foster, M., & Johnson, S.E. (Eds.), (1996). Occupational therapy and physical dysfunction: Principles, skills and practice. 4th ed. New York: Churchill Livingston

Turner, A., Foster, M., & Johnson, S. E. (1997). Glossary. In A. Turner, M. Foster, & S. E. Johnson (Eds.), *Occupational therapy and physical dysfunction: Principles, skills and practices* (4th ed., p. 873). New York: Churchill Livingstone.

Turner, A., & MacCaul, C. (1996). The therapeutic use of activity. In A. Turner, M. Foster, & S. E. Johnson (Eds.), *Occupational therapy and physical dysfunction: Principles, skills and practices* (4th ed., pp. 125-157). New York: Churchill Livingstone.

Unsworth, C. (1999). Glossary of terms. In C. Unsworth (Ed.), *Cognitive and perceptual dysfunction: A clinical reasoning approach to evaluation and intervention* (pp. 473-484). Philadelphia: F. A. Davis.

Upham, E. G. (1918a). *Training of teachers for occupational therapy for the rehabilitation of disabled soldiers and sailors*. (Federal Board for Vocational Education Bulletin no. 6). Washington, DC: Government Printing Office.

Upham, E. G. (1918b). *Ward occupations in hospitals* (Federal Board for Vocational Education, Reeducation Series no. 4). Washington, DC: Government Printing Office.

Upham, E. G. (1919). Occupational therapy and the trained nurse. *Modern Hospital, 12*, 210-212.

Walker, L. O., & Avant, K. C. (1995). *Strategies for theory construction in nursing* (3rd ed.). Norwalk, CN: Appleton & Lange.

Wantanabe, S. (1968). Four concepts basic to the occupational therapy process. *American Journal of Occupational Therapy 22*, 439-445.

Warren, H. H. (1974). Self-perception of independence among urban elderly. *American Journal of Occupational Therapy*, *28*(6), 329-336.

Watson, D. E. (1997). *Task analysis: An occupational performance approach*. Bethesda: American Occupational Therapy Association.

West, W. L. (1969). The growing importance of prevention. *American Journal of Occupational Therapy, 23*(3), 226-231.

White, R. (1971). The urge toward competence. *American Journal of Occupational Therapy*, *25*(6), 271-274.

White, R.W. (1974). Strategies of adaptation: An attempt to systematic description. In S. V. Coelho, D. A. Hamburg, & J. E. Adams (Eds.), *Coping and adoption* (pp. 47-68). New York: Basic Books.

White, V. K. (1986). Promoting health and wellness: A theme for the eighties. *American Journal of Occupational Therapy*, *40*(11), 743-748.

Whiteford, G. E., & Wilcock, A. A. (2000). Cultural relativism: Occupation and independence reconsidered. *Canadian Journal of Occupational Therapy*, *67*(5), 324-336.

Wiemer, R. B. (1972). Some concepts of prevention as an aspect of community health. *American Journal of Occupational Therapy* 26(1), 1-9.

Wilcock, A. A. (1998). *An occupational perspective of health.* Thorofare, NJ: SLACK Incorporated.

Willard, H. S., & Spackman, C. S. (1947). *Principles of occupational therapy*. Philadelphia: J. B. Lippincott.

Williamson, G. G. (1997). Coping and young children with motor deficits. In J. D. Noshpitz (Ed.), *Handbook of child and adolescent psychiatry. Vol. 1: Infants and preschoolers: Development and syndromes* (pp. 439-452). New York: John Wiley & Sons.

Wolman, B. B. (1989). *Dictionary of behavioral science* (pp. 2nd ed). San Diego: Academic Press.

Woodside, H. (1976). Dimensions of the occupational behaviour model. *Canadian Journal of Occupational Therapy,* *43*(1), 11-14

World Health Organization. (2000). *International classification of functioning, disability and health. Prefinal draft, Full version.* Geneva, Switzerland: Author.

Yerxa, E.J. (1996), The social and psychological experience of having a disability. In L.W. Pedretti (Ed), Occupational therapy: Practice skills for physical dysfunction, (4th ed. pp. 253-274). St Louis: Mosby.

Zeitlin, S., Williamson, G. G., & Szczepanski, M. (1988). *Early coping inventory: A measure of adaptive behavior* (manual). Bensenville, IL: Scholastic Testing Service.

Zemke, R., & Clark, F. (Eds.) (1996). *Occupational science: The evolving discipline*. Philadelphia: F. A. Davis.

Zimmerman, M. E. (1957). Ideas for independence. *Crippled Child, 34*(5), 7-8.

INDEX